VESICULAR & PARTICULATE DRUG DELIVERY SYSTEMS

VESICULAR & PARTICULATE DRUG DELIVERY SYSTEMS

Editor

Dr. R.S.R. MURTHY

M.Pharm., Ph.D.,
Professor of Pharmaceutics,
Pharmacy Department,
M.S. University of Baroda,
Gujrat.
Presently Director, ISF College of Pharmacy,
Moga, Punjab.

CAREER Publications

VESICULAR & PARTICULATE DRUG DELIVERY SYSTEMS

First Edition: March 2010

ISBN: 978-81-88739-56-1

Published by:
Nishad Deshmukh
CAREER Publications

Reg. Office:
432/B, Deshmukh Bunglow,
Vakil Wadi,
Nashik,
Maharashtra,
India,
Pincode: 422 001.

Communication Address:
First Floor,
Kaveri Smruti,
Ashok Stambh,
Nashik,
Maharashtra,
India,
Pincode: 422 001.
Phone: (0253) 2311422, 2576175
Visit us: publications@careerandyou.com
www.careerandyou.com

Pune Office:
First Floor,
Gokhale Building,
Tilak Road,
Pune,
Maharashtra,
India,
Pincode: 411 030.
Phone: (020) 24497602

Printed in India at Spectrum Offset, Satyam Estate, Erandwane, Pune. Maharashtra

Typesetting & Layout: IBH Process Solutions

Price: Rs. 1200/-

Preface

There has been keen interest in the development of a novel drug delivery system with aims to deliver the drug at a rate needed by the body during the period of treatment, and also to direct the active entity to the site of action. Even though, at present, no available drug delivery system behaves ideally achieving all the lofty goals, a sincere attempt is under way to achieve them through different novel approaches in drug delivery. Among them encapsulation or entrapment of the drug in vesicular or micro/nanoparticulate structures is one such system widely investigated actively over the last three to four decades. These systems are designed with possibility to prolong the existence of the drug in systemic circulation, and reduce the toxicity, if selective uptake can be achieved.

Biological membranes form the ubiquitous delimiting structures that surround and compartmentalize all cells and organelles. The bilayer arrangement of lipids is perhaps the only organizational feature that is common to all biological membranes. Numerous theoretical models of membrane structure have appeared since the publication of the cell theory in 1839. Experimental models provide insight into the motional dynamics and static structures of some isolated compartments of biological membranes. Lipid vesicles are just one type of the many experimental models of biomembranes although developed for basic research, many technological innovations have arisen from the applications of these models. Hence, lipid vesicular systems have evolved as a successful tool not only in immunology, membrane biology, diagnostic techniques, but also have become the vehicle of choice in drug delivery and genetic engineering. Vesicles are also playing a major role in modeling biological membranes and in the transport and targeting of active medicinal agent.

Many limitations identified in conventional chemotherapy like ineffective permeation across bio-membranes, lack of selective uptake leading to very high volume of distribution in the body could be overcome by use of vesicular drug delivery systems. The phagocytic uptake of the systemic delivery of the drug-loaded vesicular delivery system provides an efficient method for delivery of drug directly to the site of infection, leading to reduction of drug toxicity with no adverse effects. PEGylated vesicular structures are designed to prolong the existence of the drug in systemic circulation in order to facilitate selective uptake and perhaps to reduce unwanted systemic toxicity.

Consequently a number of vesicular drug delivery systems such as liposomes, niosomes, transfersomes, and pharmacosomes were developed. In addition, other colloidal systems like, micelle, micro emulsions, multiple emulsions and cellular systems like resealed erythrocytes are considered important in drug delivery. Advances have since been made in all these areas of drug delivery, leading to the development of systems that allow drug targeting, and the sustained or controlled release of conventional medicines.

Particulate systems, such as micro-particles, nano-particles, dendrimers etc could be used for site-specific and sustained delivery of drugs. Such delivery systems will likely modify the disposition of drugs at the target site, sustain drug release, reduce toxicity to the other tissues, and increase intracellular levels of the drugs. Advent of nanotechnology paved the way to develop various nanoparticulates prepared out of polymers, lipids, inorganic substances like calcium phosphate, silicates and from carbon nanotubes.

Dendrimers are a novel class of polymeric materials which are highly branched, spherical, mono-disperse macromolecules with a well de?ned globular structure and high functionality. The interior cavities of dendrimers surrounding the core and the core to which the dendrons are attached are well suited for host-guest interaction and encapsulation of guest molecules. The utility of the internal void volume of dendrimers to encapsulate hydrophobic guest molecules and drugs has been demonstrated.

The focus of this book is to bring out the theoretical principles in design, preparation and scale up problems, quality control and application, including safety aspects of these systems. The chapters dealt here are of interest for graduate and post graduate students as their curricular text and as a reference material. The practical problems in scale up and regulatory issues of delivery systems, discussed in most of the chapters are of value for corporate research and development and quality assurance scientists also.

Editor would be happy to receive any suggestions, constructive criticisms etc. from our valued readers so as to improve up on the subject matter and to include more research and developments out comes in the chapters dealt here in our forth coming revisions and editions.

Editor personally acknowledges the efforts, inputs and suggestions rendered by his co-authors of this book, Mr. Nishad Deshmukh and Ms Swati Jadhav of M/s Career Publications for their untiring efforts in bringing out this publication.

Prof. R. S. R. Murthy

Contents

Contributors

Name & designation	Contact details	Chapter/section
Dr. R.S.R.Murthy, M.Pharm, PhD, Professor of Pharmaceutics	Pharmacy department M.S.University of Baroda, Kalabhavan Vadodara Presently Director, ISF College of Pharmacy, Moga, Punjab	Liposomes, Niosomes Micro particles in drug delivery, Nanoparticles Resealed erythrocytes, Micellar drug delivery systems, Dendrimers
Dr, Krutika Sawant, M.Pharm, PhD Reader in Pharmaceutics	Pharmacy department M.S.University of Baroda, Kalabhavan Vadodara	Micro particles in drug delivery: Introduction, general methods of preparation, drug loading, drug release kinetics from microparticles
Dr. Harivardhan Reddy Lakkireddy Pharmaceutical Sciences Department	Sanofi-aventis Research & Development Paris, France	Nanoparticles, Bio-distribution, therapeutic applications
Dr. B. Ashwin Rao, M.Pharm, PhD General Manager (R&D)	M/s Alembic Limited Alembic Road, Vadodara	Liposomes: Characterization, stability, surface modification, production and scale-up.
Dr. Rajesh Kesarala, M.Pharm. PhD Professor of Pharmaceutics	Profesor of Pharmacy ISF College of Pharmacy, Moga, Punjab	Micro particles in drug delivery: Characterization, selected polymeric microparticles magnetically modulated microparticles
Dr. Gour Mukharjee, M.Pharm., PhD Head- NDDS Group Jubilant Organosys Ltd.,	NOIDA	Microemulsions
Dr. Rakesh Kumar Sharma, M.Pharm, PhD, FIC, FABMS Head-CBRN Defence Institute of Nuclear Medicine and Allied Sciences	Brig SK Mazumdar Road, Delhi	Micro particles in drug delivery: Pharmacokinetics and applications
Dr. Pradip K Ghosh Project Manager-Generics Dr. Reddy's Laboratories ltd.		Microemulsions
Prudhvi Raju, Hamsaraj, Vivek & Neha	Research scholors, Pharmacy department	Liposomes: pH sensitive liposomes Micellar drug delivery systems Dendrimers

1

Liposomes

Prof. R.S.R. Murthy, M.PHARM, PhD
Dr. Ashwin Rao, M.PHARM, PhD
Mr. Hamsaraj Karanth, M.PHARM
Dr. K. Vivek, M.PHARM, PhD

CONTENTS

1. INTRODUCTION

A liposome is a spherical vesicle with a membrane composed of a phospholipid and cholesterol (CHOL) bilayer. Liposomes can be composed of naturally-derived phospholipids with mixed lipid chains (like egg phosphatidylethanolamine [PE]), or of pure surfactant components like dioleolylphosphatidylethanolamine (DOPE). Liposomes, by definition, contain a core of aqueous solution; lipid spheres that contain no aqueous material are called micelles.

Liposomes are used for drug delivery due to their unique properties. A liposome encapsulates a region of aqueous solution inside a hydrophobic membrane; dissolved hydrophilic solutes cannot readily pass through the lipids. Hydrophobic chemicals can be dissolved into the membrane, and in this way liposome can carry both hydrophobic molecules and hydrophilic molecules. To deliver the molecules to sites of action, the lipid bilayer can fuse with other bilayers such as the cell membrane, thus delivering the liposome contents. By making liposomes in a solution of DNA or drugs (which would normally be unable to diffuse through the membrane), they can be (indiscriminately) delivered past the lipid bilayer.

Liposomes can also be designed to deliver drugs in other ways. Liposomes that contain low (or high) pH can be constructed such that dissolved aqueous drugs will be charged in solution (i.e., pH is outside the drug's p*I* range). As pH naturally neutralises within the liposome (protons can pass through a membrane), the drug will also be neutralised, allowing it to freely pass through a membrane. These liposomes work to deliver drug by diffusion rather than by direct cell fusion. Another strategy for liposome drug delivery is to target endocytosis events. Liposomes can be made in a particular size range that makes them viable targets for natural macrophage phagocytosis. These liposomes may be digested while in the macrophage's phagosome, thus releasing the drug. Liposomes can also be decorated with opsonins and ligands to activate endocytosis in other cell types.

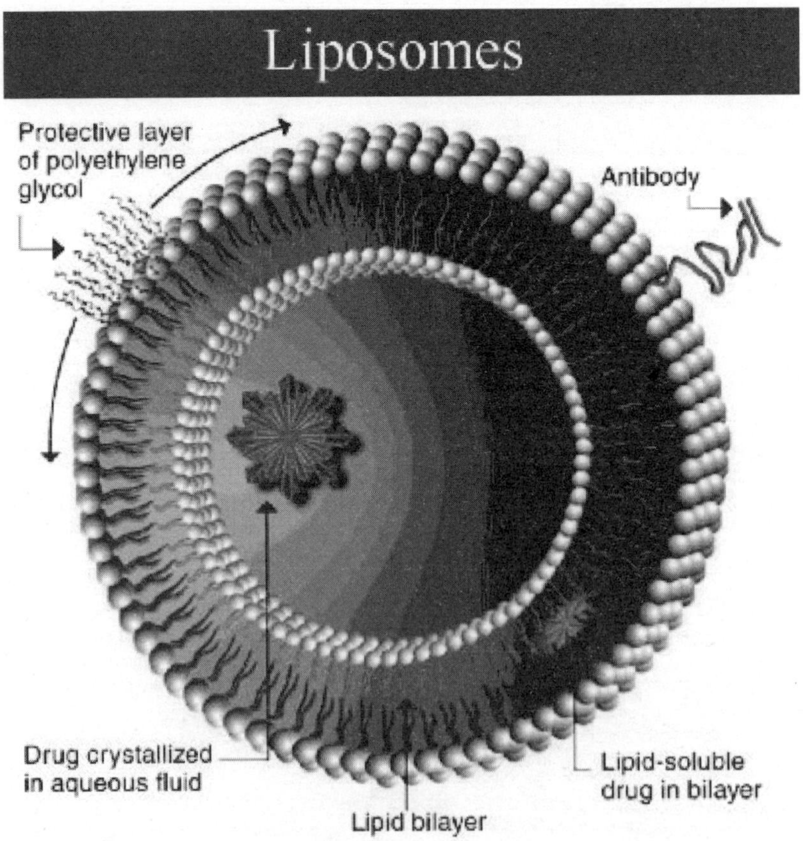

Fig. 1. Structure and composition of liposome. (Reprinted From Adv. Drug Deliv. Rev., 58(14) Torchilin VP: Multifunctional Nanocarriers, 1532–55, 2006, with permission from Elsevier) *(1)*.

Another interesting property of liposomes is their natural ability to target cancer. The endothelial wall of all healthy human blood vessels are encapsulated by endothelial cells that are bound together by tight junctions. These tight junctions stop any large particle of blood from leaking out of the vessel in the system. Tumor vessels do not contain the same level of seal between cells and are diagnostically *leaky*. This ability is known as the enhanced permeability and retention (EPR) effect. Liposomes of certain sizes can rapidly enter tumor sites from the blood, but are bound by the endothelial wall in healthy tissue vasculature. Anti-cancer drugs such as doxorubicin are currently being marketed in liposome delivery.

Liposomes can be created by sonicating phospholipids in water. Low shear rates create multi-lamellar liposomes (MLV), which have many layers like an onion. Continued high-shear sonication tends to form smaller unilamellar liposomes. In this technique, the liposome contents are same as the contents of aqueous phase.

Further advances in liposome research allows liposomes to avoid detection by the body's immune system, specifically, the cells of reticuloendothelial system (RES). These liposomes are known as "stealth liposomes", and are constructed with polyethylene glycol (PEG) studding the outside of the membrane. PEG coating, which is inert in the body, allows for longer circulatory life for the drug delivery mechanism. However, research currently seeks to investigate at what amount of PEG coating the PEG actually hinders binding of the liposome to delivery site. In addition to a PEG coating, most stealth liposomes also have some sort of biological species attached as a ligand to liposome in order to enable binding via a specific expression on the targeted drug delivery site. These targeting ligands could be monoclonal antibodies (making an immunoliposome), vitamins, or specific antigens. Targeted liposomes can target nearly any cell type in body and deliver drugs that would naturally be systematically delivered. Naturally toxic drugs can be much less toxic if delivered only to diseased tissues. Figure 1 shows structure and composition of liposome generally used for drug or gene delivery.

2. COMPOSITION OF LIPOSOME

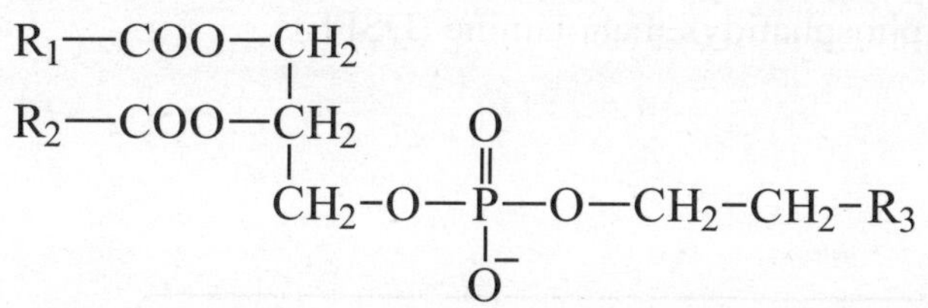

Fig. 2. General structure of phospholipids.

2.1. Lipids

Lipid is the major component of liposomes. Among the lipids, phospholipids are the amphoteric lipids capable of forming bilayer and hence are the integral part of liposomal system.

2.1.1. Phospholipids

A phospholipid has two acyl chains linked to a headgroup by means of a glycerol-backbone. Figure 2 shows the structural formula of a phospholipid, where R_1 and R_2 are saturated or unsaturated acyl chains and R_3 is the polar head group. The polar head groups are used for classification, i.e., to distinguish between different phospholipids like; phosphatidylcholines (PCs), PEs, etc.

2.1.1.1. Natural Phospholipids

Natural phospholipids are hydrogenated soybean phospholipids, egg phospholipids and sphingomyelin (SM) from milk or egg.

Main Structure : di-acyl-phosphatidylcholine

R_1COO, R_2COO:

C12~C20 fatty acid residue group

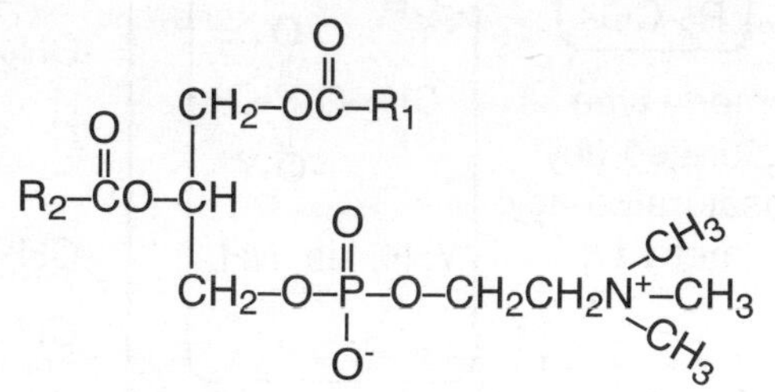

Main structure: sphingomyelin

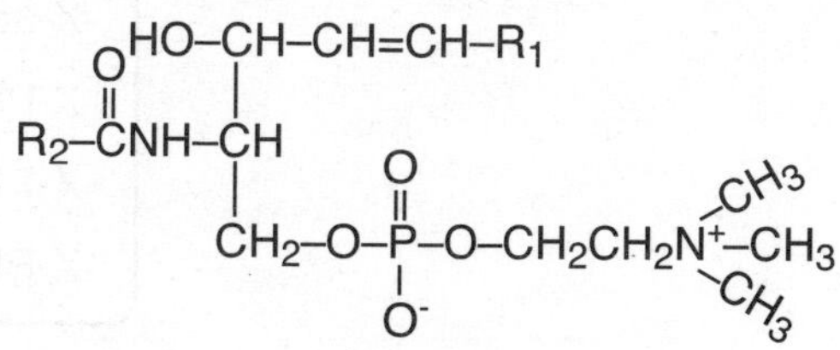

2.1.1.2. *Synthetic Phospholipids: Classification*

2.1.1.2.1. Phosphatidylcholine

1. Saturated acyl groups: symmetric type: didecanoyl phosphatidylcholine (DDPC), dilauroyl phosphatidylcholine (DLPC), dimyristoyl phosphatidylcholine (DMPC), dipalmitoyl phosphatidylcholine (DPPC) and distearoyl phosphatidylcholine (DSPC).
2. Unsaturated acyl groups: symmetric type: dioleoy-l phosphatidylcholine (DOPC), dilinoleoyl phosphatidylcholine and dierucoyl phosphatidylcholine.
3. Saturated acylgroups: asymmetric type: 1-myristoy-l-2-palmitoyl phosphatidylcholine, 1-myristoyl-2-stearoyl phosphatidylcholine, 1-palmitoyl-2-myristoyl phosphatidylcholine, 1-palmitoyl-2-stearoyl phosphatidylcholine, 1-stearoyl-2-myristoyl phosphatidylcholine and 1-stearoyl-2-palmitoyl phosphatidylcholine.
4. Mixed acyl groups: asymmetric type: 1-palmitoyl-2-oleoyl phosphatidylcholine (POPC) and 1-stearoyl-2-oleoyl phosphatidylcholine.
5. Lyso lipids: 1-myristoyl-lysophosphatidylcholine, 1-palmitoyl-lysophosphatidylcholine and 1-stearoyl-lysophosphatidylcholine.

2.1.1.2.2. Phosphatidylglycerol

1. Saturated acyl groups: symmetric type: dilauroyl phosphatidylglycerol, dimyristoyl phosphatidylglycerol (DMPG), dipalmitoyl phosphatidylglycerol (DPPG) and distearoyl phosphatidylglycerol (DSPG)—all these available as Na and NH_4 salts.
2. Unsaturated acyl groups: symmetric type: dioleoyl phosphatidylglycerol (DOPG) and dierucoyl phosphatidylglycerol.
3. Mixed acyl groups: asymmetric type: 1-palmitoyl-2-oleoyl phosphatidylglycerol.

2.1.1.2.3. Phosphatidic Acid

1. *Saturated acyl groups*: symmetric type: dilauroyl phosphatidic acid, dimyristoyl phosphatidic acid (DMPA), dipalmitoyl phosphatidic acid (DPPA) and distearoyl phosphatidic acid.
2. *Unsaturated acyl groups*: symmetric type: diloleoyl phosphatidic acid (DOPA) and dierucoyl phosphatidic acid.

2.1.1.2.4. Phosphatidylethanolamine

1. *Saturated acyl groups*: symmetric type: dilauroyl phosphatidylethanolamine, dimyristoyl phosphatidylethanolamine (DMPE), dipalmitoyl phosphatidyl ethanolamine (DPPE) and distearoyl phosphatidylethanolamine (DSPE).

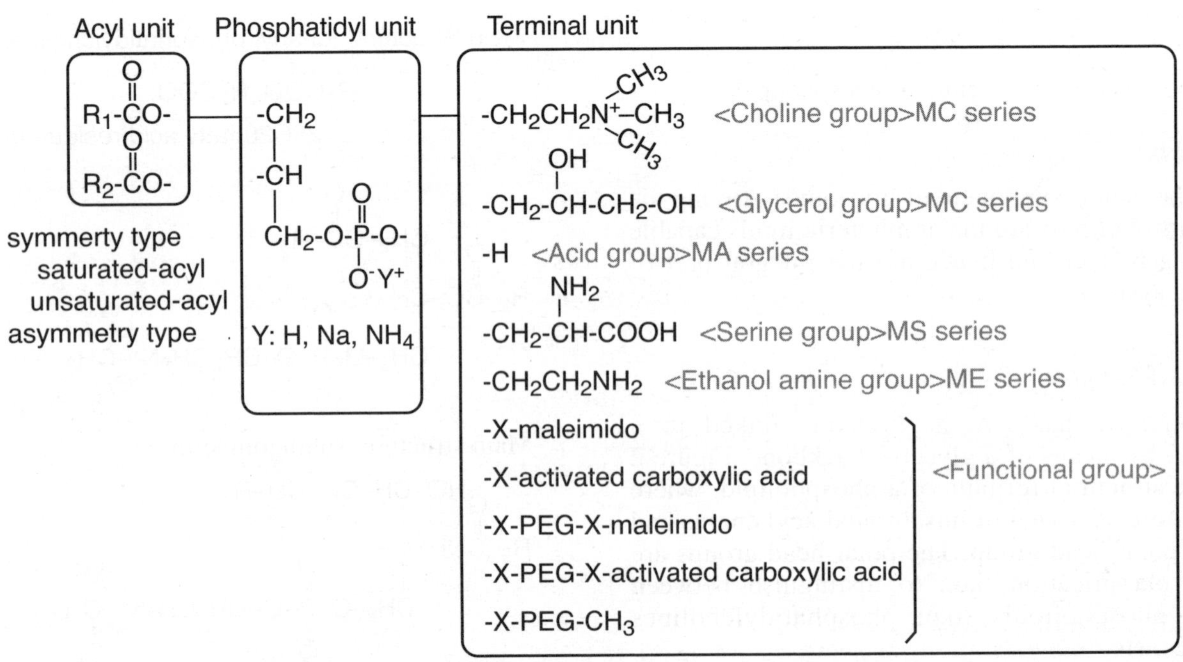

2. *Unsaturated acyl groups*: symmetric type: DOPE and dierucoyl phosphatidyl ethanolamine.
3. *Mixed acyl groups*: asymmetric type: 1-palmitoyl-2-oleoyl phosphatidyl ethanolamine.

2.1.1.2.5. Phosphatidylserine

1. *Saturated acyl groups*: symmetric type: dilauroyl phosphatidylserine, dimyristoyl phosphatidylserine (DMPS), dipalmitoyl phosphatidylserine (DPPS) and distearoyl phosphatidylserine.
2. *Unsaturated acyl groups*: symmetric type: dioleoyl phosphatidylserine (DOPS).

2.1.2. Cationic Lipids

Cationic lipids are of great importance in DNA and gene delivery. Most of the cationic lipids are trimethyl ammonium derivatives of fatty acids and the cationic charge is due to ammonium ion. Some cationic lipids used in the formulation of liposomes for delivery of genes and drugs, are listed below.

2.1.2.1. Stearyl Amine

2.1.2.1.1. DOTMA

DOTMA, a well-known cationic lipid is chemically *N*-(1,[2,3-dioleoyloxy]propyl)-*N,N,N*-trimethylammonium chloride (DOTMA). DOTMA by itself or in 1:1 combination with DOPE, sold under the tradename LIPOFECTIN® (Gibco/BRL: Life Technologies, Inc., Gaithersburg, MD), formulated into liposomes demonstrated efficient delivery of nucleic acids to some types of cells *(2)*.

2.1.2.1.2. DOTAP

Another commercially available cationic lipid is 1,2-bis(oleoyloxy)-3,3-(trimethylammonia) propane (DOTAP), which differs from DOTMA only in that the oleoyl moieties are linked via ester, rather than ether bonds to the propylamine. DOTAP is believed to be more readily degraded by target cells.

2.1.3. Other Cationic Lipids

Other related group of cationic lipids differ from DOTMA and DOTAP in that one of the methyl groups of the trimethylammonium group is replaced by a hydroxyethyl group. Compounds of this type are similar to the Rosenthal Inhibitor (RI) of phospholipase A which has stearoyl esters linked to the propylamine core *(3)*. The dioleoyl analogs of RI are commonly abbreviated as dioleoyl Rosenthal inhibitor (DORI)-ether and DORI-ester, depending on the linkage of the fatty acid moieties to the propylamine core. The hydroxy group can be used as a site for further functionalisation, for example, by esterification to carboxyspermine.

Another class of compounds is disclosed by Behr and co-workers *(4)*, where in carboxyspermine has been conjugated to two types of lipids. 5-Carboxyspermylglycine dioctadecylamide (DOGS) and dipalmitoylphosphatidylethanolamine 5-carboxy spermylamide (DPPES). Both DOGS and DPPES have been used to coat plasmids, forming a lipid aggregate complex that provides efficient transfection. The compounds are claimed to be more efficient and less toxic than DOTMA for transfection of some cell lines. DOGS is available commercially as TRANSFECTAM™ (Promega, Madison, Wis.)

Lipopolylysine, formed by conjugating polylysine to DOPE, has been reported to be especially effective for transfection in the presence of serum, a condition likely to be encountered *in vivo (5)*.

2.1.4. Cationic CHOL Derivatives

A cationic CHOL derivative (DC–CHOL) has been synthesised and formulated into liposomes in combination with DOPE *(6)*. The liposomes formulated with DC–CHOL provides more efficient transfection and lower toxicity than DOTMA-containing liposomes for some cell lines.

Lipids used generally in liposome preparations are listed in Table 1 along with their properties.

2.1.5. PEG Phospholipids and Others for Long Circulation

PEG or polyglycerine attached phospholipids can be applied for formulating liposomal drugs for prolonged circulation *in vivo*. There are three types of chemistry linking PEG with the lipid polar PE group as shown below.

2.1.5.1. Non-Charged PEGylated Lipid

1. PEG phospholipids: like DSPE–PEG (Table 2).
2. Polyglycerine phospholipids and new derivatives.
3. PEG neutral lipids:
   a. Diacylglycerol (DAG) PEG: Distearoyl $CH_3(CH_2)_6COO^-$ (PEG mol.wt.2000, 5000).
   Dipalmitoyl $CH_3(CH_2)_{14}COO$ (PEG mol.wt.2000).
   Dimyristoyl $CH_3(CH_2)_{12}COO$ (PEG mol.wt.2000).
   b. CHOL PEG derivatives: mol. wt. 1000, 2000, 5000—CHOL PEG for charge sensitive drugs.

Table 1. List of Lipids Generally Used in Liposome Preparation

Name	Carbons: unsaturation	Transition temperature (T_c [°C])	Net charge at pH 7.4
		Neutral lipids	
DLPC	12:0	–1	0
DMPC	14:0	23	0
DPPC	16:0	41	0
DSPC	18:0	55	0
DOPC	18:1	–20	0
DMPE	14:0	50	0
DPPE	16:0	63	0
DOPE	18:1	–16	0
		Anionic lipids	
DMPA sodium	14:0	50	–1.3
DPPA sodium	16:0	67	–1.3
DOPA sodium	18:1	–8	–1.3
DMPG sodium	14:0	23	–1
DPPG sodium	16:0	41	–1
DOPG sodium	18:1	–18	–1
DMPS sodium	14:0	35	–1
DPPS sodium	16:0	54	–1
DOPS sodium	18:1	–11	–1
DOPE–Glutaryl.	18:1	~–10	–2
Tetramyristoyl cardiolipin	14:0	59	–2
DPPE–mPEG-2000 sodium	16:0	N/A	–1
DPPE–mPEG-5000 sodium	16:0	N/A	–1
DPPE–carboxy PEG-2000 sodium	16:0	N/A	–2
		Cationic lipids	
DOTAP chloride salt	18:1	~–0	+1

2.1.5.2. FUNCTIONALISED PHOSPHOLIPIDS

1. Activated phospholipids:

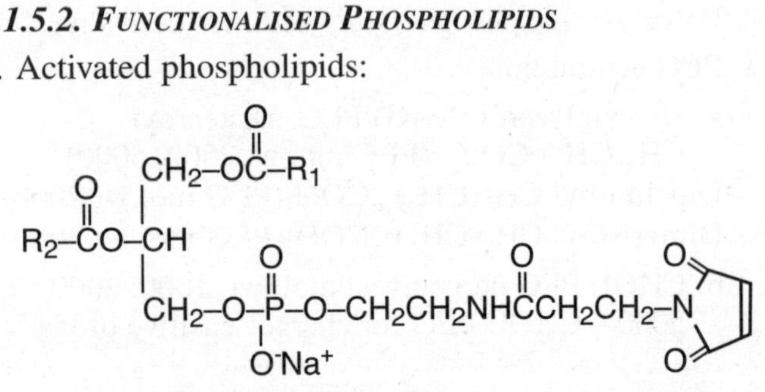

Maleimido (MAL) derivative for SH group reaction

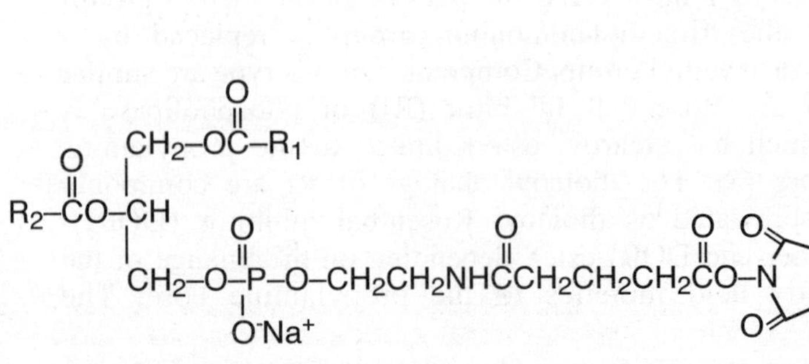

Activated carboxylic acid (NHS) for NH_2 group reaction

Table 2. List of PEG–Lipids With Their Structure and Molecular Weight

PEG–lipid	*Molecular weight (mol wt)*	*Structure*
DSPE–polyglycerine	700	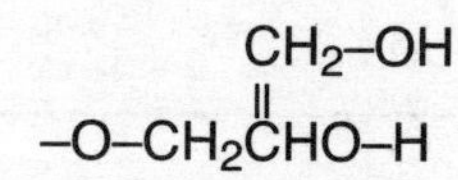
DSPE–multi-arm PEG	2000	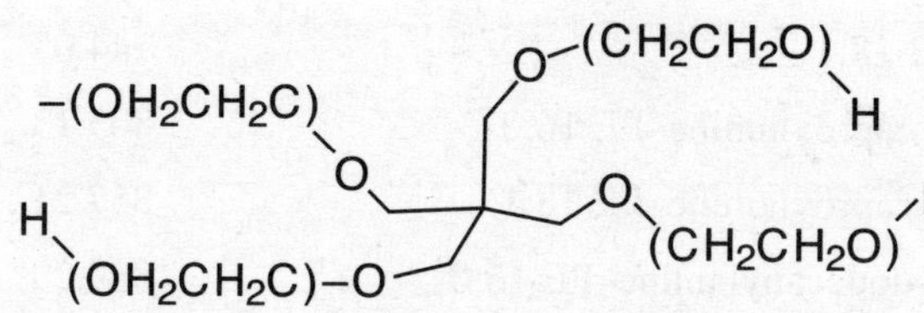
DSPE–comb-shaped PEG	12,000	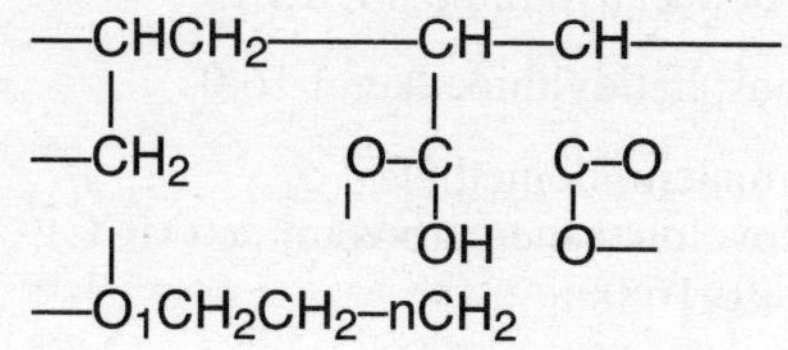

2. Activated PEG phospholipids:

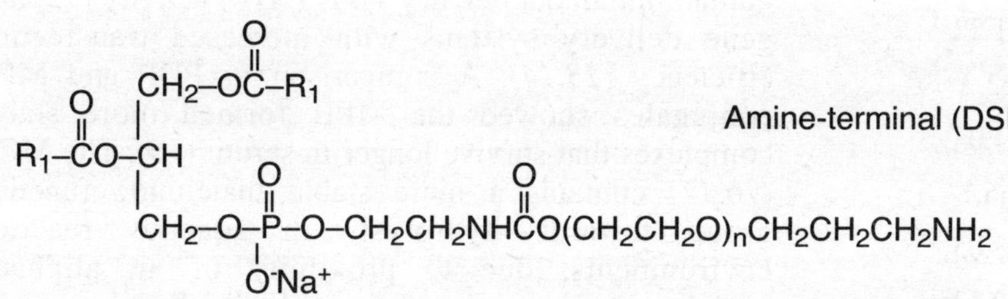

Amine-terminal (DSPE-PEG-NH_2)

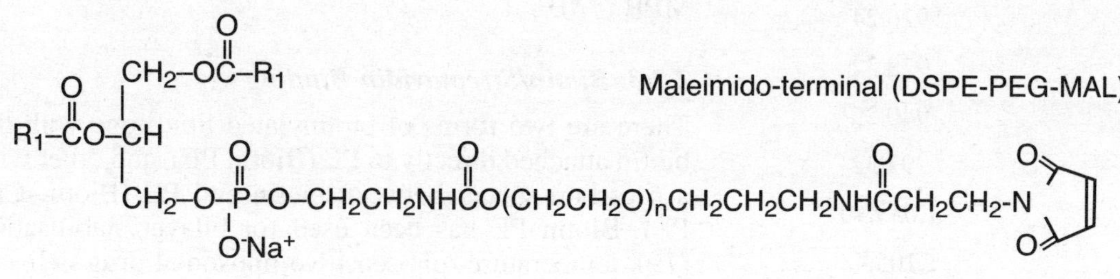

Maleimido-terminal (DSPE-PEG-MAL)

Lipids listed in Table 3 are a group of compounds designed to act as “membrane anchors” for ligands. A variety of functional groups are available to covalently attach various ligands. Each group of compounds is available with a saturated or unsaturated hydrophobic group so the transition temperature of the “anchor” can be defined.

2.2. Conjugation of Proteins/Peptides/Drugs to Liposomes

Numerous lipids exist for covalent or non-covalent attachment of proteins, peptides, or drugs to the liposome surface. Most of these lipids fall into three major classes of functionality: conjugation through amide bond formation, disulphide or thioether formation, or biotin/streptavidin binding.

Table 3. List of Lipids Used for Conjugation of Proteins/Peptides/Drugs to Liposomes

Product acyl composition	*Molecular weight (mol wt)*
PE 16:0	691.97
PE 18:1	744.05
N-caproylamine–PE 16:0	805.13
N-caproylamine–PE 18:1	857.21
N-dodecanylamine–PE 16:0	889.29
N-dodecanylamine–PE 18:1	941.37
Phosphatidylthioethanol 16:0	731
N-maleimidomethyl-cyclohexane-carboxamide (MCC)–PE 16:0	928.24
N-MCC–PE 18:1	980.32
N-maleimido-phenyl-butyramide (MPB)–PE 16:0	955.2
N-MPB–PE 18:1.	1,007.27
N-pyridyl-dithiopropionate (PDP)–PE 16:0.	911.22
N-PDP–PE 18:1.	963.3
N-succinyl–PE 16:0	814.03
N-succinyl–PE 18:1	866.1
N-glutaryl–PE 16:0	828.05
N-glutaryl–PE 18:1	880.13
N-Dodecanoyl–PE 16:0	926.24
N-dodecanoyl–PE 18:1	978.32
N-biotinyl–PE 16:0	940.25
N-biotinyl–PE 18:1	992.32
N-biotinyl cap–PE 16:0	1,053.40
N-biotinyl cap–PE 18:1	1,105.48
Phosphatidyl(ethylene glycol)16:0	714.94
Phosphatidyl(ethylene glycol)18:1	767.01

2.2.1. Amide Conjugation

Phospholipids with either amine or carboxyl functional groups for conjugation with proteins/peptides, or drugs containing amine, carboxyl, or hydroxy groups. Carboxyacyl derivatives of PE have been used to achieve high (up to 60%) coupling efficiency of antibodies to the surface of preformed liposomes *(7)*. Various acyl chain lengths ranging from 4 to 22 carbons were utilised in the study, with optimum coupling efficiency being achieved with a chain length of 12 carbons (1,12-dodecanedicarboxylate). More recently, it has been demonstrated that conjugation of an antibody to *N*-glutaryl PE prior to mixing with DOPE/DOPA successfully produced target-sensitive immunoliposomes *(8)*.

2.2.2. Disulphide/Thioether Conjugation

Several lipids for disulphide (PDP–PE) or thioether (MPB–PE or MCC–PE) conjugation of thio-containing proteins or peptides. The maleimide-containing lipid, MPB–PE, has been used to couple the homing device glu-plasminogen to liposomes without loss of activity or interference with its fibrin-binding/homing capacity *(9)*. Also, this compound successfully formed antibody-conjugated echogenic liposomes for ultrasonic image enhancement, specifically for the detection and characterisation of atherosclerosis *(10)*. These lipid derivatives have also been used for delivery of prodrugs with anti-tumoral activity *(11)*, drug carriers with anti-human immunodeficiency virus (HIV) activity *(12)* and gene delivery systems with increased transfection efficiency *(13,14)*. A comparison of PDP and MPB conjugates showed the MPB formed more stable complexes that survive longer in serum *(15)*. The MCC *(16,17)* contains a more stable maleimide function group towards hydrolysis in aqueous reaction environments, due to proximity of an aliphatic cyclohexane ring rather than aromatic phenyl group of MPB *(18)*.

2.2.3. Biotin/Streptavidin Binding

There are two forms of biotinylated lipid: one with the biotin attached directly to PE (Biotin PE), and other with a 6-carbon spacer between biotin and PE (Biotin–Cap PE). Biotin PE has been used for bilayer stabilisation *(19)*, temperature-/pH-sensitive liposomal drug delivery *(20)*, tumor imaging *(21)*, two-dimensional (2D) crystallisation on lipid bilayers *(22–24)* and immobilisation of liposomes on gel beads for chromatographic analysis of drug-partitioning *(25)*. Its use for *in vivo* targeting applications utilising liposomes containing monosialoganglioside (GM_1) or PEG lipid derivatives has been demonstrated *(26)*. However, it was later shown that the Biotin–Cap PE derivative was superior in these applications because the spacer arm extended the biotinyl group out from the membrane

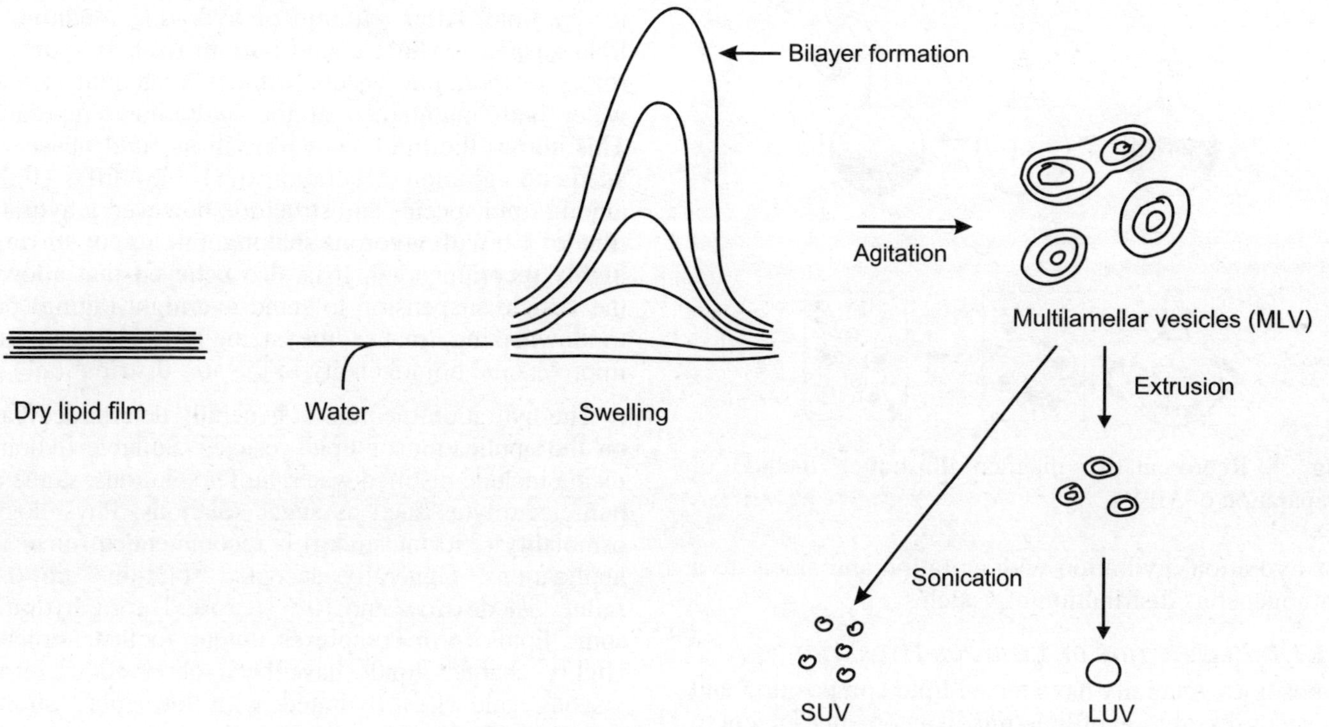

Fig. 3. Mechanism of liposome formation.

surface *(27)*. Steric hindrance at the surface due to inclusion of large bulky amphiphiles such as GM_1 or PEG–PE inhibits optimal vesicle binding to streptavidin which could be alleviated by using Biotin–Cap PE.

2.2.4. Mechanism of Vesicle Formation

Liposomes (lipid vesicles) are formed when thin lipid films or lipid cakes are hydrated and stacks of liquid crystalline bilayers become fluid and swell (Fig. 3). The hydrated lipid sheets detach during agitation and self-close to form large multi-lamellar vesicles (LMV), which prevents interaction of water with the hydrocarbon core of bilayer at the edges.

Once these particles have formed, reducing the size of particle requires energy input in the form of sonic energy (sonication) or mechanical energy (extrusion).

3. PREPARATION OF LIPOSOMES

Liposomes can be prepared by several methods, most simple like hand shakes method to highly complex involving pH gradient method. Similarly, the equipment required may be as simple as a flask to high pressure homogeniser. However, method selection for preparation depends on various parameters like type of liposomes, size, composition, property of components particularly lipids and scales of preparation, etc. However, there are few basic methods which are generally adopted with necessary modifications to prepare different types of liposomes.

3.1. Preparation of MLVs and Small Unilamellar Vesicles (SUVs)

3.1.1. Thin Film Hydration Method

The method, probably the first technique developed for preparation of basic liposomes which are generally MLVs, is represented in Fig. 4. Properties of lipid formulations can vary depending on the composition (cationic, anionic and neutral lipid species); however, same preparation method can be used for all lipid vesicles regardless of composition. The general elements of the procedure involve preparation of lipid

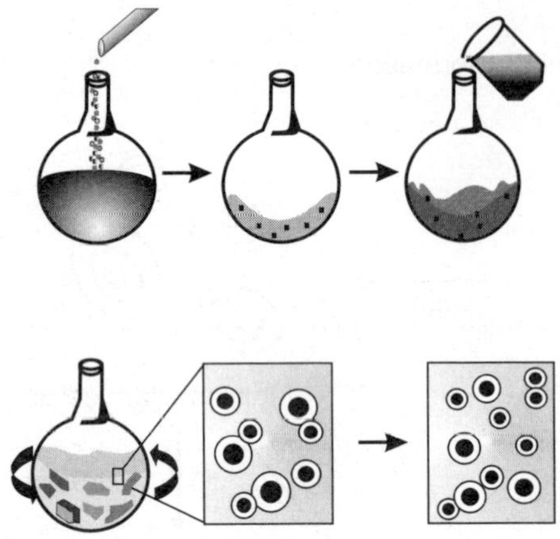

Fig. 4. Representative diagram illustrating method of preparation of MLVs.

for hydration, hydration with agitation and sizing to a homogeneous distribution of vesicles.

3.1.1.1. Preparation of Lipid for Hydration

Liposomes generally have mixed lipid composition and so needs dissolution of lipid mix in an organic solvent to assure a homogeneous mixing of lipids. Usually this process is carried out using chloroform or chloroform: methanol mixtures. Generally, lipid solutions are prepared at 10–20 mg lipid/mL organic solvent, although higher concentrations may be used if the lipid solubility and mixing are acceptable. The lipid solution is then subjected to evaporation to yield a lipid film. For small volumes of organic solvent (<1 mL), the solvent may be evaporated using a dry nitrogen or argon stream in a fume hood while for larger volumes, the organic solvent should be removed using a rotary evaporator to get a thin lipid film on the sides of a round bottom flask. The lipid film is thoroughly dried to remove residual organic solvent by placing the vial or flask on a vacuum pump overnight. If the use of chloroform is objectionable, an alternative is to dissolve the lipid(s) in tertiary butanol or cyclohexane. The lipid solution is transferred to containers and frozen by placing the containers on a block of dry ice or swirling the container in a dry ice–acetone or alcohol (ethanol or methanol) bath. The frozen lipid cake is placed on a vacuum pump and lyophilised until dry (1–3 d depending on volume) and is stored in frozen state in a tightly closed container until ready to hydrate.

3.1.1.2. Hydration of Lipid Film/Cake

Hydration of dry lipid film/cake is accomplished by adding an aqueous medium to the container of dry lipid and agitating. The temperature of hydrating medium should be above the gel-liquid crystal transition temperature (T_c) of lipid with highest T_c before adding to dry lipid. After addition of hydrating medium, the lipid suspension in a round bottom flask is spun on a rotory evaporation system without a vacuum in warm water bath maintained at the hydrating temperature. This allows the lipid to hydrate in its fluid phase with adequate agitation. Hydration time may differ slightly among lipid species and structure, however, a hydration time of 1 h with vigorous shaking, mixing, or stirring is highly recommended. It is also believed that allowing the vesicle suspension to stand overnight (aging) prior to downsizing, makes the sizing process easier and improves the homogeneity in the size distribution.

The hydration medium is generally determined based on the application of lipid vesicles. Suitable hydration media include distilled water, buffer solutions, saline and non-electrolytes such as sugar solutions. Physiological osmolality (290 mOsm/kg) is recommended for *in vivo* applications. Generally accepted solutions are 0.9% saline, 5% dextrose and 10% sucrose. During hydration, some lipids form complexes unique to their structure. Highly charged lipids have been observed to form a viscous gel when hydrated with low ionic strength solutions. The problem can be alleviated by addition of salt or by downsizing the lipid suspension. Poorly hydrating lipids such as phosphatidylethanolamine have a tendency to self aggregate upon hydration. Lipid vesicles containing more than 60 mol% phosphatidylethanolamine form particles having a small hydration layer surrounding the vesicle. As particles approach one another they adhere and form aggregates, as there is no hydration repulsion to repel the approaching particle. The aggregates settle out of solution as large flocculates which will disperse on agitation but reform on storage.

The product of hydration is generally a LMV with each lipid bilayer separated by a water layer. The spacing between lipid layers is dictated by composition with polyhydrating layers being closer together than highly charged layers which separate based on electrostatic repulsion. Once a stable, hydrated LMV suspension has been produced, the particles can be downsized by a variety of techniques, including sonication or extrusion.

3.1.1.3. Sizing of Lipid Suspension

3.1.1.3.1. Sonication

Disruption of LMV suspensions using sonic energy (sonication) typically produces SUV with diameters in range of 15–50 nm. The most common instrumentation for preparation of sonicated particles is bath and probe tip sonicators. Cup-horn sonicators, although less widely used, have successfully produced SUV. Probe tip sonicators deliver high-energy input to the lipid suspension but suffer from overheating of the lipid suspension causing degradation. Sonication tips also tend to release titanium particles into the lipid suspension which must be removed by centrifugation prior to use. For these reasons, bath sonicators are the most widely used instrumentation for preparation of SUV. Sonication of LMV dispersion is accomplished by placing a test tube containing the suspension in a bath sonicator (or placing the tip of the sonicator in the test tube) and sonicating for 5–10 min above T_c of the lipid. The lipid suspension should begin to clarify to yield a slightly hazy transparent solution. The haze is due to light scattering induced by residual large particles remaining in suspension. These particles can be removed by centrifugation to yield a clear suspension of SUV. Mean size and distribution is influenced by composition and concentration, temperature, sonication time and power, volume and sonicator tuning. Because it is nearly impossible to reproduce the conditions of sonication, size variation between batches produced at different times is not uncommon. Also, due to the high degree of curvature of these membranes, SUV are inherently unstable and will spontaneously fuse to form larger vesicles when stored below their phase transition temperature.

3.1.1.3.2. Extrusion

Lipid extrusion is a technique in which a lipid suspension is forced through a polycarbonate filter with a defined pore size to yield particles having a diameter near the pore size of the filter used. Prior to extrusion through the final pore size, LMV suspensions are disrupted either by several freeze–thaw cycles or by prefiltering the suspension through a larger pore size (typically 0.2–1.0 μm). This method helps prevent the membranes from fouling and improves the homogeneity of size distribution of final suspension. As with all procedures for downsizing LMV dispersions, the extrusion should be done at a temperature above the T_c of the lipid. Attempts to extrude below the T_c will be unsuccessful as the membrane has a tendency to foul with rigid membranes which cannot pass through the pores. Extrusion through filters with 100 nm pores typically yields large unilamellar vesicles (LUV) with a mean diameter of 120–140 nm. Mean particle size also depends on lipid composition and is quite reproducible from batch to batch.

The particle size distribution of unilamellar vesicles prepared by extrusion is a function of the number of passes through extruder membrane. Hydrated lipid solutions will initially form LMVs. After the initial pass through a membrane, the particle size distribution will tend towards a bimodal distribution. After sufficient passes through the membrane, a unimodal, normal distribution is obtained. A minimum of 11 passes through the extruder membrane is recommended for most lipids *(28,29)*.

3.1.1.4. Method Involving Injection of Water Immiscible Solvent

Alternative "two phase" methods for preparing liposomes with higher encapsulation is developed based on injection of water immiscible solvents containing a mixture of bilayer forming lipids into an aqueous medium. These methods can produce relatively uniform, unilamellar and oligolamellar vesicles with encapsulation efficiencies of about 20% and 45%, presumably due to the formation of relatively large unilamellar structures.

3.1.1.4.1. Ether Injection Method

The ether injection method provides a means of preparing liposomes by slowly introducing a solution of lipids dissolved in diethyl ether into warm aqueous solution of material to be encapsulated at about 55–60°C or under reduced pressure under stirring. A syringe type infusion pump may be used for the purpose (Fig. 5). Vaporisation of ether leads to formation of single layer vesicles. Depending on the conditions used, the vesicle size ranges from 50 to 200 nm.

3.1.1.4.2. Fluorocarbon Injection Method

To overcome the hazards presented by diethyl ether, flurocarbons like Freon 21 ($CHFCl_2$) is an excellent alternative, which is an excellent solvent for phospholipids, water immiscible and boils at low temperature (9°C). Hindjani *et al.* rather than injecting the lipid solution into warm water, improvised the method by infusing the lipid solution in fluorocarbon into cool water under low pressure and manipulating the solvent evaporation by increasing pressure or temperature *(30)*. This method was able to accomplish solvent stripping at a low temperature *(30)*.

3.1.1.5. Method Involving Injection of Water Miscible Solvent

Using fairly safe water miscible solvent like ethanol, glycerol and polyglycols is an alternative solvent injection approach. In this method, during infusion the solvent containing lipid is diluted by an excess amount of the aqueous phase. As solvent power is reduced due to dilution, liposome is formed. The major drawback in this method is removal of solvent. However, such solvent can be removed by diafiltration to limit of acceptable residual volume.

3.1.1.5.1. Ethanol Injection Method

This is an alternative method that avoids both sonication and exposure to high pressure *(31)*. Lipid mixture is

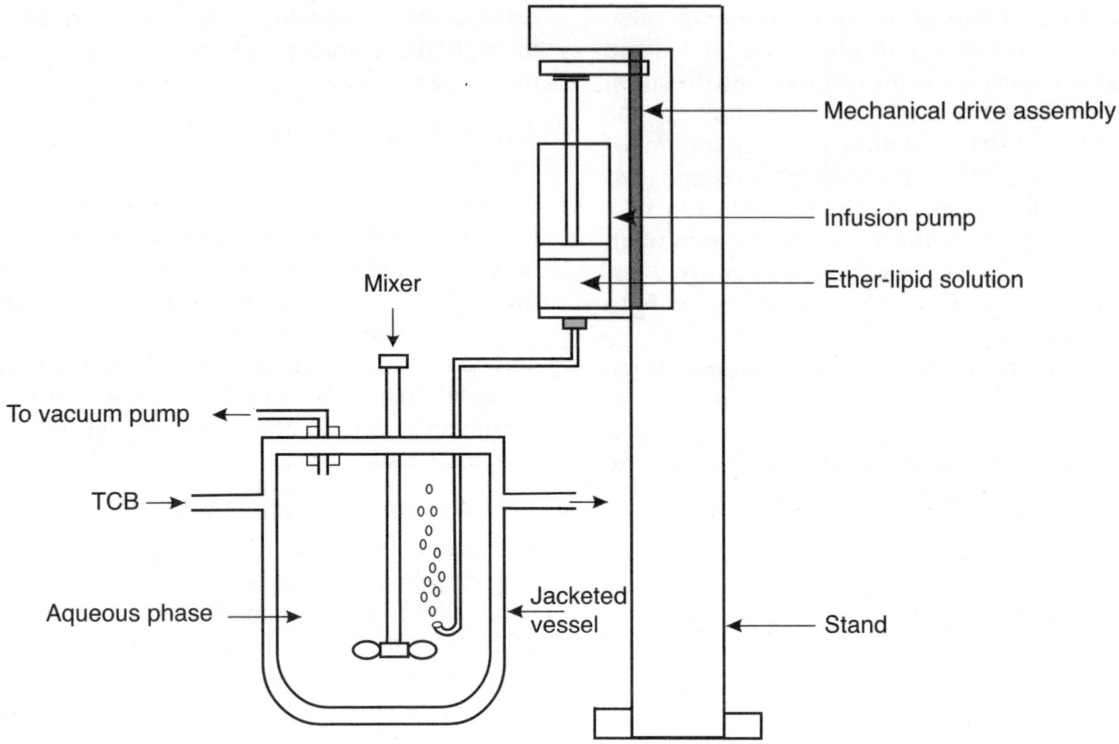

Fig. 5. A Syring type infusion pump used to prepare liposome by ether injection method.

dissolved in ethanol and rapidly injected in to an excess of buffer solution. SUVs are spontaneously formed. The procedure is simple and rapid and suitable for protein drugs that denature under drastic conditions of sonication or exposure to high pressure. Unfortunately, this method produces comparatively dilute suspensions of SUVs. The concentration of ethanol in the final product should not exceed 10–20% by volume as at higher concentration, SUVs tends to grow in size after formation. Residual ethanol is generally removed by ultrafiltration because vacuum distillation pose problems since the partial vapour pressure of ethanol in low residual concentration is small compared to that of water. The other disadvantage of ethanol is that even at low residual concentration there is a loss of activity of biologically active macromolecules.

3.1.1.5.2. Alternative Water Miscible Solvents

Polyhydric alcohols such as glycerol, polyglycerols, propyleneglycol and ethyleneglycol as well as glyceroesters such as monocetin are claimed to adequately solubilise lipids and form liposomes on mixing with large excess of aqueous volume *(32)*. Because these solvents are relatively safe, they can be left in formulations in small concentrations and in fact would stabilise liposomal suspension from sedimentation. Presence of these solvents has an additional advantage during freeze drying as cryoprotectants.

3.2. Preparation of LMVs

LMVs and also MLVs are prepared by lyophilising (freeze-drying) lipid mixtures dissolved in a non-polar organic solvent. The method involves the following steps;

- Dissolve the lipids in chloroform.
- Combine the lipids in the appropriate ratio.
- Carefully evaporate the organic solvent using a dry nitrogen stream.
- Re-suspend the lipid mixture in cyclohexane. If the mixture is not completely soluble in cyclohexane, add a small amount of ethanol (1–2% of cyclohexane volume). Do not use too much ethanol as the solution will not freeze with excessive ethanol present.
- Freeze the cyclohexane solution using dry ice.
- Quickly place the frozen mixture on a high vacuum system (lyophilisation system). The sample should remain frozen until it is completely dry; if the sample begins to thaw, either the vacuum is not strong enough or there is too much ethanol present. A thawed sample will not produce a white powder and it may bump or foam out of the vial.
- Leave the sample on vacuum system for 3–5 h (depending on how much cyclohexane was used) or until the sample is completely dry.

- Suspend the lipid mixture in aqueous buffer and allow mixture to hydrate above the transition temperature of lipid for 30–60 min (vortexing occasionally).

This procedure yields large multi-lamellar vesicles (LMV or MLV) *(33)*. For water soluble compounds to be entrapped, the same protocol is followed except the compound is dissolved in aqueous buffer used to reconstitute the dry lipid and the external compound (not encapsulated) is removed by gel filtration.

3.3. Preparation of LUVs (Intermediate Size)

LUVs refer to vesicles bounded by a single bilayer membrane that are above 100 nm in diameter. However, some authors have referred liposome of size between 50 and 100 nm as large *(34)*. LUVs provide a number of advantages as compared to MLVs, including high encapsulation of water soluble drugs, economy of lipids and reproducible drug release rates. But LUVs are perhaps the most difficult types of liposomes to produce and are also sensitive to external influences particularly while in circulation in the body. Two primary methods are used to produce LUVs, one involving detergent dialysis and the other by formation of water in oil emulsion. Intermediate sized LUVs can also be generated from MLV dispersions by sequential extrusion through polycarbonate membranes of small pore size under high pressure. Freeze–thaw cycling *(35)*, slow swelling in non-electrolytes *(36)*, dehydration and rehydration *(37)* and dilution or dialysis of lipids in presence of chaotropic ions *(38)* are the other techniques adoptable for preparing large/intermediate sized unilamellar vesicles.

3.3.1. Detergent Dialysis Method

This method utilises radically different approach of removing detergent molecules from aqueous dispersion of phospholipids/detergent mixed micelles. As the detergent is removed, the micelles become progressively richer in phospholipids and finally coalesce to form closed, single bilayer vesicles. Drawbacks of this method are leakage and dilution of drug during liposome formation, high cost, difficulty in removal of last traces of detergent and quality control. Detergents generally used are Triton X-100. The method involves preparation of micellar dispersion of phospholipids and detergent in aqueous system in which the drug is dissolved/solubilised. The micellar dispersion is then subjected to one of the following methods to remove the detergent.

3.3.1.1. Detergent Dialysis

Detergent dialysis as a method of preparation of liposome was first introduced by Kagawa and Racker in 1971 *(39)*. Detergents commonly used for this purpose are the one with relatively high critical micelle concentration like bile salts, octylglucoside, etc. and this property facilitates their removal. Milsmann *et al.* *(40)* optimised the conditions for the removal of detergent with a flow through dialysis cell of the type illustrated in Fig. 6. The procedure results in the formation of homogenous population of single layered vesicles with mean diameters of 50–100 nm.

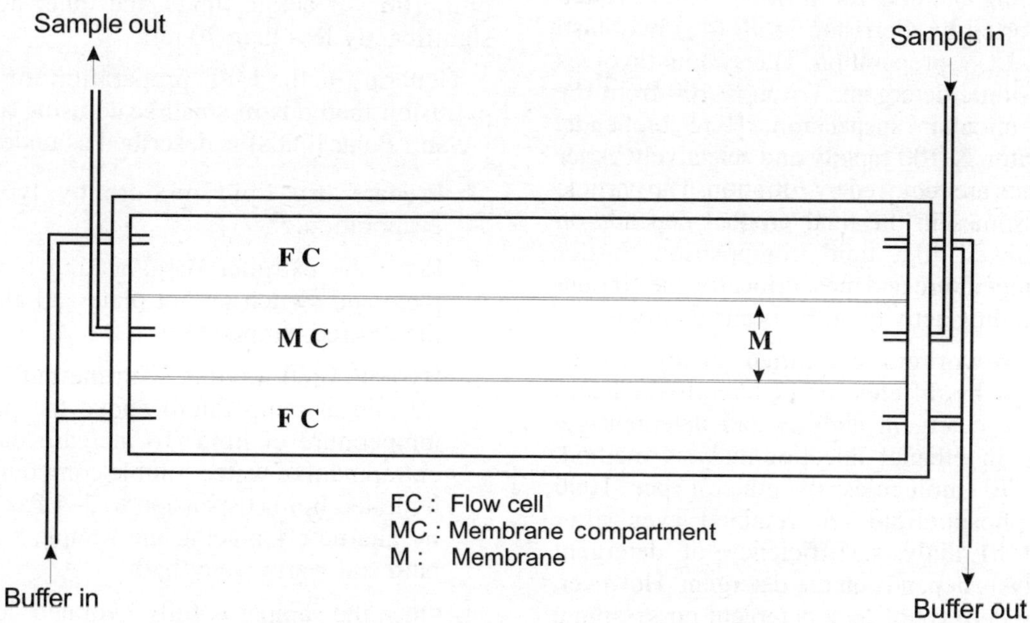

Fig. 6. Flow through dialysis cell for removal of detergent.

Wim Jiskoot *et al.* *(41)* prepared fairly homogeneous liposome dispersions with mean diameters ranging from 100 to more than 200 nm from mixed micellar solutions, containing constant octyl glucoside and egg PC concentrations and varying amounts of CHOL and/or a charged compound, by dilution followed by dialysis. The particle size was found dependent on CHOL content and surface charge, and could be reproducibly controlled by adjustment of dilution rate. Liposomes with a mean diameter less than 100 nm were also obtained, but were heterodispersed and unstable. The incorporation of charged compounds was monitored by micro-electrophoresis. ^{31}P-Nuclear magnetic resonance (NMR) measurements indicated that liposomes were unilamellar. Dialysis appeared to be more convenient than washing to remove octyl glucoside.

3.3.1.2. Column Chromatography

The formation of 100 nm, single layered phospholipids vesicles during removal of deoxycholate by column chromatography has been reported by Enoch and Strittmater *(42)*. The method involves mixing phospholipids, in the form of either small sonicated vesicles or a dry lipid film, with deoxycholate at a molar ratio of 1:2, respectively. Subsequent removal of detergent during passage of the dispersion over a Sephadex G-25 column results in the formation of uniform 100 nm vesicles that are readily separable from small sonicated vesicles.

3.3.1.2.1. Biobeads

Another promising method for forming reconstituted membranes reported by Gerristen *et al.* (43) may also be applicable to LUV preparation. The system involves removal of non-ionic detergent, Triton X-100 from the detergent/lipid micellar suspension. Here biobeads, SM-2 absorb Triton X-100 rapidly and selectively. After removal, the beads are removed by filtration. The particle size of the liposomes in the final product depends on conditions followed like lipid composition, buffer composition, temperature and most critically, the amount and detergent binding activity of the beads themselves.

Allen and co-workers examined efficiency of detergent removal by different procedures like ethanol injection-dialysis, detergent dialysis and detergent-gel filtration (211). In ethanol injection-dialysis method, approximately 70 molecules of ethanol per 1000 molecules of phospholipid are retained even after extensive (150 h) dialysis. Efficiency of detergent removal by dialysis depends on the detergent. However, even for sodium deoxycholate, a detergent possessing a large critical micelle concentration, there are approximately 7 molecules of deoxycholate per 1000 molecules of phospholipid retained by the bilayer even after extensive (310 h) dialysis. Detergent removal by gel filtration (Sephadex G-200 or G-50) of deoxycholate, cholic acid and Triton X-100 is more efficient than removal by dialysis; as few as 10 molecules of deoxycholate are retained per 100 molecules of phospholipid after one column passage, taking only a few hours. Ethanol was less efficiently removed by one passage over a Sephadex column than by extensive dialysis. Removal of Triton X-100 by passage over, or dialysis against, Biobeads SM-2 resulted in a similar level of detergent retention to that found by passage over Sephadex G-200 or G-50.

3.3.2. Extrusion Method

MLV suspensions rich in acidic lipids, such as phosphatidylserine and phosphatidylglycerol tend to have large inter-bilayer space due to electrostatic repulsive forces. Hence, they have large aqueous space both at internal aqueous core and also in between the bilayer. When such vesicles are repeatedly extruded through very small pore-diameter polycarbonate membrane (80–100 nm), under high pressure (up to 800 psi), they become progressively smaller in diameter up to 60–80 nm after about 5–10 passes. More over, with repeated extrusion, the vesicles tend to become single layered due to peeling. For this method to produce truly single layered, the aqueous core should be greater than 70 nm diameter, which is possible in case of liposome with high proportion of acidic lipids while, in liposome with neutral lipids or with low proportion of acidic lipids, the inner aqueous core is significantly less than 70 nm.

General method of preparation of liposome by extrusion methods in small scale using a mini extruder (Avanti Polar lipids) is described as under:

1. Prepare dry lipid mixture by lyophilisation or evaporation.
2. Place the extruder stand/heating block onto a hot plate and switch on hot plate and allow it to reach the desired temperature.
3. Hydrate lipid mixture with the buffer for less than 30 min at temperature above the phase transition temperature of lipid. To increase the efficiency of entrapment of water-soluble compounds, subject the hydrated lipid suspension to 3–5 freeze/thaw cycles by alternately placing the sample vial in a dry ice bath and warm water bath.
4. Once the sample is fully hydrated, load the sample into one of the gas-tight syringes and carefully place

into one end of the Mini-Extruder. To reduce the dead volume, pre-wet extruder parts by passing a syringe full of buffer through the extruder; discard the buffer.

5. Place empty gas-tight syringe into other end of the Mini-Extruder. Make sure the empty syringe plunger is set to zero.
6. Check temperature of heating block before placing the assembled extruder apparatus into heating block. The temperature must be less than 80°C, otherwise syringes will be damaged.
7. Insert fully assembled extruder apparatus into the extruder stand. Allow temperature of the lipid suspension to equilibrate with temperature of the heating block (~5–10 min).
8. Gently push the plunger of filled syringe until the lipid solution is completely transferred to alternate syringe. Gently push the plunger of alternate syringe to transfer the solution back to the original syringe. Repeat these steps a minimum of four times (total of 10 passes through membrane). In general, more the passes through membrane, the lipid solution becomes more homogenous.
9. The final extrusion should fill the alternate syringe. This is to reduce the chances of contamination with larger particles or foreign material.
10. After the final extrusion, remove the Mini-Extruder from heating block. Remove filled syringe from the extruder and inject lipid solution into a clean sample vial and store at 4°C. Do not freeze. Vesicle solutions are not stable in aqueous media for more than 3–4 d when stored at 4°C. Storage of vesicle solutions at higher temperatures and pH less than 5 or more than 8 may reduce the lifetime of the vesicle suspension.

4. REVERSE PHASE EVAPORATION (REV) TECHNIQUE

This method involves the preparation of water-in-oil (W/O) emulsion of phospholipids and buffer in excess organic phase followed by removal of organic phase under reduced pressure *(44)*. Emulsification of two phases is usually brought about by sonication or by any other mechanical means. Removal of organic phase causes the formation of phospholipids coated droplets of water to coalesce and eventually form a viscous gel. Removal of the final traces of solvent under high vacuum or mechanical disruption (such as vortexing) results in collapse of the gel forming smooth suspension of LUVs. However, with some compositions, the transition from emulsion to LUV suspension is so rapid that the intermediate gel phase goes unnoticed. A representative diagram showing phases during the liposome formation by REV technique is shown in Fig. 7. This method can give the entrapment efficiency up to 65%.

To prepare REV type liposomes, the phospholipids are first dissolved in an organic solvent such as diethylether, isopropylether or their mixture with chloroform. Emulsification is accomplished easily, particularly when the density of the organic solution matches with the buffer solution and hence, the organic solvent with low density like ether (0.7), is mixed with solvent of high density like trichloro fluoro methane (1.4) to produce a solvent system. The aqueous phase containing the material to be entrapped is added to the lipid solution in a ratio of 1:3 for ether and 1:6 for isopropylether:chloroform mixture. The two phases are sonicated for few minutes to form W/O emulsion. The organic phase is carefully removed under partial vacuum in a rotary evaporator at 20–30°C and pressure maintained at about 500 psi for the removal of the bulk of organic phase and then lowered cautiously to remove the traces.

Principle disadvantage of this method is the exposure of material to be entrapped to organic solvent and mechanical agitation which may cause denaturation of proteins. However, there are reports where biologically active molecules like RNA and various enzymes have also been encapsulated without loss of activity.

LUV and oligolamellar vesicles are formed when an aqueous buffer is introduced into a mixture of phospholipid and organic solvent and the organic solvent is subsequently removed by evaporation under reduced pressure. These vesicles can be made from various lipids or mixtures of lipids and have aqueous volume to lipid ratios that are 30 times higher than sonicated preparations and four times higher than MLV. Most importantly, a substantial fraction of the aqueous phase (up to 65% at low salt concentrations) is entrapped within the vesicles, encapsulating even large macromolecular assemblies with high efficiency. Thus, this relatively simple technique has unique advantages for encapsulating valuable water-soluble materials such

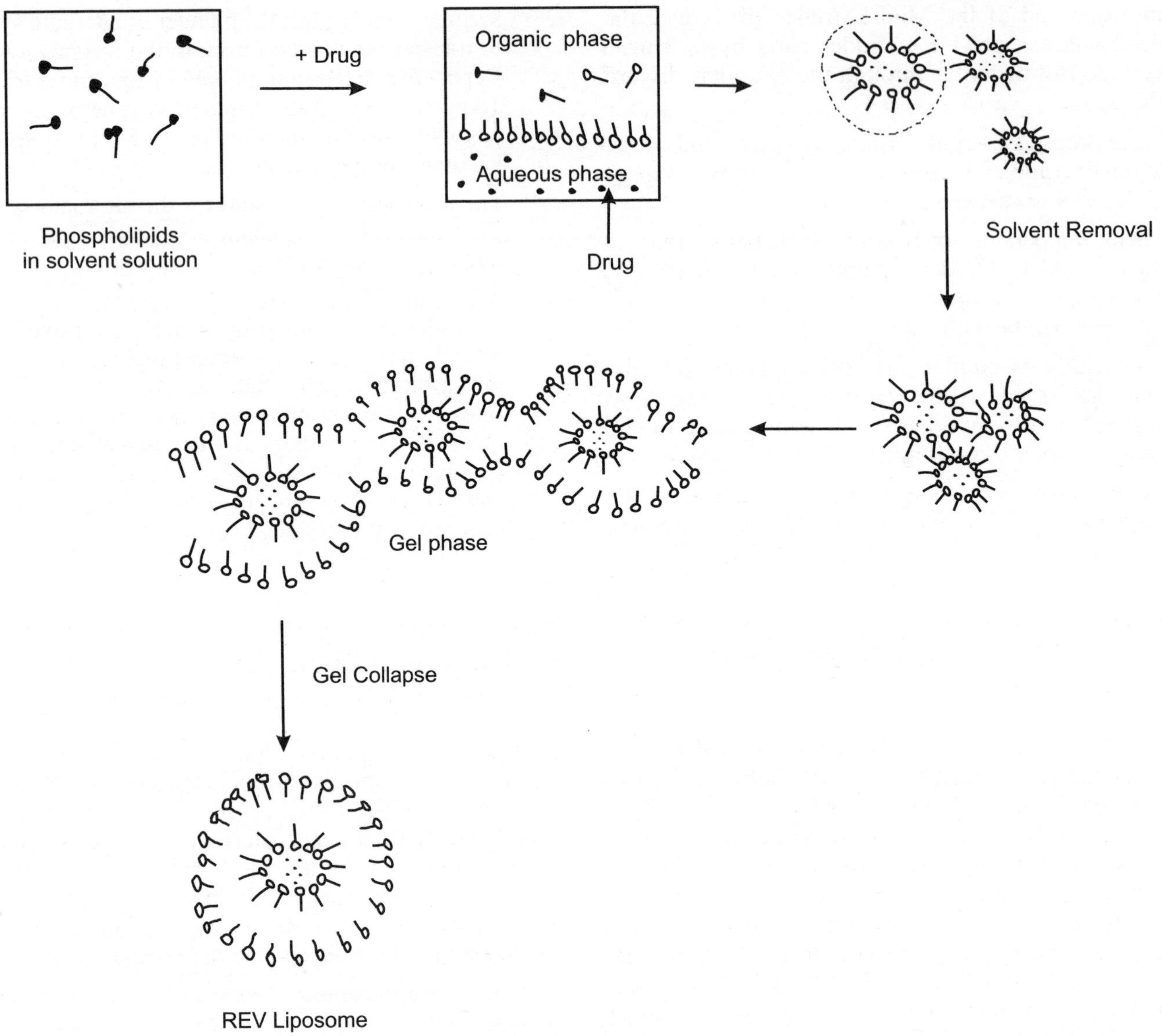

Fig. 7. A representative diagram showing phases during the liposome formation by REV technique.

as drugs, proteins, nucleic acids and other biochemical compounds. The preparation and properties of the vesicles are described in detail.

Cortesi *et al.* describes the use of different organic solvents, namely ethanol, ethyl acetate and mixtures of ethanol/ethyl acetate, for the production of liposomes by the REV technique using retinyl acetate and sodium cromoglycate as model drugs *(45)*. The association yield for hydrophilic drug and the encapsulation yield for hydrophilic model drug were found, in all the liposome preparations, to be satisfactory. In particular, the use of more polar organic solvents (with respect to diethyl ether) appears to enhance the encapsulation of the hydrophilic drug, sodium cromoglycate. The author proposed the use of alternative organic solvents to diethyl ether with the aim of reducing toxic problems associated with the presence of residual traces of organic solvents in final liposome formulation.

Sallie *et al.* compared several lipid reconstitution methods in transferring the predominant thylakoid lipid, monogalactosyldiglyceride (MG), to the aqueous phase *(46)*. They reported a REV method that employs Freon 11 as a lipid solvent capable of successfully hydrating MG in spinach (*Spinacia oleracea* L.) at room temperature within minutes. Using this method it is possible to force an equal weight mixture of MG and digalactosyldiglyceride into small bilayer vesicles without formation of inverted micellar 'lipidic particles' in the membranes.

4.1. A Single-Step Method of Liposome Preparation

All the liposome preparation protocols, which involve drug encapsulation are multi-step processes, i.e., they consist of several steps of preparation and homogenisation. The conditions of converting all lipids into vesicles smaller than 200 nm in a single step was worked out by Zawada by replacing ultrasonication with mechanical stirring of buffer and solution of lipids in a low-boiling point organic solvent or solvents and the process be carried out at a temperature higher than the temperature of the gel/fluid phase transition (T_c), and higher than the boiling point of the organic solvent(s). For many lipid membrane compositions, the products of preparation contain a dominant fraction of unilamellar vesicles (<200 nm) and a fraction of much larger multivesicular or MLV, easily separated by simple centrifugation at 15000*g*. If PEG–PE or cholesteryl palmitate are additional membrane components, multi-vescular or MLVs are virtually absent in the final product, of a single-step process and all the used lipids are quantitatively converted into vesicles smaller than 200 nm in diameter *(47)*.

4.2. Methods of Controlling Liposome Size

Three possible approaches have been explored for achieving defined particle size distribution of liposomes:

1. Fractionation of desired size from a heterogeneous population.
2. Homogenisation of a poly-disperse distribution.
3. Extrusion of a heterogeneous preparation through various membranes of known pore diameter to yield liposome with average size that bear some relationship to the rated pore diameter of the extruding membrane.

4.2.1. Fractionation

Two methods have become popular for fractionating defined sized liposomes from a heterogeneous population; centrifugation and size exclusion chromatography (SEC). Both the techniques are used for the enrichment of product with the desired particle size.

4.2.1.1. Centrifugation

Sedimentation of liposomes under the influence of centrifugal force is related to the particle size and density and thus offers method to isolate liposomes of desired particle size range. Large liposomes composed of neutral lipids such as PC can easily be pelleted at fairly low gravitational force. Under proper conditions, smaller liposomes will remain in the supernatant and thus may be isolated from large liposomes. This technique is suitable for small batches but fail to find their use in the commercial manufacture. Another disadvantage particularly for very small liposomes of size generally less than 500 nm is the requirement for spinning at high gravitational force for longer duration of time for fractionation. Such conditions may be achievable only in ultracentrifugation where the capacity of such instrument is limited.

4.2.1.2. Size Exclusion Chromatography

Preparative scale chromatography has also been applied to isolate liposomes of fairly homogenous sizes particularly for separating SUVs from larger liposomes. Typically, Sepharose 4B is used for this purpose *(48)*. As the column is washed with buffer, larger liposomes elute in the void volume while SUV appear with the included volume. The sharper peak eluting with the void volume represent larger liposomes while, the other broader peak occurring within the included volume of the column, represent SUV. Larger pore size chromatographic media have been used in a similar fashion to fractionate population of larger particles. Strict controls are required to avoid microbial contamination of the gel bed.

4.2.2. Homogenisation

Homogenisation has proven as a useful tool in producing very small liposome like long circulating or for liposome entrapped with lipid soluble drugs. The process is very much similar to the one adopted for the preparation of milk or emulsion. The equipment used are generally called high pressure homogeniser which can generate vesicles of size range of 50–100 nm and workable at the pressure of 10–30 K *PSIG*. The method is amenable to scale up for industrial production. A representative diagram of such equipment is given in Fig. 8.

4.2.3. Capillary Pore Membrane Extrusion

This is a wide spread technique for the production of liposome of defined size with narrow distribution *(49)*. The technique involves extrusion of liposome suspension containing heterogeneous population of fairly large vesicles through polycarbonate membrane under pressure. Polycarbonate membranes have uniform straight-through capillary pores of defined size and normally do not bind liposomes. MLVs with a mean diameter of 260 nm were obtained by a single extrusion through 200 nm pore size polycarbonate membrane. Normally 75% retention of the encapsulated volume can be found in vesicle between 170 and 370 nm while, when extruded through 200 nm polycarbonate membrane, the average size reduces to about 190 nm with 85% of particle between 170 and 210. In practice, it is difficult to

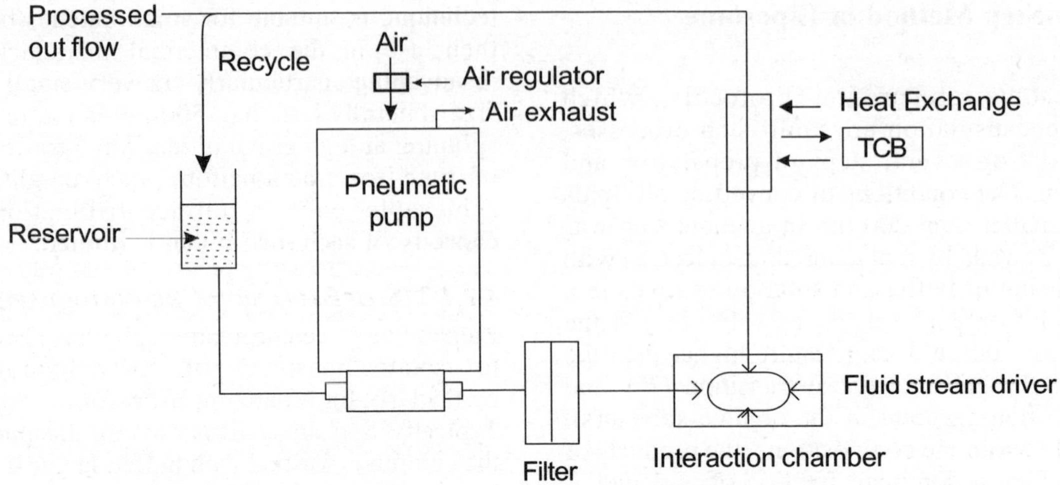

Fig. 8. Representative diagram of high pressure homogeniser.

extrude through small pore membrane (100–200 nm) when the suspension is highly concentrated. In such situation it is advisable to go for sequential extrusion starting from 1 μm membrane and finally up to 200 nm membrane. Alternatively, it can be done by increasing pressure coupled with increase in the filtration area.

4.2.4. Ceramic Extrusion

To overcome the problem of clogging generally seen with polycarbonate membrane is the use of ceramic membrane *(50)*. Extrusion of unsized liposomes through asymmetric ceramic filters yields sized liposomes with selected average size. The method overcomes problems like heat generation, low rate and output, scale up problems, risk of contamination, etc. In practice, a suspension of liposomes containing substantial portion of vesicles of particle size more than 1 μm are passed through asymmetric ceramic filters to yield vesicles of defined particle size depending on number of passages through 1 μm ceramic filter given in Table 4.

The average size of liposomes may be further reduced by passage through similar types of ceramic filters that have been rated at smaller inner-surface pore diameters.

Table 4. Influence of Number of Passages on Size of Liposomes

Number of passes	*Mean diameter (nm)*	*Standard deviation (%)*
1	301.4	36.5
2	300.7	38.1
3	259.4	32.6
4	251.8	36.2
5	239.7	34.2
6	241.8	33.4
7	233.1	33.6
8	234.6	31.1
9	233.2	33.4
10	223.5	35.1

4.3. Comparitive Study of Various Methods of Preparation

Preparation method largely determine the characteristics of liposomes particularly, size and encapsulation (Table 5). Hence, the defined types of liposome (MLV, SUV, LUV, etc.) are prepared by the specific method suited for it. An overview of the typical characteristics of liposomes prepared by various methods are given in the Table 6.

Table 5. Advantages and Inconveniences of Liposome Preparation Methods

Preparation method	*Advantages*	*Inconveniences*
Thin film hydration by mechanical shaking (MLV)	Simple and rapid	Poor encapsulation efficiency, heterogenous dispersion of MLVs, no upscaling feasibility
Ultrasonication (SUV)	Small liposomes (20 nm), homogeneity	Poor encapsulation, contamination of metallic particles, production of aerosols, warming and lipid degradation, no scale up feasibility
French press extrusion	Simple, reproducible, non-aggressive, allow high lipid concentration, high encapsulation	Not economical, need MLV to start, poor encapsulation for fragile liposomes
Extrusion through polycarbonate membrane	Rapid and reproducible, homogeneity, allow high lipid concentration, high encapsulation	Not economical, need MLV to start
Microfluidisation	High encapsulation, scale up feasibility	Not economical, need MLV to start
Ethanol injection	Homogeneity, simple, rapid, scale up feasibility	Poor encapsulation
REV	High encapsulation	Lipid exposure to ultrasonic and solvents, complicated technique, problem of low solubility of lipids in the selected solvent, up scaling difficulties
Ether infusion	High encapsulation, scale up feasibility	Poor encapsulation efficiency, lipids exposed to high temperature and solvents, heterogeneity
Lyophilisation/rehydration	High encapsulation, simple, scale up feasibility, stability	Heterogeneity, need SUV preparation
Freezing/thawing (MLV)	High encapsulation, rapid process	Need the preparation of SUV
Freezing/thawing (SUV)	Rapid process	Need the preparation of SUV, difficult to prepare in presence of neutral lipids, sugars and high concentration of divalent ions
Detergent dialysis	Homogeneity, smooth condition	Low encapsulation, lengthy process, difficult to remove the detergent

Table 6. Characteristics of Liposome Preparation Methods

Method	*Structure*	*Diameter*	*Volume encapsulated μL/μmol*	*Encapsulation (%)*	*References*
Hydration film	MLV	–	–	1.8–8.5	*51*
		–	0.5	6	*34*
		0.05–30	3	–	*52*

Continued

		0.4–5	4.1	5–15	*49*
		1.0	1.4–1.8	9–27	*53*
Ultrasonication of MLV	SUV	0.02–0.05	0.2–1.5	0.1–1.0	*33*
French press extrusion of MLV	SUV	0.02–0.08	0.2–1.5	5–25	*54*
Polycarbonate membrane extrusion of MLV (0.1 μm)	SUV	0.06–1.0	1–3	5–30	*55*
Polycarbonate membrane extrusion of MLV (1–0.2 μm)	MLV	0.05–2.0	1.8–3.7	15–60	*49*
Microfluidisation	SUV	<0.1	0.7–1.0	5–78	*33*
Ethanol injection	SUV	0.03	–	0.5	*31*
	SUV	0.12	0.4–1.5		*56*
REV	LUV	0.1–1.0	7–11	30–68	*33*
Ether infusion	LUV	0.05–0.25	13–25	2.0	*57*
Lyophilisation/ hydration	MLV	0.02–0.2	–	26–72	*51*
Freezing/thawing SUV	LUV	0.09	–	25–30	*58*
Congelation/ decongelation MLV	MLV	–	2–5	31–89	*59*
Detergent dialysis	LUV	0.6	–	12	*39*
		0.1	2.4	12	*42*
		0.04–0.18	1.75–2.4	–	*60*
		0.2–0.3	6.0–7.4	22	*61*
	SUV	0.037	0.47	–	*62*

5. DRUG LOADING

Drug molecules can interact with liposomes in several different ways depending on the drug solubility and polarity. Water-soluble drugs are usually entrapped in to aqueous cavity, while water-insoluble drugs can be solubilised in the hydrophobic part of the liposomes. Hydrophilic drugs are most simply encapsulated automatically upon hydration of the lipids with a corresponding drug solution. The non-encapsulated drug molecules are then removed by gel filtration. However, the efficiency of this method is quite low.

Several methods exist to improve loading of drug molecules. Mostly, they are simply based on the passive entrapment taking into account special geometrical considerations. At high lipid concentrations liposomes encapsulate up to 70% of the sample volume and upon dilution large fractions of drug can be encapsulated. These samples are, however, difficult to size down, and if possible, an active loading method is preferable *(63,64)*. One of the more elegant solutions is so called remote loading where the drug is loaded into preformed liposomes using different ion gradients *(65,67,71)*.

5.1. Remote Loading

Remote loading can be used for loading of weakly acidic or alkaline drug molecules. The method consists

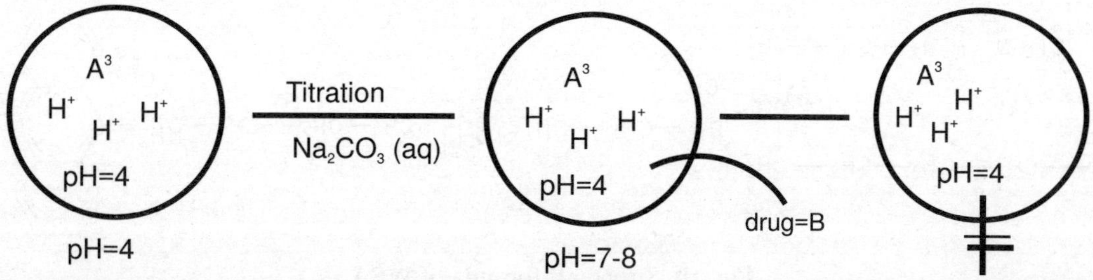

Fig. 9. The pH-gradient method, for loading of weak hydrophilic alkaline drugs. (Reprinted from Chem. Phy. Lipids. 53 (1) Madden, TD., Harrigan, PR., Tai, LC., Bally, MB., Mayer, LD., Redelemir, TE., Loughrey, HC., Tilcock, CP., Reinish, LW., Cullis, PR. The accumulation of drugs within large unilamellar vesicles exhibiting a proton gradient: a Survey 37–46, 1990, with permission from Elsevier) *(71)*.

of forced entrapment of drug molecules upon establishing certain concentration gradients between liposome interior and exterior. Molecules which can respond to these gradients must be weak bases or weak acids co-existing in aqueous solutions in neutral and charged form. Mostly the driving forces are pH gradients and electrostatic and transmembrane potential differences across the vesicle membrane. The molecules (and possibly ions in the presence of ionophores and uncoupling agents) redistribute between the interior and exterior according to the gradient *(64–66)*. These gradients, however, can dissipate and the encapsulated molecules can leak out. To bypass this disadvantage, a method which uses a specific salt, i.e., chemical potential, gradient was recently introduced *(67)*.

5.2. pH Gradient Method

The basic idea of the method is that neutral molecules are shuttled, due to the different pH between the inside and the outside of the membrane, into liposomes where they become charged. Charged drug molecules will thereby be trapped in the liposomal interior, owing to a low diffusion rate of charged molecules over the membrane. Figure 9 shows a representation of the remote loading of a weak base into pre-formed liposomes by means of the so called pH-gradient method. The pH inside the liposome is lower than the pH outside and the weak base *B*, which is in equilibrium with its protonated form, passes through the membrane in its unchanged form. Inside it is, however, protonated and thereby inhibited to leave the liposome. Although the pH-gradient loading method can accumulate large amount of acids or bases in the liposomes, a decaying pH-gradient may cause problems with premature drug leakage *(71)*. However, some drugs have been shown to have the ability to precipitate inside the liposomes at higher concentrations and so this problem becomes negligible *(70)*.

One of the methods of pH gradient drug loading patented is for loading doxorubicin by using ammonium sulphate. The method consists of encapsulating ammonium sulphate into liposomes, and after dialysis into isotonic saline or sucrose solution, a weak base, such as anti-cancer agent doxorubicin (adriamycin [ADR]), is added into the external phase and non-encapsulated drug is removed after incubation. Loading efficiencies approaching 100% were achieved *(66,67)* and it was shown that, contrary to the pH gradient loading, drug molecules do not leak from the vesicle *(67,68)*. Harrigan *et al. (66)* presented a rigorous treatment of loading/unloading of permeable neutral forms (including the pH as well as ammonium salt gradient methods as special cases) of weak bases and acids into liposomes. The same mathematical formalism can be applied to any system separated with a membrane permeable to neutral species and impermeable to charged species or, in a more general case, with differential permeability. The model can also be scaled up to many compartment systems.

5.3. Remote Loading of Boronated Agents

The boron compounds most often used in combination with liposomes are hydrophilic substances, consisting of a boron-rich carborane cage coupled to a moiety that is known to intercalate into, or interact with, DNA. One of the compounds, water-soluble acridine (WSA), is the carborane cage coupled to acridine and spermidine (Fig. 10), both known to interact with DNA *(69)*. The rationale for using DNA-intercalating/interacting compounds is that the therapeutic efficiency is substantially increased when the neutron-activated fission can take place in, or in the vicinity of, the cell nucleus. Furthermore, the retention of the compound in the tumor cell should increase if the compounds are bound to the DNA.

In order to optimise the encapsulation efficiency of WSA, two types of remote loading methods were used; the pH-gradient *(71)*, mentioned above, and the ammonium sulphate gradient *(67)*. The results show that

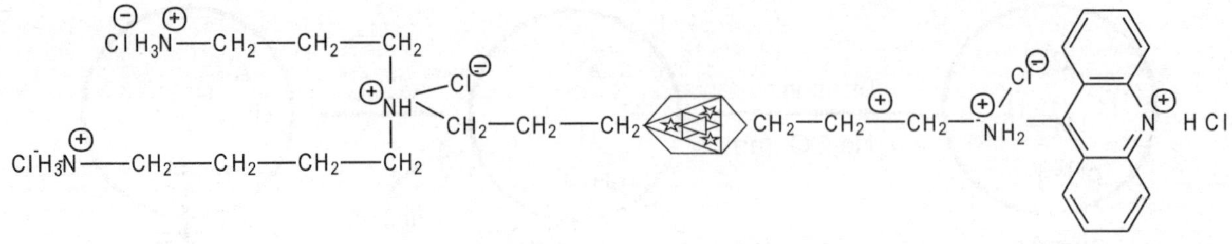

Fig. 10. Structural formula of WSA.

by using the pH-gradient method, trapping efficiencies greater than 95% can be achieved even at rather large drug-to-lipid ratios.

The high trapping efficiency obtained yielded concentrations of the drugs inside the liposomes that were two orders of magnitude higher than the solubility of the drug in the aqueous phase. At such high concentrations it is likely that the drug molecules precipitate inside the liposomes. This was confirmed by cryo-Transmission electron microscope (TEM), as shown in Fig. 11, where the dark globular spots in the liposome interior represent a drug precipitate.

The release rate of the encapsulated WSA is a very important parameter, and the stability of WSA loaded liposomes was shown to be excellent, both in buffer and in 25% human serum. For most formulations the release rate was only around 10% after 24 h at 37°C, as shown in Fig. 12. When the leakage measurements were performed in media containing human serum, no elevated leakage was observed and hence the retention of WSA during blood circulation should be rather good.

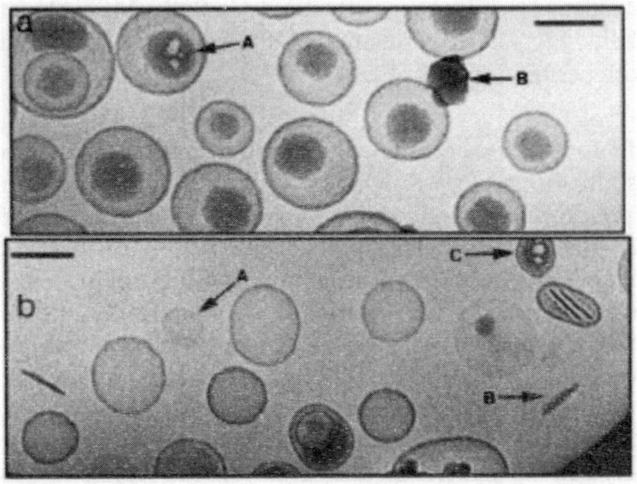

Fig. 11. Cryo-TEM micrographs of DSPC/CHOL/PEG$_{2000}$–DSPE (55/40/5) (mol%) liposome loaded with WSA using the (a) pH-gradient, (b) ammonium sulphate gradient. Arrows in (b) denote bilayer discs as observed face-on (A) and edge-on (B). Bar = 100 nm. Reproduced with permission from refs. (Reprinted from Biochim. Biophys. Acta 1151(2) Haran, G., Cohen, R., Bar, LK., Barenholz, Y. Transmembrane ammonium amphipathic weak base, 201–215, 1993, with permission from Elsevier) *(67,71)*.

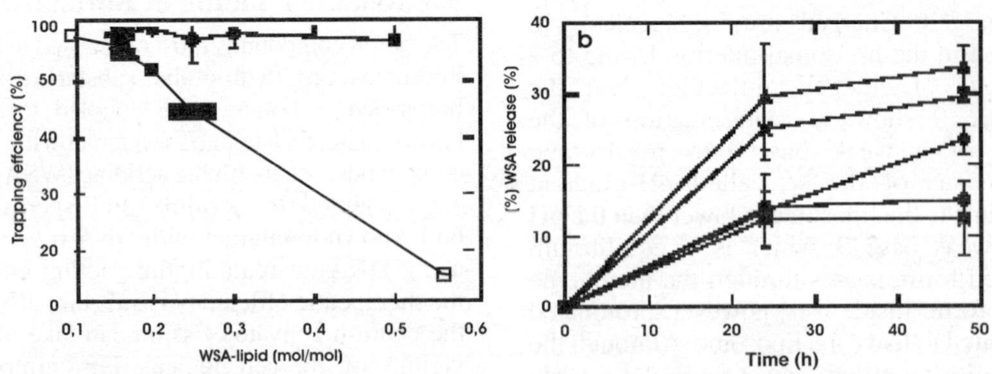

Fig. 12. (A) Trapping efficiency of WSA liposome prepared by the pH-gradient loading procedure (●) or the ammonium sulphate gradient (O). **(B)** Effect of drug-to-lipid ratio on the release of WSA at 37°C, when loaded by means of the pH-gradient method. The initial drug-to-lipid ratios (mol/mol) were 0.15:1 (●), 0.20:1 (■), 0.25:1, 0.30:1 (▲) and 0.50:1(X). Reproduced with permission from refs. (Reprinted from Biochim Biophys Acta, 1151 (2), Haran, G., Cohen, R., Bar, LK., Barenholz. Y. Transmembrane ammonium sulphate gradients in liposomes produce efficient and stable entrapment of amphipathic weak base, 201–215, 1993, with permission from Elsevier. *(67,71)*.

6. CHARACTERISATION OF LIPOSOMES

Both physical and chemical characterisation of liposomes influences their behaviour *in vivo* and *in vitro*. Several examples demonstrating the importance of proper selection of liposome structures to obtain optimum and reproducible therapeutic effects have been published *(72–74)*.

Liposomes are most commonly characterised for the following attributes:

1. Shape and lamellarity.
2. Size and size distribution.
3. Surface charge.
4. Encapsulation efficiency and entrapped volume.
5. Phase transition behaviour.

6.1. Shape and Lamellarity

Conventional microscopic techniques still remain the most popular method of ensuring the sphericity of liposomes. These techniques are explained in brief in the section on "Size and size distribution" later.

However, newer techniques have now been investigated for the determination of liposome shape.

Atomic force microscopy (AFM) is also referred to as scanning probe microscopy, is a high-resolution imaging technique that can resolve features as small as an atomic lattice in the real space. It allows researchers to observe and manipulate molecular and atomic level features.

AFM works by bringing a cantilever tip in contact with the surface to be imaged. An ionic repulsive force from the surface applied to the tip bends the cantilever upwards. The amount of bending, measured by a laser spot reflected on to a split photo detector, can be used to calculate the force. By keeping the force constant while scanning the tip across the surface, the vertical movement of the tip follows the surface profile and is recorded as the surface topography by AFM.

AFM imaging and light scattering was used to study vesicle shape and structure of unilamellar lipid vesicles consisting of egg yolk-derived PC encapsulating monomeric actin (G-actin). These studies indicated the formation of specialised structures, including an overall liposome structure transformation from spherical to torus, disc-shaped geometries and tubular assemblies *(75)*. Other reports of use of AFM to study liposomal shape are also found *(76–78)*.

A simple technique for the determination of the shape of liposomes and cationic liposome–DNA complexes is proposed using a minicapillary viscometer that requires a minimal amount of sample, in combination with a new type of viscometric measurement. The non-dimensional intrinsic viscosity (η) is related to the axial ratio, a/b, of an ellipsoid. This method of measurement is practical in the study of DNA–lipid complexes, and possibly other particles including liposomes and bioactive polymers. Almost perfect sphericity of DPPC–DPPG liposomes was expressed by the axial ratios, a/b, of 1.14 (prolate) and 1.16 (oblate), whereas DNA–DOTAP lipoplexes have ratios of 3.7 (prolate) and 4.9 (oblate). The deviation of shape from perfect sphere is thus expressed quantitatively in more than two significant figures *(79)*.

On the basis of the average number of bilayers present, liposomes can be classified as unilamellar (containing only one bilayer), oligolamellar (from 2 to 5 bilayers) and multilamellar (>5 bilayers). The lamellarity of liposomes influences the encapsulation efficiency, to a great extent the efflux rate of liposomally encapsulated material, and the fate of a drug after cellular uptake.

6.1.1. Estimation of Number of Lamelle

It is not possible to determine the exact number of lamellae in a liposome population. An estimate of the lamellarity can be obtained from the value of E, the entrapped volume (the equation for this parameter has been discussed in the section on "Encapsulation efficiency and entrapped volume"). If the calculated E is low compared to the experimental E, the sample contains a significant proportion of SUVs or MLVs *(80)*.

Lamellarity in liposomes has historically been measured by ^{31}P-NMR. In this technique, the signals are recorded before and after the addition of a non-permeable broadening agent such as Mn^{2+}. Manganese ions interact with the outer leaflet of the outermost bilayer. Thus, a 50% reduction in NMR signal means that the liposome preparation is unilamellar and a 25% reduction in the intensity of original NMR signal means that there are two bilayers in liposome *(81)*.

Freeze-fracture electron microscopy is used for examining samples in "face on" view. The sample is frozen rapidly (cryofixed), then fractured by simply breaking or by using a microtome while maintained at liquid nitrogen temperature. The cold fractured surface (sometimes "etched" by increasing the temperature to about 100°C for several minutes to let some ice sublime) is then shadowed with platinum or gold at an average angle of 45° in a high vacuum evaporator. A second coat of carbon, evaporated normal to the average surface plane is often performed to improve stability of the replica coating. The specimen is returned to room temperature and pressure, and then the extremely fragile "pre-shadowed" metal replica of the fracture surface is released from the underlying biological material by careful chemical digestion. The still-floating replica is thoroughly washed from residual chemicals, carefully fished up on EM grids, dried then viewed in the TEM, freeze-fracture techniques have been used for lamellarity observations of liposomal samples. However, the frequency of cross-fracture is highly variable and thus, no quantitative estimate of lamellarity is possible *(34)*.

Other techniques, which have been investigated for the study of lamellarity, include negative staining electron microscopy (described in the section on "Size and size distribution"), trinitrobenzenesulphonic acid method *(80)* (which is based on the extent of interaction of 2,4,6–trinitrobenzenesulphonic acid with membrane bilayers) and small angle X-ray scattering *(81)*. Combinations of these methods have also been used *(82)*.

6.2. Size and Size Distribution

Size of liposomes is extremely important not only from the point of administration and stability but also because size is one of the most important parameters determining the fate of liposomes in the body. The size distribution of liposomes is often difficult to estimate because no one technique can monitor all the sizes present. The major techniques used can be divided into microscopy techniques, light scattering techniques and other techniques.

6.2.1. Microscopy Techniques

These include:

6.2.1.1. Light Microscopy

If the liposomes are large enough, they can be observed with a light microscope and size can be determined using an optical scale.

6.2.1.2. Electron Microscopy

Electron microscopy techniques used for the purpose of estimating particle size of liposomes include:

6.2.1.2.1. Negative Staining Electron Microscopy

Negative stain electron microscopy utilises an electron-opaque substance to surround liposomes. The stain surrounds and penetrates the biological structure, giving contrast between the liposomes and the background against which it is viewed.

6.2.1.2.2. Bare Grid Electron Microscopy

It is possible to observe a specimen in the native state by rapidly freezing fine samples in liquid and embedding them directly in a thin film of amorphous ice. In other words, an unstained specimen embedded in ice is observed in the hydrated state as it is.

6.2.1.2.3. Freeze-Fracture Electron Microscopy

This technique has already been described earlier in the section on "Shape and lamellarity".

6.2.1.3. Atomic Force Microscopy

AFM has already been described earlier. In a report, diameters of vesicles in solution estimated from two different vesicle concentrations using AFM are not close to those reported by electron microscope studies but are close to those reported by dynamic light scattering studies *(83)*.

6.2.1.4. Scanning Tunneling Microscopy (STM)

The STM is a type of electron microscope that shows three-dimensional (3D) images of a sample. In the STM, the structure of a surface is studied using a stylus that scans the surface at a fixed distance from it. An extremely fine conducting probe is held close to the sample. Electrons tunnel between the surface and the stylus, producing an electrical signal. The stylus is extremely sharp, the tip being formed by one single atom. It slowly scans across the surface at a distance of only an atom's diameter. The stylus is raised and lowered in order to keep the signal constant and maintain the distance. This enables it to follow even the smallest details of the surface it is scanning. Recording the vertical movement of the stylus makes it possible to study the structure of the surface atom by atom. A profile of the surface is created, and from that a computer-generated contour map of the surface is produced. Liposomes have been sized using this technique *(84)*.

6.2.2. Light Scattering Techniques

These techniques include:

6.2.2.1. Dynamic Light Scattering

This technique is also known as photon correlation spectroscopy. It is an extremely rapid and simple method to analyse liposome size in the range of 3 nm–3 μm. This technique involves the measurement of diffusion co-efficient of colloidal particles through analysis of the time dependence of intensity of fluctuations in scattered laser light due to the Brownian motion of particles in solution or suspension. Small liposomes diffuse more rapidly than larger liposomes and the fluctuation of scattered light intensity varies accordingly *(85)*. Advantages of these methods include the reduction in time required for obtaining such information and the minimal preparatory steps required while processing the samples. Disadvantages of the techniques include the expensive systems used for such determinations and the chances of misleading results being obtained for heterogeneous systems exhibiting bimodal or more complex size distributions *(86)*.

6.2.2.2. Turbidity Measurements

This technique is a rapid and non-disruptive method of measuring particle size and is more useful for following relative size changes of liposomes when quantitative particle size distribution measurements are not required. Changes in liposome size can be determined by either measuring the changes in absorbance with a spectrophotometer or preferably by measuring the changes in fluorescence using the same wavelength of excitation and emission. A linear response should be achieved with liposomes ranging in size upto 500 nm. It is possible to obtain the absolute rather than the relative size by measuring the scatter at several angles and at several concentrations *(87)*.

6.2.3. Miscellaneous Techniques

Many other techniques have been investigated especially for obtaining approximate particle size distributions:

6.2.3.1. Size Exclusion Chromatography

SEC is also known as gel permeation chromatography. It is a chromatographic method in which particles are separated based on their size, or in more technical terms, their hydrodynamic volume. The underlying principle of SEC is that particles of different sizes will elute (filter) through a stationary phase at different rates. This results in the separation of a solution of particles based on size. Provided that all the particles are loaded simultaneously, particles of the same size should elute together. SEC has been demonstrated for measuring the particle size of liposomes *(88)*.

6.2.3.2. High-Performance Gel Exclusion Chromatography (HPGEC)

HPGEC is an improvement of the gel permeation technique wherein gel chromatography is coupled with high-performance liquid chromatography (HPLC). Sample detection is by optical density measurement. The column is pre-saturated with phospholipids before analysis of each sample *(89)*.

6.2.3.3. Field-Flow Fractionation (FFF)

Flow FFF is one of a family of FFF techniques where particles or macromolecules are separated in a thin rectangular channel by applying an appropriate field (e.g., flow, electrical and thermal) orthogonal to the channel flow, which under normal operating conditions results in longer retention times for larger macromolecules or colloids. Fractions eluting from the FFF chamber may be fed continuously to a detector for analysis. Quantitative analyses of particle size distribution of liposomes were performed in 30–60 min by exponential-field sedimentation FFF *(90)*. Asymmetric flow FFF in series with multi-angle static light scattering was used to study the size distribution of liposomes encapsulating haemoglobin *(91)*.

Combinations of size distribution measurement techniques have also been used. Ingebrigtsen *et al. (92)* have used SEC in conjunction with photon correlation spectroscopy as well as enzymatic PC assays. Results using such combinations of techniques appear to give more reliable and reproducible estimates of the particle size than one technique alone.

6.3. Surface Charge

Liposomes may be neutral, negative or positively charged depending on the lipid used in the liposome preparation. The impact of charge on *in vivo* behaviour of liposomes is discussed later in this chapter.

Charge determination of liposomes is generally done by means of capillary zone electrophoresis. This technique helps in charge determination of liposomes based on their size to charge ratio (which determines the electrophoretic mobility) in the interior of a small capillary filled with an electrolyte.

The size-dependent electrophoretic migration and separation of liposomes was demonstrated and studied in capillary zone electrophoresis. It was shown that size-dependent migration is primarily a function of κR, where κ^{-1} is the thickness of the electric double layer (which can be derived from the ionic strength [I] of the buffer) and R is liposome radius *(93)*. Individual liposome measurements by capillary electrophoresis with post-column laser-induced fluorescence detection facilitated the determination of liposome property distributions, 2D plots, and an improved characterisation of a liposomal preparation *(94)*. Psyher and Hayes have elucidated the possible effects of applied field strength, bilayer rigidity and surface charge on the behaviour of liposomes during electrophoretic studies by monitoring the electrophoretic mobilities of liposome populations while varying the applied potential, ionic strength of the medium, and the surface charge and CHOL content of liposomes *(95)*.

Other techniques have also been investigated as a means of obtaining an estimate of the surface charge of liposomes.

Aqueous two-phase partitioning systems have been demonstrated as useful aids in understanding liposomal charge. Aqueous two-phase partition is a technique that separates substances, on the basis of differences in surface properties, by partitioning the cells between two immiscible, aqueous solutions of polymers. The two aqueous polymer solutions most commonly used are dextran and PEG, which when mixed at certain concentrations, form the two immiscible phases. The upper phase is rich in PEG and is relatively more hydrophobic than lower phase, which is rich in dextran. Depending upon the salt composition of the phase system, the system can also be made charge sensitive. Such systems have been reported for understanding the behaviour of charged liposomes *(96,97)*.

The surface potential of the membranes (liposomes) was calculated from the partition co-efficient of methylene blue dye between the membrane and the bulk phase. The effects of charge density of membrane and of ionic strength on the surface potential were also studied *(98)*.

6.4. Encapsulation Efficiency and Entrapped Volume

Encapsulation efficiency of the liposomal sample is a particularly important characteristic. A high encapsulation efficiency of a population of liposomes will avoid the need to separate unentrapped material, which more often than not involves the use of time consuming and tedious techniques. An encapsulation efficiency of about 90% is considered to be satisfactory since the remaining 10% of free material can act as the loading dose *(82)*.

In order to estimate the encapsulation efficiency, the free drug needs to be separated from the entrapped drug. Separation procedures are described below in general and must be modified for specific uses.

6.4.1. Minicolumn Centrifugation

Sephadex G-50 is swelled in an appropriate buffer and packed into a 1-mL syringe plugged with a Whatman filter. This minicolumn is then centrifuged to remove excess buffer. Then a small quantity of undiluted liposome sample is carefully added to the minicolumn. Centrifugation of the minicolumn and collection of eluate affords liposomes and entrapped drug. Buffer is then added to rinse the minicolumn. The eluate obtained after centrifugation of minicolumn at this stage should not contain any drug. A second rinsing with buffer is then used to collect free drug *(80)*.

6.4.2. Protamine Aggregation

This method is useful for neutral or negatively charged liposomes. However, the free drug should not be precipitated by protamine. An appropriate volume of protamine solution (10 mg/mL) is added first to a sample of liposomes followed by centrifugation at a low rpm. The precipitated liposomes are pelletised and the supernatant contains free drug that can be estimated. The entrapped drug can be estimated by lysing the pelletised liposomes by use of, for example, Triton X-100 to lyse the liposomes. The analytical method for estimating the drug should be capable of avoiding interference from lipid components, protamine or Triton X-100 *(80)*.

6.4.3. Ultracentrifugation

The ultracentrifuge is a centrifuge optimised for spinning a motor at very high speeds, capable of generating acceleration as high as 1,000,000 G (9800 km/s^2). At this force of gravity, the liposomes are separated as a pellet from the unentrapped drug which is present in the supernatant. Gradient separations, in which the tubes are filled from top to bottom with an increasing concentration of a dense substance such as Ficoll or sucrose in solution, can also be perfomed. This is a very common method of separation of unentrapped drug. Reports also suggest the simplicity of this method over other methods *(99)*.

6.4.4. Special Markers

Markers can be used to optimise entrapment in the early stages of product development. Examples of such markers include Arsenazo III (a dye which complexes with calcium which shifts its absorption from 560 nm to peaks at 606 and 660 nm) *(80)*, carboxyfluorescein (CF) and calcein (the use of which involves utilisation of their self quenching properties at high concentrations) *(80,100)*.

6.4.5. Dialysis

The technique of dialysis involves the separation of unentrapped drug from liposomal drug by means of a semipermeable membrane. The pore size (in terms of the mol wt) of the membrane determines the solute, which can cross the membrane.

Various methods available to separate non-encapsulated drug from LUV have been compared. The non-encapsulated drug was separated by: filtering through Centrifree tubes, passing through gel (Sepharose-4B and Sephadex G-25M), passing through minicolumn, ficoll density gradient, protamine aggregation or dialysis. The dialysis method was found to be unsuitable for separation of non-encapsulated drug due to equilibration of encapsulated drug as the free drug was dialysed. The upper limit for lipid concentration was 5 mg/mL using the Centrifree method. Separation using gel chromatography led to dilution of liposome preparation. Minicolumn and density gradient techniques did not lead to sample dilution; however, the minicolumn method was tedious. The time required for separation of liposomes by protamine aggregation was longer for neutral liposomes. Thus it was concluded that Centrifree was the fastest method to estimate encapsulation; the density gradient method was ideal to separate non-encapsulated drug; and protamine aggregation was least expensive method to estimate encapsulation efficiency *(101)*.

In an excellent review, factors that affect encapsulation of drugs in liposomes such as liposome size and type, charge on the liposome surface, bilayer rigidity, method of preparation, remote loading, addition of ion pairing, and complexing agents and characteristics of drug to be encapsulated have been dealt with *(102)*.

The entrapped volume of liposome preparations is normally expressed as the trapped volume per lipid and can vary from 0.5 μL/μmol for some multi-lamellar systems and SUVs to as much as 30 μL/μmol for certain LUVs *(86)*.

For intermediate to LUV, the radius (*r*) is large relative to the thickness of membrane and the entrapped volume (*E*) is given by the equation

$$E = (1/3)\, A \cdot r$$

where *A* is the area of membrane occupied by one mole of lipid. *E* is calculated by measuring the average radius of liposomes.

The best procedure to measure the entrapped volume of liposomes is a direct measurement of water. The liposome sample is centrifuged for 6 h at 200,000*g* to form a tight pellet. After decanting the supernatant, the pellet is re-suspended with deuterium oxide (D_2O). The D_2O quickly equilibriates with entrapped water. The peak height of a NMR is then related to standards consisting of known amounts of H_2O in D_2O *(80)*.

Trapped volumes are usually determined experimentally by preparing liposomes in an aqueous medium containing non-permeable radioactive solute such as [^{22}Na] or [^{14}C] inulin. The trapped proportion of solute is determined by removing external radioactivity by centrifugation, dialysis or gel filtration and determination of residual radioactivity per lipid *(103)*.

A method for determining the aqueous internal volume of small unilamellar liposomes has been proposed. The method is based on an equilibrium uptake of hydrogen iodide by liposomes. After chromatographic separation of liposomes from external solution, the membrane is solubilised and the amount of captured iodide is determined using an ion selective electrode *(104)*.

Chloride has been used as a convenient marker ion for measurement of entrapped volume using solute entrapment because the ubiquity of Cl^- in physiological buffers eliminates pre-labeling with exogenous markers and because minute concentrations of trapped chloride are well detectable in the presence of large extra-vesicular nitrate concentrations *(105)*.

An electron spin resonance (ESR)-stopped flow technique has been developed and employed for the simple and rapid determination of internal volumes of biomembrane vesicles and liposomes. A vesicle suspension containing a neutral and membrane-permeable spin label, 2,2,6,6-tetramethyl-4-oxopiperidine-1-oxyl (TEMPONE), was mixed in the stopped-flow apparatus with an isotonic solution of relatively impermeable line broadening agents, potassium tris(oxalato)chromate(III) or potassium ferricyanide, and an ESR spectrum was recorded. From the relative intensity of sharp triplet signal due to TEMPONE in the aqueous space within vesicles, the determination of internal aqueous volume was straightforward. Using this technique, it is possible to measure intra-vesicular volumes in 0.1 s *(106)*.

6.5. Phase Transition Temperature

The phase transition temperature is defined as the temperature required to induce a change in lipid physical state from the ordered gel phase, where the hydrocarbon chains are fully extended and closely packed, to the disordered liquid crystalline phase, where the hydrocarbon chains are randomly oriented and fluid.

Differential scanning calorimetry (DSC) widely used for phase transition studies. ^{31}P NMR has also been used for phase transition studies (Kruijjf *et al.* 1975). The phase heterogeneity of giant unilamellar dinervonoylphosphocholine vesicles in the course of main phase transition has been investigated by confocal fluorescence microscopy observing the fluorescence from the membrane incorporated lipid analog, 1-palmitoyl-2-(*N*-4-nitrobenz-2-oxa-1,3 diazol) amino-caproyl-*sn*-glycero-3-phosphocholine *(107)*. Changes in shape and size of DPPC liposomes at phase transition at 41.5°C have been monitored by light microscopy. All liposomes change size or shape at the transition and those with simple topologies such as spheres and cylinders can be readily measured *(108)*. The effect of 2,4-dichlorophenol on the structures and phase transitions of fully hydrated 1,2-dipalmitoyl-*sn*-glycero-3-phosphocholine (DPPC) liposomes was studied using Fourier transform-Raman spectroscopy *(109)*.

The composition of bilayer is perhaps the most important determinant of phase transition tempertature. Above the gel to liquid crystalline phase transition temperature, liposomes prepared from saturated lecithins with 14 or more carbon atoms per acyl chain exist as stable bilayers, which are practically impermeable to ions. An enhanced release of trapped potassium from liposomes was demonstrated in the vicinity of transition temperature. The extent of increase, however, depend strongly on the length of paraffin chain *(110)*. ^{31}P NMR spectra of unsonicated liposomes consisting of PCs of varying chain length and unsaturation have been investigated. In liquid crystalline state the ^{31}P NMR liposome spectra are similar for both saturated and unsaturated PCs, demonstrating that the motion of polar headgroup is not sensitive to fatty acid composition in disordered liquid crystalline state. Below hydrocarbon phase transition temperature there is a marked increase in the linewidth of ^{31}P NMR liposome spectra, indicating a reduction in motion of polar headgroup. The addition of equimolar concentrations of CHOL to PC eliminates phase transition effects experienced by polar headgroup. The motion of polar headgroup is then very similar to that obtained in the liquid crystalline state for pure PC bilayers. In liquid crystalline state the motion of polar headgroup in the phosphate region is insensitive to changes in the available area per phosphatidycholine molecule *(111)*. The addition of lysolipid to DPPC bilayers dramatically enhances the amount of, and speed at which, encapsulated markers or drugs are released at the gel-to-liquid, already leaky, phase transition through leaky interfacial regions between still solid and melting liquid phases *(112)*.

The entrapment of solutes in bilayer also determines the phase transition temperature. Non-polar drugs can perturb the phase transition behaviour of synthetic PCs; polar drugs have no such effect. Thus, in presence of non-polar drugs such as vinblastine sulphate and actinomycin D, the DSC profile of dimyristoylphosphatidylcholine is markedly altered, with a broadening of major peak and appearance of a second peak at lower temperature *(113)*. DSC showed progressive decrease and broadening of the phase transition temperature of DPPC with increasing fraction of cationic lipid DOTAP (*N*-(1-[2,3-dioleoyloxy]propyl)- *N*,*N*,*N*-trimethylammonium), in the range of 0.4–20 mol%. The anionic lipid DOPG had similar effects on DPPC membrane fluidity *(114)*.

Phase transition determination is very important for *in vivo* behaviour. Permeability changes are most marked at or near the phase transition temperature. Liposomal membranes with their lipids in the gel state are still permeable to water. The rate of water permeation changes drastically on passing the transition temperature. The water permeation has different activation energies above and below the transition temperature, respectively, indicating that the diffusion process takes place by different mechanisms *(110)*. It has been shown that for the plasma-induced dissolution of unsonicated liposomes, which is most probably achieved by interaction with (apo) lipoproteins, the presence of phase boundaries is required *(115)*. Membrane fusion is promoted by defects created in the bilayer due to the vicinity of lipid phase transition, lateral phase separation or domain generation, high local membrane curvature, osmotic or electric stress in or on the membrane; the addition of amphiphats or macromolecules which insert themselves into the membrane, freezing or other mechanical membrane perturbation have similar effects *(116)*.

Phase transition temperatures also assume relevance for dry membrane conservation which is important when liposomes have to be stabilised, for example, by lyophilisation. Two prevailing theories for dry membrane preservation are the water replacement hypothesis and glass formation. A manifestation of water replacement hypothesis is the ability of sugars to depress dry membrane main phase transition temperatures (T_c). DSC was employed to test the effects of sugars (trehalose, α-lactose, maltose and glucose) on the T_cs of slowly frozen, lyophilised liposomes prepared from hydrogenated egg phosphatidylcholine, DPPC and POPC. For each lyophilised phospholipid membrane, the disaccharides caused significant T_c reduction to at least 14°C less than the hydrated membrane T_cs *(117)*. It has been proposed that if calorimetric criteria are appropriately established using a proper reference lipid sample, the quality and stability of a liposomal preparation, which has a distinct thermogram, can be assessed by DSC *(118)*.

7. SPECIALISED LIPOSOMES

7.1. Surface Modified Liposomes (Long-Circulating Liposomes [LCLs] or Stealth Liposomes)

Until recently, the therapeutic use of liposomes had been limited mainly to delivery of drugs to mononuclear phagocyte system (MPS), for example, manipulation of macrophage function and treatment of diseases involving macrophages like leishmaniasis. However, this scenario changed with the advent of what are known as sterically stabilised liposomes, which show prolonged residence times in body.

7.1.1. Immune System

The human body has ability to resist almost all types of organisms or toxins that tend to damage the tissues and organs, which is called immunity. Immunity is further divided into innate immunity and acquired immunity. Innate immunity involves use of processes such as phagocytosis (by neutrophils and macrophages of RES), and defences such as acid secretions of stomach and digestive enzymes, skin and chemical compounds in the blood such as lysozyme, basic polypeptides and the complement complex for the defence of the body against invading organisms.

Acquired immunity is largely mediated by the lymphoid tissues of body, which are located most extensively in the lymph nodes, in the spleen, submucosal areas of gastrointestinal (GI) tract and in bone marrow. Acquired immunity can be humoural immunity (where circulating antibodies are produced by B-lymphocytes of lymphoid tissue which are globulin molecules that are capable of attacking the invading agent, also known as immunoglobulins (Igs) or cell-mediated immunity (where large numbers of activated lymphocytes are formed by T-lymphocytes of the lymphoid tissue that are specifically designed to destroy foreign agent.)

7.1.2. Phagocytosis and Opsonisation

The main obstacle to the successful use of liposomes as drug delivery systems is process of phagocytosis (if the phenomenon of formation of specific antibodies against the components of liposomes, a rare occurrence, is to be disregarded).

In body, neutrophils and monocytes are major populations of cells involved in body immunity. The neutrophils are mature cells that can attack and destroy such agents even in the circulating blood. However, the blood monocytes are immature cells that have very little ability to fight with injurious agents. However, once they enter the tissues, they swell to, too much larger sizes to become macrophages. While mainly these cells are mobile, a large portion of these macrophages become attached to the tissues and remain attached for months or perhaps even years unless they are called upon to perform specific protective functions. When appropriately stimulated, the fixed macrophages can break away from their attachments and become mobile macrophages. The combination of mobile macrophages and fixed tissue macrophages is collectively called the RES. The tissue macrophages in various tissues differ in appearances and they are known by different names: Kupffer cells in liver; tissue macrophages in lymph nodes, spleen and bone marrow; alveolar macrophages in the alveoli of lungs; tissue histocytes in subcutaneous (s.c.) tissues and microglia in brain. The term MPS has been proposed to replace RES.

The most important function of neutrophils and macrophages is phagocytosis. Phagocytosis involves two selective procedures:

1. If surface of a particle is rough, the likelihood of phagocytosis is increased.
2. Most natural substances of the body have protective coats that repel phagocytes. Dead tissues and foreign particles frequently have no protective coats and many are also strongly electrically charged, which also makes them susceptible to phagocytosis.

Opsonisation: This is a process whereby materials absorb to a foreign surface in such a way as to prepare the surface for recognition as foreign and thus for phagocytosis by the MPS. The word opsonin is of Greek origin and means a relish, a seasoning or a sauce. It has often been quoted as being 'the preparation of a meal'. The materials involved in opsonisation are known as opsonins. Opsonins are poorly defined plasma factors, which bind to foreign particles and promote phagocytosis. The opsonins facilitate attachment of phagocyte to antigen by forming a bridge between the phagocyte and antigen. These opsonins can be specialised or non-specific. Specialised opsonins contain at least one receptor-recognisable site and often more than one binding site (so that they can cross-link). They also play important roles in immune response regulation and may alter vascular permeability. Specialised opsonins bind to antigen expose receptor-recognisable sites and, thus mediate further immunocomplexes interaction with cells. The latter process depends on factors such as number and type(s) of incorporated opsonin molecules. Those immunocomplexes, which contain a small number of opsonin molecules, are known to circulate for hours and even days while others are immediately arrested by phagocytes (e.g., in liver, spleen bone narrow or lungs). Thus, phagocytosis is triggered faster by multiple rather than single opsonin-receptor interactions *(119)*.

Major specialised opsonins of normal blood include:

1. Igs: which have already been discussed before.
2. Complement: Complement is a collective term to describe a system of about 20 different proteins that work to eliminate micro-organisms and other antigens from blood. This task is achieved by complement co-operation with cells that express complement receptors and, often, with antibodies and other opsonins. Proteins of complement have historically assigned numbers, which do not completely correspond to the sequence of their actions, for example, C2, C3, C4, etc, many of which are enzyme precursors. All these are present normally among the plasma proteins that leak out of the capillaries into tissue spaces. The enzyme precursors are normally inactive but they can be activated through either the classical pathway (an antigen–antibody reaction) or the alternate pathway (without the intermediation of an antigen–antibody reaction). Since the alternate pathway does not involve an antigen–antibody reaction, it is one of the first lines of defense against invading agents.
3. Fibronectins: Fibronectins are large proteins abundant in plasma and extra-cellular matrix. Fibronectin is believed to participate in hepatic uptake of particulates *(119)*.

Minor or non-specific opsonins are proteins present in blood in small concentrations. Some minor opsonins are acute-phase proteins (i.e., their concentration in plasma increases as a result of inflammation or trauma). Most of minor opsonins are lectins, for example, conglutinin *(120)*. Other minor opsonins include mannose-binding protein, lipopolysaccharide binding protein *(121)*, vitronectin *(122)*, serum amyloid P-component *(123,124)*, C-reactive protein *(125)* and tuftsin *(126)*.

Recently the presence of 'organ-specific' opsonins has been proposed by Moghimi and Patel, 1988 *(144)*. It has been suggested that phagocytosis is regulated by the presence and balance between two groups of blood components: opsonins, which promote phagocytosis and dysopsonins, which suppress the process. IgA and secretory IgA are the best-known dysopsonins *(126)*.

From the above discussion, it can be seen that the opsonisation process is a consequence of multiple adsorption and displacement processes, probably involving conformational changes, which ultimately lead to the final opsonisation process. The net effect of opsonisation is to make the particle surface more hydrophobic and it is reasonable to assume that this may be the probable reason for phagocytosis. This has been proved by a simple model in which contact angles of different biological substances were measured and it was claimed that the difference in contact angle between the phagocytic cells and bacterial cells would define whether phagocytosis will occur or not.

7.1.3. Strategies for Prolonged In Vivo Residence

Phagocytosis in the body needs to be avoided in order for liposomes to stay in body for a prolonged period of time. This can be achieved through use of various strategies. The surface chemistry of liposome (particle) will undoubtedly play a major role in determining the biodistribution of liposome. Allen wrote "if you want to be invisible, look like water' *(127)*. The hydrophobicity/hydrophilicity of surface affects the attractive forces experienced by particle, thereby influencing the opsonisation process and interaction forces that govern adhesion of particle to the cell. Particles with hydrophilic surfaces, upon which water molecules can readily absorb, have longer blood half lives.

The surface charge has been recognised for many years as an important determinant of particulate clearance from circulation. Biological particles are usually negatively charged whilst administered carrier systems can be positively or negatively charged and that charge can be changed as a consequence of changes in fluid. Charged particles are surrounded by associated charged species of opposite charge creating the electrical double layer. When a charged carrier and a biomolecule are in close proximity, their associated charged layers will overlap. If two materials have same charge, this will cause repulsion but if they are of opposite charges then this will result in attraction. The Derjaguin, Landau, Verwey and Overbeek (DLVO) theory can be used to describe the net interaction between two particles of the same charge as they approach each other. In plasma, the ionic strength is such that a secondary minimum is probable, and thus materials of same charge will exhibit net attraction in this region. At short distances of separation, different forces dominate and in this region, it is the surface nature, which becomes important. It is a general view that negative surface charge increases the clearance of particulates from the circulation, relative to neutral or positively charged ones *(126)*. Particles with neutral surfaces seem most appropriate with regard to blood persistence *(128)*.

Liposome size plays an important role in determining their biodistribution. There is an inverse relationship between liposome size and the rate at which they are distributed to MPS cells such as Kupffer cells. Larger liposomes have dramatically more rapid clearance into MPS cells than smaller liposomes. A kinetic model has been proposed where large liposomes are removed from circulation by cells predominantly situated in intravascular space, for example, Kupffer cells in liver and fixed macrophages in spleen. However, disposition of very small liposomes is a function of uptake of cells of both the intra- and extra-vascular space. Two parallel pathways have been proposed to account for the difference in hepatic uptake rates between large and very small liposomes. Large liposomes are deposited in a high affinity, low capacity saturatable system, predominantly involving Kupffer cells. It was suggested that the smaller liposomes avoid, to some extent, the first pathway but are removed by a low affinity, high capacity system involving the parenchymal cells *(129)*.

Several studies have also shown the importance of bilayer rigidity in prolonging circulation time of liposomes *(130–133)*.

It has to be borne in mind that any one of these strategies alone may not be adequate for preventing uptake of liposomes by the cells of MPS. Appropriate combinations of two or more of these strategies will, in most cases, ensure that liposomes will not be sequestered by the cells of MPS.

7.1.4. Studies in Prolonged Blood Residence

It was found that inclusion of CHOL results in an enhanced structural stability of liposomes in serum, resulting in a relatively prolonged circulation time as compared with CHOL-free liposomes *(134)*. Careful studies by several investigators of the dependence of uptake on lipid components as well as other liposome properties led to one of the first major advances in prolonged blood residence. These studies led to the finding that small (≤100 nm in diameter) electrically neutral, rigid (composed with fully saturated lipids below their phase transition and a high CHOL content) liposomes can exhibit prolonged circulation, but only at moderately high doses and probably by saturation of uptake mechanism with a relatively small portion of the injected dose *(135)*.

A reduction in MPS uptake was achieved by inclusion of special lipids contributing to changes in their surface properties. Initially, incorporation of relatively small amounts of materials like purified glycolipids such as GM_1, hydrogenated phosphatidylinositol and sulphatides was found to improve MPS avoidance *(132,133,136,137)*. The use of phospholipids having a high melting temperature such as SM and DSPC leads to further increase in circulation time of GM_1 containing liposomes *(132)*. The activity of GM_1, in prolonging the circulation time is restricted to a relatively narrow size range *(138)*. Optimum liposome size for prolonged circulation ranges from 70 to 200 nm in average diameter. The larger liposomes have an increased tendency to accumulate in spleen *(139,140)*, whereas the smaller liposomes accumulate in liver very efficiently *(138)*. In contrast, this size dependent accumulation in spleen and liver is less profound for liposomes containing no GM_1. The preferential accumulation of GM_1 containing large and small liposomes in spleen and liver, respectively, can be attributed to the anatomical structure of these organs in addition to their lower affinity to RES, in particular, the Kupffer cells of liver. Because GM_1 containing liposomes show the reduced affinity to liver Kupffer cells, they have an increased chance to stay in circulation. When liposomes are large enough (>300 nm in diameter), they are retained by the splenic sinusoidal filter, thus resulting in enhanced accumulation in spleen. On the other hand, sufficiently small liposomes (>70 nm in diameter) can extravasate to liver parenchyma through the holes (~100 nm in average diameter) located in the fenestrae of liver sinus, thus resulting in enhanced accumulation in liver. Thus, the mechanisms responsible for the biodistribution of small and large liposomes are basically different. The highest circulation level of GM_1 containing liposomes can be obtained using liposomes of appropriate size, i.e., between 70 and 200 nm in diameter; the total uptake of these liposomes by the spleen and liver is minimised *(141)*. GM_1 has been used with success by Gabizon and Papahadjopoulos in tumor targeting *(133)* and in immunoliposomes (i.e., antibody-directed liposomes) *(142,143)*. However, the use of GM_1 in various types of immunoliposomes with triggered release mechanism results in reduced sensitively to the appropriate environmental change *(137)*.

The prolonged systemic circulation effect of GM_1 was suggested to be related to reduction in opsonisation brought about through increasing surface hydrophilicity (a sterically hindered negative charge on sialic acid), suppression of complement dependent phagocytosis and a barrier effect of carbohydrate chains *(126)*. The stabilising effect of gangliosides depends on number of sialic acid residues: the higher order the ganglioside, greater the activity in enhancing the stability of liposomes. However, among various gangliosides, GM_1 is unique in terms of having a strong activity in prolonging the circulation time of liposomes; other gangliosides such as GD_{1a} and GT_{1b} exhibit little or no activity *(141)*. A liposome agglutination assay was used to assess the degree of steric barrier produced on liposome surface by GM_1 *(143)*. The study indicated that the steric barrier activity of GM_1 is weaker than that of PEG 2000–PE; however, its activity in prolonging the circulation time of liposomes is greater than that of PEG 2000–PE. The above two findings, in conjunction, indicate that stabilising effect of GM_1 via steric barrier provided by the oligosaccharide residue is probably not a major mechanism in prolonging the circulation time of liposomes. The mechanism of high melting phospholipids in improving the circulation time of GM_1 containing liposomes has been attributed to increased bilayer rigidity, as a result of diminished rotational and translational diffusions of the lipids at the physiological temperature and thus the enhanced stability of liposomes. However, membrane rigidity is not a strong requirement in liposome construction for prolonged circulation *(141)*.

It was first suggested by Moghimi and Patel *(144)* that dysopsonins might be involved in decreased phagocytosis of rigid liposomes especially by Kupffer cells. Supporting evidence is available to support this theory *(145,146)*.

The use of GM_1 was followed by findings that a hydrophilic polymer–lipid conjugate, PEG–PE, can provide similar or even better protection from uptake with little dependence on liposome composition *(147–150)*. Research today is concentrated on liposomes coated with PEG as a means of MPS avoidance. Commonly referred to as sterically stabilised liposomes or LCLs, this new type of liposome is sometimes referred to as a stealth liposome. Alternative coinages include "cryptosomes" and "ninjasomes"; which one of these will survive the test of time remains to be seen *(151)* PEG possesses an ideal array of properties for use in liposomes: chiefly, low toxicity and extremely low immunogenicity and antigenicity *(152)*. For drug delivery, PEG coated liposomes have several advantages *(135,153)*.

1. Prolonged circulation independent of the bilayer physicochemical properties, thereby permitting separate control of drug loading/leakage and blood circulation.
2. Plasma pharmacokinetics independent of lipid dose, thereby simplifying dose escalation.
3. Compatibility with ligands or other chemical functionalities at the outer surface of PEG coating.
4. Ease of preparation and use without modification of many well-known liposome methodologies.
5. Amenable to pharmaceutical product regulatory requirements.
6. Economy (as compared with the use of GM_1).

Most of the PEG–lipids used for preparation of LCLs are prepared by derivatisation of PEs, which act as an anchor to graft the PEG chain to liposome surface. Monomethyl ether of PEG (mPEG) is often used for conjugation. It is particularly useful when multiple chains of polymer have to be linked to the intended substrate. Due to its structural simplicity and possession of only one derivatisable end group, the use of mPEG minimises cross-linking possibilities and leads to improved homogeneity of conjugates. Figure 13 shows various reagents used for derivatisation of PE and the end products so obtained *(152)*.

The chlortriazine approach to preparation of PEG–PE is not attractive due to the toxicity of reagent and its degradation products. The presence of slightly reactive chloride in PE conjugate with (Fig. 13A) is another drawback of this method.

Klibanov and co-workers *(147)* used succinimidyl (succinimidylsuccinate–PEG) (Fig. 13B) derived from mPEG-5000 for preparation of mPEG–succinamide–dioleoyl-PE. Succinate ester linkage present in this conjugate is known to undergo hydrolysis under physiological conditions *(152)*. Parr and co-workers *(154)* convincingly demonstrated that this type of conjugate readily releases free mPEG-OH after few hours of incubation at 37°C in mouse serum.

Urethane linked mPEG–PE conjugates were obtained by reacting mPEG oxycarbonylimidazole (Fig. 13C) or succinimidyl carbonate (SC) SC–PEG (Fig. 13D) with distearoyl-PE *(155,156)*. The reagent (D), being more reactive, allows preparation of mPEG–DSPE within 10–15 min at 45°C. Urethane linkages are quite stable and thus are more attractive than other linkages *(152)*.

DSPE conjugates derived from m-PEG tresylate (Fig. 13E) of mol wt 5000 were prepared for formulation of LCLs *(157,148)*. Instead of using a PEG–lipid

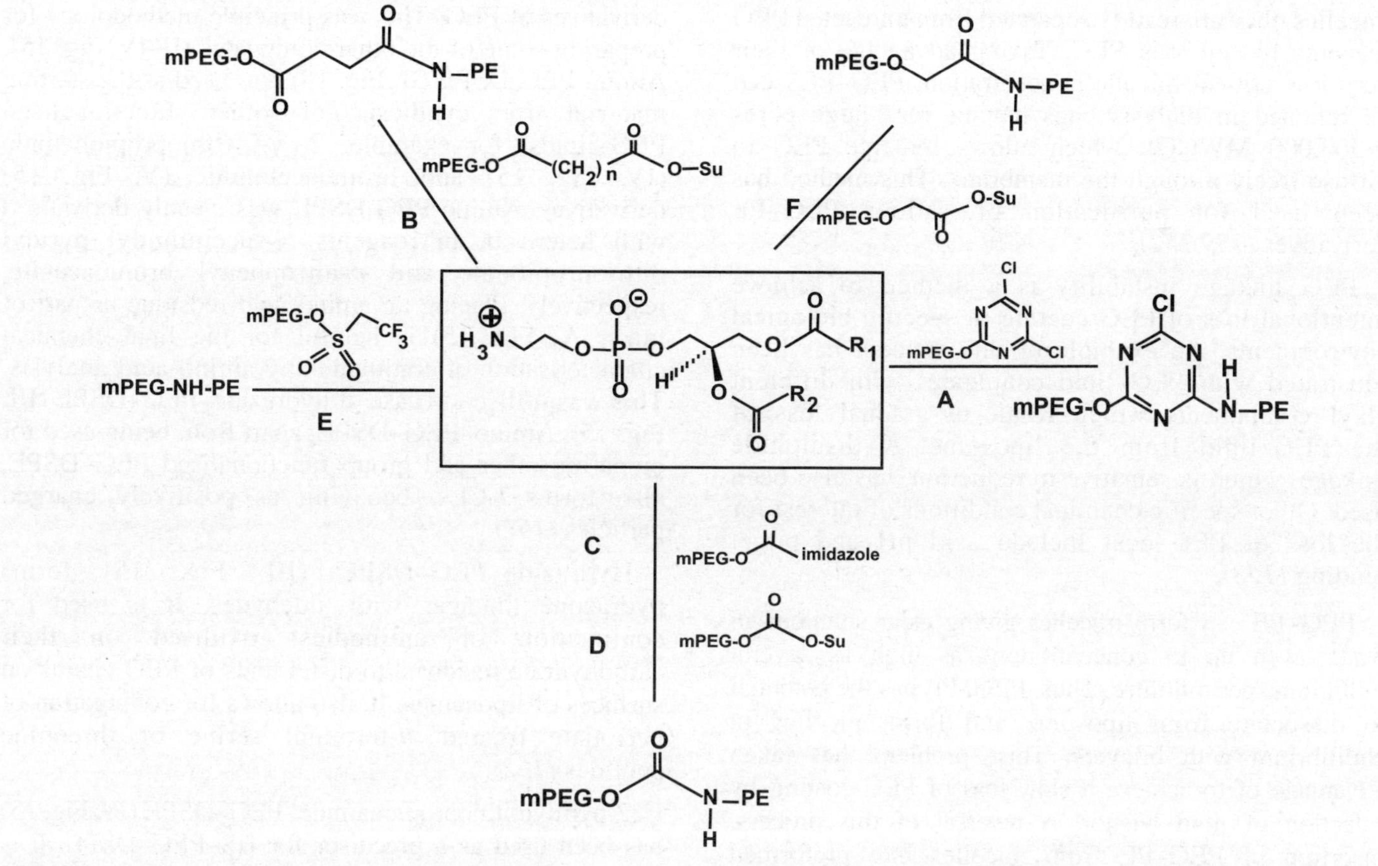

Fig. 13. Various reagents used for derivatisation of PE and end products. (Reprinted from Advanced drug delivery review, 16, Zalipsky, S., Chemistry of polyethylene glycol conjugates with biological active molecules, 157–182, 1995, with permission from Elsevier) *(152)*.

conjugate to form liposomes, Senior and co-workers *(72)* modified surface amino groups of DSPC–DPPE (dipalmitoyl-PE)–CHOL vesicles with mPEG-tresylate. The attractive feature of this approach is in its selective grafting of polymer on the exterior of residues. It avoids the presence of mPEG residues inside the liposomes. However, the difficulty in substituting all available amino groups of PE residues and the formation of an asymmetrical lipid bilayer might be undesirable in some situations.

Amide-liked mPEG–DSPE was prepared by coupling (Fig. 13F) to the amino group of PE *(158)*.

Herron *et al. (159)* used direct grafting of mPEG residues on liposomes by preparing maleimido-PE-containing vesicles which were then reacted with a thiol derivative of polymer.

Examples of mPEG conjugates with other lipids (non-PE) include attachment of phosphatidic acid directly to mPEG-OH using 2,6,6-triisopropylbenzene-sulfonyl chloride-mediated coupling in pyridine *(158)*. Oxidation of the diol residue of DSPG with periodate followed

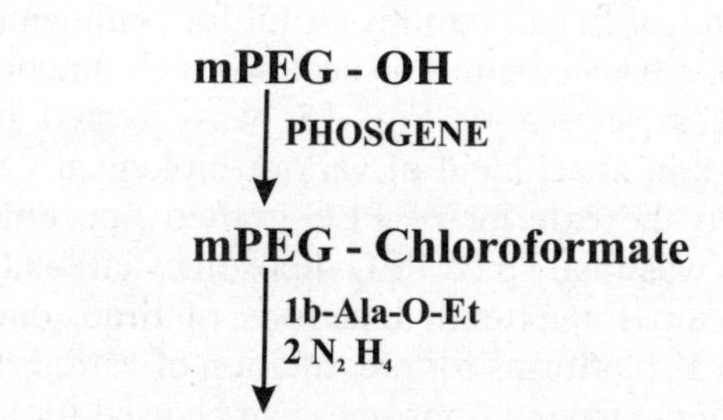

Fig. 14. Oxidation of the diol residue of DSPG with periodate followed by reaction with m-PEG hydrazide.

by reaction with mPEG-hydrazide (Fig. 14) led to a hydrazone-linked mPEG–lipid. For some applications, it might be useful to have an acid-labile hydrazone linkage connecting the conjugate components *(152)*.

The PEG–lipid conjugates can be purified from the conjugation reaction mixtures by silica gel chromatography. Because conjugates exist in water almost exclusively as micelles, they are readily separated from unreacted PEG reagents by aqueous SEC. Taking advantage of their very low critical micelle concentration, PEG–PES can be retained in dialysis bags having very large pores (>300,000 MWCO), which allows for free PEG to diffuse freely through the membrane. This method has been used for purification of various PEG–PE derivatives *(139,152)*.

PEG linkage instability is a method to achieve intentional loss of PEG coating in specific biological environments. An example of this concept has been illustrated with PEG–lipid conjugates with different alkyl components which result in gradual loss of the PEG–lipid from the liposome. A disulphide linkage, which is sensitive to reduction, has also been used. Other specific chemical conditions of interest for the loss of PEG coat include acid pH and target binding *(153)*.

PEG–PE can form micelles giving clear solutions in water even up to concentrations as high as several milligrams per millilitre. Thus, PEG–PE has the potential to dissociate from liposome and form micelles in equilibrium with bilayers. This 'problem' has taken advantage of to achieve a slow loss of PEG-coating by selection of lipid anchor. A reversal of this process, insertion of PEG–PE from micelles into preformed liposomes, also has been used as a means to prepare liposomes with a PEG coating *(153)*.

Introduction of PEG–PE replacing the distal methoxy with chemical functionalities useful for conjugation is an important advancement. The need for such functionalised PEG lipids, shown in Fig. 15, was created by their usefulness in attachment of various biologically relevant ligands to the exterior of PEG-grafted liposomes. The rationale was that, since PEG–liposomes circulate in the bloodstream for extended periods of time, one could use them as platforms for presentation of various ligands. Such ligand-carrying liposomes can be used for a variety of applications, most notably for receptor-mediated targeting. Some of the end group functionalised PEG–lipids have already been successfully used in various conjugation protocols resulting in attachment of Ig, peptides and other ligands to the distal ends of liposome-grafted PEG chains *(152)*.

Carboxy–PEG–DSPE was prepared by coupling *bis*-carboxyl–PEG to amino group of PE followed by isolation of desired product (I, Fig. 15) by silica gel chromatography. It has been used for conjugation of plasminogen to liposomes for targeting to fibrin. Longevity in plasma circulation was well preserved *(148,160)*. It is very convenient, however, to synthesise functionalised PEG–lipids from suitable hetero or bi derivatives of PEG. This was principle methodology for preparing some of the other conjugates (II–IV, Fig. 15). Amino-PEG-DSPE (II, Fig. 15) was used as the starting material for synthesis of other functionalised PEG–lipids, for example, 2-pyridylthiopropionamide (IV, Fig. 15) and bromoacetamide (V, Fig. 15) derivatives. Amino-PEG-DSPE was cleanly derivatised with hetero or bi reagents *N*-succinimidyl pyridyl dithiopropionate and *p*-nitrophenyl bromoacetate, respectively. Placing an amino acid redsidue as part of linker A (Fig. 15) is helpful for the final chemical characterisation of conjugates by amino acid analysis. This was utilised in case of hydrazide–PEG–DSPE (III, Fig. 15). Amino–PEG–DSPE, apart from being used for preparing other end group functionalised PEG–DSPE, also forms LCLs, behaving as positively charged particles *(161)*.

Hydrazide–PEG–DSPE (III, Fig. 15) forms hydrazone linkages with aldehydes. It is used for conjugation of antibodies, oxidised on their carbohydrate residues, to distal ends of PEG chains on surfaces of liposomes. It also allows for conjugation of periodate treated *N*-terminal serine or threonine peptides *(152)*.

2-pyridyldithiopropionamide–PEG–DSPE (IV, Fig. 15) has been used as a precursor for HS–PEG–DSPE. It is very efficient for attachment of maleimide-containing antibodies to end groups of PEG on liposomal surfaces. It is used for binding HS-containing ligands through disulphide linkage *(129)*.

Bromoacetate-PEG-DSPE (V, Fig. 15) is an efficient moiety for thioether-forming reactions with HS-ligands. It is utilised for Fab-SH attachment to end groups of PEG chains on liposomes *(152)*.

Linker B in most of the above cases (Fig. 15) was a stable urethane linker formed by reacting PE with an appropriate SC PEG derivative (SC–PEG–X) where X represents a functional residue or a protected form thereof. It is possible and in some cases might be advantageous, to design a linker with a well-defined lability. This might allow further control of *in vivo* properties of relevant conjugated liposomes *(152)*.

PEG–CHOL conjugates have been studied for preparing LCLs *(162–165)*. Inhibition of fluid phase endocytic process is attributed to binding of PEG–CHOL to cells plasma membrane inducing a decrease in surface hydrophobicity of cells, resulting in a marked decrease in extent of phagocytic ingestion.

A new amphiphilic PEG derivative, *p*-nitrophenylcarbonyl-PEG-1,2-dioleoyl-*sn*-glycero-3-phosphoethanolamine (pNP–PEG–DOPE), readily incorporates into

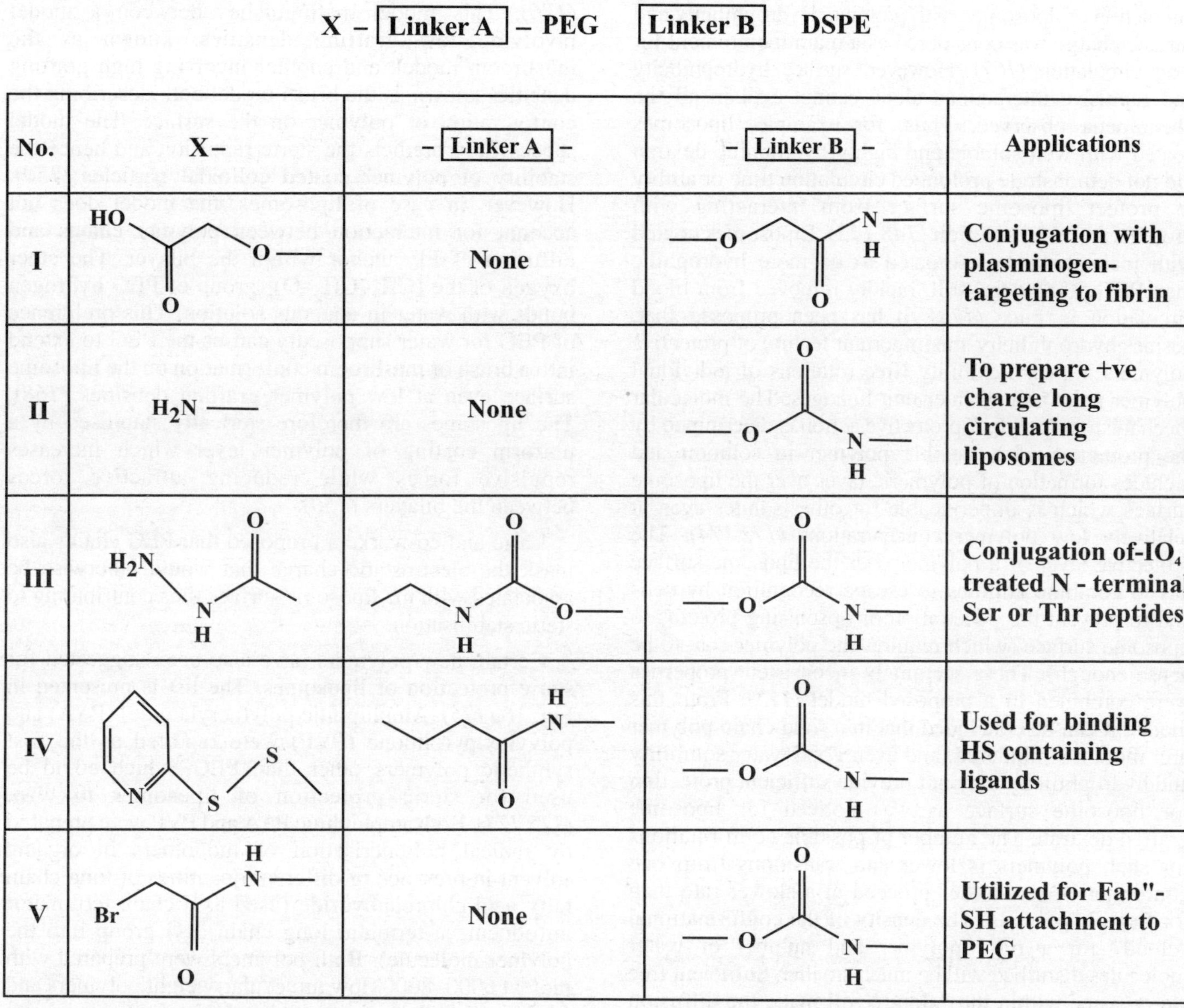

Fig. 15. Attachment of various biologically relevant ligands to the exterior of PEG-grafted liposomes (Reprinted from Advanced drug delivery review, 16, Zalipsky, S., Chemistry of polyethylene glycol conjugates with biological active molecules, 157–182, 1995, with permission from Elsevier) *(152)*.

liposomes via its PE residue, and easily binds primary amino group-containing ligands via its water-exposed pNP groups, forming stable and non-toxic urethane (carbamate) bonds. The reaction between the pNP group and ligand amino group proceeds easily and quantitatively at pH around 8.0, and remaining free pNP groups are promptly eliminated by spontaneous hydrolysis. Therefore, pNP–PEG–DOPE could serve as a very convenient tool for protein attachment to the distal ends of liposome-grafted PEG chains *(166)*.

The mechanism of PEG protective action is under continuous investigation *(148,149,167–169)*. The general opinion is that, on biological level, coating liposomes with PEG sterically hinders interactions of blood components with liposome surface. This slows down inhibition of liposome destruction by lipoproteins and prevents liposome interaction with opsoinins resulting in fast capture of liposomes by the RES. To confirm this, reduced binding of plasma proteins with PEG liposomes was demonstrated *(127,149,170,171)*. The role of supposed inhibition of opsonisation of PEG liposomes in the prolongation of their circulation time also seems evident *(72)*. Less evident is the mechanism by which PEG (or similar polymers) prevents opsonisation and interaction of liposomes with proteins. Hydrophilicity and surface charge was considered as a main requirement for long circulation *(167)*. However, surface hydrophilicity and repulsive interactions alone cannot explain all the phenomena observed. Thus, for example, liposomes coated with well soluble and highly hydrophilic dextran did not demonstrate prolonged circulation time or ability to protect liposome surface from interacting with proteins from the solution *(148,172)*. Liposomes coated with maltopentaose, estimated to be more hydrophilic than PEG 5000 were, still, rapidly removed from blood circulation in mice *(173)*. It has been proposed that, besides hydrophilicity, the important feature of protective polymers is their flexibility (free rotations of individual polymer units around inter-unit linkages. The molecular mechanism of polymer protective action is determined by the properties of a flexible polymer in solution and includes formation of polymeric layer over the liposome surface which is impermeable for other solutes even at relatively low polymer concentrations *(172,174)*. The protective layer of a polymer over the liposome surface has to combine abilities to escape recognition by cells and to prevent the penetration of opsonising proteins to liposome surface (which requires the polymer coat to be dense enough). These seemingly inconsistent properties were combined in a proposed model *(175)*. From this model, it can be concluded that in a rigid chain polymer unit motion is hindered, and even good water solubility and hydrophilicity may not provide sufficient protection for liposome surface as was noticed for liposome grafted dextran. The number of possible conformations for such polymers is lower and transitions from one conformation to another proceed at a slower rate than for flexible polymer. The density of the conformational "cloud" for a rigid polymer and number of water molecules disturbed will be much smaller. Sufficient free water space within the "cloud" will make the diffusion of plasma proteins towards the liposome surface still possible. So, to serve as an effective liposome protector even at relatively low concentration of the surface-immobilised macromolecules, the polymer has to combine hydrophilicity (solubility) and flexibility (which is characteristic of, e.g., PEG). A flexible polymer forms a high density conformational cloud. A rigid polymer of the same length forms a broad but loose and thus permeable cloud *(172)*.

It has been proposed that the transient, flexible and rapidly changing structure of PEG makes difficult the modeling of an antibody around it by the immune system *(150)*.

The conformation of PEG on liposome surface has been predicted using model of interactions between polymer-coated surfaces developed by De Gennes *(176)*. This model distinguishes between a model involving low grafting densities, known as the mushroom model, and another involving high grafting densities known as the brush model both describing the configuration of polymer on the surface. The model successfully predicts the steric repulsion and hence the stability of polymer coated colloidal particles *(150)*. However, in case of liposomes, the model does not account for interaction between polymer chains and diffusion of PE anchor within the bilayer. The ether oxygen of the $(CH_2–CH_2–O)_n$ group of PEG hydrogen bonds with water in aqueous solution. This preference of PEG for water supposedly causes the PEG to extend into a brush or mushroom conformation on the liposome surface even at low polymer grafting densities *(168)*. The liposomes are therefore sterically stabilised by a uniform coating of polymer layer which increases repulsive forces while reducing attractive forces between the bilayers *(150)*.

Lasic and co-workers proposed that PEG chains also mask the electrostatic charge that would otherwise be associated with the liposome surface thus contributing to steric stabilisation.

Certain new polymers have also been suggested for steric protection of liposomes. The list is presented in Fig. 16 *(175)*. Amphiphilic poly(acrylamide) (PAA) and polyvinylpyrolidone (PVP) were reported as the first synthetic polymers other than PEG, which could be used for steric protection of liposomes *in vivo*. *(175,177)*. Both amphiphilic PAA and PVP were prepared by radical polymerisation of monomers in organic solvent in presence of different quantities of long chain fatty acid chloroanhydride (used as a chain terminator introducing a terminal long chain acyl group into the polymer molecule). Both polymers were prepared with mol wt 6000–8000 (low molecular-weight polymers and 12,000–15,000 Da high molecular weight polymers). As a terminal hydrophobic anchor, these polymers contained either a palmityl or a dodecyl group. It was shown that amphiphilic derivatives of PAA and PVP provide effective protection to liposomes *in vivo* similar to PEG–PE *(147,177)*.

Other amphiphilic polymers with well soluble and flexible hydrophilic moiety such as amphiphilic poly(acryloylmorpholine) (PAcM), branched PEG in which two PEG chains are attached to a single hydrophobic phospholipid group (PEG 2) and phospholipid attached PVP have also been successfully used as liposome steric protectors *in vivo* *(172)*. Amphiphilic PEG2, PAcM and PVP were prepared in two steps. In the first step, carboxyl-terminated polymers were synthesised. In the second step, carboxyl-terminated polymers were modified with PE.

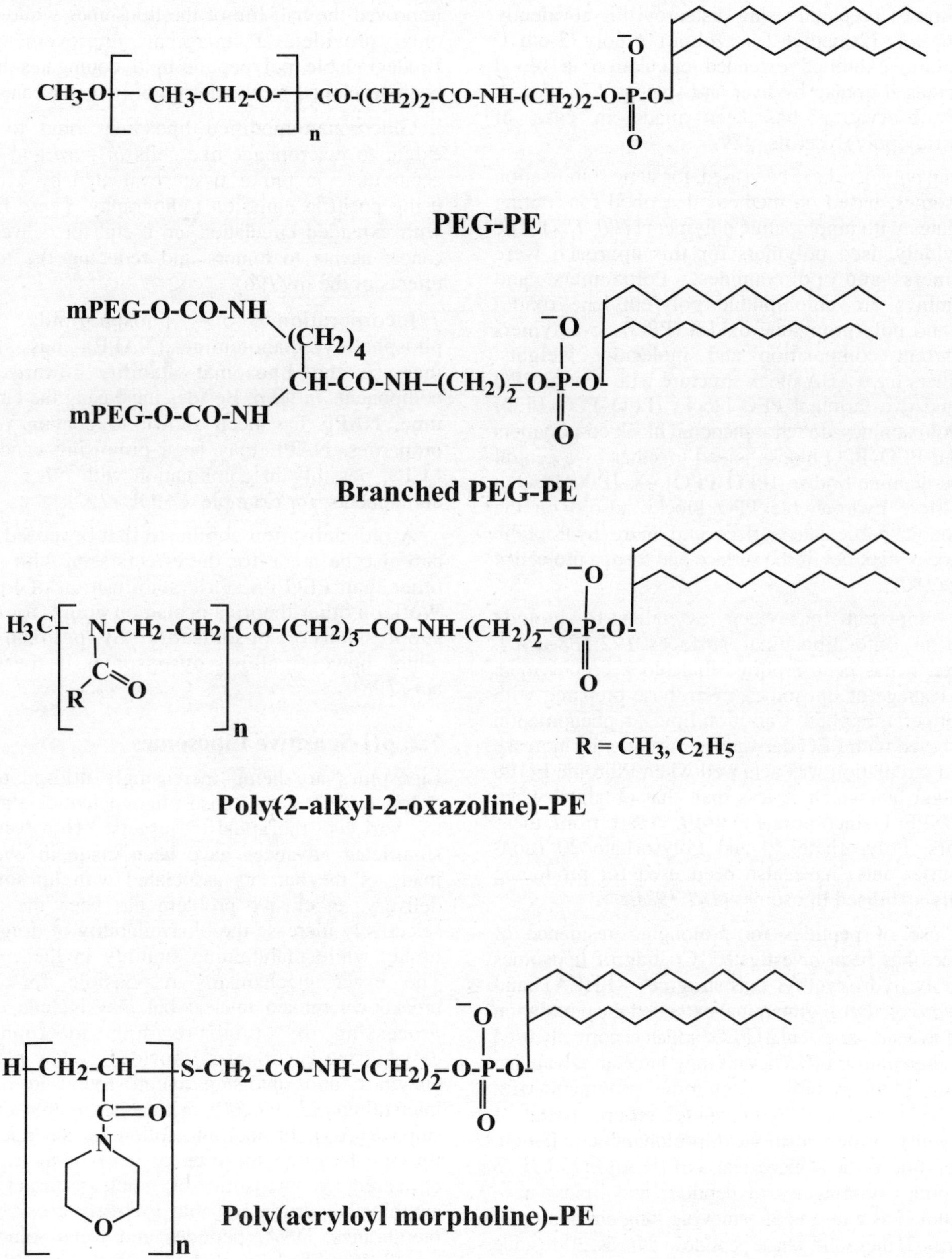

Fig. 16. Some polymers suggested for steric protection of liposomes.

Liposomes prepared using distearoyl-PE covalently linked to poly (2-methyl-2-oxazoline) or poly (2-ethyl-2-oxazoline) exhibited extended circulation in blood and decreased uptake by liver and spleen *(175,178)*. A similar observation has been made in case of phosphatidylpolyglycerols *(179)*.

Certain polymers have been used, for steric stabilisation of liposomes, based on methods described for coating particulates with amphipathic polymers *(180–187)*. The most widely used polymers for this approach were poloxamers and poloxamines. Poloxamers and poloxamines are amphiphthic poly(ethylene oxide) (PEO) and poly(propylene oxide) (PPO) co-polymers of different composition and molecular weights. Poloxamers have ABA block structure with central PPO block and two terminal PEO blocks (PEO–PPO–PEO) while Poloxamines are tetrafunctional block co-polymers with four PEO–PPO blocks joined together by a central ethylene diamine bridge ($[PEO–PPO]_2$–X–$[PPO-PEO]_2$) *(126)*. More hydrophobic PPO blocks adsorb on the hydrophobic particulate surface and more hydrophilic PEO blocks stick out of the surface and form a protective coating *(180)*.

This approach has been extended to include adsorption onto liposomal surfaces *(72,188–190)*. However, it has been reported that block co-polymers induce leakage of liposomes, even those prepared with high temperature phase transition lipids, a phenomenon not observed with PEG derivatives. A moderate increase in blood circulation was achieved when Pluronic F-108 was added but which is less than that obtained when PEG–DSPE is incorporated *(169)*. Apart from these polymers, Polysorbate 80 and Polysorbate 20 (non-ionic surfactants) have also been used for producing sterically stabilised liposomes *(191,192)*.

The use of peptides for prolonging residence of liposomes has been investigated. Coating of liposomes with poly(hydroxyethyl-L-asparagine) (PHEA) and poly(hydroxyethyl-L-glutamine) extended the circulation half-life to a similar extent as PEG, which is normally used for the preparation of LCL and they have an advantage of being biodegradable. Glutamine polymers with a hydroxypropyl or a hydroxybutyl group instead of hydroxyethyl group also yield prolonged circulation, however, not to the same extent as PHEA/G *(193,194)*. Lipopeptides (conjugates of peptides and lipids) have been studied as a means of achieving long circulation in liposomes. Using solid-phase peptide synthesis, 30-residue random libraries were synthesised consisting of a random sequence of glycine, β-alanine and γ-aminobutyric acid. The libraries were coupled to stearic acid (SA) or PE. The liposomes modified with library-PE greatly improved the half-life of the liposomes while PEG–SA only provided a marginal improvement *(195)*. Biodegradable polypeptide-lipid conjugates have also been developed for the design of polymer-coated LCL.

Glucuronate-modified liposomes bind to a lower extent to macrophage-like cells *in vitro* and passively accumulate in tumor tissue evaluated by a technique using positron emission tomography. These liposomes with extended circulation are useful for delivering anti-cancer agents to tumors and reducing the toxic side effects of the m *(196)*.

Incorporation of phospholipid, *N*-acyl-phosphatidylethanolamine (NAPE), has shown to increase the liposomal stability towards plasma components *in vitro*. Besides increasing the circulation-time, NAPE has been shown to contain fusiogenic properties. NAPE may be a promising candidate for LCLs, possibly in combination with other stabilising components, for example, CHOL *(197)*.

A rationalisation similar to that proposed for PEG can also be made for the effects seen with polymers other than PEG on steric stabilisation of liposomes. Work on other theories is also on going, for example, suppression of opsonisation by poloxamine 908 which however allows dysopsonins in the serum to act *(198)*.

7.2. pH-Sensitive Liposomes

Liposomes are being increasingly utilised to deliver drugs, enzymes, antisense oligonucleotides, and genes to various therapeutic targets. However, while significant advances have been made in overcoming many of the barriers associated with liposomal drug delivery, an elusive problem has been the ability to selectively increase the bioavailability of drug at target tissue, while maintaining stability in the circulation. The exact mechanisms responsible for liposome breakdown remain unclear but may include lysosomal processing by tumor-residing macrophages, a destabilising environment provided by low pH, lipases, enzymes, and oxidising agents found in the tumor interstitium *(73,199,200)*, or catalysis by free ammonium sulphate *(63)*. In addition, following the release from liposomal carrier, the drug or gene often needs to be delivered to cytosolic or nuclear targets. While amphipathic drugs are able to freely cross biological membranes, DNA, peptides and water-soluble drugs are likely to be excluded completely from the cell or trapped in internal organelles.

To overcome these problems, a variety of approaches have been employed; including complexation of DNA with

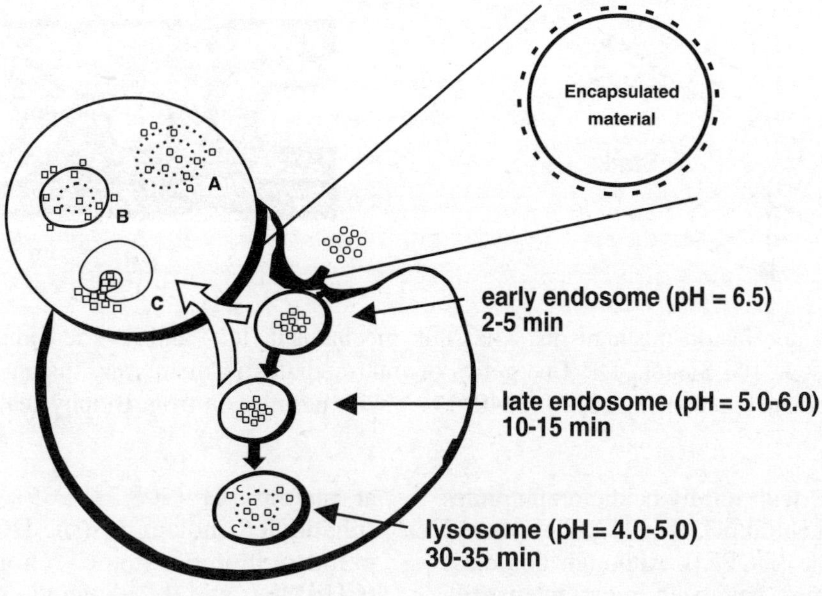

Fig. 17. Hypothetical mechanisms of internalization and intracellular delivery of pH-sensitive liposomes. (Reprinted from Cell, 32 Straubinger, R.M., Hong, K., Friend, DS., and Papahadjopoulos, D. Endocytosis of liposomes and intracellular fate of encapsulated molecules: encounter with a low PH compartment after internalization in coated vesicles, 1069–1079, 1983, with permission for Elsevier) *(217)*.

cationic lipids *(201–203)*, the design of thermo-sensitive liposomes (TSLs) capable of releasing their contents in response to small changes in temperature *(204–206)* and development of pH-sensitive liposomes *(207–209)*. The approach and the focus is use of pH-sensitive liposomes to release their contents into the cytoplasm following endocytosis. This approach relies on selective destabilisation of liposomes following acidification of the surrounding medium. The initial rationale for design of pH-sensitive liposomes was to exploit the acidic environment of tumors to trigger destabilisation of liposomal membranes *(210)*. However, the sites of greatest acidity in tumors are often the most distant from tumor microvasculature, where liposomes often fail to reach *(211–213)*. In addition, the pH of tumor interstitium rarely declines less than pH 6.5 and therefore, makes it technically difficult to engineer liposomes that become disrupted in such a narrow window of pH. Endosomes and lysosomes, on the other hand, can reach values less than 5.0 *(214–216)* and liposomes can be internalised by cells on the tumor periphery.

One fate of liposomes upon reaching the target tissues is their recognition and uptake by endocytes *(217)*. However, upon uptake by the cell, thcy arc cvcntually delivered to lysosomes (Fig. 17) *(214)*, where liposome and its contents may be degraded by various hydrolases and peptidases *(218,219)*.

The result can be diminished or lost biological activity of delivered drug or macromolecule. pH-sensitive liposomes have been designed to circumvent this problem by releasing their contents prior to reaching lysosomes and at least partly, into the cytosol, where they can diffuse to their cytosolic or nuclear targets. Endosomes and lysosomes are acidified by proton-translocating ATPases *(215,220)* to an average pH 5.0 of approximately *(215)*, but which can be as low as 4.6 in macrophages *(214,216)*. pH-sensitive liposomes release their contents into the cytosol by one, or a combination, of several potential mechanisms. These liposomes can be induced to undergo a pH-induced fusion of liposomal membranes with endosomal membranes, directly releasing liposomal contents into cytosol. Alternatively, liposomes can become destabilised and cause destabilisation of endosomal membranes, resulting in leakage of drug or liposomal "cargo" into cytosol. In case of certain encapsulated molecules, pH-sensitive liposomes may also become destabilised and release their contents solely inside the endosome, where amphipathic molecules may diffuse across endosomal membranes and other molecules (anti-folates and nucleoside analogues) may be translocated by membrane transporters located in the endosomal membrane *(221–224)*.

Four basic classes of pH-sensitive liposomes have been described. The first class combines *polymorphic lipids*,

Fig. 18. Proposed membrane fusion mechanisms. The stalk mechanism (left) and inverted micellar intermediate (IMI). (Reprinted from Biophys. J., 65, Siegel., DP. Energetics of intermediates in membrane fusion: comparison of stalk and inverted micellar intermediate mechanisms, 2124–2140, 1993, with permission from Biophysical Society) *(247)*.

such as unsaturated PEs, with mildly acidic amphiphiles that act as stabilisers at neutral pH. (e.g., 1,2 dioleyl-*sn*-3 phosphatidylethanolamine [DOPE]). Although this class of pH-sensitive liposomes has been most intensively studied, it may prove to be least useful for *in vivo* drug delivery due to the effects of serum components on formulation stability or pH-sensitivity, and their rapid clearance from circulation. The second class includes liposomes composed of "caged" lipid derivatives *(225–228)* (e.g., *N*-maleylphosphatidyl ethanolamine derivatives *(226)* or alkylether bonds *(227)* "Caged" PEG–lipid conjugates). Acid-induced hydrolysis of specifically engineered chemical bonds results in an increased presence of membrane destabilising lipid components in liposome membrane, and thus increased permeability to encapsulated solutes. A third class of pH-sensitive liposomes utilises pH-sensitive peptides or reconstituted fusion proteins to destabilise membranes at low pH *(229–233)* (e.g., influenza virus with fusion peptide HA2, Semliki Forest virus with fusion peptide E1, diptheria toxin B fragment with α-Helices TH8 and TH9, tetanus toxin and synthetic peptides like GALA [peptide of 30 amino acid with repeat sequence of glutamic acid-alanine-leucine-alanine], EGLA [an endoglucanase peptide designated EGLA-I with the sequence GLFL GLA EGLA EGLA EGLA EGLA…]). The fourth and most current class of pH-sensitive liposomes uses pH-titratable polymers to destabilise membranes following change of the polymer conformation at low pH *(203,209,234–237)* (e.g., polycations like poly(L-lysine), poly(L-histidine, poly(ethylenimine). Polyanions like polyacrylic acid derivatives, succinylated poly(glycidols) and co-polymers of *N*-isopropylacrylamide [NIPAM]). All four classes offer unique advantages and disadvantages that may vary in importance depending on the desired application.

7.2.1. Mildly Acidic Amphiphiles

Mildly acidic amphiphiles can be combined with unsaturated PEs, such as DOPE to form stable liposomes at neutral pH *(208,238,239)*. *N*-succinyldioleoylphosphatidylethanolamine (suc-DOPE), oleic acid (OA), palmitoylhomocysteine, cholesteryl hemisuccinate (CHEMS), and 1,2-dioleoyl- or 1,2-dipalmitoyl-*sn*-3-succinylglycerol (DOSG or DPSG) are a few of the stabilisers that have been used to prepare pH-sensitive liposome formulations *(204,207,240–245)*. The most common feature of these lipids is net negative charge at neutral pH that allows it to stabilise DOPE-containing membranes. Liposomes composed of these lipids can stably encapsulate highly water-soluble drugs, peptides, or nucleic acids at neutral pH. However, in a mildly acidic environment such as that found in the lumen of endosomes or lysosomes, the stabiliser becomes protonated, resulting in membrane destabilisation and the formation of non-bilayer structures that are important intermediates in membrane fusion *(246–248)*.

7.2.2. Mechanistic Rationale for pH-Induced Destabilisation

Several groups have demonstrated that such polymorphic phases as inverted hexagonal (H_{II}) and lipidic particles are important intermediates in membrane fusion *(246,248)*. Lipids with relatively small head groups relative to their fatty acyl chains are accommodated into these highly curved fusion intermediates such as stalk or inverted micellar intermediates (Fig. 18) *(247)*.

Unsaturated PE, DAG and phosphatidic acid (at low pH and in presence of calcium) have weakly hydrated head groups and thus fit into this class of lipids. These lipids form a hexagonal phase (H_{II}) rather than a lamellar phase, which is formed by lipids such as PC or many of the acidic amphiphiles *(249)*. Bilayer forming lipids, such as PC, have an approximately equivalent molecular area in their head group and acyl chains and thus a more cylindrical shape. A final class of lipids includes detergents and lysolipids which have only a single hydrophobic chain and thus, a conical molecular shape. Theoretical calculations support data showing that PE-containing membranes promote fusion while membranes containing primarily bilayer-forming lipids inhibit fusion. Mixtures of anionic lipids and PE fuse at low pH or in presence of Ca^{2+} *(243,244,250)*, while substituting bilayer forming lipids, such as PC, for PE inhibits fusion. Thus, one can theoretically form pH-sensitive membranes by mixing lipids with an average molecular shape that favours the lamellar phase at neutral pH, but which reverts to an average shape consistent with hexagonal phases at acidic pHs. Protonation of an acidic amphiphile in theory accomplishes this goal by reducing the effective molecular area in headgroup.

For pH-sensitive liposomes, when the amphiphile is in the charged form, it stabilises the lipid in bilayer form by increasing effective hydration in the interfacial region due to charge repulsion and preventing aggregation. Since aggregation, or close apposition of membranes, is the first step in the fusion process *(251)*, this is inhibitory towards fusion. However, upon protonation of stabiliser, the interfacial region is dehydrated and opposing membranes come in close approximation *(243,252)*. Additionally, intra-membrane electrostatic repulsive interactions, due to charged stabiliser, disrupt critical hydrogen bonds between neighbouring PE molecules *(253,254)* and prevent the formation of fusion competent non-bilayer structures. This stabilisation is lost upon protonation of ionised group or upon Ca^{2+} binding, both of which result in dehydration of interfacial region. pH-sensitive liposomes can thus be induced to fuse in response to decreasing pH and increasing Ca^{2+}. Calcium can also produce lateral phase separations of lipids in membranes containing negatively charged lipids *(255,256)*. However, the kinetics of phase separation are slow compared to fusion *(257)*, suggesting another mechanism, such as the ability of Ca^{2+} to form a dehydrated trans complex between opposing bilayers that facilitates membrane fusion *(243)*, is responsible for observed effect of Ca^{2+}.

7.2.3. pH-Sensitive Fusion and Leakage of Stabilised PE Liposomes

Of the various formulations examined, CHEMS:DOPE and OA:DOPE liposomes have been the most extensively studied. Contents leakage assays are routinely used to measure membrane destabilisation in response to external stimuli such as pH. These assays employ either liposome-encapsulated self-quenched fluorophores, or fluorophores encapsulated with collisional quenchers, and determine the amount of leakage by observing increase in quantum efficiency of these fluorophores upon leakage and dilution of the probes. PE:CHEMS (7:3) liposomes are sensitive to leakage of an aqueous contents marker less than pH 5.5 *(244,252)*. OA:PE liposomes are considerably more sensitive to pH, releasing their contents less than pH 6.5 *(243)*. Mixing of lipid component of opposing membranes is an important criterion for membrane fusion *(258)*. In addition to the effect of pH, a synergistic effect of Ca^{2+} and pH was observed on membrane fusion *(243,244)*. Engineering liposomes with different pH-sensitivities may allow both the location of solute release within the endocytic pathway and the liposomal delivery kinetics. Ca^{2+} and low pH decrease the barrier to aggregation by reducing the hydration at membrane surface and by decreasing repulsive electrostatic interactions.

The role of non-bilayer structures in fusion or destabilisation of pH-sensitive liposomes was studied. OA:DOPE *(259)*, CHEMS:DOPE *(260)* and suc-DOPE:DOPE *(261)* membranes were shown to undergo an acid induced transition from bilayer to the H_{II} form. Freeze-fracture electron microscopy confirmed the appearance of lipidic particles and hexagonal structures *(259,260)*. Non-bilayer intermediates appear important in the transition to a fusion competent state and Ca^{2+}, pH and lipid composition are important factors leading to the acquisition of this state.

pH-sensitive liposomes have been used to deliver cytotoxic agents, such as methotrexate and cytosine arabinoside or ara-C to cultured cells *(223,262)*. Other drugs, such as methotrexate, doxorubicin and *N*-(phosphonacetyl)-L-aspartic acid (PALA) are able to withstand the degradative enzymes present in intra-cellular organelles and even increase their cytotoxicity following internalisation *(263–268)*. This is possibly due to an increase in release of drug from the carrier following breakdown of liposomal membrane in late endosomes or lysosomes *(199,207,219,269)*. It is suggested that the increased activity may also be due to limited drug diffusion away from the cells following internalisation *(270)*. Immuno-targeted pH-sensitive liposomes were able to increase the cytotoxicity of ara-C above that of free ara-C and ara-C delivered via pH-insensitive liposomes *(262)*. Diptheria toxin (DTA) delivered to cytosol of cultured cells using pH-sensitive liposomes *(241,259,271–273)*.

The efficiency of delivery is likely to be dependent on mechanism of release from liposome, as well as physicochemical properties of entrapped solute. For example, amphipathic drugs such as doxorubicin would be expected to redistribute rapidly throughout the cell, following release from the liposome. Drugs such as methotrexate and ara-C would be expected to reach cytoplasm faster than non-transported molecules. However, both rate of release, position of release within the endocytic pathway, and rate of degradation of ara-C are all likely to play a role in the efficiency of its transport to cytoplasm. All of these factors must be taken into consideration while designing a pH-sensitive delivery system.

pH-sensitive liposomes have been used to deliver antigens like ovalbumin to antigen presenting cells (APC) for processing via the major histocompatibility complex-I pathway *(274–276)*.

An additional concern when using liposomes *in vivo* is their stability in presence of human plasma or serum. For liposomes to be used effectively *in vivo*, they must quantitatively retain their contents, while in the circulation *(277)*. Some liposome preparations have been shown to be destabilised and release their contents in the presence of serum or plasma *(277,278)*. This serum induced destabilisation was exquisitely sensitive to lipid composition of liposome. Several factors have been implicated in the destabilisation of liposomes in plasma or serum, including complement mediated lysis *(279–281)* and destabilisation by HDL *(282–284)*. DOPE:OA liposomes were shown to be unstable in presence of mouse and human plasma, most likely due to extraction of the OA stabiliser from the membrane by albumin *(278,285)* or transfer to other membranes *(286)*. The addition of CHOL resulted in an increase in plasma stability, but also in a concomitant decrease in the acid-sensitivity of contents leakage *(285)*. In contrast, other pH-sensitive liposome formulations have been shown to be stabilised by human plasma. SUVs composed of OA:DOPE or OA:DOPE:CHOL were stabilised to pH- induced leakage by pre-incubation in presence of human plasma *(285,287)*. pH-sensitive liposome formulations containing DOPE and the double-chain amphiphile 1,2-palmitoyl-3-succinylglycerol (DPSG) were significantly more stable in presence of plasma than OA-containing liposomes, but showed a similar decrease in acid-sensitivity following pre-incubation in presence of plasma *(259)*. In order to effectively develop a liposomal drug delivery system, the effects of serum on liposomal stability require careful investigation.

7.2.4. Alternative Strategies Under Acidic Conditions to Generate Fusogenic Liposomes

While the development of pH-sensitive liposomes has been correlated normally with inclusion of DOPE in liposomal formulations, other strategies have also been investigated.

7.2.5. Use of Novel pH-Sensitive Lipids

Inference obtained with a new type of pH-sensitive liposome formulation, composed of egg yolk phosphatidylcholine (EPC) liposomes bearing succinylated poly(glycidol), a PEG derivative having carboxyl groups, proved that under weakly acidic conditions fusion ability of liposomes increases *(235)*. This has been shown to result in intensive and diffuse cytoplasmic fluorescence as a consequence of intra-cellular delivery of calcein. It is concluded according to the observations, that polymer-modified liposomes, upon endocytosis by CV-1 cells, transfer their content into cytoplasm by fusing with the endosomal membrane *(308)*. Recently this strategy has been utilised to target anti-BCG antibody-bearing pH-sensitive liposomes to tumor cells expressing BCG antigen *(288)*. More recently, three different techniques have been engaged to generate pH-sensitive liposomes in the absence of DOPE *(289–291)*. Formulations with cationic/anionic lipid combinations were shown to be highly efficient vehicles for intra-cellular drug and gene delivery. Liposomes composed of EPC, dimethyldioctadecylammonium bromide (DDAB), CHEMS and Tween-80 (25:25:49:1, mol/mol) were shown to stably entrap calcein at pH 7.4 and undergo destabilisation and irreversible aggregation under acidic pH. These liposomes showed improved retention of pH-sensitivity in presence of serum, compared to pH-sensitive liposomes containing DOPE *(290)*. One more hopeful strategy consisted of preparing anionic pH-sensitive liposomes composed of diolein/CHEMS (6:4). The outcome proves that these liposomes are stable at physiological pH, however undergo rapid aggregation and efficiently release encapsulated calcein at pH 5.0. Complexes formed upon association of developed liposomes with DNA–protamine mixtures maintained their transfection activity in media containing up to 50% fetal bovine serum, on the contrary to what was observed for DOPE-containing liposomes *(289)*. Hopeful results in terms of pH-sensitivity and resistance to serum were also gained using a novel liposome formulation composed of PC, CHEMS, oleyl alcohol (OAlc), Tween-80 *(291)* and a monostearoyl derivative of morpholine *(292)*. The above formulation showed much better retention of its pH sensitive properties in presence of 10% serum, compared with DOPE-based pH-sensitive liposomes.

7.2.6. Liposomal Co-Encapsulation of Synthetic Fusogenic Peptides and Therapeutic Molecules

To promote cytosolic delivery of hydrophilic molecules with limited access to sub-cellular compartments, the liposomal co-encapsulation of therapeutic molecules with peptides has turned out to be a promising strategy. Gelonin, a type I plant toxin, represents an example of such a compound known to inactivate ribosomes and arrest protein synthesis. The failure of this compound to permeate plasma membrane and to escape efficiently from endosomes into the cytosol, leads to its rapid degradation within endosomes and lysosomes, thus compromising its anti-tumor activity. To overcome this problem, gelonin was co-encapsulated inside pH-sensitive liposomes with listeriolysin-O, the pore-forming protein that mediates escape of the intra-cellular pathogen. *Listeria monocytogenes* from the endosome into cytosol *(293)*. This technique resulted in a significant improvement on cytotoxicity of encapsulated gelonin against murine B16 melanoma cell line, compared to free gelonin or gelonin encapsulated alone in pH-sensitive liposomes. The inclusion of PEG strongly decreased the cytotoxicity of pH-sensitive formulation co-encapsulating gelonin and listeriolysin-O. It is to be noticed whether the inclusion of PEG compromises the cell uptake and/or the pH-sensitivity properties of liposomes *(293)*. A similar strategy has been explored to demonstrate that co-encapsulation of a pH-dependent fusogenic peptide (diINF-7) and diphtheria toxin *(294)*. A chain DTA in non-pH-sensitive immunoliposomes promotes cytosolic delivery of encapsulated macromolecule. This peptide (resembling the NH_2-terminal domain of influenza virus haemagglutinin HA-2 subunit) was used as functional characterisation studies showed its capability to induce fusion between liposome membranes and leakage of liposome-entrapped compounds when exposed to low pH. In addition, co-encapsulation of diINF-7 into DTA-containing immunoliposomes resulted in significantly increased cytotoxicity towards ovarian carcinoma cells, indicating that this peptide can be used to obtain cytosolic delivery of liposome entrapped drugs with poor membrane permeation capacities *(294)*.

7.2.7. Synthetic Fusogenic Peptides/Proteins with Cationic Liposomes

Immunogenicity is major problem while using pH sensitive proteins/peptides in formulation. This drawback can be over come by using cationic liposomes (lipoplexes) and polymers (polyplexes). As cationic liposome/DNA complexes are believed to enter cells primarily through endocytosis, it has been theorised that use of peptides that can destabilise endosomes or facilitate the fusion of liposome/DNA complexes with the endosomal membrane would enhance gene delivery. Incubation of COS-7 cells with a β-gal-expressing plasmid, and anionic or cationic derivatives of N-terminal peptide of HA-2 subunit of influenza virus fusion protein, haemagglutinin, in presence of Lipofectin, resulted in improvement of transfection activity by a factor of 2–7 over that of Lipofectin alone *(295)*. The degree of Transfectam (lipopolyamine)-mediated transfection of H225 human melanoma cells could be increased by up to 1000-fold (over that obtained with a sub-optimal charge-equivalent [1.5] of Transfectam/DNA) by adding the haemagglutinin-derived peptide INF6 to preformed lipoplexes *(296)*. The correlation of the pH-sensitive peptide GALA *(297,229)* with DOTAP/DOPE (1:1) liposomes before complexation with plasmid DNA resulted in a significant enhancement in luciferase expression in COS-7 cells, which depended on the cationic liposome/DNA (+/–) charge ratio *(298)*. The capacity of certain peptides to cause endosomal destabilisation due to their fusogenic properties may also be extended to proteins. Actually studies on methods of gene delivery mediated by transferrin associated lipoplexes performed indicated that besides triggering internalisation of complexes, transferrin may also play a role in the cytoplasmic delivery of DNA by facilitating endosome destabilisation *(299)*. Indeed, transfection experiments carried out with cells pre-treated with drugs that prevent acidification of endosomal lumen (bafilomycin A1 and chloroquine) demonstrated that a significant inhibition was observed not only in the levels of transfection activity, but also in the extent of release of complexed DNA into the cytoplasm, as assessed by fluorescence microscopy. Contradictory to the observation of diffused cytoplasmic fluorescence in absence of lysosomotropic drugs, treatment of cells resulted in punctate fluorescence restricted to intra-cellular organelles, suggesting that complexed DNA was incapable to escape from endosomes. Also, recent studies on kinetics of the initial steps involved in lipoplex–cell interactions suggest that association of transferrin to lipoplexes increases the extent of fusion with endosomes. Generally, these results support the hypothesis that transferrin acquires fusogenic properties under acidic conditions by exposure of hydrophobic domains, thus facilitating endosomal disruption and intra-cellular release of DNA *(299,300)*. Alarmed by these results and by previous reports describing the ability of albumin to promote membrane fusion under acidic conditions *(301,302)*, studies by Plank *et al.* *(303)* showed that albumin could also function as a fusogenic protein that destabilises endosomes under acidic conditions, thus enhancing intra-cellular gene delivery and transfection activity.

7.2.8. pH-Sensitive Polymers with Liposomes

In the recent years, a number of studies have confirmed the potential of alkylated NIPAM co-polymers to provide pH-sensitivity to liposomes. Complexation of hydrophobically modified co-polymers of NIPAM (either randomly or terminally alkylated) with EPC/CHOL liposomes resulted in an improvement of *in vitro* release of both highly-water soluble markers and amphipathic drugs upon acidification *(236,237,304,311)*. Randomly alkylated NIPAM anchored liposomes containing ara-C were shown to mediate a higher cytotoxicity towards J774 macrophage-like cells as compared with non-pH-sensitive liposomes *(237)*. Recently, different NIPAM based co-polymers were synthesised and estimated in terms of their ability to give pH sensitivity, serum stability and steric stabilisation to liposomes *(237,305,306)*. Terminally alkylated NIPAM co-polymer coating promotes steric stabilisation of liposomes, as a result leading to prolonged blood circulation *(311)*. However, as this effect was still considered insufficient for *in vivo* purposes, co-incorporation of PEG–lipid derivatives into the liposomal surface was evaluated. As anticipated, a considerable increase in blood circulation time was observed, blood clearance profiles being essentially analogous to that observed for stealth liposomes without NIPAM. Similar to earlier observations, the stabilising effect of PEG noticeably reduced the liposome pH-sensitivity contributed by the co-polymers *(305,307)*.

pH-sensitive LCLs have also been proposed as a means of using the long circulation of liposomes for effective targeting. Addition of PEG–PE to the membrane of pH-sensitive liposomes composed of CHEMS and DOPE conferred steric stability to the vesicles *(307)*. Succinylated poly(glycidol), a PEG derivative having carboxyl groups, has also been proposed as a means of preparing pH sensitive LCLs *(308)*. Liposomes composed of DOPE, 1,2-dipalmitoylsuccinyl glycerol (DPSG) and PEG-derived PE (DSPE–PEG, up to 5%) were pH sensitive, plasma stable and had a long circulation time in the blood *(309)*. NIPAM co-polymers have been demonstrated to provide a steric barrier that is dependent on pH *(306,310)*. pH-sensitive liposomes were prepared using a terminally-alkylated co-polymer of NIPAM and methacrylic acid (MAA) and PEG phospholipid derivative *(311)*. Simoes and co-workers *(312)* have provided an excellent review on the topic.

7.2.9. Thermo-Sensitive Liposomes

Liposomes could be used effectively as a drug delivery vehicle if it is possible to deliver their contents selectively to the predetermined target which could be a particular organ/cells or an anatomical site. Several types of liposome formulations have been explored for this purpose; such as those bearing carbohydrate determinants (lectins), monoclonal antibodies, glycoprotein and antigens with a view of targeting the liposomes to selective tissues or anatomical sites *(313–316)*. However, most of these formulations have one or the other limitations in achieving all objectives for target delivery due to several reasons such as antigenicity of ligands, inability of drug to reach the appropriate cellular compartment in active form and presence of endothelial or other histological barrier between liposome and its cellular binding site. Development of an ideal liposome carrier system for target delivery is continued till date out of which, temperature sensitive (TSL) is one of them.

The use of heat-sensitive liposomes for selective drug delivery was first suggested two centuries ago *(317)*. Liquid-crystalline transition temperature (T_c) of liposome is a characteristic property and is dependent on composition of the bilayer membrane. At temperatures well below their T_c, liposomes are relatively stable, but as T_c is approached, the phase transition of their membrane renders them "leaky" for small molecules. Liposomes with a T_c, a few degrees above body temperature can therefore be used for local drug delivery if the target zone is heated locally.

TSLs as a delivery system were developed by Yatvin *et al. (204)*, Weinstein *et al. (317)* and others *(318–320)* using a mixture of synthetic lipids such as DPPC and DSPC that exhibits a gel to sol transition at temperature few degrees above the physiological temperature, a range easily obtainable by local hyperthermia. It was postulated that such liposomes would remain reasonably stable in the vascular system at normal body temperature (37°C), and when passing through heated area they would release their contents when the transition temperature is attained. TSLs are extensively investigated for their potential to release anti-tumor drugs in response to hyperthermia occurring in the heated regions. Udupa *et al.* have also reported the therapeutic efficacy of this unique and attractive strategy against sarcoma-180 tumors *(321)*.

Release rate of drugs from TSL was also found dependent on lipid composition and the method of preparation. Kim *et al. (322)* prepared temperature sensitive MLVs of egg PC by either reverse-phase evaporation or film hydration method, and DOPE liposomes by detergent removal. Their temperature-dependent release behaviours were investigated in presence of co-polymer of *N*-isopropyl acrylamide and octadecylamine (poly[NIPAM-*co*-ODA]) or co-polymer of *N*-isopropyl acrylamide, acrylic acid and octadecylamine (poly[NIPAM-*co*-AA-*co*-ODA]) using calcein a fluorescence probe. By a temperature jump from 17 to 40°C, crossing the transition temperature of poly(NIPAM-*co*-ODA), approximately 29°C, the release from reverse-phase evaporation vesicles (REVs) containing the polymer in 270 s increased in a saturation manner until the mixing ratio of polymer to lipid was 0.1, where degree of release was approximately 55%. For film hydration vesicles (FHVs), the release pattern with polymer to lipid ratio was similar to that of REVs, but the degree of release under same conditions was much less than in case of REVs, even though both are composed of same phospholipid. Since the bilayers of REVs are less in number, and more closely stacked with each with other than those of FHVs, the defect in bilayers of REVs would be induced more easily by a thermal contraction of polymer. For DOPE liposomes, the degrees of releases under same conditions as in the REVs and the FHVs of egg PC were more than 80%. The extensive release is probably because DOPE liposomes disintegrated into non-bilayer structure. On the other hand, in temperature-dependent release from liposomes mixed with either poly(NIPAM-*co*-ODA) or poly(NIPAM-*co*-AA-*co*-ODA), of which the transition temperatures are approximately 29°C and 37°C, respectively, REVs and FHVs started to release significantly around the transition temperature of each polymer. However, for DOPE liposomes the temperature where liposomes start to release, is not clear and an appreciable amount of calcein released below transition temperature. Therefore, REVs and FHVs are expected to be more favourable than DOPE liposomes when off-on behaviour of release at a certain temperature is desired. Of the egg PC liposomes, REVs would be a better choice than FHVs in aspects of degree of release.

7.2.9.1. Thermo-Sensitive Polymers in Site Specific Drug Delivery

Modulation of drug release behaviour of thermo-sensitive sterically stabilised liposomes by exposure to hyperthermic condition have bearing on the strategies adopted for controlled release of drugs at specific site of the body. Such a study conducted by Gaber *et al.* *(206)* and Wu *et al.* *(323)*, indicated that hyperthermia can be used to selectively enhance both delivery and rate of release of drugs from TSLs to targeted tissues. The study included *in vivo* fluorescence video microscopy to measure extravasation of liposomes, as well as release of their contents, in a rat skin flap window chamber containing a vascularised mammary adenocarcinoma under defined thermal conditions (34, 42 and 45°C, respectively). Images of tissue areas containing multiple blood vessels were recorded via a SIT camera immediately before, and for up to 2 h after i.v. injection of two liposome populations with identical radiolabeled (Rh-PE) lipid composition. The calculated intensity of liposome contents (DOX) in the interstitial space was negligible at 34°C, and increased by 38- and 76-fold, when the tumor was heated at 42°C and 45°C for 1 h, respectively.

Efforts are in progress to focus on the development of a new thermal-sensitive drug delivery system, specifically for local control of solid tumors. Needham *et al.* *(324)* describe a new lipid formulation containing doxorubicin that has been optimised for both mild hyperthermic temperatures (39–40°C) that are readily achievable in clinic and rapid release times of drug (tens of seconds). This new liposome, in combination with mild hyperthermia, was found to be significantly more effective than free drug or with conventional liposome formulations in reducing tumor growth in a human squamous cell carcinoma xenograft cell line (FaDu). The study was successful in producing 11 of 11 complete regressions lasting up to 60 days post-treatment.

Long circulating TLSs have also been proposed. The novel lipid 1,2-dipalmitoyl-*sn*-glycero-3-phosphoglyceroglycerol (DPPGOG), which is closely related to naturally occurring 1,2-dipalmitoyl-*sn*-glycero-3-phosphoglycerol, in combination with 1,2-dipalmitoyl-*sn*-glycero-3-phosphocholine and 1,2-distearoyl-*sn*-glycero-3-phosphocholine provides long-circulating TLSs with favourable properties under mildly hyperthermic conditions (41–42°C) *(325)*. Doxorubicin (DOX) has been delivered by encapsulation in long-circulating, TSLs (180–200 nm), prepared from DPPC/DSPC (9:1 [m/m]) and 6 mol% of ganglioside GM_1 (GM_1) *(326)*. Enhanced delivery of doxorubicin (DOX) to a solid tumor subjected to local hyperthermia was achieved by using long-circulating, TSLs composed of DPPC/DSPC (9:1, m/m) and 3 mol% amphipathic PEG in colon 26-bearing mice. Inclusion of 3 mol% of distearoyl phosphatidylethanolamine derivatives of PEG (DSPE–PEG, amphipathic PEG) with a mean molecular weight of 1000 or 5000 in DPPC/DSPC liposomes resulted in decreased RES uptake and a concomitant prolongation of circulation time, affording sustained increased blood levels of liposomes *(327)*. DOPC/CHOL liposomes with encapsulated Pluronic F127 molecules made stealth using distearoyl (PEG 5000) PE (DSPEG 5000PE) have also been investigated as temperature sensitive LCLs. The interaction of Pluronic F127 with the lipid bilayer at elevated temperature causes release of encapsulated contents *(328)*.

Ning *et al.* *(329)* examined the possibility that hyperthermia would accelerate drug release from LCLs, and enhance their anti-tumor activity. Liposomes prepared by thin film hydration technique were tested for anti-tumor efficacy against RIF-1 tumor in C3H mice in which, hyperthermia was induced by ultrasound apparatus and a water bath heating system and were evaluated by tumor growth delay assay. Results of *in vitro* drug release experiments demonstrated that increase in temperature from 37 to 41°C resulted in about a six fold increase in doxorubicin (DOX) release in a 1h period. Further increase in temperature to 43°C, resulted in only a modest additional drug release. Drug uptake studies showed that local hyperthermic treatment immediately following the drug administration dramatically enhanced stealth liposome-encapsulated doxorubicin (S-DOX) uptake by tumors, but did not do so for free DOX. The anti-tumor efficacy study confirmed the hypothesis that addition of hyperthermia to the treatment of RIF-1 tumors with doxorubicin encapsulated in LCLs would enhance anti-tumor effects.

Studies by Kong *et al. (330)* reported the tumor drug concentrations, drug distributions and therapeutic efficacies achieved by three fundamentally different liposomes, non-TSL (NTSL), traditional TSL (TTSL) and low-temperature sensitive liposome (LTSL); free doxorubicin (DOX); and saline in combination with hyperthermia (HT) compared directly in a human tumor xenograft model. NTSL is a non-thermo-sensitive liposome in physiological temperature range, TTSL is a traditional thermo-sensitive liposome that triggers in range of approximately 42–45°C and releases drug over approximately 30 min, and LTSL is a new low temperature sensitive liposome that triggers in range of approximately 39–40°C and releases drug in a matter of seconds. Athymic nude mice bearing FaDu human tumor xenograft were given a single i.v. dose of 5 mg/kg of DOX (free drug or liposome encapsulated), and the tumors were then heated to either 34°C or 42°C for 1 h at 34°C. All treatment groups were similar, achieving low concentrations of DOX (0–4.5 ng/mg). At 42°C, the LTSL (25.6 ng/mg) achieved highest DOX concentration ($P < 0.04$), but all three liposomal formulations (7.3–25.6 ng/mg) were higher than saline or DOX (0–0.7 ng/mg; $P < 0.02$). LTSL + HT was also the only group that resulted in significant amounts of DNA-bound DOX (silver nitrate-extractable fraction; $P < 0.02$). Overall, the LTSL + HT group showed the largest DOX concentration, the highest and most pervasive DOX fluorescence, and the most anti-tumor effect. Thus, HT-triggered liposomal drug release may account for the largest differential therapeutic effect and demonstrates the importance of rapid drug release from drug carriers at tumor site.

7.2.9.2. Paramagnetic TSLs

Magnetic resonance (MR)-thermometry methods are used for guidance and control of thermal therapies such as thermal ablation or regional hyperthermia but, they are limited to measurement of temperature changes and, thus, cannot be used to assess absolute temperature values. Paramagnetic TSLs are investigated as innovative contrast agents offering the potential to overcome these limitations *(331)*. They are composed of a gadolinium- or manganese-based compound enclosed by a phospholipid membrane with a distinct gel-to-liquid crystalline phase transition temperature (T_c). At this temperature, the phospholipid membrane changes from a gel-phase to a liquid-crystalline phase which is associated with an increased transmembrane permeability towards solutes and water. Under these conditions, both types of paramagnetic TSLs demonstrate a significant increase in longitudinal (T_1) relaxivity, attributed to release of paramagnetic material from the liposome and/or to the increased water exchange rate between liposome interior and exterior. Paramagnetic TSLs have already been successfully studied in animal models and have demonstrated a clear correlation between tissue temperature changes and signal intensity changes in magnetic resonance imaging.

8. STABILITY OF LIPOSOMES

To be pharmaceutically useful, liposomes should be stable in some form (perhaps dehydrated) for a satisfactory period of time, for example, 2 yr preferably at room temperature. An estimate of stability of liposomes can be obtained from an Arrhenius plot constructed using stability studies at accelerated temperatures and humidity conditions. These studies should generally be carried out at temperatures below the phase transition temperature of phospholipids to avoid a break in the Arrhenius plot. Due to this reason, initial predictions of stability and the influence of formulation factors upon stability may involve prolonged studies.

Possible stability problems include:

8.1. Loss of Entrapped Drug

Drug loss is less of a problem if the drug has a very low or a very high log P_{oct} value. Very water-soluble drugs (log P_{oct} < (0.3) remain in inner aqueous compartment of liposome. Drugs with intermediate solubility (1.7 < log P_{oct} < 4) are a major problem because they partition easily between the lipid and water phases and are lost from liposomes. These drugs are only trapped in the liposomes if they form a complex with membrane lipids. Lipid soluble drugs (log P_{oct} > 5) are entrapped almost completely in the lipid bilayer of liposome *(85)*. However, the stability of SUVs may be compromised as entrapment of drugs in bilayer promotes fusion of liposomes. For all drugs, entrapment stability is better in MLVs than unilamellar vesicles. Addition of CHOL to liposome formulations decreases the permeability of bilayers to entrapped drugs. Stability is enhanced when the lipid portion of phospholipid has long acyl chains. Methods to determine the loss of drug from liposomes are dependent upon the specific drug and its location in the liposome. In order to estimate the loss of entrapped drug, separation procedures discussed earlier in the section on "Encapsulation efficiency and entrapped volume" are generally utilised.

8.2. Change in Liposome Structure Including Particle Size Distribution and Aggregation/Fusion of Liposomes

The techniques described in the section on "Characterisation of liposomes" are also generally useful in monitoring the stability of liposomes. As mentioned earlier, the presence of hydrophobic molecules increases slow, spontaneous fusion of SUVs to form LUVs. Charged phospholipids in liposomes reduce aggregation and facilitate initial liposome hydration. In early stages of product development, fusion can be easily monitored using a fluorescence marker. This method is based upon the mixing of markers originally present in either membranes or entrapped volume in different sets of liposomes. Mixing of markers upon liposome fusion leads to a change in the sample fluorescence. Examples of such markers include terbium citrate–sodium dipicolinate, calcein/cobalt/ethylenediamine tetra acetic acid (EDTA), etc. *(332)*.

8.3. Chemical Instability of the Liposomes and the Entrapped Drug

Liposome instability is mainly in part due to the instability of phospholipids and CHOL. Most common mechanisms of phospholipid degradation are oxidation of fatty acids and hydrolysis of ester bonds linking fatty acids to the glyceryl backbone. The oxidation of fatty acids is initiated by abstraction of hydrogen from the lipid chain. Double bonds present in acyl chains of polyunsaturated lipids render these chains particularly susceptible to oxidation.

Oxidation of phospholipids can be minimised by using one or more of the following techniques:

1. Use of completely or partially hydrogenated lipids.
2. Addition of an anti-oxidant.
3. Protection of phospholipids from light.
4. Storage in an oxygen free atmosphere.
5. Addition of EDTA to chelate any traces of heavy metal ions.

The hydrolysis of ester bonds normally occur before oxidation and leads to the formation of lyso compounds such as lysolecithin. These compounds can cause changes in the properties of bilayers such as an increase in permeability. These reactions are temperature sensitive with higher temperatures causing greater hydrolysis. They are also pH-dependent with a pH of maximum stability of around 6.5.

Lyophilisation (freeze-drying) is an excellent method to extend the shelf life of compounds with stability problems in aqueous media. The lyophilised product is re-constituted prior to administration. Lyophilisation and reconstitution can be achieved without a significant effect on liposome size, release properties and trapping ability. Cryoprotectants such as sucrose, lactose or trehalose are normally required, with trehalose being the most effective. In anhydrous state, trehalose preserves liposome structure by replacing the water molecules normally bound to the phospholipid headgroups. When lyophilised liposomes are reconstituted, water quickly replaces the sugar molecules and liposomes appear to reseal before significant leakage of entrapped contents can occur. The ratio of cryoprotectant agent to lipid appears to be critical with the least loss of entrapped drug occurring at a 3:1 ratio of trehalose to lipid. It may also be helpful to entrap cryoprotectant agent in liposomes as well as in suspending medium. Charged liposomes seem to be more stable to lyophilisation than neutral liposomes *(86)*.

9. LIPOSOMAL PHARMACO-KINETICS

Pharmacokinetics of liposome is of special interest as drugs entrapped in liposome behave differently than the free drug in body at all sites-absorption, distribution, metabolism and elimination. It is this property that leads the liposome as one of the most potential carrier for drug delivery for various applications such as; absorption modification, protection of drug from rapid metabolism, accumulation in desired site, avoidance of unwanted site and also to control the release of drug entrapped in a specific domain and at a desired rate. Pharmacokinetic information of liposomal formulation are very useful in interpreting changes in the pharmacodynamic characters of free drug when entrapped in such a carrier and subsequently be exploited to design system for site specific drug delivery.

As a drug delivery system, liposomes can significantly alter the pharmacokinetics and pharmacodynamics of entrapped drugs, for example, by enhancing drug uptake, delaying rapid drug clearance, and reducing drug toxicity. Liposomes are also known to sustain the release of entrapped drug(s) and to decrease the mucociliary clearance of drug(s) because of their surface viscosity. Therefore, more effective and sustained systemic absorption of a drug would be attained by administering the drug containing liposomes in respiratory tract.

Under ideal conditions, intravenous (i.v.) injection of liposome formulation could carry the entrapped drug safely in circulation; accumulate in predetermined site, organ, tissue or cell and release drug at a desired rate for maximum therapeutic benefit. However, the path of liposome in circulation is not so smooth as it encounters various hurdles listed below:

1. Engulfed by phagocytes and clear them from circulation before they reach the desired site.
2. Loose drug by leakage during circulation totally or partially in the blood.
3. Rupture due to mechanical stress during circulation.
4. Preferentially adsorb or interact with blood components and hence dumping in an unwanted domain.

Above problems are to be well addressed during the formulation development and so liposomes are required to under go rigorous pharmacokinetic tests to confirm their efficacy. Pharmacokinetics of liposome varies significantly with the route of administration, hence would also provide ample scope for manipulation in designing systems based on the therapeutic necessity.

9.1. PharmacoKinetics of Liposome Following I.V. Administration

Liposome being a vesicular system behaves as particles in almost all respects and so the liposome formulation is termed as dispersion. Particles including microorganisms in circulation present a disposition pattern as represented in Fig. 1. Size of liposomes ranges from 190 A° to several microns. Although they are distributed in a similar manner, their distribution to some tissues are restricted due to structural barriers of capillaries and endothelium. Based on structure and continuity of endothelium and its basal lamina, capillaries are classified into three main types: continuous, fenestrated and discontinuous (sinusoids) capillary beds. Studies on trans-capillary migration of liposomes (particularly SUVs and MLVs) under normal conditions reports that the liposomes larger than 600 A° in diameter have little access to tissues containing continuous capillaries normally found in skeletal, cardiac and smooth muscles, lungs, skin, subcutaneous tissues and mucus membranes. Larger liposomes (>0.5 μm in diameter) are confined to intra-vascular space and as a result the phagocytic cells in blood and RES located primarily in liver, spleen and bone marrow, are major organs involved in uptake of large liposomes *(136,333)*. Thus, very low fraction of large liposome could reach the extravascular space *(129,334)*. However, excess dose of large liposomes in experimental animals showed higher levels of liposome in blood with not much increase in concentration in organs like liver and spleen beyond a limit. This indicates the presence of saturable uptake process for large liposomes by tissues *(129,335)* and is mathematically described as non-linear, capacity limited elimination process following Michaelis-Menten kinetics where rate of clearance of liposomes from the blood (V) is given by the equation:

$$V = \frac{V_{max} C}{K_m + C} + K'C$$

where, V_{max} is the maximum velocity of clearance by non-linear pathway, C is concentration of liposome in the blood, K is Michaelis-Menten constant (equal to concentration of liposome in blood at half-maximal velocity). $K'C$ denotes a non-saturable process, such as clearance due to extravasation or uptake by liver hepatocytes.

Small liposomes (<0.1 μm in diameter) are eliminated by phagocytosis and uptake by liver parenchymal cells. Both these parallel pathways decides the pharmacokinetic biodistribution of liposomes in the body. Uptake by liver parenchymal cells has been hypothesised to be pinocytic (fluid phase endocytic) and follows non-saturable linear kinetics.

9.1.1. Phagocytic Uptake of Liposomes in Blood

Interaction of liposomes injected intravenously with blood components is well reviewed by Frezard *et al.* *(336)*. Liposomes normally interact with at least two distinct groups of plasma proteins *(337)*: (1) plasma high density lipoproteins and (2) so called opsonins, which (by adsorbing onto the surface of vesicles) mediate their endocytosis by MPS macrophages. The rate of liposome clearance from blood circulation will therefore depend on the ability of opsonins to bind to liposome surface and can be manipulated through the appropriate selection of liposome characteristics *(338,339)*. For instance, "fluid" vesicles are removed more rapidly from blood circulation than "rigid" ones. It was suggested that opsonins did not adsorb as avidly on vesicles with rigid bilayers. Clearance from blood stream is also influenced by surface charge *(340)* and by vesicle size. The longest half-life is obtained when liposomes are relatively small (diameter <0.05 μm) and carry no net surface charge. However, regardless of time of liposome persistence within the vascular system, much of an injected dose is taken up by MPS macrophages, ending up in lysosomal apparatus. There, liposomes are disrupted within lysosomes, the solute is released locally and, depending on its nature, can either remain in lysosomes be transferred into cytoplasm or diffuse out from cells.

Fetterly and Straubinger *(341)* studied altered biodistribution of paclitaxel-containing liposomes administered intravenously (40 mg/kg) as either MLV liposomes composed of phosphatidylglycerol/PC (L-pac) or in the Cremophor EL/ethanol vehicle (Cre-pac) in rats. The pharmacokinetic parameters determined from blood and tissue samples showed similar AUC for blood for both the formulations while the AUC for various tissues was formulation-dependent. For bone marrow, skin, kidney, brain, adipose and muscle tissue, the AUC was statistically higher for Cre-pac. For spleen, a tissue of RES that is important in clearance of liposomes, the area under curve (AUC) was statistically higher for L-pac. Apparent tissue partition co-efficients (K_p) for bone marrow (a tissue in which paclitaxel exerts significant toxicity), K_p was fivefold greater for paclitaxel in Cre-pac indicating the contribution of liposomal formulations of paclitaxel in reducing paclitaxel toxicity.

Studies by Swenson *et al.* *(342)* showed that gentamicin sulphate encapsulated in liposomes composed solely of egg PC and administered via i.v. injection to rats and mice resulted in higher and more prolonged activity in organs rich in reticuloendothelial cells (especially spleen and liver). In acute septicemia infections in mice, the liposomal formulation showed enhanced prophylactic activity. In a model of murine salmonellosis, liposomal gentamicin greatly enhanced survival when given as a single dose (10 mg/kg) at 1 or 2 day after infection as well as up to 7 day before infection.

Prolonged survival of liposomes in the circulation is required when these are designed to act on non-MPS tissues, within the vascular system, extravascularly through leaky capillaries or as circulating slow drug release systems. Recent works have shown that coating the liposome surface with PEG and other hydrophilic polymers *(343)*, or chemically modifying the hydrophobic part of phospholipids *(344,345)*, have shown substantial prolongation of half-life of liposomes in blood. These liposomes have a propensity to accumulate in implanted tumors at levels compared to other non-MPS tissues.

9.1.2. Sterically Stabilised Liposomes

Research today is concentrated on liposomes coated with PEG as a means of MPS avoidance. Commonly referred to as sterically stabilised liposomes or LCLs, this new type of liposome is sometimes referred to as a stealth liposome *(151)*. PEG possesses an ideal array of properties for use in liposomes *(152)*. For drug delivery, PEG coated liposomes have several advantages *(135,153)*.

1. Prolonged circulation independent of bilayer physicochemical properties thereby permitting separate control of drug loading/leakage and blood circulation.
2. Plasma pharmacokinetics independent of lipid dose thereby simplifying dose escalation.
3. Compatibility with ligands or other chemical functionalities at the outer surface of PEG coating.
4. Ease of preparation and use without modification of many well known liposome methodologies.
5. Amenable to regulatory requirements of pharmaceutical product.
6. Economy (as compared with use of GM_1).
7. Very low toxicity, low immunogenicity and antigenicity.
8. Excellent solubility in aqueous solutions.
9. Non-biodegradable, yet readily excretable after administration.

10. Excellent pharmacokinetic and biodistribution behaviour.
11. Readily available in a variety of molecular weights.
12. Inertness of polyether backbone in chemical reaction conditions.

MPS uptake and prolongation of circulation times of sterically stabilised liposomes prepared using PEG and other such moieties depend on polymer molecular weight. Decreasing the molecular weight (or chain length) of PEG to less than 750 Da increases clearance from circulation *(155,156,327)*. However, increasing the molecular weight of PEG above 1000 Da did not further increase the survival times of liposomes in circulation. Incorporation of PEG-1000 or PEG-2000 into liposomes resulted in higher blood levels compared with PEG-5000. This effect appeared to be sensitive to liposome concentration with fluid liposomes containing higher molecular weight PEG polymers (5000 or 12000 Da) showing higher blood levels than similar liposomes containing lower molecular weight polymers *(346,347)*. Sterically stabilised liposomes also distribute into MPS tissues but at a slower rate and to a lesser extent than plain liposomes *(127,132,147–149,155,159,348)* There is also increased distribution of these liposomes into tumors *(129,349)* and into areas of infection *(129,135,350)*.

The major route of elimination of liposomes is by the cells of MPS. The clearance of sterically stabilised liposome follows first order elimination (log-linear) kinetics while clearance of plain liposomes follows saturation-type, Michaelis-Menten pharmacokinetics *(348)*. It was proposed that there are two distinct elimination systems. A high affinity, low capacity saturable system likely corresponds to the recognition and binding of liposome by cells of MPS. A low affinity, high capacity system also appears to exist. This system is undoubtedly multifaceted and likely contains components of lipid metabolism, new MPS cell recruitment, binding site turnover and recycling and uptake into other tissues. The elimination of sterically stabilised liposome by this system appears to be slower than the capacity of this system to "turnover". The low affinity, high capacity system may also be saturable but only at very high lipid doses *(348)*. Sterically stabilised liposome ultimately localise in liver and spleen, but at a reduced rate and with decreased total uptake *(129)*.

The blood residence half-life and organ distribution of recombinant human tumor necrosis factor (TNF)-α encapsulated in sterically stabilised liposomes, were investigated by Van Der Veen *et al. (351)* in rats bearing a soft tissue sarcoma in hind leg. The pharmaco-kinetics of TNF-α were markedly altered after encapsulation in liposomes, with a 33-fold increase in mean residence time of TNF-α in blood, and a concomitant 14-fold increase in the area under plasma concentration vs. time curve for liposomal TNF-α. These sterically stabilised liposomes resulted in a marked increase in localisation of cytokine in tumor measured as total uptake over time. However, peak TNF-α concentration levels in tumor were not significantly enhanced compared with free TNF-α. Schettini *et al. (352)* demonstrated significant increase of antimony concentration in bone marrow and delay in antimony elimination following administration of multiple dose regimen of a liposomal formulation of meglumine antimoniate (LMA) in dogs. Treatment with LMA significantly reduced the number of dogs positive for parasites compared to controls.

Although several reports stressed the advantages of sterically stabilized liposomes (SSL) in the delivery of anti-cancer agents, the findings that SSL can reduce acute and chronic toxicities of doxorubicin (DOX) with the possible advantages for efficacy accelerated research on SSL for commercial exploitation. Many methods of loading DOX in SSL were worked out like pH and ion gradient method. The plasma pharmacokinetics of S-DOX was evaluated in several species including rats, dogs and also in humans. All species investigated showed a prolonged circulation, which is essentially insensitive to dose. In humans plasma levels of DOX following i.v. administration of 'Doxil' (Sterically stabilised DOX preparation), show a half-life of 40–60 h *(349,353)*. This amount to, by calculation, about 10% of the injected dose is still in plasma even 1 week after the administration. Interestingly, despite prolonged higher plasma levels, estimates of free DOX in plasma reported are quite low indicating the intactness of SSL and providing slow release of drug. A further reduction in the release rate of drug was reported when fully hydrogenated lipids along with CHOL used to form a rigid bilayer with the encapsulated DOX as a gel inside. The plasma pharmacokinetics of DOXIL® evaluated in 42 patients with acquired immuno-deficiency syndrome (AIDS)-related Kaposi sarcoma (KS) who received single doses of 10 or 20 mg/m^2 administered by a 30-min infusion are presented in Table 7.

DOXIL displayed linear pharmacokinetics over a range of 10–20 mg/m^2. Disposition occurred in two phases after administration, with a relatively short first phase (≈5 h) and a prolonged second phase (≈55 h) that accounted for majority of the area under curve (AUC); While at a 50 mg/m^2 dose, it is reported to be non-linear with longer elimination half-life and lower clearance compared with a 20 mg/m^2 dose. The exposure (AUC) is thus expected to be more than proportional at a 50 mg/m^2 dose when compared with the lower doses.

Table 7. Pharmacokinetic Parameters of DOXIL® in Patients with AIDS-Related Kaposi Sarcoma

Parameter (units)	*Dose (mg/m²)*	
Dose	10	20
Peak plasma concentration (μg/mL)	4.12 ± 0.215	8.34 ± 0.49
Plasma clearance (L/h/m²)	0.056 ± 0.01	0.041 ± 0.004
Steady state volume of distribution (L/m²)	2.83 ± 0.145	2.72 ± 0.120
AUC (μg/mL h)	277 ± 32.9	590 ± 58.7
First phase (λ_1) half-life (h)	4.7 ± 1.1	5.2 ± 1.4
Second phase (λ_1) half-life (h)	52.3 ± 5.6	55.0 ± 4.8

$N = 42$; mean ± standard error

In contrast to pharmacokinetics of doxorubicin, which displays a large volume of distribution, ranging from 700 to 1100 L/m², the small steady state volume of distribution of DOXIL® shows that it is confined mostly to vascular fluid volume. Plasma protein binding of DOXIL® has not been determined; the plasma protein binding of doxorubicin is approximately 70%.

Tissue distribution studies were conducted using KS lesions and normal skin biopsies at 48 and 96 h post-infusion of 20 mg/m² DOXIL® in 11 patients. The concentration of DOXIL® in KS lesions was a median of 19 (range, 3–53) times higher than in normal skin at 48 h post-treatment. Allen and Hansen *(348)* have reported 100-fold increase in concentration in the tissue distribution of two different formulations of stealth liposomes, i.e., sphingomyelin:egg phosphatidylcholine:cholesterol:monosialoganglioside (SM:PC:-CHOL:GM_1) 1:1:1:0.2 and SM:PC:CHOL: PEG distearoylphosphatidylethanolamine (PEG[1990]–DSPE) 1:1:1:0.2, when compared them with the tissue distributions seen for a conventional liposomal formulation (PC:CHOL, 2:1) which is avidly removed from circulation by the cells of MP system.

The biodistribution and pharmacokinetics of ^{111}In-DTPA-labeled PEGylated liposomes in tumor-bearing nude mice was studied by Harrington *et al. (354)* to examine possible applications of PEGylated liposome-targeted anti-cancer therapies. Following an i.v. injection of 100 μL of ^{111}In-DTPA-labeled PEGylated liposomes, containing 0.3$\tilde{7}$ 0.74 MBq of activity, tumor uptake was found maximum at 24 h at 5.5 ± 3.0% ID/g. Significant reticulo-endothelial system uptake was demonstrated with 19.3 ± 2.8 and 18.8 ± 4.2% ID/g at 24 h in the liver and spleen, respectively. Other sites of appreciable deposition were kidney, skin, female reproductive tract and to a lesser extent the GI tract. There was no indication of cumulative deposition of PEGylated liposomes in lung, central nervous system, musculoskeletal system, heart or adrenal glands.

The pharmacokinetics and distribution in tissue of 2′,3′-dideoxyinosine (ddI) encapsulated in sterically stabilised liposomes have been evaluated by Harvie *et al. (355)* in rats. Most of the sterically stabilised liposomes concentrated in spleen with a peak level at 24 h after their i.v. injection. An extended half-life in plasma was observed for sterically stabilised liposomes (14.5 h) compared with that of conventional liposomes (3.9 h). The systemic clearance of ddI incorporated in sterically stabilised liposomes was 180 times lower than that of the free drug.

9.2. Pharmacokinetics of Liposome Following Subcutaneous Administration

The behaviour of preparations given by alternative parenteral routes, such as the intra-peritoneal (i.p.), s.c. or intra-muscular (IM) route, is influenced by distribution of liposome size and their lipid composition and will also depend on route of injection *(356)*. A proportion of liposomes enter the lymphatic system and, eventually, the blood circulation where they behave as if given intravenously. However, whereas liver, spleen and bone marrow take up nearly all liposomes given by i.v. route, they will account for a much smaller proportion if s.c. or IM route is used (Fig. 19). The remainder (up to 80% of liposomes) is retained at the site of injection and attacked by infiltrating macrophages or intercepted in the local lymph nodes.

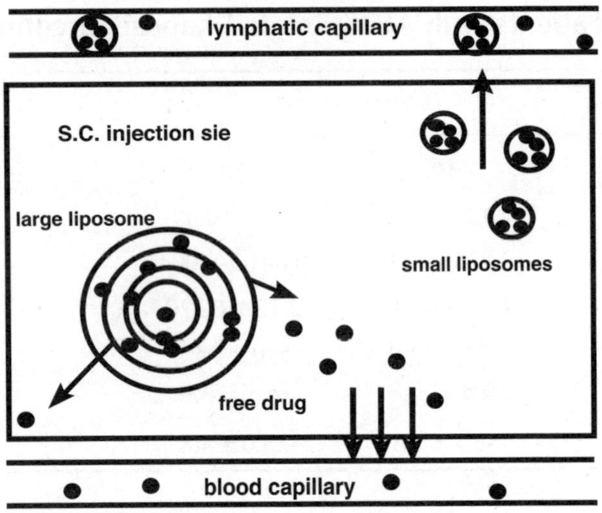

Fig. 19. Distribution of liposomes administered by s.c. route. (Reprinted from Adv. Drug Deliv. Rev. 50, Oussoren, C. and Storm, G. Liposomes to target the lymphatics by subcutaneous Administration, 143–156, 2001, with permission from Elsevier) *(360)*.

After s.c. injection, the sustained mechanism of release from liposomes is not clearly explained, but some theories have been postulated. Researchers speculate that liposomal structure can be destabilised because of various factors, and the drug is absorbed in a free form *(357,358)*. Moreover, Kim and Han *(359)* suggested that liposomes injected by the s.c. route entered into the lymphatics and only drug released from liposomes diffused directly into the systemic circulation. Decisive factors influencing lymphatic absorption and lymph node uptake of s.c. administered liposomes as cited by Oussoren and Storm *(360)* in their review are liposome size and the anatomical site of injection. Generally, other factors such as lipid composition, charge and presence of a hydrophilic PEG-coating on the liposome surface do not substantially affect lymphatic absorption and lymph node uptake of s.c. administered liposomes. Studies on intranodal fate of liposomes demonstrate that phagocytosis by macrophages is most important mechanism for lymph node uptake of liposomes. The observation of relatively high uptake of liposomes in regional lymph nodes after s.c. administration has stimulated research on lymphatic targeting of liposomes for diagnostics and therapeutic applications.

Kadir *et al.* described that once injected; liposomes remain in the structure of tissue, forming a compressed depot from which the drug is released slowly *(361)*. Studies by Yapar and Levent Bas showed that C_{max} of liposome encapsulated ampicillin (LEA) was lower than that of the free ampicillin (FA). After s.c. administration, liposome acted as a local depot, and so showed slower release, lower C_{max} and long-lasting concentrations of active agent in the serum compared with administration of free form. The low C_{max} and serum concentrations after s.c administration of LEA may cause a reduction in dose-dependent side effects of drug *(362,363)*. The study also showed longer $T_1/2\beta$ and mean residence time (MRT) higher V_d and lower clearance of LEA than those of FA. These results suggest that liposome encapsulated drug formulations provide longer effective concentrations in serum.

9.3. Pharmacokinetics of Liposome Following Intra-Tracheal and Pulmonary Administration

Pulmonary route of administration offers several advantages over the conventional GI pathway, including large surface area, extensive vasculature, easily permeable membrane, and low intra- and extra-cellular enzymatic activity *(364)*. Recent clinical and pre-clinical reports reveal that delivery of peptide drugs such as leuprolide acetate and insulin is feasible through pulmonary route *(365)*.

Intra-tracheal administration of tobramycin in liposomes was associated with marked changes in pharmacokinetics of drug in the lung and an apparent trend for a prolonged efficacy against *Bacillus Cepacia*. These results support the hypothesis that inhalation of liposomal tobramycin may improve the management of chronic pulmonary infections caused by resistant bacteria in patients with cystic fibrosis *(366)*.

The pulmonary distribution and clearance of ^{99m}Tc-labeled beclomethasone dipropionate (Bec), DLPC and DPPC liposomes delivered using Aerotech jet nebuliser in 11 healthy volunteers were studied using gamma scintigraphy. Both liposome aerosols had a suitable droplet size (mass median aerodynamic diameter 1.3 μm) and allowed deep pulmonary deposition. Progressive clearance of both ^{99m}Tc-labeled Bec liposomes was seen: 24 h after inhalation, 79% of originally deposited radioactivity of DLPC liposomes and 83% of that of DPPC liposomes remained in lungs indicating that both liposome formulations are suitable for nebulisation, although aerosol clouds were more efficiently made from the DLPC liposome suspension.

The encapsulation of aminoglycosides (gentamicin, amikacin and tobramycin) in liposomes resulted in altered pharmacokinetics and biodisposition as compared with the conventional formulations *(367,368)*. Recently, the intra-tracheal administration of a liposomal formulation of tobramycin in rats decreased its systemic exposure and adverse effects. Although less toxic, the relative efficacy of tobramycin administered as the conventional and liposomal formulations against pulmonary infection of *Pseudomonas aeruginosa* remains to be determined *in vivo (369).*

9.4. Pharmacokinetics of Liposome Following Topical Administration

Verma and Fahr *(370)* studied influence of ethanol mixed with a commercially available lipid mixture, NAT 8539, to improve the topical delivery of cyclosporin A (CyA). The vesicles formed from this solution ranged from 56.6 to 100.6 nm in diameter, depending on the amount of ethanol added in formulation. CyA vesicles containing 10% and 20% ethanol showed statistically enhanced deposition of CyA into the stratum corneum, as compared with vesicles prepared without ethanol. The results showed advantages of topical delivery of problematic molecules like CyA using liposomes as a tool for treatment of inflammatory skin diseases like psoriasis, atopic dermatitis and diseases of hair follicle like alopecia areata, etc.

One of the possibilities for increasing skin absorption or permeation of drugs is the use of nano-/sub-micron vesicular systems. Classic liposomes are of little value as carriers for drug delivery via the skin because they do not deeply penetrate it. Only specially designed liposomes have been shown to be capable of achieving enhanced delivery. The incorporation of some additives such as anionic surfactants and ethanol can fluidise the phospholipid bilayers, thus increasing the depths to which liposomes can penetrate into the intercellular pathways of skin. Hair follicles are also important for the enhancement of transdermal liposomes *(371).*

A positively charged liposomal formulation for topical administration of acyclovir (ACV) was investigated by Chetoni *et al. (372)* in comparison with a commercial ACV ointment, by determining the pharmacokinetic profile of drug in aqueous humour of rabbits after topical administration. ACV liposomal dispersion (LIPO–ACV) produced a significantly higher drug concentration in aqueous humour with respect to three reference formulations containing the same ACV concentration. The aqueous humour ACV concentration maintained by LIPO–ACV during plateau was in upper range of ID (50) s (0.01–0.7 μm/mL) reported for Herpes simplex type 1. *In vitro* release tests through a cellophane membrane substantiated the concept that positively charged liposomal formulations owe their efficacy to interactions with positively charged corneal epithelium.

9.5. Liposome in Imaging

Liposome, specifically stealth liposome, by virtue of its *in vivo* pharmacokinetic behaviour show great potential to be developed as carrier for contrast agents for imaging. Non-invasive *in vivo* assessment of the transport kinetics of carrier-based therapeutics was conducted by Zheng *et al. (373)* using liposome loaded with contrast-enhancing agents such as iodine and gadolinium. The study evaluated the *in vivo* pharmacokinetics, in both mice and rabbits, of a liposome-based computed tomography (CT) and MR contrast agent previously developed by the group. A linear relationship was found between iodine and gadolinium concentrations found in rabbit plasma by HPLC and inductively coupled plasma spectroscopic (ICP) assays and the signal enhancement obtained in rabbit aorta in CT and MR using circular regions of interest over all time points. This pilot study demonstrated the potential of employing CT and MR imaging for longitudinal *in vivo* mapping of contrast agent containing liposomes.

Utility of sterically stabilised liposomes (stealth liposomes) in tumor scintigraphy was investigated by studying its biodistribution and accumulation in target tissue after radiolabeling with Technetium-99m (^{99m}TC) *(374).* Conventional and stealth liposomes containing methotrexate prepared by lipid film hydration method were radiolabeled using reduced ^{99m}Tc. The biodistribution studies carried out in mice bearing Ehrlich ascites tumor after i.v. administration, showed prolonged circulation in blood and significant increase in accumulation in tumor for the sterically stabilised liposomes compared with conventional liposomes.

9.6. Pharmacokinetics of Liposomes and Target Delivery

A novel arginine-glycine-aspartate (RGD) lipopeptide for targeting of liposomes to integrin-expressing endothelial and melanoma cells was developed by Peter Hölig *et al. (375).* A high-affinity peptide (RGD10) constrained by only one disulphide bond was used to generate novel lipopeptides composed of a lipid anchor, a short flexible spacer and peptide ligand conjugated to the spacer end. Incorporation of RGD10 lipopeptides into liposomes resulted in specific and efficient binding of liposomes to integrin-expressing cells. *In vivo* experiments applying doxorubicin-loaded RGD10 liposomes in a C26 colon carcinoma mouse model demonstrated improved efficacy compared with free doxorubicin and untargeted liposomes.

Treatment of cancer through co-administration of anti-cancer drugs and multi-drug resistance (MDR) modulators as a strategy to overcome drug resistance has been extensively explored. However, success has been limited by pharmacokinetic interactions because of non-specific blockade of P-glycoprotein (P-gp) in normal tissues or inability to reach relevant concentrations clinically. Using i.v. administrations, the effects of verapamil (VER) either free (FV) or liposome co-encapsulated with DOX (DARSLs) on the pharmacokinetics and tissue distribution characteristics of DOX either as free (FD) or liposome-encapsulated (LD) were evaluated in normal rats. FV increased ($P < 0.05$) the plasma AUC of free DOX (FD) while LD had significantly prolonged systemic exposure and slow tissue distribution of DOX. Liposomal DOX with free verapamil and DARSLs shared similar DOX pharmacokinetics but the latter showed slower DOX distribution in most tissues studied and slower ($P < 0.05$) DOX biliary transport. The addition of VER into LD in these two preparations significantly increased the AUC ($P < 0.01$) and reduced the clearance ($P < 0.01$) of DOX when compared to LD. Specifically, DARSLs reduced initial DOX distribution to heart ($P < 0.05$) corresponding to initial alleviation ($P < 0.05$) of bradycardia when compared with other DOX with VER preparations. In conclusion, liposomal co-encapsulation of DOX with VER has promise of significant therapeutic advantages, and should be explored further in therapeutic studies with animal tumor xenograft models.

10. CLINICAL APPLICATIONS OF LIPOSOMES

Liposomes are used as carriers for drugs and antigens. The primary reason for this is that they can serve several different purposes (Table 8). Liposomes can direct a drug to a certain target. Liposomes can also prolong duration of drug exposure, acting as a slow-release reservoir. As liposomes can solubilise lipophilic compounds, this solubilising potential can be used to inject poorly water-soluble, lipophilic compounds intravenously. If a fast pharmacological response is desired, then 'fragile' liposomes with 'fluid' bilayers should be selected. Considering this list of applications and the existing literature, it is clear that liposomes provide an extremely flexible drug carrier modality with many potential applications and an impressive track record as a carrier system.

Liposomes are developed as a new drug delivery system when an existing formulation is not satisfactory and reformulation in liposomes offers clear benefits with respect to targetability, therapeutic efficacy and safety compared to existing formulations. Lack of specificity in pharmacologically active agents is an obstacle to their effective use in biological research and medicine. Any approach enabling the drug to reach its target selectively and in a controlled fashion would contribute to the elimination of problems inherent in conventional methods. One such approach was the development of a non-toxic and biodegradable carrier capable of delivering a variety of substances of biological interest directly to the site of action and subsequently allows performing their task. It has been well established that liposomes can meet many of these requirements. Encouraging results of liposomal drugs in the treatment or prevention of a wide spectrum of diseases in experimental animals and in human, indicate that more liposome-based products for clinical and veterinary applications may be forthcoming *(379)*. These could include treatment of skin and eye diseases, anti-microbial and anti-cancer therapy, metal chelation, enzyme and hormone replacement therapy, vaccine and diagnostic imaging, etc. Below, we discuss some of the liposome applications with realistic prospects of being developed for clinical use.

10.1. Targeting with Liposomes

10.1.1. 'Conventional' Liposomes

Liposomes can be used for site-specific delivery of drugs. Figure 20 depicts schematically the four basic types of liposome 'surface make-up' (non-surface-modified). Liposomes either disintegrate in the bloodstream ('fluid state' liposomes) or they circulate and are picked up predominantly by macrophages (Kupffer cells) in liver and also in spleen. The rate and extent of their uptake depends on bilayer rigidity, liposome size and dose (small liposomes with rigid bilayers tend to circulate for a number of hours). This predominant uptake by macrophages has been used to deliver anti-microbial agents effectively to these macrophages when they are infected with intra-cellular pathogens. Dramatic improvements in therapeutic potential have been reported *(151,380)*. Another therapeutic goal that has been identified is the possibility of delivering immuno-modulating agents (e.g., muramyl dipeptide or tripeptide) to enhance the anti-tumor and anti-viral activity of macrophages.

Table 8. Reasons to Use Liposomes as Drug Carriers

Purpose	*Strategy*	*Examples*	*References*
Protection	Liposome-encapsulated drugs are inaccessible to metabolising enzymes; conversely, body components are not directly exposed to the full dose of drug	Erythrocytes or tissues at the injection site. Reduction of haemolytic effects of drugs by liposome encapsulation and the protection against local irritation on intra-dermal, s.c. or IM injection of a tissue-irritating drug	*376*
Solubilisation	Liposomes may solubilise lipophilic drugs that would otherwise be difficult to administer intravenously	–	–
Duration of action	Liposomes can prolong drug action by slowly releasing the drug in body	Anti-malarial drug chloroquine or the radical scavenger superoxide dismutase	*377*
Directing potential	Targeting options change the distribution of drug through the body	Dose limitation of cytotoxic drug doxorubicin is its (irreversible) damage to heart muscles and it's encapsulation in liposome greatly reduces drug exposure to the heart and thereby its cardiotoxicity	–
Internalisation	Liposomes are endocytosed or phagocytosed by cells, opening up opportunities to use 'liposome-dependent drugs'	Lipid-based structures (not necessarily liposomes) are also able to bring plasmid material into cell through same mechanism	–
Amplification	Liposomes can be used as adjuvants in vaccine formulations	–	–

10.1.2. 'Stealth' Liposomes

Coating liposomes with PEG reduces the rate of uptake by macrophages ('stealth' effect) and leads to a prolonged presence of liposomes in circulation and consequently ample time for these liposomes to escape from circulation through a leaky endothelium. This stealth principle has been used to develop the successful doxorubicin-loaded liposome product that is currently marketed as Doxil® or Caelyx® for treatment of solid tumors. Recently, impressive therapeutic improvements were described by using corticosteroid-loaded liposomes in experimental arthritic models. By far the most attention regarding the application of LCLs has been on their potential to escape from blood circulation. However, these LCLs may also act as a reservoir for prolonged release of a therapeutic agent. Woodle *et al.* reported on a remarkably long pharmacological action of vasopressin when formulated in LCLs *(150)*.

10.1.3. pH-Sensitive Liposomes

There are many potential applications for pH-sensitive liposomes in treating human diseases. One of the primary uses of pH-sensitive liposomes is in avoiding degradation in lysosomes following internalisation and in increasing access to cytosolic or nuclear targets. DNA, oligonucleotides, and some drugs, such as ara-C, are labile under the conditions found in lysosomes and are also highly water-soluble and thus less permeable to biological membranes. These types of therapeutics are ideal for a triggerable release system such as the pH-sensitive liposomes.

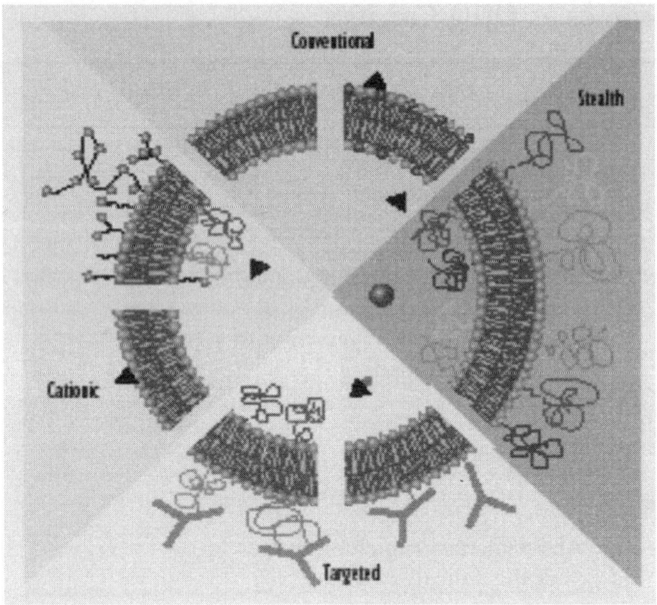

Fig. 20. Schematic diagram showing four basic types of liposome. (Reprinted from Pharmaceutical Science & Technology Today, 1, Storm, G. and Crommelin, DJA. Liposomes quo vadis, 19–31, 1998, with permission from Elsevier) *(378)*.

The usefulness of pH-sensitive liposomes has been well exhibited in a wide variety of applications. These include: (1) the transport of fluorescent probes to estimate the efficacy of different liposome compositions and also to explain the mechanisms involved in intra-cellular trafficking, (2) the effective delivery of neoplastic drugs or recombinant proteins, (3) the intra-cellular transport of antigens, targeting at intra-cellular pathways involved in processing and presentation of antigens and enhancing the immune response to tumor cells and (4) the intra-cellular transport of genetic material for application in gene and antisense therapies. A large extent of work has been dedicated to improve therapeutic efficacy of drugs entrapped in pH-sensitive liposomes, to confer tissue and cell specificity by directing the liposomes to cell surface receptors. Different ligands have been coupled covalently to liposome surface or to distal end of PEG–lipid conjugates for this purpose. These ligands comprise monoclonal antibodies against the H-2K^k receptor (expressed in several types of tumor cells) *(381)*, E-selectin (on activated vascular endothelial cells) *(382)*, CD-19 (on B-lymphoma cells) *(383)*, CD3 (on T-leukaemia cells) *(384)*, P-glycoproteins (on endothelial cells) *(385)* and BCG antigen *(288)*. The folate receptor targeted pH-sensitive liposomes via coupling of folic acid to distal end of PEG molecules have been recently used to deliver neoplastic drugs like methotrexate, doxorubicin *(386)*, ara-C *(290,291)* for cancer therapy and plasmid DNA *(290,387,388)*. pH-sensitive liposomes have been revealed to be less effective than cationic liposomes to mediate intra-cellular gene delivery into mammalian cells under the same experimental conditions *(389)*. Different methods have been developed recently, to avoid the limitations of pH-sensitive liposomes for nucleic acid delivery. These approaches share an identical strategy that basically consists of, complexing preformed pH-sensitive liposomes with plasmid DNA pre-condensed with a cationic polymer *(289,290,384,386,390)*. These strategies were further optimised by promoting nuclear entry of DNA, which was achieved by incorporation of a nuclear targeting sequence into plasmid DNA *(390)*. The approach of intra-cellular delivery of antisense oligonucleotides and ribozymes to inhibit virus production in HIV-infected macrophages derived from human peripheral blood monocytes has been assessed *(391,392)*. As these liposomes circulate for prolonged periods and can localise in lymph nodes after i.v. or s.c. injection *(393)*, they may be useful for the delivery of antisense molecules to lymph nodes where active HIV replication takes place *(394,395)*. As reported earlier, other fusogenic liposome formulations exhibiting long circulation times have also been utilised for nucleic acid delivery. Programmable fusogenic vesicles (PFV), formerly revealed for delivery of mitoxantrone (LEM), are liposomes composed of DOPE, CHOL, DODAC and an exchangeable PEG–ceramide conjugate. PFV have also been assessed as carriers for the intra-cellular delivery of antisense oligonucleotides.

10.1.4. Liposomes With 'Homing' Devices

An important consideration is how to make liposome uptake tissue or cell-specific. Figure 20 shows liposomes with antibodies attached covalently to the surface of the liposomes. Most work on liposome targeting has focused on antibodies or antibody fragments attached to the surface but other homing devices have been considered as well *(396)*. For example, plasminogen-coated liposomes were designed to reach fibrin clots specifically (plasminogen has an affinity for fibrin) in order to deliver fibrinolytics. More recently, reports have appeared on arginine-glycine-aspartic acid (RGD) peptide-driven targeting of liposomes to endothelial cells in order to block angiogenesis *(397)*. Saccharide-directed targeting has also been described, for example, use of saccharide antennae (including galactose) to direct liposomes to hepatocytes. Targeted liposomes should have ready access to the target site and should not be taken up by macrophages before encountering their target tissue or cells. Therefore, nowadays, stealth technology is often combined with attachment of a homing device to the terminal end of PEG chain that is exposed to aqueous medium. Specific attachment of targeted liposomes to their target has been successful; however, hard and convincing experimental data on therapeutic advantages is scarce.

10.1.5. Strategies of Liposome Drug Targeting

There has been investigation into how liposome targeting can lead to tissue-specific therapeutic effects. Upon interaction with the target cell, a number of approaches have been proposed and some of these have proven to offer therapeutic advantages in animal models. The more successful approaches so far are discussed as follows.

10.1.5.1. Strategy One

The immunoliposomes interact with a cell surface receptor that is endocytosed, leading to immunoliposome internalisation upon immunoliposome–cell interaction. For successful action of liposome-associated drug, escape from the endosome is often required as many drugs are inactivated when endosome matures from the endosomal state into a lysosome. For endosomal escape, fusogenic peptides (often derived from viruses such as influenza virus) have been proposed, or, alternatively, pH-dependent liposomes are used that destabilise endosomal membrane when the pH level drops.

10.1.5.2. Strategy Two

An effective strategy developed by Koning and co-workers is based on the selective binding of immunoliposomes that contain a lipophilic prodrug *(398)*. This prodrug is transferred selectively from the cell bound immunoliposomes into target cell. Subsequently, the prodrug is converted in lysosome into active drug. From lysosome, it leaks into the cytoplasm and maybe even to the outside of cell, causing a so-called ‘bystander effect’.

10.1.5.3. Strategy Three

In antibody-dependent enzyme prodrug therapy, a prodrug is converted only at sites where its converting enzyme is delivered. Site-specific delivery of enzyme is performed by using a site-specific antibody. To make target site enzyme delivery more efficient, enzymes can be attached to immunoliposomes. Now, many enzyme molecules can be delivered to target site on one targeted immunoliposome.

10.1.6. Cancer Therapy

Cytotoxic drugs could cause death of normal as well as malignant cells due to non-specific distribution of drug throughout body, thereby giving rise to a variety of toxic side effects. Entrapment of these drugs into liposomes resulted in altered tissue distribution of drug, with its enhanced uptake in organs rich in mononuclear phagocytic cells (liver, spleen and bone marrow) and decreased uptake in kidney, myocardium and brain. When coated with hydrophobic agents, they also increased circulation lifetime, thus enhancing drug deposition in infected tissues and tumors. Encapsulation in liposomes also offered protection for drugs from the drug metabolic degradation. Various studies have demonstrated accumulation of liposomes in certain tumors in a higher concentration than found in normal tissues *(399,400)*. One or more of the following factors may account for this:

1. Higher endocytic activity of some tumor cells combined with augmented local permeability of capillaries allowing the passage of small liposomes, a phenomenon also described as “enhanced permeability and retention effect”, which can facilitate liposome uptake.
2. Diffusion of drugs from liposomes either during circulation or after they have been lodged in tissues adjacent to tumors, followed by preferential drug entry into tumor mass.
3. Liposomes may be phagocytosed by circulation monocytes, which subsequently migrate to tumors.
4. Sustained release effect of liposomes may enhance the drugs cytotoxic effect. Passive targeting of LCLs to tumor tissues may be useful for delivering cancer chemotherapeutic agents to the target tumors, since there is a positive correlation between the circulation time of liposomes and their localisation in tumors.

Many research efforts have been directed towards improving the safety profile of anthracycline cytotoxics, doxorubicin (DOX) and daunorubicin (DNR), along with vincristine (VCR), which are associated with severe cardiotoxic side effects, although acute GI effects and other toxicities may also occur. Liposomal entrapment of these drugs showed reduced cardiotoxicity, dermal toxicity and better survival of experimental animals compared with the controls receiving free drugs *(399)*. Such beneficial effects of liposomal anthracyclines have been observed with a variety of liposomal formulations regardless of their lipid composition provided that lipids used high CHOL concentration or phospholipids with high phase transition temperature (T_c) are conducive to drug retention by the vesicles in systemic circulation *(401)*.

DOX is a potent antineoplastic agent active against a wide range of human cancer including lymphomas, leukaemia and solid tumors. However, administration of this drug produces acute toxicity in the form of bone marrow depression, alopecia and oral ulceration *(402–404)*. DOX entrapped in stealth liposomes shows reduced non-specific toxicity and maintains or enhances anti-cancer effect. DOX hydrochloride constitutes first liposomal product (Doxil™) licensed in the United States. The lipid matrix and an internal buffer system combine to keep virtually all the DOX encapsulated in liposome during circulation with no free drug thus reducing toxic effects *(68,405)*. Decreased toxic effects of DOX allow administration in a dose higher than the *LD*50 without acute toxicity. Liposomes extravasate from endothelium of tumor tissues and reside around tumor cells where they release the drug into interstitial fluid. Therapeutic effect was therefore, achieved by a slow and sustained release of drug at target site. Encapsulation of DOX in stealth liposomes showed significant accumulation, enhanced therapeutic efficacy and reduced toxic effect against human pancreatic carcinoma AsPC-implanted into nude Swiss mice compared to DOX suspension. Increased penetration and a long presence with a slow drug release from liposomes in tumor account for the enhanced therapeutic effects *(406)*.

A new liposome formulation containing DOX developed *(324,407)*, in combination with mild hyperthermia, was found to be significantly more effective than free drug or current liposome formulations for reducing tumor growth in a human squamous cell carcinoma xenograft line. Similarly, Ishida *et al. (383)* developed pH-sensitive liposomes, targeted at the CD19 epitope on B-lymphoma cells, which showed enhanced DOX delivery into nuclei of the target cells and increased cytotoxicity compared to non-pH-sensitive liposomes. Moreover, a unique liposomal formulation of DOX (TLC D-99) recently developed was found active against AIDS related KS and resulted in improved safety and efficacy profile, and the response is dose-dependent *(408)*.

Ten Hagen and co-workers *(409)* reported that systemic administration of low-dose TNF-α augments the anti-tumor activity of a liposomal formulation of DOX. In addition, a significant increase of liposomal drug in tumor tissue was observed when TNF-α was co-administered. The anti-tumor effects against solid tumors, such as Meth A sarcoma, MH-134 hepatoma and colon 26 adenocarcinoma, were examined after intra-tumoral administration of liposomes and TNF solution. The anti-tumor effects of liposomes against solid tumors were superior to those of TNF solution. In particular, the anti-tumor effect of positively charged liposomes was superior to that of negatively charged liposomes and TNF solution. Further, positively charged liposomes containing a higher dose of TNF could be administered without killing the mice because of reduced side effects *(410)*.

10.1.7. Immunoliposomes

Liposomal anti-cancer drugs via specific ligands against antigens expressed on malignant cells could specifically target and improve the therapeutic effectiveness as well as reduce adverse side effects associated with chemotherapy. Immunoliposomes conjugated with S5A8 monoclonal antibody, an anti-idiotype antibody to 38C13 murine B-cell lymphoma, when loaded with DOX exhibited a long circulation time and showed more effectiveness for prolonging the survival of mice bearing 38C13 tumor than non-targeted liposomal DOX or free DOX plus empty immunoliposomes *(411)*. Lopes de Menezes *et al. (412)* reported that targeted monoclonal antibody, anti-CD19, liposomes containing DOX may be selectively cytotoxic to malignant B cells expressing CD19 surface antigens, compared with DOX entrapped in non-targeted stealth liposomes/free DOX, and may be useful for selective elimination of circulating malignant B cells *in vivo*. Neuroblastoma (NB) tumor over-expresses the disialoganglioside (GD) at cell surface, but not normal tissues (2). Anti-GD (2) whole antibodies aGD (2) or their corresponding Fab fragments were covalently coupled to stealth immunoliposomes (aGD [2]-SIL or Fab'-SIL) containing DOX and showed higher cytotoxicities than untargeted liposomes. Fab'-SIL encapsulated DOX formulations led to total inhibition of metastatic growth of human NB in a nude mouse metastatic model *(413)*. Furthermore, long-term survivors were obtained when treated with Fab'-SIL encapsulated DOX but not among untreated mice and those treated with free anti-GD (2) Fab' fragments or free-DOX. Fab'-SIL containing DOX also prevented the establishment and metastatic growth of tumor cells in different organs *(414)*.

DOX also plays an important role in treatment of breast cancer, both in the adjuvant and metastatic settings. However, the benefits of conventional DOX in terms of anti-tumor activity are limited by its therapeutic index. PEGylated liposomal DOX provides tumor-targeted efficacy without many of the toxicities associated with conventional DOX, including myelosuppression, alopecia, nausea and vomiting and most importantly, cardiac toxicity. It has also demonstrated efficacy in combination with other agents or modalities, including cyclophosphamide, paclitaxel, docetaxel, gemcitabine, vinorelbine and hyperthermia. Examples of anti-cancer liposomal formulation along with their efficacy is given in Table 9.

Table 9. Efficacy Study of Some Anti-Tumor Agents Encapsulated in Liposomes

Drug	*Formulation*	*Activity*	*References*
Doxorubicin (DOX)	PEGylated liposome	Treatment of breast cancer due to higher efficacy and favourable safety profile	–
Hexadecyl phosphocholine	Sterically stabilised liposomes	Improved anti-tumor activity in breast carcinoma in nude mice compared with conventional hexadecyl phosphocholine liposomes or free hexadecyl phosphocholine	*415*
Cisplatin	LCLs	Prolonged circulation time and enhanced tumor uptake in different mouse tumor models	–
Daunorubicin (DNR)	Liposomes	Significantly increased clinical efficacy in treatment of advanced cutaneous T-cell lymphoma	*416*
DNR and carboplatin with etoposide	Liposomes	Used to treat children with recurrent high-grade glioma after surgery and with progressive teratoid/rhabdoid tumor. Showed encouraging results with only little and transient hematological toxicity	*417*
Vincristine (VCR)	Liposomes	VCR entrapped in liposomal gel showed superior anti-tumor activity compared to conventional VCR against human small cell lung carcinoma LXFS 650 and human mammary carcinoma MX1	*418*
ADR	Magnetic liposomes	Effectively deliver ADR to osteosarcoma, Os515, implanted with a magnet, as well as to the lungs, a common site of osteosarcoma metastases	*419,420*
Melphalan	Thermo-sensitive SUVs	*In vivo* efficacy of liposome-encapsulated melphalan in combination with hyperthermia was higher than that of an equivalent concentration of free melphalan with or without heating	*421*
Sarcolysine	Liposomes attached with a saccharide (lectin) vector	Increased level of vectored liposome binding to malignant cells by 50–80% as compared to liposomes without vector	*422*
Mannobiose mono arachidic acid esters	Modified liposomes	Modification did not affect the distribution of liposomes to kidney, lungs, or thymus, it increased the distribution to liver and spleen	–
Mannobiose mono fatty acid esters	Liposomes	Targeting of liposomes on Kupffer's and other macrophages	–
LEM	Liposome	Significantly decreased toxicity, which showed altered pharmacokinetics and enhanced efficacy	*424*

Continued

Dipalmitoyl derivative of 5-fluoro-2'-deoxyuridine	Liposomes	The parent drug was released intracellularly and showed a much stronger inhibition of CC531 cell growth *in vitro* than in non-targeted liposomes	*398*
Etoposide	Liposomes	Delayed tumor growth, increase in maximum tolerated dose and lesser degree of myelo-suppression than the animals treated with non-liposomal etoposid	*425*
Etoposide	pH-sensitive liposomes	Showed excellent stability at pH 7.4 and underwent rapid destabilisation upon acidification	–
Cytosine-β-D-arabinofu-ranoside (Ara c)	pH-sensitive liposomes	Folate receptor (FR) expression was amplified in many types of human tumors. Shown to mediate the internalisation of folate-derivatised liposomes into an acidic intra-cellular compartment	*291*
Ara C	FR-targeted oleyl alcohol-based pH-sensitive liposomes	Showed 17-times higher FR-dependent cytotoxicity in cancer cells compared to Ara c delivered via FR-targeted non-pH-sensitive liposomes	*291*
Boron CHOL-carborane conjugate	Liposomes	Delivered sufficient levels of boron to 9L rat glioma cells *in vitro*. Liposomes containing high levels of exogenous natural ceramide lipid in bilayer showed anti-tumor activity *in vivo* against the J774 ascites tumor model	*426,427*
All-*trans*-retinoic acid (ATRA)	Liposomes (L-ATRA)	L-ATRA showed a favourable pharmaco-kinetic profile for effective treatment of acute promyelocytic leukaemia or other retinoid-responsive cancers	*428*
c-myb antisense oligodeoxynucleotides	Immunoliposomes	Enhanced toxicity towards targeted cells while shielding non-targeted cells from antisense effects. May be efficacious for delivery of drugs with broad therapeutic applications to tumor cells	*429*
Anti-CD19	Charge neutralised - liposome antisense oligodeoxynucleotides (asODN)	Effective in delivering an asODN to a multi-drug-resistant human B-lymphoma cell line *in vitro*, decreasing the activity of P-glycoprotein. No such activity was observed for non-targeted liposomes and free asODN	*430,431*
Teniposide and paclitaxel	octadecyl phosphor-choline and ET-18-OCH_3 liposomes	Enhanced *in vitro* cytotoxic activity against leukaemic cells was found	–

Photodynamic therapy (PDT) as a cancer treatment is notable for its quite low side effects in comparison with those of chemotherapy and radiotherapy. However, the accumulation of porphyrin derivatives used in PDT in tumor tissues is rather low. Therefore, the benzoporphyrin derivative monoacid ring A (BPD-MA) was encapsulated in LCLs to enhance targeting to tumors. Tumor regression in mice bearing Meth A sarcoma and complete tumor curing were observed when these liposomes were injected and laser-irradiated, as compared to BPD-MA solution or BPD-MA entrapped in conventional liposomes. These results suggest that a LCLs formulation of photo-sensitive agents is useful for PDT *(432)*. Some commercial liposomal anti-tumor products currently undergoing clinical trials are compiled in Table 10.

Table 10. Some Commercial Liposomal Anti-Tumor Products in Clinical Trials

Cancer type	*Company*	*Therapeutic agent*	*Study phase*
Breast	NeoPharma/Pharmacia	Doxorubicin	III
Breast	Liposome company	Doxorubicin	III
Breast	NeoPharma/Pharmacia	Paclitaxel	II/III
Leukaemia (AML)	Aronex Pharmaceuticals/ Abbott laboratories	Nystatin	II
Lung	Aronex pharmaceuticals	Platinum	II
Lung (NSCLC)	Biomira	Vaccine (BLP 25)	IIb
Lung (SCLC)	OSI pharmaceuticals	Topisomerase inhibitor	II
Lymphoma (NHL)	Antigenic Inc	ATRA	II
Lynphoma (NHL)	NeXstar	Daunorubicin	II
Relapsed NHL	Inex Pharmaceuticals	Vincristin	III
Ovarian	Gilead Sciences	Topisomerase inhibitor	II
Prostrate	NeoPharma/Pharmacia	Doxorubicin	III
Skin	AGI Dermatics	Endonuclease V (T4N5)	Applied

AML, acute myeloid leukaemia; BLP 25, commercial name for liposomal vaccine by Biomira Inc, UK; NSCLC, non-small cell lung cancer; NHL, non-Hodgkins lymphomas; SCLC, small cell lung cancer.

10.1.8. Anti-Microbial Therapy

It is a well-known fact that liposomes are able to localise in liver and spleen, specially the RES component, where many pathogenic microorganisms reside; they can be therefore used for targeting of antibiotics on these organs. Treatment of mycobacterial infections differs from that of other bacterial diseases because of complex lipid-rich cell protective envelope possessed by the mycobacteria. In addition, mycobacteria are facultative intra-cellular parasites, which generally cause a more chronic type of disease. To be effective, anti-mycobacterial drugs must be able to penetrate the host macrophage, infected intra-cellular sites. They should have reduced toxicity and be effective at low doses to allow prolonged therapy *(399,433)*.

Some important reports on the efficacy of liposomal anti-tubercular drugs is summarised in Table 11.

The current treatment of AIDS patients infected with *M. avium* complex (MAC) micro-organisms is ineffective, probably because the organism resides intracellularly, mostly in monocytes. Liposomal encapsulation of aminoglycosides increases the therapeutic index of this class of antibiotics by increasing aminoglycosides concentration at the site of infection and/or by reducing the toxicity of these drugs *(380)*. Effective treatment of MAC in mice was achieved with liposomal amikacin due to delayed clearance of drug in liposomes (MiKasome^{TM}) thus prolonging plasma and tissue residence and *in vivo* activity against extra-cellular infections, including *Klebsiella pneumoniae* and *P endocarditis (445,446)*. Similarly, encouraging results were previously obtained with liposomal ampicillin in treatment of *L. monocytogenes (350)*, liposomal cefalothin against *Salmonella typhimurium (447)*, liposomal benzyl penicillin in *Staphylococcus aureus* infection in mice *(448)* and with liposomal dihydrostreptomycin against intra-cellular *S. aureus (449)*.

Another group of microbial diseases, severe disseminated fungal infections, has benefited substantially from the use of liposomes as drug delivery system. Polyene antibiotics such as amphotericin B (AmB) and nystatin are useful in systemic fungal infections such as candidosis and aspergillosis. AmB selectivity of action is due to its higher affinity for the

Table 11. Efficacy of Anti-Tubercular Drug Encapsulated Liposomes

Drug	*Preparation*	*Efficacy study*	*References*
Gentamicin	Liposome	Alters tissue distribution of gentamicin when given by IV to rabbits; however, IM administration resulted in sustained release providing prolonged plasma concentrations of drug	*434,435*
Gentamicin	TLC G-65 (liposomal gentamicin preparation)	Showed higher activity alone and in combination of rifapentine when evaluated in the beige mouse model of disseminated *Mycobacterium avium* infection.	*436*
Rifabutin	Liposomes	Resulted in a significant enhancement of activity against *M. avium* infection compared to free rifabutin	*437*
Rifampin	Liposomes and tustin grafted liposome	The anti-tubercular activity was increased. A further increase in activity was observed when the macrophage activator tetrapeptide tuftsin was grafted on the surface of drug-loaded liposomes	*438*
Clarithromycin	Liposome	More effective than free form against *M. avium* intra-cellular infections *in-vivo*, and the use of a combination therapy with ethambutol could further enhance the efficacy	*439*
Clarithromycin + Gentamicin	Clarithromycin + TLC G-65 (liposome)	The activity of clarithromycin in combination with TLC G-65 was similar to that of either agent alone	*435*
Clofazimine + Gentamicin	Clofazimine + TLC G-65 liposome	Improved activity of TLC G-65 with respect to spleen, while ethambutol improved the activity with respect to liver	*436*
Ciprofloxacin	Liposome	Increases the circulation half-life of drug when given by IV in mice, due to enhanced delivery of drug to the liver, spleen, kidneys and lungs	*440*
Streptomycin and chloramphenicol	Liposome	Showed enhanced activity against *Escherichia coli* in the cells of J774 murine macrophage	*441*
Streptomycin sulphate	Liposome	Demonstrated a higher accumulation in liver and spleen than free drug. Furthermore, streptomycin liposomes, when administered in two IV injections, caused greater reduction of colony forming unit in spleen, lungs and liver, than free drug given in a much higher dose by IM route	*442,443*
Ciprofloxacin or azithromycin	Liposome	Showed increased cellular delivery of these antibiotics and efficiency of intra-cellular targeting was sufficient to mediate enhanced anti-mycobacterial effects	*444*

ergosterol of fungal membranes, although it binds with CHOL as well *(450)*. The conventional amphotericin B (CAB) therapy, fungizone, a mixed colloidal dispersion of AmB with deoxycholate as surfactant, is associated with toxicity problems *(451)*. The most serious adverse effect of CAB therapy is nephrotoxicity, although clinical efficacy is also limited by a high incidence of haematological adverse effects *(452)*. Data from both animal and human studies clearly indicate significant reduction in both renal and haematological toxicity with liposomal formulations of AmB in comparison to CAB *(453,454)*. Among the three lipid-based formulations of AmB commercially introduced; (1) lipid-based AmB preparations, AmB lipid complex (Abelcet®), (2) AmB colloidal dispersion (Amphotec® or Amphocil®) and (3) liposomal AmB (AmBisome®), AmBisome® is effective in treating both intra-cellular (leishmaniasis and histoplasmosis) and extra-cellular (candidosis and aspergillosis) systemic infections. Because of its low toxicity at the organ level, i.v. AmBisome® can be safely delivered in a markedly high dose for the treatment of systemic fungal infections. AmBisome® appears to localise at sites of infection in brain (cryptococcosis, aspergillosis and coccidioidomycosis), lungs (blastomycosis, paracoccidioidomycosis and aspergillosis) and kidneys (candidosis) in animal models, delivering AmB, which remains bioavailable in tissues for several weeks following treatment *(455)*. A large number of clinical trials have confirmed the effectiveness of AmBisome® in majority of patients with invasive or superficial fungal infections *(456–458)*, in patients with moderate-to-severe histoplasmosis associated with AIDS.

The improved anti-fungal therapy with liposomal AmB resulted in incorporation of nystatin into liposomes *(459–461)*. Furthermore, lipid-based formulations of hamycin, miconazole and ketoconazole have been developed *(462)*. Besides their anti-fungal use, liposomal polyene antibiotics are expected to disrupt HIV because the lipid envelope of HIV has a higher CHOL concentration than most normal human cells *(463)*. *In vitro* screening indicated that liposomal nystatin is effective to suppress the expression of HIV at concentrations that are not toxic to uninfected cells *(464)*.

Using the mannosyl-fucosyl receptors on macrophages, mannosylated liposomes loaded with an indigenous drug, andrographolide, were made to target this anti-leishmanial drug to treat experimental leishmaniasis in the hamster model. These liposomes were found to be most potent in reducing the parasitic burden in the spleen as well as in reducing hepatic and renal toxicity *(465)*.

Similarly, liposomes encapsulated with an antimonial drug, meglumine antimoniate, showed significant reduction in liver parasite burdens in animals treated with these liposomes compared to control animals treated with free meglumine antimoniate in hamsters experimentally infected with *Leishmania chagasi*. A. This novel liposome-based meglumine antimoniate formulation appears to be promising as a pharmaceutical product for the treatment of visceral leishmaniasis *(336)*.

10.1.9. Gene Therapy

A number of systemic diseases are caused by lack of enzymes, factors due to missing or defective genes. Gene delivery systems are designed to control the location of administered therapeutic genes within the patient's body. Successful *in vivo* gene transfer may require: (1) condensation of plasmid and its protection from nuclease degradation, (2) cellular interaction and internalisation of condensed plasmid, (3) escape of plasmid from endosomes (if endocytosis is involved) and (4) plasmid entry into cell nuclei *(466)*. Gene therapy methods involve introduction of genetic material into patient's cells to synthesise therapeutic protein.

Administration of genes to patients may be virally or non-virally mediated. As viruses represent a highly suitable vector for gene transfer, several viruses including retrovirus, adenovirus, adeno-associated-virus and herpes virus have been investigated for their potentials in gene delivery. However, there is always potential risk that the viruses would become replication competent and therefore infectious, immune and may also cause inflammation. The drawbacks associated with use of viral vectors, particularly, those related to safety problems, have prompted investigators to develop alternative methods of gene delivery. Out of many approaches, cationic lipid-based systems (cationic liposomes, plasmid–liposome complex, etc.) has been extensively investigated due to many advantages they have over viral based vectors *(467)*. They are: (1) these complexes are relatively non-immunogenic because they lack proteins, (2) liposomes or lipid complexes can be used for transfection of large-sized genetic material and (3) viruses, unlike plasmid liposome complexes, may replicate and cause infection.

Cationic liposomes are usually composed of cationic lipid derivatives and a neutral phospholipid such as DOPE *(468)*. Widely accepted cationic liposome formulations are lipofectin, lipofectamine, transfectace, transfectam and DC–CHOL 3BN-(*N,N*-dimethylaminoethane) carbamoyl–CHOL. Cationic liposomes based on DOTMA, such as lipofectin, and several other types have demonstrated success both in *in vitro* and *in vivo* gene delivery *(469,470)*.

The negatively charged genetic material, for example, plasmid, is generally complexed with cationic lipids by electrostatic interactions. Plasmid liposome complexes are thought to enter the cells through fusion with plasma or endosome membrane *(471)*. These liposomes were found more effective in transfecting genes than micelles of same lipid composition, thus suggesting a role for bilayer structure in facilitating transfection. In addition, the transfection efficiency of liposome-delivered genes was highly dependent upon the lipid composition, lipid/DNA ratio, particle size of liposome–DNA complex and cell lines used *(472)*.

Targeting potentials of DNA–liposome complexes are extensively studied. Different ratios of DNA phosphate to polyethylenimine amine were used to encapsulate and deliver chloramphenicol acetyl transferase to liver cells. Luciferase expression plasmids are encapsulated in cationic, neutral and anionic liposomes with galatocerebroside amount fraction of 8% for targeting on the hepatocyte asialoglycoprotein receptor. All liposome formulations demonstrated increased transfection efficiency and significantly lower toxicity compared with non-encapsulated polyethylenimine complexes and thus these formulations represent feasible systems for optimising *in vivo* delivery systems to hepatocytes *(473)*. Liposomes composed of DPPC, soybean-derived sterylglucoside mixture (SG) and CHOL, showed greater accumulation in hepatocytes than in non-parenchymal cells after i.v. injection *(474)*. Kawaura and co-workers *(475)* studied the effect of GM_1 containing cationic liposomes with cationic CHOL on liposome mediated gene transfection into mammalian culture cells. They found that both cationic liposomes with either a cationic CHOL derivative of a hydrophobic amino head group (I) and a hydrophilic amino head group (II) promoted the transfection of luciferase plasmids (pGL3) into HeLa and CHO-K1 cells more than the control cationic liposomes without GM_1.

Liposomes consisting of *O,O′*-ditetradecanoyl-*N*-(α-trimethyl ammonioacetyl) diethanolamine chloride (DC-6-14) as a cationic lipid, phospholipid and CHOL showed effective gene transfection activity in cultured cells. Surface charge on DC-6-14 liposome–DNA complexes were found dependent on the ratio of DNA to liposomes and ζ-potential of complexes. Surface charge of these liposomes determine their biodistribution pattern, i.e., positively charged complexes showed immediate lung accumulation whereas negatively charged complexes did not show such accumulation. *(476)*. Transfer of interferon β gene via cationic liposomes has been found to induce regression of malignant glioma suggesting the feasibility and safety of interferon β gene therapy, which may become an important treatment option for patients with malignant glioma *(477)*. Transfection efficiency of ultra-deformable cationic liposome/DNA complexes and their retention time within the organs was studied by Kim and co-workers *(478)* by applying formulation onto hair-removed dorsal skin of mice. The study demonstrated that genes were transported into several organs for 6 days when applied once onto intact skin.

The main problem of cationic liposomes seems to be a lack of organ or cell selectivity. Therefore, application of cell-specific targeting technology to cationic liposomes would improve *in vivo* gene delivery and reduce unexpected side effects. Both liver parenchymal and non-parenchymal cells exclusively express large numbers of high-affinity asialoglycoprotein and mannose receptors, respectively. Receptor mediated gene delivery systems are able to introduce foreign DNA into specific cell types *in vivo (479)*.

The transfection efficiency of transferrin conjugated cationic (Tf-DDAB) liposomes was found to be much higher than that of unconjugated cationic liposomes. Target-oriented Tf-DDAB liposomes were proven to be very efficient in DNA delivery into cervical cancer cells in culture *(480)*.

The presence of blood-brain barrier (BBB) hinders gene therapy of brain. Shi and Pardridge *(481)* reported that i.v. administration of a 6- to 7-kb expression plasmid encoding either luciferase or β-galactosidase in neutral PEGylated immunoliposomes expressed an exogenous gene in brain. Such liposomes are conjugated with the OX26 mAb *(481)* peptidomimetic mAb *(482)* to the rat transferrin receptor, which enables targeting of the plasmid DNA on brain via endogenous BBB transferrin receptor. These studies indicate that tissue-specific gene expression in brain is possible after i.v. administration of a non-viral vector with combined use of gene targeting technology and tissue-specific gene promoters *(482)*. This neutral liposome formulation, unlike cationic liposomes, is stable in blood and does not result in selective accumulation in lungs. Nabel *et al. (483)* studied Allovectin–7™, a gene transfer liposomal product for the treatment of metastatic melanoma, renal cell and colorectal carcinoma. They demonstrated that intra-lesional injection of Allovectin–7™ can be given safely and showed anti-tumor activity in some patients. Yoshida *et al. (477)* studied the transfer of interferon beta gene via cationic liposomes in patients with malignant glioma and found that liposomal formulation induced regression of experimental glioma. The study indicated the feasibility and safety of interferon β gene therapy, which may help treat the patients with malignant glioma.

The clinical significance of hydroxyapatite as a bone substitute has become apparent in recent years and bone morphogenetic protein (BMP), a substance that induces bone formation, has attracted much attention. Ono *et al. (484)* created a bone defect on rabbit cranium and treated it with the *BMP-2* gene (cDNA plasmid) combined with cationic liposomes as a vector and confirmed the clinical usefulness of gene therapy for bone formation. Anti-sense oligodeoxynucleotides (ODNs) possess a great potential as sequence-specific therapeutic agents but needs sufficient concentration of intact. ODN must bypass membrane barriers and access the cytosol and nucleus for ODNs to be therapeutically effective. Mathew *et al. (485)* designed a liposome-based formulation that utilises listeriolysin O (LLO), the endosomolytic haemolysin from *L. monocytogenes*, to mediate escape of ODN from endocytic compartments into cytosol and trafficked to nucleus efficiently. Delivery without LLO resulted in sequestration of

ODN in vesicular compartments leading to little inhibition of intercellular adhesion molecule-1 expression, which supports the LLO requirement of efficient cytosolic delivery using this system. It has been demonstrated that LLO-mediated escape of ODN from intra-cellular vesicles is an effective approach to achieve full therapeutic antisense activity in cultured macrophages.

10.1.10. Liposomes in Immunology

Allison and Gregoriadis *(486)* found that liposome encapsulation of antigens resulted in elevated antibody titres in comparison to free antigen. This interesting observation opened the field for study of immuno potentiating properties of liposomes. Earlier, the common adjuvants used for experimental immunisation in laboratory animals were Freund's complete and incomplete adjuvants (complete Freund's adjuvants and incomplete Freund's adjuvants), which are composed of a W/O emulsion with or without heat killed mycobacteria. Though these adjuvants evoke high level and long lasting immunity, they are not suitable for use in humans since they cause formation of granulomas at the site of injection. Other adjuvants such as alum, aluminium hydroxide and calcium chloride used in humans are also not free from disadvantages. During the course of investigation for a safe and effective adjuvant for use in human, liposomes were found to have a decided advantage over the afore-mentioned adjuvants since they are prepared from biodegradable phospholipids which do not produce granulomas *(487)*. In addition, liposomes protect the entrapped antigens from hypersensitivity reactions *(486)*.

Liposomes have also been shown to potentiate DNA mediated vaccination. IM immunisation of mice with DNA encoding the S region of hepatitis B antigen entrapped into cationic liposomes has led to improved humoural and cell mediated immunity, as compared to naked DNA or DNA complexed with preformed similar liposomes. It is assumed that immunisation with liposomes entrapped plasmid DNA involves APC, either locally or in regional draining lymph nodes *(486)*.

10.1.10.1. Effect of Surface Charges of Vesicles

The effect of surface charge on the immuno potentiating activity of liposomes was first observed by Allison and Gregoriadis *(486)*. It was found that inoculation of diptheria toxoid in negatively charged liposomes elicited significantly higher antibody levels than when entrapped in neutral or positively charged liposomes. But recently the effectiveness of positively charged liposomes in producing significant levels of antibodies have been demonstrated *(488)*. The antibody titres obtained with lysozyme entrapped in positively charged liposomes has been found to be higher than neutral, negatively charged liposomes. Though the exact mechanism of action of positively charged liposomes is not understood, it is clear that these liposomes interact differently with cells *in vivo* in comparison to neutral and negatively charged liposomes possibly eliciting a cell-mediated immunity. There is a possibility that the positive charge may hamper the fusion of vesicles with lysosomes, thus allowing protection and prolonged exposure of the entrapped antigen to immune system.

10.1.10.2. Effect of Sites of Association of the Antigen With Liposome Vesicles

There are a number of ways by which proteins can be associated with liposomes and this depends upon the physicochemical properties of proteins. Water-soluble molecules may be entrapped within the aqueous compartments between lipid lamellae whereas hydrophobic proteins may interact with lipid bilayers *(489)*. Further, amphipathic substances may be associated with lipid bilayers; at the same time their hydrophilic tails may project on the surface of liposomes. Recent interest has been centred on the effect of modes of association of antigen with liposomes on antibody production. Van Rooijen and Van Nieuwmegen *(490,491)* reported comparable antibody titres elicited by human serum albumin and bovine γ-globulin adsorbed on and entrapped within the liposomal vesicles. Subsequently, it was postulated that only those ligands that are exposed on the liposome surface are immunogenic. However, internalising of a number of antigens in liposomes was also reported to induce antibody production *(486,492)*. It was also observed that trypsinisation of liposome encapsulated antigens does not reduce or abolish the immunological response.

Viral antigens are mostly membrane proteins and were found to associate with aqueous compartments as well as the lipid membranes in liposomes. Such a polypeptide derived from Hepatitis B surface antigen incorporated in liposomes showed higher antibody titres when administered in guinea pigs than antigen administered in aluminium gel *(493)*. The immunogenicity of surface expressed antigens has been further demonstrated using human LS174T colon tumor cell membranes incorporated in vesicles *(494)*.

Proteins, as described earlier could be associated with the liposomes by covalent linkage with vesicles. However, the effect of such an association on immuno potentiation by liposomes has not been extensively investigated. Shek and Heath *(495)* reported that, bovine serum albumin (BSA) covalently linked to the surface of preformed unilamellar vesicle composed of PC, CHOL and *N*-(4-maleimidophenyl butyryl) phosphatidyl ethanolamine has been found to be immunogenic.

10.1.10.3. Effect of Size and Structure of Liposomes

The size and structure of liposomes is anticipated to affect the immunogenicity of liposome associated antigens. However, comparative studies of immunogenicity of antigens associated with different preparations of liposomes are not available. Most of the immunological studies on liposomes have been carried out using MLVs. Recently the differences in MLV and unilamellar liposomes of comparable size in promoting antibody response to a protein antigen has been analysed *(495)*. Results obtained with the negatively charged liposomes prepared from dimyristoyl-lecithin indicate that unilamellar vesicles (ULVs) are more effective than MLVs in promoting an immune response to the entrapped BSA.

10.1.10.4. Effect of Lipid Composition

Most of the liposomal vesicles for immunological studies have been prepared from egg lecithin, CHOL and a negatively charged phospholipid, diacetyl phosphate or phosphatidic acid. In order to introduce a positive charge, stearylamine is used. The molar ratio of lipids used in preparation of liposomes which promotes effective antibody production is usually 7:2:1 of egg leicthin, CHOL and charged lipid, respectively *(486)*. Egg lecithin or PC is the most important ingredient of liposomes used for adjuvant activity. In contrast to phosphatidyl inositol, phosphatidyl glycerol and phosphatidic acid, PC is a very poor antigen *(496)*. However an immune response against PC is induced when lipid A is incorporated in liposomes *(497)*.

Liposomes prepared from SM have been reported to be more effective in eliciting an immune response to incorporated antigen than liposomes from phsophatidylcholine *(498,499)*. There is a striking difference in the T_c of these lipids (PC, 8–15°C and SM, 42°C) and it is suggested that high immunological response by SM liposomes may be due to their greater stability. Liposomes composed of DPPC and DSPC (T_c 41.4–54.9°C, respectively) have also been reported to be more effective immunogens than those prepared from egg lecithin *(500)*. It is postulated that these liposomes may have greater bilayer stability at physiological temperature and may thus persist longer *in vivo* than egg lecithin.

10.1.10.5. Effect of Route of Administration

For potentiating an immunological response to liposome-associated antigens, animals may be immunised intravenously, intraperitoneally, intramuscularly or subcutaneously. A strong primary immune response is induced by i.v. administration of liposome-associated antigens *(486,501)*. However, the response does not persist and may not show a secondary induction. In contrast, IM and s.c. route elicit higher concentration of antibodies *(486,502)* on secondary immunisation. Liposome-associated antigens are injected through i.p., to induce a substantial antibody production *(503,504)*. Significant stimulation of immune system is observed when liposomes are injected subcutaneously intramuscularly or intraperitoneally. It is possible that liposomes injected by these routes will remain at the site of injection for a long period. Thus liposomes exert their adjuvant effect bý retaining a 'depot' of an antigen at the site of injection *(489)*. However, the adjuvant action is not entirely physical. Some interaction between liposome and cells of the immune system has been reported *(500)*. The appearance of activated mononuclear phagocytes and increased specific activities of several lysosomal hydrolases in these cells by a single liposomal sensitisation in mice *(492)* indicates that liposomes may affect the reticuloendothelial function directly by activating phagocytic cells.

10.1.10.6. Effect of Sugars on Surface of Liposomes

It is well established that macrophages possess recognition sites for sugars such as mannose, galactose and fucose *(505)*. Liposomes carrying terminal galactose and mannose residues are specifically recognised by lecithin-like molecules present on plasma membranes of macrophages of parenchymal and non-parenchymal tissues *(506)*. A recent study of immunological response of sugar grafted liposomes shows that antigen entrapped liposomes bearing galactose on the surface induce an immune response comparable to sugar-free neutral liposomes. However, the immune response by mannose-coupled liposomes is almost equal to that of free antigen *(507)*. Based on these results, it is postulated that s.c. administration of liposomes facilitates a receptor mediated uptake by peritoneal macrophages and macrophages derived from bone marrow by a recognition system specific for mannose.

10.1.10.7. Liposomes as Carriers of Antigens

In addition to their adjuvant effect, liposomes have been recognised as efficient carriers of antigens in recent years. Haptens such as dinitrophenyl and phosphorylcholine groups are generally inserted in liposomes by coupling them to one of the phospholipids used in liposome preparation *(508)*. The most obvious advantages of the use of liposomes as carriers are easy biodegradability and low immunogenicity of liposomes compared to protein carriers, thus eliminating the need to remove carrier specific antibodies. These potentials of liposomes attracted extensive research in production of antibodies to a number of haptens. This approach for obtaining specific antibodies has been extended to molecules of clinical interest such as hormones, drugs and vitamins, etc. For example, anti-L-thyroxine antiserum has been produced with liposomes sensitised with L-thyroxine derivative of PE *(509)*. In addition, extensive studies on the immunogenic properties of haptenated liposomes have been carried out using tripeptide enlarged haptens such as 3-(*p*-azobenzene arsonate)-*N*-acetyl-L-tyrosylglycylglycine and *N*-(2,4-dinitrophenyl)-β-alanylglycylglycine *(510)*. Wood and Kabat *(511)* showed the production of anti-glycolipid antibodies and Das *et al.* *(512–514)* reported the production of antibodies against sugars such as mannose, galactose and *N*-acetyl-D-glucosamine using liposomes as carriers. The carrier effect of liposomes to protein antigens has also been reported *(515)*.

The immuno adjuvant activity of liposomes to associated antigens may be enhanced further by incorporation of immuno modulators. Studies carried out with endotoxin and lipid-A show an enhanced adjuvant effect to antigen in association with liposomes *(490,499)*. However, further increase in adjuvant activity is observed when antigen and immunomodulator are incorporated in the same liposomes. Another compound possessing immune potentiating activity is *N*-acetylmuramyl-L-alanyl-D-isoglutamine (muramyl dipeptide [MDP]). Encapsulation of MDP in liposomes enhances its effectiveness in producing an immune response against antigen compared with the unencapsulated MDP *(516)*. In addition, encapsulation of MDP in liposomes reduces the amount of drug needed for protection against infections *(517)*. Liposome-encapsulated MDP has been found to activate macrophages more efficiently *in vitro* than free MDP *(518)*. This property to activate macrophages has been further extended *in vivo* for the destruction of spontaneous lymph node and visceral metastasis *(518)*. Lymphokines like macrophage-activating factor (MAF) have a short life and after injection into circulation they rapidly bind to serum proteins. Moreover, preparations of MAF are antigenic and therefore their repeated injections may not be possible. Encapsulation of MAF in liposomes prevents these undesirable side effects at the same time induces an efficient macrophage activation *(519)*.

11. PRODUCTION AND SCALE UP

Reports on liposomes have mainly focused on the formulation aspects and dealt with laboratory preparations only with the result that very few papers concentrated on the production aspects of liposomes such as scale up and sterilisation.

11.1. Methodology

Generally, being sterile products, liposomes are processed in a sterile area. While theoretically all the methods proposed for liposome preparation can be used for large scale production, some methods have gained faster acceptance at the industrial scale due to their simplicity and ease of scale up as compared to other methods.

Various aspects of process development work pertinent to aseptic process techniques for liposomes have been reviewed *(520)*.

A pH gradient across liposome bilayers was established in order to load a model drug (orciprenaline sulphate) into liposome vesicles. This method of liposome loading resulted in yields as high as 80–85% encapsulation. An eight-step process was designed to scale up the process and was evaluated. In this process a diafiltration technique was successfully used to remove excess orciprenaline sulphate present in external medium. Finally, drug-loaded liposomes were lyophilised using lactose as an internal and external liposomal cryoprotectant *(520)*.

A new scalable liposome production system has been presented, based on the ethanol injection technique. The principal item herein is the crossflow injection module. The system permits liposome manufacture regardless of production scale, as scale is determined only by free disposable vessel volumes. Once the parameters are defined, an easy scale up can be performed by just changing the process vessels. These vessels are fully steriliseable and all raw materials are transferred into sanitised and sterilised system via 0.2 μm filters to guarantee an aseptic production. Liposome size can be controlled by local lipid concentration at injection point depending on process parameters like injection pressure, lipid concentration and injection rate. Compared with other technologies like film method, which is normally followed by size reduction through high-pressure homogenisation, ultrasonication or extrusion, no mechanical forces are needed to generate homogeneous and narrow distributed liposomes. Another important advantage of this method is the suitability for entrapment of different drug substances such as large hydrophilic proteins by passive encapsulation, small amphiphilic drugs by a one step remote loading technique or membrane association of antigens for vaccination approaches *(521,522)*.

A dialysis method for preparation of large volumes of stable and homogeneous bilayer liposomes under sterile conditions was developed. The equipment consists of a disposable haemodialysis capillary dialyser connected to two reservoirs through which the micelle/liposome solution is pumped in a closed circuit. The detergent is removed by a countercurrent flow of dialysis buffer. Homogeneous, detergent free liposome preparations totaling 100 mL with lipid concentrations ranging from 5 to 25 mg/mL can be prepared within 2–4 h *(523)*.

Two types of equipments, which are nowadays commonly used for reproducible production of liposomes need to be mentioned here.

The Microfluidiser® is patented equipment which contains electric-hydraulic modules that provide power to double-acting intensifier pumps. Intensifier pumps amplify the hydraulic pressure and, in turn, impart that pressure to the input product streams to create high velocity and high-shear product flow. Each intensifier pump is designed to supply the desired pressure at a constant rate to product stream. As the pump travels in one direction, it drives the product at constant pressure through one or more interaction chambers. Within each chamber are specially designed fixed-geometry microchannels through which the product accelerates to high velocities, creating shear and impact forces having orders of magnitude greater than any other conventional means as the product stream impinges upon itself and on wear-resistant surfaces, bringing about desired results, including uniform particle and droplet size reduction (often sub-micron), deagglomeration, etc. As intensifier pump continues its travel in one direction, a series of check valves allow product to be drawn into opposite end of pump. As intensifier pump completes its stroke, it reverses direction and the new volume of product is pressurised repeating the process. This creates a near-constant flow of product at constant pressure through the interaction chamber. Upon exiting the interaction chamber, the product may be directed through an optional heat exchanger, re-circulated through the system for further processing or directed externally to the next step in the process.

Microfluidics manufactures two levels of microfluidiser material processors; laboratory and scale up production units which can offer pressures ranging from 250 to 40,000 psi and capable of processing samples ranging from 100 mL to a gallon. All models of microfluidiser are available with Clean-In-Place and Steam-In-Place options. In general, important guidelines for processing liposomes by microfluidiser include use of higher pressures (15,000 psi and up) and multiple passes (1–5). Processing temperatures generally are kept between 35 and 40°C. The product is cooled on the final pass (http://www.microfluidicscorp.com; accessed on 9/9/2007).

A variety of factors were evaluated in order to establish the characteristics of liposomes obtained with a high-pressure homogeniser (microfluidiser 110S). Responses obtained by variation of two groups of factors were studied–first, the inlet pressure of homogeniser, the times that the samples were processed (cycles) and the bulk ionic strength and second, the phospholipid (P) and ethanol concentrations. Mean liposome diameter decreases with increasing inlet pressure, number of cycles and ethanol concentration and increases raising ionic strength. No phospholipid concentration effect was observed. The variation of entrapped volume of liposomes upon cycles and pressure has a similar behaviour to diameter. Within the studied variable range, microfluidisation does not increase phospholipid oxidation index, nor does it significantly alter the phospholipids concentration *(524)*. Large scale production and testing of DC–CHOL cationic liposomes by microfluidisation has been described *(525)*. These liposomes were produced in a good manufacturing practice (GMP) acceptable manner to a 500 mL batch size and were shown to be sterile. Further, when stored at 4°C, DC–CHOL liposomes retained their original size, remained suspended in solution and retained activity for a period exceeding 1.5 yr *(525)*.

The second type of equipment useful in scale up and manufacturing of liposomes is the emulsiflex manufactured by Avestin. This equipment is based on principle of dynamic high-pressure homogenisation. Here, a high-pressure pump pushes product through an adjustable homogenising valve or a membrane of specific pore size to emulsify, homogenise, filter and extrude materials. The membranes usually are polycarbonate membranes of varied pore sizes, which are commercially available. Submicron particles with diameters less than 50 nm and an extremely narrow size distribution can be achieved. The emulsiflex range is available in models with capabilities for handling from 3 L (C3) to about 1000 L/h (C1000) with a maximum pressure of upto 30,000 psi or 2000 bar (www.avestin.com; accessed on 9/9/2007).

11.2. Sterilisation

It was suggested that sterilisation of liposomes by heating was practicable as well as that by filtration, if the liposomes were prepared as follows: the charged liposomes made of lipids with low peroxide values were dispersed in a sugar or polyol solution adjusted to pH 6.5, where the amount of dissolved oxygen was minimised. An ionic water-soluble drug had to be encapsulated in the oppositely charged liposomes *(526)*. Liposome stability and oxidation were studied under autoclaving conditions. It was shown that after preliminary air removal from a liposome sample there was no lipid oxidation (malonaldehyde *bis*[dimethyl acetate] was used as a control) and liposome content leakage during autoclaving. However, in another study, the autoclaving cycle was found to cause massive loss of hydrophilic, non-bilayer interacting compounds; under those conditions "free" drug removal or drug encapsulation should be performed after autoclaving step *(527)*.

The possibilities and limitations of γ-irradiation as a sterilisation method for non-frozen, frozen and freeze-dried liposomes have been investigated. The degradation of trehalose limits the use of freezing or freeze-drying liposome dispersions as a way to minimise irradiation damage *(528)*.

MLVs incorporating CF were calibrated through polycarbonate membranes of 0.1, 0.2 or 0.4 μm pore size. After removal of unencapsulated material, the vesicles were passed through 0.2 μm sterilising filters constituted of polycarbonate, cellulose acetate or polyvinylidene fluorure. The liposomes were readily filtered without significant change in vesicle size and loss of phospholipids *(529)*.

11.3. Patents and Established Technologies on Liposome Production

A method for preparing liposomes with a water-soluble, biologically active compound using lyophilisation was disclosed in US patent no. 4,311,712 to Evans, *et al.* in 1980. The disclosed methods are not particularly suitable for aqueous soluble materials and requires mixture of biologically active material with an organic solvent. Felgner *et al.* (EP 172 007 B) also describe a technique incorporating an organic solvent. It was also known that liposomes and their contents may be relatively unstable in aqueous dispersion. Accordingly, an attempt to increase relatively short storage life of certain liposomal products by dehydrating the dispersion has been the focus of several liposome preparation methods. For example, the aqueous dispersion of encapsulated material was lyophilised to form a stable powder which can be stored for a long period and from which, with an aqueous medium, a liposome dispersion can be reconstituted (*see* Schneider, *et al.* US patent no. 4,229,360). US patent no. 4,515,736 (D. Deamer) also describes an encapsulation method in which liposome dispersions are dried in presence of material to be encapsulated. As the solution is dried to a highly viscous concentrated mixture, the individual liposomes fuse to form multilamellar structures which capture the material to be encapsulated between the lipid lamellae. Upon rehydration, lipid vesicles form which encapsulate the material. Crowe *et al.* (US patent no. 4,857,319) describe a method for preserving liposomes involving freeze-drying a mixture containing lipid vesicles, the material to be encapsulated and a disaccharide preserving agent. Later invention disclosed to encapsulate a material while avoiding the need to subject that material to such rigorous manipulations as lyophilisation, thereby decreasing the possibility of physically inactivating or degrading the material to be encapsulated.

Mayer *et al.* (US patent no. 5,077,056) describe a liposome preparation method involving the use of small ions to produce gradients which enhance the retention of charged biologically active agents, and optionally involving subjecting liposome and biologically active agents to a freeze–thaw process during encapsulation procedure to produce "freeze and thaw multilamellar vesicles" (FATMLV). The FATMLV method requires that freezing and thawing be done in the presence of material to be entrapped. A new patent (US patent no. 6,855,296) issued to Martin T Baker and William A Heriot in 2005 (Assignee M/s Optime therapeutics Inc) describes a new method of producing liposomes using an in-line mixing system. The liposomes produced by this method find utility in numerous therapeutic applications. Some of the technologies and production methods patented for the production of liposomes are listed below in Tables 12 and 13.

Table 12. List of Technologies and Production Methods Patented for the Production of Liposomes

Patent no.	*Author*	*Title of the patent/details*
US 4,235,871 (1980)	D. Paphadjopoulus and F. Szoka	Method of encapsulating biologically active materials in lipid vesicles
US 4,394,372 (1983)	J.L.Taylor	Process for making lipid membrane structures
US 4,508,703 (1985)	G.Redziniak and A. Meybeck	Production of pulverulent mixtures of lipidic and hydrophobic constituents
US 4,522,803 (1985)	R.P.Lenk, *et al*	Stable plurilamellar vesicles, their preparation and use
US 4,529,561 (1985)	C.A.Hunt and D. Paphadjopoulus	Method for producing liposomes in selected size range
US 4,608,211 (1986)	R.M.Hindjani, *et al.*	Process for preparing lipid vesicles by vapourisation of solvents
US 4,621,023 (1986)	G.Redziniak and A. Meybeck	Method of homogenising dispersions of hydrated lipidic lamellar phases and suspensions obtained by the said method
US 4,687,661 (1987)	H.Kikuchi and H.Yamauchi	Method for producing liposomes
US 4,737,323 (1988)	F.J.Martin and J.K.Morano	Liposome extrusion method
US 4,752,425 (1988)	F.J.Martin and G. West	High-encapsulation liposome processing method
US 4,781,871 (1988)	G. West and F.J.Martin	High-concentration liposome processing method
US 5.192,549 (1993)	Y. Barenolz and G. Haran	Method of amphiphatic drug loading in liposomes by pH gradient
US 5,264,221 (1993)	Tagawa, Toshiaki, *et al.*	Drug containing protein bonded liposome
US 5,855,910 (1999)	GW Ashley, RC MacDonald, M Shida	Cationic phospholipids for transfection
US 5,935,599 (1999)	E.J.Dadey	Polymer associated liposome delivery system and methods of manufacturing the same
US 5,939,096 (1999)	C. Stephane and B. Yechezkel	Liposome drug-loading method and composition
US 5,945,121 (1999)	Muneyoshi Kato, *et al.*	Liposome eye drops
US 5,958,378 (1999)	J.C.Waldrep, *et al.*	High dose liposomal aerosol formulations containing cyclosporin A or budesonide
US 5,965,156 (1999)	Richard T. Proffitt, *et al.*	Amphotericin B liposome preparation
US 6,045,824 (2000)	Sinil Kim, *et al.*	Sustained release liposomal anaesthetic composition
US 6,090,955 (2000)	Regine reszka, *et al.*	Liposome-encapsulated taxol, its preparation and its use
US 6.221,385 (2001)	Frederic Camu, *et al.*	Freeze-dried liposome encapsulated amphiphilic drug compositions and a process for the preparation there of
US 6,334,999 (2002)	Kapil Mehta, *et al.*	Liposomal aerosols for delivery of chemotherapeutic retinoids to the lungs
US 6,346,233 (2002)	Knight J. Vernon, *et al.*	Composition for treating cancer via liposomal aerosol formulation containing taxol
US 20040156889 (2004)	Hu, Ning, *et al.*	Method of drug loading in liposomes by gradient
CA 2506749	Hu, Ning, *et al.*	Method of drug loading in liposomes by gradient

Table 13. Established Patented Technologies for Liposomes

Technology	*Company*	*Year*	*Details*
"Neo lipid™"	Neo pharma	2000	
Zilip's liposomal technology	Zilip, USA	–	Utilises PEGylated liposomes free of biologicals, which have a longer half-life and have been used successfully with other approved products
NanoSorb™	BioPharma Scientific, San Diego, CA 92121	–	Mimics our body's own strategy in creating submicron sized liposomes as carriers for otherwise poorly soluble, and therefore poorly absorbed, nutrients
LCM technology (brandname "Filmix®")	Cavitation-Control Technology, Inc. (Cav-Con), USA	–	Lipid-coated microbubble for diagnosis and therapy

REFERENCES

1. **Torchilin, VP.** Multifunctional nanocarriers. *Adv. Drug Deliv. Rev.* 2006;58(14):1532–1555.
2. **Felgner, PL. and Ringold, GM.** Cationic liposome-mediated transfection. *Nature* 1989;337(6205):387–388.
3. **Rosenthal, AF. and Geyer, RP.** A synthetic inhibitor of venom lecithinase A. *J. Biol. Chem.* 1960;235:2202–2206.
4. **Behr, JP., Demeneix, B., Loeffler, JP., and Perez-Mutul, J.** Efficient gene transfer into mammalian primary endocrine cells with lipopolyamine-coated DNA. *Proc. Natl. Acad. Sci. USA* 1989;86:6982–6986.
5. **Zhou, XH., Klibanov, AL., and Huang, L.** Lipophilic polylysines mediate efficient DNA transfection in mammalian cells. *Biochim. Biophys. Acta* 1991;1065(1):8–14.
6. **Gao, X. and Huang, L.** A novel cationic liposome reagent for efficient transfection of mammalian cells. *Biochim. Biophys. Res. Comm.* 1991;179:280–285.
7. **Kung, VT. and Redemann, CT.** Synthesis of carboxyacyl derivatives of phosphatidylethanolamine and use as an efficient method for conjugation of protein to liposomes. *Biochim. Biophys. Acta* 1986;862:435–439.
8. **Zhao, L., Meyer, JD., Rittmann-Grauer, L., and Manning, MC.** Use of circular dichroism spectroscopy in determining the conformation of a monoclonal antibody prior to its incorporation in an immunoliposome. *J. Pharm. Biomed. Anal.* 1997;16:507–513.
9. **Heeremans, JL., Kraaijenga, JJ., Los, P., Kluft, C., and Crommelin, DJ.** Development of a procedure for coupling the homing device glu-plasminogen to liposomes. *Biochim. Biophys. Acta* 1992;1117:258–264.
10. **Demos, SM., Onyuksel, H., Gilbert, J., et al.** In vitro targeting of antibody-conjugated echogenic liposomes for site-specific ultrasonic image enhancement. *J. Pharm. Sci.* 1997;86:167–171.
11. **Crosasso, P., Brusa, P., Dosio, F., et al.** Antitumoral activity of liposomes and immunoliposomes containing 5-fluorouridine prodrugs. *J. Pharm. Sci.* 1997;86:832–839.
12. **Kamps, JA., Swart, PJ., Morselt, HW., et al.** Preparation and characterization of conjugates of (modified) human serum albumin and Liposomes: drug carriers with an intrinsic anti-HIV activity. *Biochim. Biophys. Acta* 1996;1278:183–190.
13. **Kichler, A., Remy, JS., Boussif, O.,** Efficient gene delivery with neutral complexes of lipospermine and thiol-reactive phospholipids. *Biochem. Biophys. Res. Commun.* 1995;209:444–450.
14. **Legendre, JY., Trzeciak, A., Bohrmann, B., Deuschle, U., Kitas, E., and Supersaxo, A.** Dioleoylmelittin as a novel serum-insensitive reagent for efficient transfection of mammalian cells. *Bioconjug. Chem.* 1997;8:57–63.
15. **Martin, FJ. and Papahadjopoulos, D.** Irreversible coupling of immunoglobulin fragments to preformed vesicles. *J. Biol. Chem.* 1982;257:286–288.
16. **Hashida, S. and Ishikowa, E.** Use of normal IgG and its fragments to lower the non-specific binding of Fab5-enzyme conjugates in sandwich enzymes immunoassay. *Anal. Lett.* 1985;18(b9):1143–1155.
17. **Dewey, RE., Timothy, DH., and Levings III, CS.** A mitochondrial protein associated with cytoplasmic male sterility in the T cytoplasm of maize. *Proc. Natl. Acad. Sci.* 1987;84:5374–5378.
18. **Hermanson, GT.** Bioconjugate Techniques. Academic Press, Inc. 1996, 505 p.
19. **Wright, SE. and Huang, L.** Bilayer stabilization of phosphatidylethanolamine by N-biotinylphosphatidylethanolamine. *Biochim. Biophys. Acta* 1992;1103:172–178.

20. **Ferraretto, A., Sonnino, S., Soria, MR., and Masserini, M.** Characterization of biotinylated liposomes sensitive to temperature and pH: new tools for anti-cancer drug delivery. *Chem. Phys. Lipids* 1996;82:133–139.
21. **Ogihara-Umeda, I., Sasaki, T., Toyama, H., Oda, K., Senda, M., and Nishigori, H.** Rapid tumor imaging by active background reduction using biotin-bearing liposomes and avidin. *Cancer Res.* 1994;54:463–467.
22. **Darst, SA., Ahlers, M., Meller, PH., et al.** Two-dimensional crystals of streptavidin on biotinylated lipid layers and their interactions with biotinylated macromolecules. *Biophys. J.* 1991;59:387–396.
23. **Hemming, SA., Bochkarev, A., Darst, SA., et al.** The mechanism of protein crystal growth from lipid layers. *J. Mol. Biol.* 1995;246:308–316.
24. **Qin, H., Liu, Z., and Sui, SF.** Two-dimensional crystallization of avidin on biotinylated lipid monolayers. *Biophys. J.* 1995;68:2493–2496.
25. **Yang, Q., Liu, XY., Ajiki, S., Hara, M., Lundahl, P., and Miyake, J.** Avidin-biotin immobilization of unilamellar liposomes in gel beads for chromatographic analysis of drug-membrane partitioning. *J. Chromatogr. B Biomed. Sci. Appl.* 1998;707:131–141.
26. **Loughrey, HC., Ferraretto, A., Cannon, AM., et al.** Characterization of biotinylated liposomes for *in vivo* targeting applications. *FEBS Lett.* 1993;332:183–188.
27. **Corley, P. and Loughrey, HC.** Binding of biotinated-liposomes to streptavidin is influenced by liposomes composition. *Biochim. Biophys. Acta.* 1994;1195, 27:149–156.
28. **Subbarao, NK., MacDonald, RI., Takeshita, K., and MacDonald, RC.** Characteristics of spectrin-induced leakage of extruded, phosphatidylserine vesicles. *Biochim. Biophys. Acta* 1991;1063:147–54.28.
29. **MacDonald, RC., MacDonald, RI., Menco, BP., Takeshita, K., Subbarao, NK., and Hu, LR.** Small-volume extrusion apparatus for preparation of large, unilamellar vesicles. *Biochim. Biophys. Acta* 1991;1061:297–303.
30. **Hindjani, RM., Ribier, A., and Maurelli, MM.** Process for preparing lipid vesicles by vaporisation of solvents, US. Patent 4.608,211,1986.
31. **Batzri, S. and Korn, ED.** Single bilayer liposomes prepared without sonication. *Biochim. Biophy. Acta* 1973;298:1015–1019.
32. **Kikuchi, H. and Yamauchi, H.** Method for producing liposomes, U.S. Patent 4, 687, 661, 1987.
33. **Szoka, F. Jr. and Papahadjopoulos, D.** Comparative Properties and methods of preparation of lipid vesicles (liposomes). *Ann. Rev. Biophys. Bioeng.* 1980;9:467–508.
34. **Cullis, PR., Hope, MJ., Bally, MB., Madden, TD., Mayer, LD., and Janoff, AS.** Liposomes as pharmaceuticals in liposomes from biphysics to therapeutics. (Ostro, MJ., ed.), Marcel Dekker, New York, 1987, pp. 39–72.
35. **Kasahara, M. and Hinkle, PC.** Reconsitution and purification of the D-glucose transporter from human erythrocytes. *J. Biol. Chem.* 1977;252(20):7384–7390.
36. **Reeves, JP. and Dowben, RM.** Formation and properties of thin walled vesicles. *J. Cell. Physiol.* 1969;73(1):49–60.
37. **Shew, RL. and Deamer, DW.** A novel method for encapsulation of macromolecules in liposomes. *Biochim. Biophys. Acta* 1985;816(1):1–8.
38. **Oku, N. and MacDonald, RC.** Solubilization of phospholipids by chaotropic ion solutions. *J. Biol. Chem.* 1983;258(14): 8733–8738.
39. **Kagawa, Y. and Racker, E.** Partial resolution of the enzymes catalyzing oxidative phosphorylation XXV. Reconstitution of vesicles catalyzing Pi—adenosine triphosphate exchange. *J. Biol. Chem.*1971;246:5477–5487.
40. **Milsmann MH., Schwendener, RA., and Weder, HG.** The preparation of large single bilayer liposomes by a fast and controlled dialysis. *Biochim. Biophys. Acta* 1978;512(1):147–155.
41. **Jiskoot, W., Teerlink, T., Beuvery, EC., and Crommelin, DJA.** Preparation of liposomes via detergent removal from mixed micelles by dilution. *Pharm. World Sci.* 1986;8(5):259–265.
42. **Enoch, HG. and Strittmatter, P.** Formation and properties of 1000-A-diameter, single-bilayer phospholipid vesicles. *Proc. Natl. Acad. Sci. USA* 1979;76(1):145–149.
43. **Gerristen, WJ., Verkleij, AJ., Zwall, RFA., and Van Deenan, LLM.** Freeze-fracture appearance and disposition of band 3 protein from the human erythrocyte membrane in lipid vesicles. *Eur. J. Biochem.* 1978;85(1):255–261.
44. **Szoka, F. and Papahadjopoulos, D.** Procedure for preparation of liposomes with large internal aqueous space and high capture by reverse-phase evaporation. *Proc. Natl. Acad. Sci.* 1978;75(9):4194–4198.
45. **Cortesi, R., Esposito, E., Gambarin, S., Telloli, P., Menegatti, E., and Nastruzzi, C.** Preparation of liposomes by reverse-phase evaporation using alternative organic solvents. *J. Microencapsul.* 1999;16:251–256.
46. **Sprague, SG. and Staehelin, LA.** A rapid reverse phase evaporation method for the reconstitution of uncharged thylakoid membrane lipids that resist hydration. *Plant Physiol.* 1984;75(2):502–504.
47. **Zawada, Z.** A single-step method of liposome preparation. *Cell Mol. Biol. Lett.* 2004;9(4A):603–615.
48. **Huang, C., Mason, JT., and Levin, IW.** Raman spectroscopic study of saturated mixed-chain phosphatidylcholine multilamellar dispersions. *Biochem.* 1983;22(11):2775–2780.
49. **Olson, F., Hunt, CA., Szoka, FC., Vail, WJ., and Papahadjopoulos, D.** Preparation of liposomes of defined size distribution by extrusion through polycarbonate membranes. *Biochim. Biophys. Acta* 1979;557(1):9–23.
50. **Martin, FJ. and Morano, JK.** Liposome extrusion method, United States Patent, 4,737,323, 1988.
51. **Kirby, CJ. and Gregoriadis, G.** Preparation of liposomes containing factor VIII for oral treatment of haemophilia. *J. Microencapsul.* 1984;1(1):33–45.
52. **Lichtenberg, D. and Barenholz, Y.** Liposomes: preparation, characterization, and preservation. *Methods Biochem. Anal.* 1988;33:337–462.

53. **Mayhew, E., Lazo, R., Vail, WJ., King, J., and Green, AM.** Characterization of liposomes prepared using a microemulsifier. *Biochim. Biophys. Acta* 1984;775(2):169–174.

54. **Lekkes, I.** The use of French Pressed vesicles for efficient incorporation of bioactive macromolecules and carriers in vitro and in vivo, in Liposomes Technology, (Gregoraidis, G., ed.), CRC Press, Boca Raton, Florida, 1984, pp. 51–65.

55. **Hope, MJ., Madden, TD., Bally, MB., Cullis, PR., Schieren, HP., Janoff, AS.** Protection of large unilamellar vesicles by trehalose during dehydration: retention of vesicle contents. *Biochim. Biophys. Acta* 1985;817(1):67–74.

56. **Kremer, JM., Esker, MW., Pathmamanoharan, C., and Wiersema, PH.** Vesicles of variable diameter prepared by a modified injection method. *Biochem.* 1977;16(17):3932–3935.

57. **Deamer, D. and Bangham, AD.** Large volume liposomes by an ether vaporization method. *Biochim. Biophys. Acta* 1976;443(3):629–634.

58. **Pick, U.,** Liposomes with large trapping capacity prepared by freezing and thawing of sonicated phospholipid mixtures. *Arch. Biochim. Biophys.* 1981;212:186–194.

59. **Mayer, LD., Hope, MJ., Cullis, PR., and Janoff, AS.** Solute distributions and trapping efficiencies observed in freeze-thawed multilamellar vesicles. *Biochim. Biophys. Acta* 1985;817(1):193–196.

60. **Zumbuehl, O. and Weder, HG.** Liposomes of controllable size in the range of 40 to 180 nm by defined dialysis of lipid/detergent mixed micelles. *Biochim. Biophys. Acta* 1981;640(1):252–262.

61. **Mimms, LT., Zampighi, G., Nozaki, Y., Tanford, C., and Reynolds, J.** Phospholipid vesicle formation and transmembrane protein incorporation using octyl glucoside. *Biochem.* 1981;20(4):833–840.

62. **Brunner, J., Skrabal, P., and Hauser, H.** Single bilayer vesicles prepared without sonication. Physico-chemical properties. *Biochim. Biophys. Acta* 1976;455(2):322–331.

63. **Lasic, DD.** Liposomes: From Physics to Applications, Elsevier: Amsterdam, 1993.

64. **Deamer, DW., Prince, RC., and Crofts, AR.** The response of fluorescent amines to pH gradients across liposome membranes. *Biochim. Biophys. Acta* 1972;274(2):323–335.

65. **Lee, HC. and Forte, JG.** A study of H+ transport in gastric microsomal vesicles using fluorescent probes. *Biochim. Biophys. Acta* 1978;508(2):339–356.

66. **Harrigan, PR., Wong, KF., Redelmeier, TE., Wheeler, JJ., and Cullis, PR.** Accumulation of doxorubicin and other lipophilic amines into large unilamellar vesicles in response to transmembrane pH gradients. *Biochim. Biophys. Acta* 1993;1149(2):329–338.

67. **Haran, G., Cohen, R., Bar, LK., and Barenholz, Y.** Transmembrane ammonium sulfate gradients in liposomes produce efficient and stable entrapment of amphipathic weak bases. *Biochim. Biophys. Acta* 1993;1151(2):201–215.

68. **Lasic, DD., Frederik, PM., Stuart, MC., Barenholz, Y., and McIntosh, TJ.** Gelation of liposome interior. A novel method for drug encapsulation. *FEBS Lett.* 1992;312(2–3):255–258.

69. **Soloway, AH., Tjarks, W., Barnum, BA., et al.** The chemistry of neutron capture therapy. *Chem. Rev.* 1998;98(6):2389–2390.

70. **Li, X., Hirsh, DJ., Cabral-Lilly, D., et al.** Doxorubicin physical state in solution and inside liposomes loaded via a pH gradient. *Biochim. Biophys. Acta* 1998;1415(1):23–40.

71. **Madden, TD., Harrigan, PR., Tai, LC., et al.** The accumulation of drugs within large unilamellar vesicles exhibiting a proton gradient: a survey. *Chem. Phys. Lipids* 1990;53(1):37–46.

72. **Senior, J. and Gregoriadis, G.** Is half-life of circulating liposomes determined by changes in their permeability. *FEBS Lett.* 1982;145:109–114.

73. **Storm, G., Steerenberg, PA., Emmen, F., Vanborguumwaalkes, M., and Crommelin, DJA.** Release of doxorubicin from peritoneal macrophages exposed in vivo to doxorubiicn-containing liposomes. *Biochem. Biophys. Acta* 1988;965:136–145.

74. **Goren, D., Gabizon, A., and Barenholz, Y.** The influence of physical characteristics of liposomes on their pharmacological behaviour. *Biochim. Biophys. Acta* 1990;1029:285–294.

75. **Palmer, AF., Philip, W., and Jonathan, N.** Atomic force microscopy and light scattering of small unilamellar actin-containing liposomes. *Biophy. J.* 2003;85:1233–1247.

76. **Egawa, H. and Furusawa, K.** Liposome adhesion on mica surface studied by atomic force microscopy. *Langmuir* 1999;15:1660–1666.

77. **Jass, J., Tjärnhage, T., and Puu, G.** From liposomes to supported, planar bilayer structures on hydrophilic and hydrophobic surfaces: an atomic force microscopy study. *Biophys. J.* 2000;79:3153–3163.

78. **Thomson, NH., Collin, I., Davies, MC., et al.** Atomic force microscopy of cationic liposomes. *Langmuir* 2000;16:4813–4818.

79. **Sun, Y., Li, X., Duzgunes, N., Takaoka, Y., Ohi, S., and Hirota, S.** The shape parameter of liposomes and DNA-lipid complexes determined by viscometry utilizing small sample volumes. *Biophys. J.* 2003;85(2):1223–1232.

80. New, RRC. Characterization of liposomes in Liposomes: A practical approach, (New, RRC., ed.), Oxford University Press, New York, 1990, pp. 105–161.

81. **Jousma, H., Talsma, T., Spies, F., Joosten, JGH., Junginger, HE., and Crommelin, DJA.** Characterization of liposomes: the influence of extrusion of multilamellar vesicles through polycarbonate membranes on particle size, particle size distribution and number of bilayers. *Int. J. Pharm.* 1987;35:263–274.

82. **Talsma, H., Jousma, H., Nicolay, K., and Crommelin, DJA.** Multilamellar or multivesicular vesicles. *Int. J. Pharm.* 1987;37:171–173.

83. **Kanno, T., Yamada, T., Iwabuki, H., et al.** Size distribution measurement of vesicles by atomic force microscopy. *Anal. Biochem.* 2002;309(2):196–199.

84. **Mozafari, MR., Reed, CJ., Rostron, C., Kocum, C., and Piskin, E.** Construction of stable anionic liposome-plasmid particles using the heating method: a preliminary investigation. *Cell Mol. Biol. Lett.* 2002;7(3):923–927.

85. **Defrise-Quertain, Chatelain, FP., Delmelle, M., and Ruysschaert, J.** Model studies for drug entrapment and liposome stability, in Liposome Technology: Incorporation of Drugs, Proteins and Genetic Material, (Gregoriadis, G., ed.), CRC Press, Boca Raton, 1984, pp. 1–17.

86. **Betagiri, GV., Jenkins, SA., and Parsons, DL.** Stability of liposomes in Liposome Drug delivery Systems, (Betagiri, GV., Jenkins, SA., and Parsons, DL., eds.), Technomic Publishing Co, Inc., Lancaster, 1993, pp. 29–46.

87. **Strauss, G.** Freezing and thawing of liposome suspensions, in Liposome Technology: Preparation of Liposomes, (Gregoriadis, G., ed.), CRC Press, Boca Raton, pp. 197–219.

88. **Ruysschaert, T., Marquel, A., Duteyrat, J., Lesieur, S., Winterhalter, M., and Fournier, D.** Liposome retention in size exclusion chromatography, BMC Biotechnology, 2005;5:11, through http://www.biomedcentral.com/1472-6750/5/11, 09-09-2006.

89. **Lesieur, S., Grabielle-Madelmont, C., Paternostre, MT., and Ollivon, M.** Size analysis and stability study of lipid vesicles by high-performance gel exclusion chromatography, turbidity and dynamic light scattering. *Anal. Biochem.* 1991;192:334–343.

90. **Kirkland, JJ., Yau, WW., and Szoka, FC.** Sedimentation field flow fractionation of liposomes. *Science* 1982;215(4530):296–298.

91. **Arifin, DR. and Palmer, AF.** Determination of size distribution and encapsulation efficiency of liposome-encapsulated haemoglobin blood substitutes using asymmetric flow field-flow fractionation coupled with multi-angle static light scattering. *Biotechnol. Prog.* 2003;19(6):1798–1811.

92. **Ingebrigtsen, L. and Brandl, M.** Determination of the size distribution of liposomes by SEC fractionation, and PCS analysis and enzymatic assay of lipid content. *AAPS PharmSciTech.* 2002;3(2):E7.

93. **Radko, SP., Stastna, M., and Chrambach, A.** Size-dependent electrophoretic migration and separation of liposomes by capillary zone electrophoresis in electrolyte solutions of various ionic strengths. *Anal. Chem.* 2000;72(24):5955–5960.

94. **Duffy, CF., Gafoor, S., Richards, DP., Admadzadeh, H., O'Kennedy, R., and Arriaga, EA.** Determination of properties of individual liposomes by capillary electrophoresis with postocolumn laser-induced fluorescence detection. *Anal. Chem.* 2001;73(8):1855–1861.

95. **Pysher, MD. and Hayes, MA.** Examination of the electrophoretic behavior of liposomes. *Langmuir* 2004;20(11):4369–4375.

96. **Sharpe, PT.** The partition of charged liposomes in aqueous two-phase systems. *Mol. Cell Biochem.* 1985;68(2): 151–159.

97. **Tilcock, C., Chin, R., Veiro, J., Cullis, P., and Fisher, D.** Detection of surface charge-related properties in model membrane systems by aqueous two-phase partition. *Biochim. Biophys. Acta* 1989;986(1):167–171.

98. **Nakagaki, M., Katoh, I., and Handa, T.** Surface potential of lipid membrane estimated from the partitioning of methylene blue into liposomes. *Biochem.* 1981;20(8):2208–2212.

99. **Tortorella, D. and London, E.** Method for efficient pelleting of small unilamellar model membrane vesicles. *Anal. Biochem.* 1994;217(2):176–180.

100. **Lelkes, PI.** Methodological aspects dealing with stability measurements of liposomes *in vitro* using the carboxyfluorescein assay, in Liposome Technology: Targetted Drug Delivery and Biological Interaction, (Gregoriadis, G., ed.), CRC Press, Boca Raton, 1984, pp. 225–246.

101. **Dipali, SR., Kulkarni, SB., and Betageri, GV.** Comparative study of separation of non-encapsulated drug from unilamellar liposomes by various methods. *J. Pharm. Pharmacol.* 1996;48(11):1112–1125.

102. **Kulkarni, SB., Betageri, GV., and Singh, M.** Factors affecting microencapsulation of drugs in liposomes. *J. Microencapsul.* 1995;12(3):229–246.

103. **Hope, MJ., Bally, MB., Webb, G., and Cullis, PR.** Production of large unilamellar vesicles by a rapid extrusion procedure: characterization of size distribution and ability to maintain a membrane potential. *Biochim. Biophys. Acta* 1985;812:55–65.

104. **Furman, A. and Saygin, O.** Internal volume determination of liposomes by a rapid equilibrium technique using hydrogen iodide as a marker. *Biotechnol. Tech.* 1992;6(4):299–304.

105. **Gruber, HJ., Wilmsen, HU., Schurga, A., Pilger, A., and Schindler, H.** Measurement of intravesicular volumes by salt entrapment. *Biochim. Biophys. Acta* 1995;1240(2):266–276.

106. **Anzai, K., Higashi, K., and Kirino, Y.** Rapid determination of internal volumes of membrane vesicles with electron spin resonance-stopped flow technique. *Biochim. Biophys Acta* 1988;937(1):73–80.

107. **Metso, AJ., Zhao, H., Tuunainen, I., and Kinnunen, PKJ.** Observation of the main phase transition of dinervonoylphosphocholine giant liposomes by fluorescence microscopy. *Biochim. Biophys. Acta* 2005;1713(2):83–91.

108. **Yager, P., Sheridan, JP., and Peticolas, WL.** Changes in size and shape of liposomes undergoing chain melting transitions as studied by optical microscopy. *Biochim. Biophys. Acta* 1982;693(2):485–491.

109. **Csiszár, A., Koglin, E., Meier, RJ., and Klumpp, E.** The phase transition behavior of 1,2-dipalmitoyl-sn-glycero-3-phosphocholine (DPPC) model membrane influenced by 2,4-dichlorophenol—an FT-Raman spectroscopy study. *Chem. Phys. Lipids* 2006;139(2):115–124.

110. **Blok, MC., van der Neut-Kok, EC., van Deenen, LL., and de Gier, J.** The effect of chain length and lipid phase transitions on the selective permeability properties of liposomes. *Biochim. Biophys. Acta* 1975;406(2):187–196.

111. **Cullis, PR., De Kruyff, B., and Richards, RE.** Factors affecting the motion of the polar headgroup in phospholipid bilayers. A ^{31}P NMR study of unsonicated phosphatidylcholine liposomes. *Biochim. Biophys. Acta* 1976;426(3):433–446.

112. **Mills, JK. and Needham, D.** Lysolipid incorporation in dipalmitoylphosphatidylcholine bilayer membranes enhances the ion permeability and drug release rates at the membrane phase transition. *Biochim. Biophys. Acta.* 2005;1716(2):77–96.

113. **Juliano, RL. and Stamp, D.** Interactions of drugs with lipid membranes: characteristics of liposomes containing polar or non-polar antitumur drugs. *Biochim. Biophys. Acta* 1979;586(1):137–145.

114. **Campbell, RB., Balasubramanian, SV., and Straubinger, RM.** Phospholipid-cationic lipid interactions: influences on membrane and vesicle properties. *Biochim. Biophys. Acta* 2001;1512(1):27–39.

115. **Scherphof, G., Morselt, H., Regts, J., and Wilschut, JC.** The involvement of the lipid phase transition in the plasma-induced dissolution of multilamellar phosphatidylcholine vesicles. *Biochim. Biophys. Acta* 1979;556:196–207.

116. **Cevc, G. and Richardsen, H.** Lipid vesicles and membrane fusion. *Adv. Drug Deliv. Rev.* 1999;38(3):207–232.

117. **Mobley, WC. and Schreier, H.** Phase transition temperature reduction and glass formation in dehydroprotected lyophilized liposomes. *J. Control. Rel.* 1994;31(1):73–87.

118. **Biltonen, RL. and Lichtenberg, D.** The use of differential scanning calorimetry as a tool to characterize liposome preparations. *Chem. Phys. Lipids* 1993;64(1–3):129–142.

119. **Papisov, MI.** Modeling *in vivo* transfer of long circulating polymers (two classes of long circulating polymers and factors affecting their transfer *in vivo*). *Adv. Drug. Deliv. Rev.* 1995;16:127–139.

120. **Young, NM. and Leon, MA.** The carbohydrate specificity of conglutinin and its homology to proteins in the hepatic lectin family. *Biochem. Biophys. Res. Commun.* 1987;143:645–651.

121. **Tobias, PS., Soldau, K., Kline, L., et al.** Cross-linking of lipopolysaccharide (LPS) to CD14 on THP-1 cells mediated by LPS-binding protein. *J. Immunol.* 1993;150:3011–3021.

122. **Savill, J., Dransfield, I., Hogg, N., and Haslett, C.** Vitronectin receptor-mediated phagocytosis of cells undergoing apoptosis. *Nature* 1990;343:170–173.

123. **Pinteric, L., Assimeh, SM., Kells, DIC., and Painter, RH.** The ultrastructure of C1t, a subcomponent of the first component of complement: an EM and ultracentrifuge study. *J. Immunol.* 1976;117:79–83.

124. **Saxena, U., Nagpurkar, A., Dolphin, PJ., and Mookerjea, S.** A study on the selective binding of apoprotein B- and E-containing human plasma lipoproteins to immobilised rat serum phosphorylcholine-binding protein. *J. Biol. Chem.* 1987;262:3011–3016.

125. **Kottgen, E., Hell, B., Kage, A., and Tauber, R.** Lectin specificity and binding characteristics of human C-reactive protein. *J. Immunol.* 1992;149:445–453.

126. **Stolnik, S., Illum, L., and Davis, SS.** Long circulating microparticulate drug carriers. *Adv. Drug. Deliv. Rev.* 1995;16:195–214.

127. **Allen, TM.** The use of glycolipids and hydrophilic polymers in avoiding rapid uptake of liposomes by the mononuclear phagocyte system. *Adv. Drug. Deliv. Rev.* 1994;13:285–309.

128. **Petrak, K.** Design and properties of particulate carriers for intravacular administration, in Pharmaceutical Particulate Carriers, (Rolland, A., ed.), Marcel Dekker, Inc., New York, 1993, pp. 275–297.

129. **Allen, TM., Brandeis, E., Hansen, CB., Kao, GY., and Zalipsky, S.** A new strategy for attachment of antibodies to sterically stabilized liposomes resulting in efficient targeting to cancer cells. *Biochim. Biophys. Acta.* 1995;1237:99–108.

130. **Hwang, KJ., Luk, KFS., and Beaumier, PL.** Hepatic uptake and degradation of unilamellar sphingomyelin/cholesterol liposomes: a kinetic study. *Proc. Natl. Acad. Sci. USA* 1980;77:4030–4034.

131. **Senior, J., Delgado, C., Fisher, D., Tilcock, C., and Gregoriadis, G.** Influence of surface hydrophilicity of liposomes on their interaction with plasma protein and clearance from the circulation: studies with poly(ethyleneglycol)-coated vesides. *Biochim. Biophys. Acta* 1991;1062:77–82.

132. **Allen, TM. and Chonn, A.** Large unilamellar liposomes with low uptake into the reticuloendothelial system. *FEBS Lett.* 1987;223:42–46.

133. **Gabizon, A. and Papahadjopoulos, D.** Liposome formulations with prolonged circulatuion time in blood and enhanced uptake by tumors. *Proc. Natl. Acad. Sci.* 1988;85:6949–6953.

134. **Patel, HM., Tuzel, NS., and Ryman, BE.** Inhibitory effect of cholesterol on the uptake of liposomes by liver and spleen. *Biochim. Biophys. Acta.* 1983;761:142–151.

135. **Woodle, MC.** Sterically stabilised liposome therapeutics. *Adv. Drug. Deliv. Rev.* 1995;16:249–265.

136. **Allen, TM., Hansen, C., and Rutledge, J.** Liposomes with prolonged circulation times: factors affecting uptake by reticuloendothelical and other tissues. *Biochim. Biophys. Acta* 1989;981:27–35.

137. **Liu, D. and Huang, L.** pH-sensitive, plasma stable liposomes with relatively prolonged residence in circulation. *Bichim. Biophys. Acta.* 1990;1022:348–354.

138. **Liu, D., Mori, A., and Huang, L.** Role of liposome size and RES blockage in controlling biodistribution and tumor uptake of GM_1-containing liposomes. *Biochim. Biophys. Acta.* 1992;1104:95–101.

139. **Klibanov, AL., Maruyama, K., Beckerleg, AM., Torchilin, VP., and Huang, L.** Activity of amphipathic poly(ethylene glycol) 5000 to prolong the circulation time of liposomes depends on the liposome size and is unfavourable for immunoliposome binding to target. *Biochim. Biophys. Acta.* 1991;1062: 142–148.

140. **Liu, D., Mori, A., and Huang, L.** Large liposomes containing ganglioside GM_1 accumulate effectively in spleen. *Biochim. Biophys. Acta* 1991;1066:159–165.

141. **Mori, A., Liu, D., and Huang, L.** Novel immunoliposome targeting system avoiding reticuloendothelial cell interactions, in Drug Targeting and Delivery: Concepts in Dosage From Design, (Junginger, HE., ed.), Ellis Horwood Limited, England, 1992, pp. 26–42.

142. **Maruyama, K., Kennel, SJ., and Huang, L.** Lipid composition is important for highly efficient target binding and retention of immunoliposomes. *Proc. Natl. Acad. Sci.* 1990;87:5744–5748.

143. **Mori, A., Klibanov, AL., Torchilin, VP., and Huang, L.** Influence of the steric barrier activity of amphipathic poly (ethylene

glycol) and ganglioside GM_1 on the circulation time of liposomes and on the target binding of immunoliposomes *in vivo*. *FEBS Lett.* 1991;284:263–266.

144. **Moghimi, SM. and Patel, HM.** Tissue specific opsoinins for phagocytic cells and their different affinity for cholesterol rich liposomes. *FEBS Lett.* 1988;233:143–147.

145. **Park, YS., Maruyama, K., and Huang, L.** Some negatively charged phospholid derivatives prolong the liposome circulation *in vivo*. *Biochim. Biophys. Acta* 1992;1108:257–260.

146. **Park, YS. and Huang, L.** Effect of chemically modified GM_1 and neoglycolipid analogs of GM_1 on liposome circulation time: evidence supporting the dysopsonin hypothesis. *Biochim. Biophys. Acta* 1993;1166:105–114.

147. **Klibanov, AL., Maruyama, K., Torchilin, VP., and Huang, L.** Amphipathic polyethylene glycols effecively prolong the circulation time of liposomes. *FEBS Lett.* 1990;268:235–237.

148. **Blume, G. and Cevc, G.** Liposomes for the sustained drug release in vivo. *Biochim. Biophys. Acta* 1990;1029:91–97.

149. **Senior, JH., Trimble, KR. and Maskiewicz, R.** Interaction of positively charged liposomes with blood: implications for their applications *in vivo*. *Biochim. Biophys. Acta* 1991;1070:173–179.

150. **Woodle, MC. and Lasic, DD.** Sterically stabilised liposomes. *Biochim. Biophys. Acta* 1992;1113:171–199.

151. **Crommelin, DJA. and Schreir, H.** Liposomes, in Colloidal Drug Delivery Systems, (Kreuter, J., ed.), Marcel-Dekker, Inc., New York, 1994, pp. 73–190.

152. **Zalipsky, S.** Chemistry of polyethylene glycol conjugates with biologically active molecules. *Adv. Drug. Deliv. Rev.* 1995;16:157–182.

153. **Woodle, MC.** Poly (ethylene glycol)-grafted liposome therapeutics, In: Poly(ethylene glycol) Chemistry and Biological Applications, (Harris, JM. and Zalipsky, S., eds.), American Chemical Society, USA, 1997, pp. 60–81.

154. **Parr, MJ., Ansell, SM., Choi, LS., and Cullis, PR.** Factors influencing the retention and chemical stability of poly(ethylene glycol)-lipid conjugates incorporated into large unilamellar vesides. *Biochim. Biophys. Acta* 1994;1195:21–30.

155. **Allen, TM., Hansen, C., Martin, F., Redemann, C. and Yau-Young, A.** Liposomes containing synthetic derivatives of poly (ethyleneglycol) show prolonged circulation half-lives *in vivo. Biochim. Biophys. Acta* 1991;1066:29–36.

156. **Woodle, MC., Matthay, KK., Newman, MS., et al.** Versatility in lipid composition showing prolonged circulation with sterically stabilised liposomes. *Biochim. Biophys. Acta* 1992a;1105:193–200.

157. **Tilcock, C., Ahkong, QF., and Fisher, D.** Polymer-derivatized technitium $99m_{Tc}$-labelled liposomal blood pool agents for nuclear medicine applications. *Biochim. Biophys. Acta* 1993;1148:77–84.

158. **Parr, MJ., Bally, MB., and Cullis, PR.** The presence of GM1 in liposomes with entrapped doxorubicin does not prevent RES blockade. *Biochim. Biophys. Acta* 1993;1168:249–252.

159. **Herron, JN., Gentry, CA., Davies, SS., Wei, A., and Lin, JN.** Antibodies as targeting moieties: affinity measurements, conjugation chemistry and applications in immunoliposomes. *J. Control. Release* 1994;28:155–166.

160. **Blume, G., Cevc, G., Crommelin, MDJA., Bakker-Woudenberg, IAJM., Kluft, C., and Storm, G.** Specific targeting with poly(ethylene glycol)- modified liposomes: coupling of homing devices to the ends of the polymeric chains combines effective target binding with long circulation times. *Biochim. Biophys. Acta* 1993;149:180–184.

161. **Zalipsky, S., Brandes, E., Newmqan, MS., and Woodle, MC.** Long circulating, cationic liposomes containing amino-PEG-phosphatidyl ethsanolamine. *FEBS Lett.* 1994;353:71–74.

162. **Carrion, C., Domingo, JC., and DE Madariaga, MA.** Preparation of long-circulating immunoliposomes using PEG-cholesterol conjugates: effect of the spacer arm between PEG and cholesterol on liposomal characteristics. *Chem. Phys. Lipids* 2001;113(1–2):97–110.

163. **Vertut-Doi, A., Ishiwata, H., and Miyajima, K.** Binding and uptake of liposomes containing a poly(ethylene glycol) derivative of cholesterol (stealth liposomes) by the macrophage cell line J774: influence of PEG content and its molecular weight. *Biochim Biophys Acta* 1996;1278(1):19–28.

164. **Ishiwata, H., Sato, SB., Vertut-Doi, A., Hamashima, Y., and Miyajima, K.** Cholesterol derivative of poly (ethylene glycol) inhibits clathrin-independent, but not clathrin-dependent endocytosis. *Biochim. Biophys. Acta* 1997;1359(2):123–135.

165. **Ishiwata, H., Sato, SB., Kobayashi, S., Oku, M., Vertut-Doi, A., and Miyajima, K.** Poly (ethylene glycol) derivative of cholesterol reduces binding step of liposome uptake by murine macrophage-like cell line J774 and human hepatoma cell line HepG2. *Chem. Pharm. Bull.* 1998;46(12):1907–1913.

166. **Torchilin, VP., Levchenko, TS., Lukyanov, AN., et al.** p-Nitrophenylcarbonyl-PEG-PE-liposomes: fast and simple attachment of specific ligands, including monoclonal antibodies, to distal ends of PEG chains via p-nitrophenylcarbonyl groups. *Biochim. Biophys. Acta* 2001;1511(2):397–411.

167. **Gabizon, A. and Papahadjopoulos, D.** The role of surface charge and hydrophilic groups on liposome clearance in vivo. *Biochim. Biophys. Acta.* 1992;1103:94–100.

168. **Needham, D., McIntosh, TJ., and Lasic, DD.** Repulsive interactions and mechanical stability of polymer—grafted lipid membranes *Biochim. Biophys. Acta* 1992;1108:40–48.

169. **Woodle, MC., Collins, LR., Sponsler, E., Kossovsky, N., and Papahadjopoulos, D.** Sterically stabilised liposomes: reduction in electrophoretic mobility but not electrostatic surface potential. *Biophys. J.* 1992;61:902–910.

170. **Chonn, A., Semple, SC., and Cullis, PR.** Separation of large unilamellar liposomes from blood components by a spin column procedure: towards identifying plasma proteins which mediate liposome clearance *in vivo. Biochim. Biophys. Acta* 1991;1070:215–222.

171. **Chonn, A., Semple, SC., and Cullis, PR.** Association of blood proteins with large unilamellar liposomes in vivo: relation to circulation lifetimes *J. Biol. Chem.* 1992;267:18,759–18,765.

172. **Torchilin, VP. and Papisov, MI.** Why do polyethylene glycol-coated liposomes circulate so long ? *J. Liposomes Res.* 1994;4:725–739.

173. **Gref, R., Domb, A., Quellec, P., et al.** The controlled intravenous delivery of drugs using PEG-coated sterically stabilised nanospheres. *Adv. Drug. Deliv. Rev.* 1995;16:215–233.

174. **Torchilin, VP., Omelyanenko, VG., Papisov, IM., et al.** Poly (ethylene glycol) on the liposome surface: on the mechanism of polymer—coated liposome longevity. *Biochim. Biophys. Acta* 1994;1195:11–20.

175. **Torchilin, VP. and Trubetskoy, VS.** Which polymers can make nanoparticulate drug carriers long-circulating. *Adv. Drug. Deliv. Rev.* 1995;16:141–155.

176. **Bedu-Addo, FK. and Huang, L.** Interaction of PEG-phospholipid conjugates with phospholipid: implications in liposomal drug delivery. *Adv. Drug. Deliv. Rev.* 1995;16:235–247.

177. **Torchilin, VP., Shtilman, MI., Trubetskoy, VS., Whiteman, K., and Milstein, AM.** Amphiphilic vinyl polymers effectively prolong liposome circulation time in vivo. *Biochim. Biophys. Acta* 1994a;1195:181–184.

178. **Zalipsky, S., Hansen, CB., Oaks, JM., and Allen, TM.** Evaluation of blood clearance rates and biodistribution of poly(z-oxazoline)-grafted liposomes. *J. Pharm. Sci.* 1996;85:133–137.

179. **Maruyama, K., Okuizumi, S., Ishida, O., Yamauchi, H., Kikuchi, H., and Iwatsuru, M.** Phosphatidy polyglyceols prolong liposome circulation *in vivo*, *Int. J. Pharm.* 1994;111:103–107.

180. **Illum, L. and Davis, SS.** The organ uptake of intravenously administered colioidal particles can be altered using non-ionic surfactant (poloxamer 338). *FEBS Lett.* 1984;167:79–82.

181. **Cartensen, H., Muller, BW., and Muller, RH.** Adsorption of ethoxylated surfactants on nanoparticles. I. Characterization by hydrophobic interaction chromatography. *Int. J. Pharm.* 1991;67:29–37.

182. **Porter, CJH., Moghimi, SM., Davies, MC., Davis, SS., and Illum, L.** Differences in the molecular weight profile of poloxamer 407 affects its ability to redirect intravenously administered colloids to the bone marrow. *Int. J. Pharm.* 1992;83:273–276.

183. **Porter, CJH., Moghimi, SM., Illum, L., and Davis, SS.** The polyoxyethylene / polyoxypropylene block copolymer poloxamer 407 selectively redirects intravenously injected microspheres to sinusoidal endothelial cells of the rabbit bone marrow. *FEBS Lett.* 1992a;305:62–66.

184. **Lukowski, G., Muller, RH., Muller, BW., and Dittgen, M.** Acrylic acid copolymer nanoparticles for drug delivery: I. Characterisation of the surface properties relevant for *in vivo* organ distribution. *Int. J. Pharm.* 1992;84:23–31.

185. **Wesemeyer, H., Muller, BW., and Muller, RH.** Adsorption of ethoxylated surfactants on nanoparticles: II. Determination of adsorption enthalpy by microcalorimetry. *Int. J. Pharm.* 1993;89:33–40.

186. **Muller, RH. and Wallis, KH.** Surface modification of i.v. injectable biodegradable nannoparticles with poloxamer polymers and poloxamine 908. *Int. J. Pharm.* 1993;89:25–31.

187. **Rudt, S. and Muller, RH.** *In-vitro* phagocytosis assay of nano- and microparticles by chemiluminescence: II. Effect of surface modification by coating of particles with plolxamer on the phagocytic uptake. *J. Control. Release* 1993;25:51–59.

188. **Jamshaid, M., Farr, SJ., Kearney, P., and Kellaway, IW.** Polyoxamer sorption on liposomes: comparision with polystyrene latex and influence on solute efflux. *Int. J. Pharm.* 1988;48:125–131.

189. **Moghimi, SM. and Patel, HS.** Serum opsonins and phagocytosis of saturated and unsaturated phospholipid liposomes. *Biochim. Biophys. Acta* 1989;984:384–387.

190. **Moghimi, SM., Porter, CJH., Illum, L., and Davis, SS.** The effect of polyoxamer-407 on liposome stability and targeting to bone marrow: comparison with polystyrene microspheres. *Int. J. Pharm.* 1991;68:121–126.

191. **Kronberg, B., Dahlman, A., Carlfors, J., Karlsson, J., and Artursson, P.** Preparation and evaluation of sterically stabilized liposomes: colloidal stability, serum stability, macrophage uptake, and toxicity. *J. Pharm. Sci.* 1990;79:667–671.

192. **Kumar, S., Singh, T., Khar, RK., Sharma, SN., and Chauhan, UP.** Evaluation of sterically stabilized liposomes as a vehicle for targeting technetium-99m labelled radiopharmaceuticals. *Pharmazie* 1993;48:613–616.

193. **Metselaar, JM., Bruin, P., de Boer, LW., et al.** A novel family of L-amino acid-based biodegradable polymer-lipid conjugates for the development of long-circulating liposomes with effective drug-targeting capacity. *Bioconjug. Chem.* 2003;14(6):1156–1164.

194. **Romberg, B., Metselaar, JM., deVringer, T., et al.** Enzymatic degradation of liposome-grafted poly(hydroxyethyl L-glutamine). *Bioconjug. Chem.* 2005;16(4):767–774.

195. **Riche, EL., Erickson, BW., and Cho, MJ.** Novel long-circulating liposomes containing peptide library-lipid conjugates: synthesis and in vivo behavior. *J. Drug Target.* 2004;12(6):355–361.

196. **Oku, N. and Namba, Y.** Glucuronate-modified, long-circulating liposomes for the delivery of anticancer agents. *Methods Enzymol.* 2005;391:145–162.

197. **Vermehren, C., Hansen, HS., Clausen-Beck, B., and Frokjaer, S.** In vitro and in vivo aspects of N-acyl-phosphatidylethanolamine-containing liposomes. *Int. J. Pharm.* 2003;254(1):49–53.

198. **Moghimi, SM., Muir, IS., Illum, L., Davis, SS., and Kolb-Bachofen, V.** Coating particles with a block copolymer (poloxamine 908) suppress opsonization but permits the activity of dysopsonins in the serum. *Biochim. Biophys. Acta* 1993;1179:157–165.

199. **Soma, CE., Dubernet, C., Barratt, G., Benita, S., and Couvreur, P.** Investigation of the role of macrophages on the cytotoxicity of doxorubicin and doxorubicin-loaded nanoparticles on M5076 control cells *in vitro*. *J. Control Rel.* 2000;68(2):283–289.

200. **Martin, FJ.** In: Medical Applications of Liposomes, (Lasic, DD. and Papahadjopoulos, D., eds.), Elsevier Science B.V., New York, 1998, pp. 635–688.

201. **Xu, Y. and Szoka, FC. Jr.** Mechanism of DNA release from cationic liposome/DNA complexes used in cell transfection. *Biochem.* 1996;35:5616–5623.

202. **Zelphati, O. and Szoka, FC.** Intracellular distribution and mechanism of delivery of oligonucleotides mediated by cationic lipids. *Pharm. Res.* 1996;13:1367–1372.

203. **Hong, KL., Zheng, WW., Baker, A., and Papahadjopoulos, D.** Stabilization of cationic liposome-plasmid DNA complexes by polyamines and poly(ethylene glycol)-phospholipid conjugates for efficient *in vivo* gene delivery. *FEBS Lett.* 1997;400:233–237.

204. **Yatvin, MB., Weinstein, JN., Dennis, WH., and Blumenthal, R.** Design of liposomes for enhanced local release of drugs by hyperthermia. *Science* 1978;202:1290–1293.

205. **Gaber, MH., Hong, K., Huang, SK., and Papahadjopoulos, D.** Thermosensitive sterically stabilized liposomes: formulation and in vitro studies on mechanism of doxorubicin release by bovine serum and human plasma. *Pharm. Res.* 1995;12:1407–1416.

206. **Gaber, MH., Wu, NZ., Hong, K., Huang, SK., Dewhirst, MW., and Papahadjopoulos, D.** Thermosensitive liposomes: extravasation and release of contents in tumor microvascular networks. *Int. J. Radiat. Oncol. Biol. Phys.* 1996;36:1177–1187.

207. **Straubinger, RM., Duzgunes, N., and Papahadjopoulos, D.** pH-sensitive liposomes mediate cytoplasmic delivery of encapsulated macromolecules. *FEBS Lett.* 1985;179:148–154.

208. **Litzinger, DC. and Huang, L.** Phosphatidylethanolamine liposomes: drug delivery, gene transfer and immunodiagnostic applications. *Biochim. Biophys. Acta* 1992;1113:201–227.

209. **Meyer, O., Papahadjopoulos, D., and Leroux, JC.** Copolymers of N-isopropylacrylamide can trigger pH sensitivity to stable liposomes. *FEBS Lett.* 1998;421:61–64.

210. **Yatvin, MB., Kreutz, W., Horwitz, BA., and Shinitzky, M.** pH-sensitive liposomes: possible clinical implications. *Science* 1980;210:1253–1255.

211. **Huang, SK., Mayhew, E., Gilani, S., Lasic, DD., Martin, FJ., and Papahadjopoulos, D.** Pharmacokinetics and therapeutics of sterically stabilized liposomes in mice bearing C-26 colon carcinoma. *Cancer Res.* 1992;52:6774–6781.

212. **Dellian, M., Helmlinge, G., Yuan, F., and Jain, RK.** Fluorescence ratio imaging of interstitial pH in solid tumors: effect of glucose on spatial and temporal gradients. *Br. J. Cancer* 1996;74:1206–1215.

213. **Helmlinger, G., Yuan, F., Dellian, M., and Jain, RK.** Interstitial pH and pO_2 gradients in solid tumors in vivo: high-resolution measurements reveal a lack of correlation. *Nature Med.* 1997;3:177–182.

214. **Ohkuma, S. and Poole, B.** Fluorescence probe measurement of the intralysosomal pH in living cells and the perturbation of pH by various agents. *Proc. Natl. Acad. Sci. USA* 1978;75:3327–3331.

215. **Tycko, B. and Maxfield, FR.** Rapid acidification of endocytic vesicles containing alpha 2-macroglobulin. *Cell* 1982;28:643–651.

216. **Daleke, DL., Hong, K., and Papahadjopoulos, D.** Endocytosis of liposomes by macrophages: binding, acidification and leakage of liposomes monitored by a new fluorescence assay. *Biochim. Biophys. Acta.* 1990;1024:352–366.

217. **Straubinger, RM., Hong, K., Friend, DS., and Papahadjopoulos, D.** Endocytosis of liposomes and intracellular fate of encapsulated molecules: encounter with a low pH compartment after internalization in coated vesicles. *Cell* 1983;32:1069–1079.

218. **Huang, A., Kennel, SJ., and Huang, L.** Interactions of immunoliposomes with target cells. *J. Biol. Chem.* 1983;258:14,034–14,040.

219. **Dijkstra, J., Van Galen, M., and Scherphof, GL.** Effects of ammonium chloride and chloroquine on endocytic uptake of liposomes by Kupffer cells *in vitro*. *Biochim. Biophys. Acta* 1984;804:58–67.

220. **Anderson, RGW. and Orci, L.** A view of acidic intracellular compartments. *J. Cell Biol.* 1988;106:539–543.

221. **Plagemann, PGW., Marz, R., and Wohlhueter, RM.** Transport and metabolism of deoxycytidine and 1-beta-D-arabinofuranosylcytosine into cultured Novikoff rat hepatoma cells, relationship to phosphorylation, and regulation of triphosphate synthesis. *Cancer Res.* 1978;38:978–989.

222. **Wiley, JS., Jones, SP., Sawyer, WH., and Paterson, ARP.** Cytosine arabinoside influx and nucleoside transport sites in acute leukemia. *J. Clin. Invest.* 1982;69:479–489.

223. **Brown, PM. and Silvius, JR.** Mechanisms of delivery of liposome-encapsulated cytosine arabinoside to CV-1 cells in vitro. Fluorescence-microscopic and cytotoxicity studies. *Biochim. Biophys. Acta* 1990;1023:341–351.

224. **Kamen, BA., Smith, AK., and Anderson, RGW.** The folate receptor works in tandem with a probenecid-sensitive carrier in MA104 cells in vitro. *J. Clin. Invest.* 1991;87:1442–1449.

225. **Kirpotin, D., Hong, K., Mullah, N., and Papahadjopoulos, D.** Liposomes with detachable polymer coating: destabilization and fusion of dioleoylphosphatidylethanolamine vesicles triggered by cleavage of surface-grafted poly(ethylene glycol). *FEBS Lett.* 1996;388:115–118.

226. **Drummond, DC. and Daleke, DL.** Synthesis and characterization of N-acylated, pH-sensitive 'caged' aminophospholipids. *Chem. Phys. Lipids* 1995;75:27–41.

227. **Gerasimov, OV., Schwan, A., and Thompson, DH.** Acid-catalyzed lasmenylcholine hydrolysis and its effect on bilayer permeability: a quantitative study. *Biochim. Biophys. Acta* 1997;1324:200–214.

228. **Rui, Y., Wang, S., Low, PS., and Thompson, DH.** Diplasmenylcholine-folate liposomes: an efficient vehicle for intracellular drug delivery. *J. Am. Chem. Soc.* 1998;120: 11,213–11,218.

229. **Parente, RA., Nir, S., and Szoka, FC.** Jr. pH-dependent fusion of phosphatidylcholine small vesicles. Induction by a synthetic amphipathic peptide. *J. Biol. Chem.* 1988;263:4724–4730.

230. **Rafalski, M., Ortiz, A., Rockwell, A., et al.** Membrane fusion activity of the influenza virus hemagglutinin: interaction of HA2 N-terminal peptides with phospholipid vesicles. *Biochem.* 1991;30:10,211–10,220.

231. **Puyal, C., Maurin, L., Miquel, G., Bienvenue, A., and Philippot, J.** Design of a short membrane-destabilizing peptide covalently bound to liposomes. *Biochim. Biophys. Acta* 1994;1195:259–266.

232. **Vogel, K., Wang, S., Lee, RJ., Chmielewski, J., and Low, PS.** Peptide-mediated release of folate-targeted liposome content from endosomal compartments. *J. Am. Chem. Soc.* 1996;118:1581–1586.

233. **Bailey, AL., Monck, MA., and Cullis, PR.** pH-induced destabilization of lipid bilayers by a lipopeptide derived from influenza hemagglutinin. *Biochim. Biophys. Acta* 1997;1324:232–244.

234. **Tirrell, DA., Takigawa, DY., and Seki, K.** pH sensitization of phospholipid vesicles via complexation with synthetic poly(carboxylic acid)s. *Ann. NY Acad. Sci.* 1985;446:237–248.

235. **Kono, K., Zenitani, K., and Takagishi, T.** Novel pH-sensitive liposomes: liposomes bearing a poly(ethylene glycol) derivative with carboxyl groups. *Biochim. Biophys. Acta* 1994;1193:1–9.

236. **Zignani, M., Drummond, DC., Meyer, O., Hong, K., and Leroux, JC.** In vitro characterization of a novel polymeric-based pH-sensitive liposome system. *Biochim. Biophys. Acta* 2000;1463:383–394.

237. **Roux, E., Francis, M., Winnik, FM., and Leroux, JC.** Polymer based pH-sensitive carriers as a means to improve the cytoplasmic delivery of drugs. *Int. J. Pharm.* 2002;242:25–36.

238. **Torchilin, VP., Zhou, F., and Huang, L.** pH-sensitive liposomes. *J. Liposome Res.* 1993;3:201–255.

239. **Duzgunes, N., Straubinger, RM., Baldwin, PA., and Papahadjopoulos, D.** In: Membrane Fusion, (Wilschut, J. and Hoekstra, D., eds.), Marcel Dekker, New York, 1991, pp. 713–730.

240. **Connor, J., Yatvin, MB., and Huang, L.** pH-sensitive liposomes: acid-induced liposome fusion. *Proc. Natl. Acad. Sci. USA* 1984;81:1715–1718.

241. **Collins, D., Maxfield, F., and Huang, L.** Immunoliposomes with different acid sensitivities as probes for the cellular endocytic pathway. *Biochim. Biophys. Acta* 1989;987:47–55.

242. **Bentz, J., Ellens, H., and Szoka, FC.** Destabilization of phosphatidylethanolamine-containing liposomes: hexagonal phase and asymmetric membranes. *Biochem.* 1987;26:2105–2116.

243. **Duzgunes, N., Straubinger, RM., Baldwin, PA., Friend, DS., and Papahadjopoulos, D.** Proton-induced fusion of oleic acid-phosphatidylethanolamine liposomes. *Biochem.* 1985;24:3091–3098.

244. **Ellens, H., Bentz, J., and Szoka, FC.** H^+- and Ca^{2+}-induced fusion and destabilization of liposomes. *Biochem.* 1985;24:3099–3106.

245. **Nayar, R. and Schroit, AJ.** Generation of pH-sensitive liposomes: use of large unilamellar vesicles containing N-succinyldioleoylphos-phatidylethanolamine. *Biochem.* 1985;24:5967–5971.

246. **Verkleij, AJ.** In: Membrane Fusion, (Wilschut, J. and Hoekstra, D., eds.), Marcel Dekker, New York, 1991, pp. 155–166.

247. **Siegel, DP.** Energetics of intermediates in membrane fusion: comparison of stalk and inverted micellar intermediate mechanisms. *Biophys. J.* 1993;65:2124–2140.

248. **Chernomordik, L.** Non-bilayer lipids and biological fusion intermediates. *Chem. Phys. Lipids* 1996;81:203–213.

249. **Cullis, PR. and De Kruijff, B.** Lipid polymorphism and the functional roles of lipids in biological membranes. *Biochim. Biophys. Acta* 1979;559:399–420.

250. **Sundler, R., Duzgunes, N., and Papahadjopoulos, D.** Control of membrane fusion by phospholipid head groups. II. The role of phosphatidylethanolamine in mixtures with phosphatidate and phosphatidylinositol. *Biochim. Biophys. Acta* 1981;649:751–758.

251. **Nir, S.** In: Membrane Fusion, (Wilschut, J. and Hoekstra, D., eds.), Marcel Dekker, New York, 1991, pp. 127–153.

252. **Ellens, H., Bentz, J., and Szoka, FC.** pH-induced destabilization of phosphatidylethanolamine containing liposomes: role of bilayer contact. *Biochemistry* 1984;23:1532–1538.

253. **Hauser, H., Pascher, I., Pearson, RH., and Sundell, S.** Preferred conformation and molecular packing of phosphatidylethanolamine and phosphatidylcholine. *Biochim. Biophys. Acta* 1981;650:21–51.

254. **Boggs, JM.** Lipid intermolecular hydrogen bonding: influence on structural organization and membrane function. *Biochim. Biophys. Acta* 1987;906:353–404.

255. **Papahadjopoulos, D., Poste, G., Schaeffer, BE., and Vail, WJ.** Membrane fusion and molecular segregation in phospholipid vesicles. *Biochim. Biophys. Acta* 1974;352:10–28.

256. **Jacobson, K. and Papahadjopoulos, D.** Phase transitions and phase separations in phospholipid membranes induced by changes in temperature, pH, and concentration of bivalent cations. *Biochem.* 1975;14:152–161.

257. **Hoekstra, D.** Role of lipid phase separations and membrane hydration in phospholipid vesicle fusion. *Biochem.* 1982;21:2833–2840.

258. **Wilschut, J.** In: Membrane Fusion, (Wilschut, J. and Hoekstra, D., eds.), Marcel Dekker, New York, 1991, pp. 89–126.

259. **Collins, D., Litzinge, DC., and Huang, L.** Structural and functional comparisons of pH-sensitive liposomes composed of phosphatid ylethanolamine and three different diacylsuccinylglycerols. *Biochim. Biophys. Acta* 1990;1025:234–242.

260. **Lai, MZ., Vail, WJ., and Szoka, FC.** Acid- and calcium-induced structural changes in phosphatidylethanolamine membranes stabilized by cholesteryl hemisuccinate. *Biochem.* 1990;24:1654–1661.

261. **Nayar, R., Tilcock, CPS., Hope, MJ., Cullis, PR., and Schroit, AJ.** N-succinyldioleoyl- phosphatidylethanolamine: structural preferences in pure and mixed model membranes. *Biochim. Biophys. Acta* 1988;937:31–41.

262. **Connor, J. and Huang, L.** pH-sensitive immunoliposomes as an efficient and target-specific carrier for antitumor drugs. *Cancer Res.* 1986;46:3431–3435.

263. **Lee, RJ. and Low, PS.** Folate-mediated tumor cell targeting of liposome-entrapped doxorubicin *in vitro*. *Biochim. Biophys. Acta* 1995;1233:134–144.

264. **Park, JW., Hong, K., Carter, P., Asgari, H., Guo, LY., and Keller, GA.** Development of anti-p185HER2 immunoliposomes for cancer therapy. *Proc. Natl. Acad. Sci. USA* 1995;92:1327–1331.

265. **Heath, TD., Montgomery, JA., Piper, JR., and Papahadjopoulos, D.** Antibody-targeted liposomes: increase in specific toxicity of methotrexate-gamma-aspartate. *Proc. Natl. Acad. Sci.* 1983;80:1377–1381.

266. **Matthay, KK., Abai, AM., Cobb, S., Hong, K., Papahadjopoulos, D., and Straubinger, RM.** Role of ligand in antibody-directed endocytosis of liposomes by human T-leukemia cells. *Cancer Res.* 1989;49:4879–4886.

267. **Matthay, KK., Heath, TD., and Papahadjopoulos, D.** Specific enhancement of drug delivery to AKR lymphoma by antibody-targeted small unilamellar vesicles. *Cancer Res.* 1984;44:1880–1886.

268. **Kim, JS. and Heath, TD.** Improved in vitro growth inhibitory effect of N-(phosphonacetyl)-L-aspartic acid in immunoliposomes. *J. Control. Release* 1996;40:101–109.

269. **Drummond, DC., Meyer, O., Hong, K., Kirpotin, D., and Papahadjopoulos, D.** Optimizing liposomes for delivery of chemotherapeutic agents to solid tumors. *Pharmacol. Rev.* 1999;51:691–743.

270. **Allen, TM., Hansen, CB., and Stuart, DD.** In: Medical Applications of Liposomes, (Lasic, DD. and Papahadjopoulos, D., eds.), Elsevier Science, B. V., New York, 1998, pp. 545–565.

271. **Chu, CJ., Dijkstra, J., Lai, MZ., Hong, K., and Szoka, FC.** Efficiency of cytoplasmic delivery by pH-sensitive liposomes to cells in culture. *Pharm Res* 1990;7:824–834.

272. **Collins, D. and Huang, L.** Cytotoxicity of diphtheria toxin A fragment to toxin-resistant murine cells delivered by pH-sensitive immunoliposomes. *Cancer Res.* 1987;47:735–739.

273. **Tari, AM., Fuller, N., Boni, LT., Collins, D., Rand, P., and Huang, L.** Interactions of liposome bilayers composed of 1,2-diacyl-3-succinylglycerol with protons and divalent cations. *Biochim. Biophys. Acta* 1994;1192:253–262.

274. **Reddy, R., Zhou, F., Huang, L., Carbone, F., Bevan, M., and Rouse, BT.** pH sensitive liposomes provide an efficient means of sensitizing target cells to class I restricted CTL recognition of a soluble protein. *J. Immunol. Methods* 1991;141:157–163.

275. **Zhou, F., Rouse, BT., and Huang, L.** An improved method of loading pH-sensitive liposomes with soluble proteins for class I restricted antigen presentation. *J. Immunol. Methods* 1991;145:143–152.

276. **Lee, KD., Oh, YK., Portnoy, DA., and Swanson, JA.** Delivery of macromolecules into cytosol using liposomes containing hemolysin from Listeria monocytogenes. *J. Biol. Chem.* 1996;271:7249–7252.

277. **Senior, JH.** Fate and behavior of liposomes in vivo: a review of controlling factors. *CRC Crit. Rev. Therap. Drug Carrier Sys.* 1987;3:123–193.

278. **Connor, J., Norley, N., and Huang, L.** Biodistribution of pH-sensitive immunoliposomes. *Biochim. Biophys. Acta* 1986;884:474–481.

279. **Finkelstein, MC. and Weissmann, G.** Enzyme replacement via liposomes. Variations in lipid compositions determine liposomal integrity in biological fluids. *Biochim. Biophys. Acta* 1979;587:202–216.

280. **Chonn, A., Cullis, PR., and Devine, DV.** The role of surface charge in the activation of the classical and alternative pathways of complement by liposomes. *J. Immunol.* 1991;146:4234–4241.

281. **Mold, C.** Effect of membrane phospholipids on activation of the alternative complement pathway. *J. Immunol.* 1989;5:1663–1668.

282. **Chobanian, JV., Tall, AR., and Brecher, PI.** Interaction between unilamellar egg yolk lecithin vesicles and human high density lipoprotein. *Biochem.* 1979;18:180–187.

283. **Damen, J., Dijkstra, J., Regts, J., and Scherphof, G.** Effect of lipoprotein-free plasma on the interaction of human plasma high density lipoprotein with egg yolk phosphatidylcholine liposomes. *Biochim. Biophys. Acta* 1980;620:90–99.

284. **Scherphof, G., Roerdink, F., Waite, M., and Parks, J.** Disintegration of phosphatidylcholine liposomes in plasma as a result of interaction with high-density lipoproteins. *Biochim. Biophys. Acta* 1978;542:296–307.

285. **Liu, D. and Huang, L.** Small, but not large, unilamellar liposomes composed of dioleoylphosphatidylethanolamine and oleic acid can be stabilized by human plasma. *Biochem.* 1989;28:7700–7707.

286. **Torchilin, VP., Lukyanov, AN., Klibanov, AL., Omelyanenko, VG.** Interaction between oleic acid-containing pH-sensitive and plain liposomes. Fluorescent spectroscopy studies. *FEBS Lett.* 1992;305:185–188.

287. **Liu, D. and Huang, L.** Role of cholesterol in the stability of pH-sensitive, large unilamellar liposomes prepared by the detergent-dialysis method. *Biochim. Biophys. Acta* 1989;981:254–260.

288. **Mizoue, T., Horibe, T., Maruyama, K., et al.** Targetability and intracellular delivery of anti-BCG antibody-modified, pH-sensitive fusogenic immunoliposomes to tumor cells. *Int. J. Pharm.* 2002;237:129–137.

289. **Guo, W., Gosselin, MA., and Lee, RJ.** Characterization of a novel diolein-based LPDII vector for gene delivery. *J. Control. Release* 2002;83:121–132.

290. **Shi, G., Guo, W., Stephenson, SM., and Lee, RJ.** Efficient intracellular drug and gene delivery using folate receptor-targeted pH-sensitive liposomes composed of cationic/anionic lipid combinations. *J. Control. Release* 2002;80:309–319.

291. **Sudimack, JJ., Guo, W., Tjarks, W., and Lee, RJ.** A novel pH sensitive liposome formulation containing oleyl alcohol. *Biochim. Biophys. Acta* 2002;1564:31–37.

292. **Asokan, A. and Cho, MJ.** Cytosolic delivery of macromolecules. II. Mechanistic studies with pH-sensitive morpholine lipids. *Biochim. Biophys. Acta* 2003;1611:151–160.

293. **Provoda, CJ., Stier, EM., Lee, KD.** Tumor cell killing enabled by listeriolysin O-liposome-mediated delivery of the protein toxin gelonin. *J. Biol. Chem.* 2003;278:35,102–35,108.

294. **Mastrobattista, E., Koning, GA., van Bloois, L., Filipe, ACS., Jiskoot, W., and Storm, G.** Functional characterization of an endosome-disruptive peptide and its application in cytosolic delivery of immunoliposome-entrapped proteins. *J. Biol. Chem.* 2002;277:27,135–27,143.

295. **Kamata, H., Yagisawa, H., Takahashi, S., and Hirata, H.** Amphiphilic peptides enhance the efficiency of liposome-mediated DNA transfection. *Nucleic Acids Res.* 1994;22:536–537.

296. **Kichler, A., Mechtler, K., Behr, JP., and Wagner, E.** Influence of membrane-active peptides on lipospermine/DNA complex mediated gene transfer. *Bioconjug. Chem.* 1997;8:213–221.

297. **Subbarao, NK., Parente, RA., Szoka, FC., Jr., Nadasdi, L., and Pongracz, K.** pH-dependent bilayer destabilization by an amphipathic peptide. *Biochem.* 1987;26:2964–2972.

298. **Simoes, S., Slepushkin, V., Gaspar, R., de Lima, MC., and Duzgunes, N.** Gene delivery by negatively charged ternary complexes of DNA, cationic liposomes and transferrin or fusogenic peptides. *Gene Therap.* 1998;5:955–964.

299. **Aronsohn, AI. and Hughes, JA.** Nuclear localization signal peptides enhance cationic liposome-mediated gene therapy. *J. Drug Target.* 1998;5:163–169.

300. **Schenkman, S., Araujo, PS., Dijkman, R., Quina, FH., and Chaimovich, H.** Effects of temperature and lipid composition on the serum albumin-induced aggregation and fusion of small unilamellar vesicles. *Biochim. Biophys. Acta* 1981;649:633–647.

301. **Zanta, MA., Belguise-Valladier, P., and Behr, JP.** Gene delivery: a single nuclear localization signal peptide is sufficient to carry DNA to the cell nucleus. *Proc. Natl. Acad. Sci. USA* 1999;96:91–96.

302. **Chan, CK., and Jans, DA.** Enhancement of polylysine-mediated transferrinfection by nuclear localization sequences: polylysine does not function as a nuclear localization sequence. *Hum. Gene Ther.* 1999;10:1695–1702.

303. **Plank, C., Oberhauser, B., Mechtler, K., Koch, C., and Wagner, E.** The influence of endosome-disruptive peptides on gene transfer using synthetic virus-like gene transfer systems. *J. Biol. Chem.* 1994;269:12,918–12,924.

304. **Leroux, J., Roux, E., Le Garrec, D., Hong, K., and Drummond, DC.** *N*-Isopropylacrylamide copolymers for the preparation of pH-sensitive liposomes and polymeric micelles. *J. Control. Release* 2001;72:71–84.

305. **Roux, E., Lafleur, M., Lataste, E., Moreau, P., and Leroux, JC.** On the characterization of pH-sensitive liposome/polymer complexes. *Biomacromolecules* 2003;4:240–248.

306. **Roux, E., Stomp, R., Giasson, S., Pezolet, M., Moreau, P., and Leroux, JC.** Steric stabilization of liposomes by pH-responsive N-isopropylacrylamide copolymer. *J. Pharm. Sci.* 2002;91:1795–1802.

307. **Slepushkin, VA., Simoes, S., Dazin, P., et al.** Sterically stabilized pH-sensitive liposomes. Intracellular delivery of aqueous contents and prolonged circulation *in vivo*. *J. Biol. Chem.* 1997;272(4):2382–2388.

308. **Kono, K., Igawa, T., and Takagishi, T.** Cytoplasmic delivery of calcein mediated by liposomes modified with a pH-sensitive poly (ethylene glycol) derivative. *Biochim. Biophys. Acta* 1997;1325(2):143–154.

309. **Hong, MS., Lim, SJ., Oh, YK., and Kim, CK.** pH-sensitive, serum-stable and long-circulating liposomes as a new drug delivery system. *J. Pharm. Pharmacol.* 2002;54(1):51–58.

310. **Fattal, E., Couvreur, P., and Dubernet, C.** Smart delivery of antisense oligonucleotides by anionic pH-sensitive liposomes. *Adv. Drug Deliv. Rev.* 2004;56(7):931–946.

311. **Roux, E., Passirani, C., Scheffold, S., Benoit, JP., and Leroux, JC.** Serum-stable and long-circulating, PEGylated, pH-sensitive liposomes. *J. Control. Release* 2004;94(2–3):447–451.

312. **Simoes, S., Moreira, JN., Fonseca, C., Duzgunes, N., and DE Lima, MC.** On the formulation of pH-sensitive liposomes with long circulation times. *Adv. Drug Deliv. Rev.* 2004;56(7):947–965.

313. **Juliano, RL. and Layton, D.** Liposomes as drug delivery system, in Drug Delivery System, (Juliano, RL., ed.), Oxford University Press, Oxford, UK, 1980, pp. 189–236.

314. **Gregoriadis, G. and Neerunjun, DE.** Homing of liposomes to target cells. *Biochem. Biophys. Res. Commun.* 1975;65:537–544.

315. **Gregoriadis, G. and Ryman, BE.** Lysosomal localisation of ·fructofuranoside containing liposomes injected into rats. *Biochem. J.* 1972;129:123–133.

316. **Huang, A., Huang, L., and Knnel, SJ.** Monoclonal antibody covalently coupled with fatty acid. *J. Biol. Chem.* 1980;255:8015–8018.

317. **Weinstein, JN., Magin, RL., Cysyk, RL., and Zaharko, DS.** Treatment of solid L1210 murine tumors with local hyperthermia and temperature-sensitive liposomes containing methotrexate. *Cancer Res.* 1980;40:1388–1395.

318. **Betageri, GV., Jenkins, SA., and Parsons, DL.** Liposome Drug Delivery Systems. Informa Healthcare, 1993, pp. 101–103.

319. **Tacker, JR. and Anderson, RU.** Delivery of antitumor drug to bladder cancer by use of phase transition liposomes and hyperthermia. *J. Urol.* 1982;127:1211–1214.

320. **Zou, YY., Ueno, M., Yamagishi, M., et al.** Targeting behaviour of hepatic artery injected temperature-sensitive liposomal adriamycin on tumor-bearing rats. *Sel. Cancer Ther.* 1990;6:119–127.

321. **Rajanaresh, RA., Udupa, N., and Uma Devi, P.** Effect of macrophage activation on niosome encapsulated bleomycin in tumor bearing mice. *Ind. J. Pharmacol.* 1996;28:175–180.

322. **Kim, J-C and Kim, J.D.** Release property of temperature-sensitive liposome containing poly(N-isopropylacrylamide). *Colloids Surf. B Biointerf.* 2002;24(1):45–52.

323. **Wu, NZ., Klitzman, B., Rosner, G., Needham, D., and Dewhirst, MW.** Measurement of material extravasation in microvascular networks using fluorescence video-microscopy. *Microvasc. Res.* 1993;46(2):231–253.

324. **Needham, D., Anyarambhatla, G., Kong, G., and Dewhirst, MW.** A new temperature-sensitive liposome for use with mild hyperthermia: characterization and testing in a human tumor xenograft model. *Cancer Res.* 2000;60(5):1197–1201.

325. **Lindner, LH., Eichhorn, ME., Eibl, H., et al.** Novel temperature-sensitive liposomes with prolonged circulation time. *Clin. Cancer Res.* 2004;10(6):2168–2178.

326. **Maruyama, K., Unezaki, S., Takahashi, N., and Iwatsuru, M.** Enhanced delivery of doxorubicin to tumor by long-circulating thermosensitive liposomes and local hyperthermia. *Biochim. Biophys. Acta* 1993;1149(2):209–216.

327. **Unezaki, S., Maruyama, K., Takahashi, N., et al.** Enhanced delivery and antitumor activity of doxorubicin using long-circulating thermosensitive liposomes containing amphipathic polyethylene glycol in combination with local hyperthermia. *Pharm. Res.* 1994;11(8):1180–1185.

328. **Chandaroy, P., Sen, A., and Hui, SW.** Temperature-controlled content release from liposomes encapsulating Pluronic F127. *J. Control. Release* 2001;76(1–2):27–37.

329. **Ning, S., Macleod, K., Abra, RM., Huang, AH., and Hahn, GM.** Hyperthermia induces doxorubicin release from long-circulating liposomes and enhances their anti-tumor efficacy. *Int. J. Radiat. Oncol. Biol. Phys.* 1994;29(4):827–834.

330. **Kong, G., Anyarambhatla, G., Petros, WP., et al.** Efficacy of liposomes and hyperthermia in a human tumor xenograft model: importance of triggered drug release. *Cancer Res.* 2000;60(24):6950–6957.

331. **Lindner, LH., Reinl, HM., Schlemmer, M., Stahl, R., and Peller, M.,** Paramagnetic thermosensitive liposomes for MR-thermometry. *Int. J. Hyperthermia* 2005;21(6):575–588.

332. **Jones, GR. and Cossins, AR.** Physical methods of study in liposomes: a practical approach, (New, RRC., ed.), Oxford University Press, New York, 1990, pp. 183–220.

333. **Abra, RM. and Hunt, CA.** Liposome disposition in vivo. III. Dose and vesicle-size effects. *Biochim. Biophys. Acta* 1981;666:493.

334. **Hwang, KJ.** In: Liposomes: From Biophysics to Therapeutics, (Ostro, MJ., ed.), Marcel Dekker, New York, 1987, 109 p.

335. **Allen, TM. and Stuart, DD.** In: Liposomes: Rational Design, (Janoff, AS., ed.), Marcel Dekker, New York, 1999, 63 p.

336. **Frezard, F., Michalick, MS., Soares, CF., and Demicheli, C.** Novel methods for the encapsulation of meglumine antimoniate into liposomes. *Braz. J. Med. Biol. Res.* 2000;33:841–846.

337. **Devine, DV. and Marjan, JMJ.** The role of immuno-proteins in the survival of liposomes in the circulation. *Crit. Rev. Ther. Drug Carrier Sys.* 1997;14:105–131.

338. **Ostro, MJ.** Introduction. In: Liposomes: from Biophysics to Therapeutics, (Ostro MJ., ed.), Marcel Dekker, Inc., New York and Basel, 1987, pp. 39–72.

339. **Gregoriadis, G.** Immunological adjuvants: a role for liposomes. *Immunol. Today* 1990;11:89–97.

340. **Liu, F. and Liu, D.** Serum independent liposome uptake by mouse liver. *Biochim. Biophys. Acta* 1996;1278:5–11.

341. **Fetterly, GJ. and Straubinger, RM.** Pharmacokinetics of paclitaxel-containing liposomes in rats. *AAPS PharmSci.* 2003;5(4):32.

342. **Swenson, CE., Stewart, KA., Hammett, JL., Fitzsimmons, WE., and Ginsberg, RS.** Pharmacokinetics and in vivo activity of liposome-encapsulated gentamicin. *Antimicrob. Agents Chemother.* 1990;34(2):235–240.

343. **Lasic, DD and Papahadjopoulos, D.** Liposomes revisited. *Science* 1995;267:1275–1276.

344. **Riess, JG., Frézard, F., Greiner, J., et al.** Membranes, vesicles and other supramolecular systems made from fluorinated amphiphiles, in Handbook of Non-Medical Applications of Liposomes, (Barenholz, Y. and Lasic, D., eds.),. CRC Press Inc., Boca Raton, FL, 1995.

345. **Santaella, C., Frézard, F., Vierling, P., anf Riess, JG.** Extended *in vivo* blood circulation time of fluorinated liposomes. *Feder. Eur. Biochem. Soc. Lett.* 1993;336:481–484.

346. **Maruyama, K., Yuda, AO., Kojima, S., Suginaka, A., and Iwatsuru, M.** Prolonged circulation time in vivo of large unilamellar liposomes composed of distearoyl phosphatidyl choline and cholesterol containing amphipathic poly(ethylene glycol). *Biochim. Biophys. Acta.* 1992;1128:44–49.

347. **Maruyama, K., Yuda, T., Okamoto, A., Ishikura, C., Kojima, S., and Iwatsuru, M.** Effect of molecular weight in amphipathic polyethylene glycol on prolonging the circulation time of large unilamellar liposomes. *Chem. Pharm. Bull.* 1991;39:1620–1622.

348. **Allen, TM. and Hansen, C.** Pharmacokinetics of stealth versus conventional liposomes: effect of dose. *Biochim. Biophys. Acta* 1991;1068:133–141.

349. **Gabizon, A., Catane, R., Uzeily, B., et al.** Prolonged circulation time and enhanced accumulation in malignent exudates of doxorubicin encapsulated in polyethylene glycol coated liposomes. *Cancer Res.* 1994;54:987–992.

350. **Bakker-Woudenberg, IA., Lokerse, AF., Roerdink, F., Regts, D., and Michel, MF.** Free versus liposome-entrapped ampicillin in treatment of infection due to Listeria monocytogenes in normal and athymic nude mice. *J. Infect. Dis.* 1985;55:917–924.

351. **Van Der Veen, AH., Eggermont, AM., Seynhaeve, AL., Van Tiel, and Ten Hagen, TL.** Biodistribution and tumor localization of stealth liposomal tumor necrosis factor-alpha in soft tissue sarcoma bearing rats. *Int. J. Cancer* 1998;77(6):901–906.

352. **Schettini, DA., Costa Val, AP., Souza, LF., et al.** Pharmacokinetic and parasitological evaluation of the bone marrow of dogs with visceral leishmaniasis submitted to multiple dose treatment with liposome-encapsulated meglumine antimoniate. *Braz. J. Med. Biol. Res.* 2005;38(12)1879–1883.

353. **Northfelt, DW., Martin FJ, Kaplan, LD., et al.** Pharmacoknetics, tumor localization and safety of Doxil (Liposomal doxorubicin) in AIDS patients with kaposi's sarcoma. *Proc. Am. Soc. Clin. Oncol.* 1993;12:51.

354. **Harrington, KJ., Rowlinson-Busza, G., Syrigos, KN., Uster, PS., Abra, RM and Stewart, JSW.** Biodistribution and pharmacokinetics of ^{111}In-DTPA-labelled pegylated liposomes in a human tumor xenograft model: implications for novel targeting strategies. *Br. J. Cancer* 2000;83:232–238.

355. **Harvie, P., Désormeaux, A., Bergeron, MC., et al.** Comparative pharmacokinetics, distributions in tissue, and interactions with blood proteins of conventional and sterically stabilized liposomes containing 2',3'-dideoxyinosine. *Antimicrob. Agents Chemother.* 1996;40(1):225–229.

356. **Oussoren, C., Zuidema, J., Crommelin, DJ., and Storm, G.** Lymphatic uptake and biodistribution of liposomes after subcutaneous injection. II. Influence of liposomal size, lipid composition and lipid dose. *Biochim. Biophys. Acta* 1997;1328:261–272.

357. **Cabanes, A., Reig, F., Garcia Anton, JM., and Arboix, M.** Sustained release of liposome encapsulated enrofloxacin after intramuscular administration in rabbits. *Am. J. Vet. Res.* 1995;56:1498–1501.

358. **Ohsawa, T., Matsukawa, Y., Takakura, Y., Hashida, M., and Sezaki, H.** Fate of lipid and encapsulated drug after intramuscular administration of liposomes prepared bythe freeze-thawing method in rats. *Chem. Pharm. Bull.* 1985;33:357–377.

359. **Kim, CK. and Han, JH.** Lymphatic delivery and pharmacokinetics of methotrexate after intramuscular injection of differently charged liposome-entrapped methotrexate to rats. *J. Microencapsul.* 1995;12:437–446.

360. **Oussoren, C. and Storm, G.** Liposomes to target the lymphatics by subcutaneous administration. *Adv. Drug Deliv. Rev.* 2001;50:143–156.

361. **Kadir, F., Eling, WMC., and Crommelin, DJA.** Kinetics and prophylactic efficacy of increasing dose of liposomeencapsulated chloroquine after IM injection. *J. Control. Release* 1992;20:47–54.

362. **Eichler, HG., Gasic, S., and Korn, A.** Trägersysteme für pharmaka—neues prinzip in der pharmakotherapi. *Pharmazie* 1985;110:106–111.

363. **Elmas, M., Yazar, E., Baş, AL., Tras, B., Bayezit, M., and Yapar, K.** Comparative pharmacokinetics of enrofloxacin and tissue concentrations of parent drug and ciprofloxacin after intramuscular administrations of free and liposome encapsulated enrofloxacin in rabbits. *J. Vet. Med. B* 2002;49:507–512.

364. **Saari, M., Mika, TV., Matti, OK., Väinö, M., Turjanmaa, H., and Markku, M.** Nieminen Pulmonary distribution and clearance of two beclomethasone liposome formulations in healthy volunteers. *Int. J. Pharm.* 1999;181:1–9.

365. **Shahiwala, A. and Misra, AA.** Preliminary pharmacokinetic study of liposomal leuprolide dry powder inhaler: a technical note. *AAPS PharmSciTech.* 6(3):2005, pp. 60–64.

366. **Marier, J-F., Lavigne, J. and Ducharme, MP.** Pharmacokinetics and efficacies of liposomal and conventional formulations of tobramycin after intratracheal administration in rats with pulmonary *Burkholderia cepacia* infection. *Antimicrob. Agents Chemother.* 2002;46(12):3776–3781.

367. **Demaeyer, PE., Akodad, M., Gravet, E., P. Schietecat.** Disposition of liposomal gentamicin following intrabronchial administration in rabbits. *J. Microencapsul.* 1993;10:77–88.

368. **Fielding, RM., Lewis, RO., and Moon-McDermott, L.** Altered tissue distribution and elimination of amikacin encapsulated in unilamellar, low-clearance liposomes (MiKasome). *Pharm. Res.* 1998;15:1775–1781.

369. **Marier, JF., Brazier, JL., Lavigne, J., and Ducharme, MP.** Liposomal tobramycin against pulmonary infections of *Pseudomonas aeruginosa*: a pharmacokinetic and efficacy study following single and multiple intratracheal administrations in rats. *J. Antimicrob. Chemother.* 2003;52:247–252.

370. **Verma, DD. and Fahr, A.** Synergistic penetration enhancement effect of ethanol and phospholipids on the topical delivery of cyclosporin A. *J. Control. Release* 2004;97(1):55–66.

371. **Fang, JY., Hwang, TL., and Huang, YL.** Liposomes as vehicles for enhancing drug delivery via skin routes. *Curr. Nanosci.* 2006;2(1):55–70(16).

372. **Chetoni, P., Rossi, S., Burgalassi, S., Monti, D., Mariotti, S., and Saettone, MF.** Comparison of liposome-encapsulated acyclovir with acyclovir ointment: ocular pharmacokinetics in rabbits. *J. Ocul. Pharmacol. Ther.* 2004;20(2):169–177.

373. **Zheng, J., Liu, J., Jaffray, DA., and Allen, C.** *In vivo* tracking of liposomes using CT and MR imaging: 2006 NSTI 9th Nanotechnology conference, May 7–11th at Boston, Massachuessets.

374. **Subramanian, N. and Murthy, RSR.** Radiolabeling, biodistribution and tumor imaging of stealth liposomes containing methotrexate. *J. Alasbimn* 2003;6(22)

375. **Peter, H., Miriam, B., Tina, V., Thomas Nahde, Sven Hoffmann.** Novel RGD lipopeptides for the targeting of liposomes to integrin-expressing endothelial and melanoma cells. *Protein Engg. Des. Selection* 2004;17(5):433–441.

376. **Kadir, F., Oussoren, C., and Crommelin, DJA.** Liposomal formulations to reduce irritation of intramuscularly and subcutaneously administered drugs. Injectable drug development, techniques to reduce pain and irritation, (Gupta, PK. and Brazeau, GA., eds.), Interpharm Press, Denver, Colorado, US, 1999, pp. 337–354.

377. **Onssoren, C., Storm, G., Crommelin, DJA., and Senior, J.** Liposomes for sustained drug release, Sustained-release injectable products, (Senior, J and Radomsky, M., eds.), Interpharm Press, Engelwood, Colorado, US, 2000, pp. 137–180.

378. **Storm, G. and Crommelin, DJA.** Liposomes: quo vadis? *Pharm. Sci. Technol. Today* 1998;1:19–31.

379. **Gregoriadis, G.** Fate of injected liposomes: observations on entrapped solute retention, vesicle clearance and tissue distribution in vivo, in Liposomes as Drug Carrier: Recent Trends and Progress, (Gregoriadis, G., ed.), Wiley, Chichester, 1988, pp. 3–18.

380. **Schiffelers, R., Storm, G., and Bakker-Woudenberg, I.** Liposome-encapsulated aminoglycosides in pre-clinical and clinical studies. *J. Antimicrob. Chemother.* 2001;48:333–344.

381. **Wang, CY. and Huang, L.** pH-sensitive immunoliposomes mediate target-cell-specific delivery and controlled expression of a foreign gene in mouse. *Proc. Natl. Acad. Sci. USA* 1987;84:7851–7855.

382. **Spragg, DD., Alford, DR., Greferath, R., et al.** Immuno targeting of liposomes to activated vascular endothelial cells: a strategy for site-selective delivery in the cardiovascular system. *Proc. Natl. Acad. Sci. USA* 1997;94:8795–8800.

383. **Ishida, T., Kirchmeier, MJ., Moase, EH., Zalipsky, S., and Allen, TM.** Targeted delivery and triggered release of liposomal doxorubicin enhances cytotoxicity against human B lymphoma cells. *Biochim. Biophys. Acta* 2001;1515:144–158.

384. **Turner, C., Weir, N., Catterall, C., Baker, TS., and Jones, MN.** The transfection of Jurkat T-leukemic cells by use of pH-sensitive immunoliposomes. *J. Liposome Res.* 2002;12:45–50.

385. **Ng, K., Zhao, L., Liu, Y., and Mahapatro, M.** The effects of polyethyleneglycol (PEG)-derived lipid on the activity of target-sensitive immunoliposome. *Int. J. Pharm.* 2000;193:157–166.

386. **Ishida, T., Okada, Y., Kobayashi, T., and Kiwada, H.** Development of pH-sensitive liposomes that efficiently retain encapsulated doxorubicin (DOX) in blood. *Int. J. Pharm.* 2006;309:94–100.

387. **Reddy, JA. and Low, PS.** Enhanced folate receptor mediated gene therapy using a novel pH-sensitive lipid formulation. *J. Control. Release* 2000;64:27–37.

388. **Lee, RJ. and Huang, L.** Folate-targeted, anionic liposome entrapped polylysine- condensed DNA for tumor cell-specific gene transfer. *J. Biol. Chem.* 1996;271:8481–8487.

389. **Legendre, JY. and Szoka, FC., Jr.,** Delivery of plasmid DNA into mammalian cell lines using pH-sensitive liposomes: comparison with cationic liposomes. *Pharm. Res.* 1992;9:1235–1242.

390. **Reddy, JA., Dean, D., Kennedy, MD., and Low, PS.** Optimization of folate-conjugated liposomal vectors for folate receptor mediated gene therapy. *J. Pharm. Sci.* 1999;88:1112–1118.

391. **Duzgunes, N., Simoes, S., Slepushkin, V., et al.** Enhanced inhibition of HIV-1 replication in macrophages by antisense oligonucleotides, ribozymes and acyclic nucleoside phosphonate analogs delivered in pH-sensitive liposomes, Nucleosides Nucleotides. *Nucleic Acids* 2001;20:515–523.

392. **Konopka, K., Rossi, JJ., Swiderski, P., Slepushkin, VA., and Duzgunes, N.** Delivery of an anti-HIV-1 ribozyme into HIV infected cells via cationic liposomes. *Biochim. Biophys. Acta* 1998;1372:55–68.

393. **Allen, TM., Hansen, CB., and Guo, LS.** Subcutaneous administration of liposomes: a comparison with the intravenous and intraperitoneal routes of injection. *Biochim. Biophys. Acta* 1993;1150:9–16.

394. **Pantaleo, G. and Fauci, AS.** New concepts in the immunopathogenesis of HIV infection. *Annu. Rev. Immunol.* 1995;13:487–512.

395. **Pantaleo, G., Graziosi, C., Demarest, JF., et al.** HIV infection is active and progressive in lymphoid tissue during the clinically latent stage of disease. *Nature* 1993;362:355–358.

396. **Mastrobattista, E., Koning, GA., and Storm, G.** Immunoliposomes for targeted delivery of antitumor drugs. *Adv. Drug Deliv. Rev.* 1999;40:103–127.

397. **Mastrobattista, E., Crommelin, DJA., Wilschut, J., and Storm, G.** Targeted liposomes for delivery of protein-based drugs into the cytoplasm of tumor cells. *J. Liposome Res.* 2002;12(1–2):57–65.

398. **Koning, GA., Kamps, JA., and Scherphof, GL.** Efficient intracellular delivery of 5-fluorodeoxyuridine into colon cancer cells by targeted immunoliposomes. *Cancer Detect. Prev.* 2002;26:299–307.

399. **Gregoriadis, G.** Overview of liposomes. *J. Antimicrob. Chemother.* 1991;28:39–48.

400. **Gregoriadis, G. and Florence, AT.** Liposomes and cancer therapy. *Cancer Cells* 1991;4:144–146.

401. **Mayer, LD., Tai, LC., Bally, MB., Mitilenes, GN., Ginsberg, RS., and Cullis, PR.** Characterization of liposomal system containing doxorubicin entrapped in response to pH gradients. *Biochim. Biophys. Acta* 1990;1025:143–151.

402. **Olson, F., Mayhew, E., Maslow, D., Rustum, Y., and Szoka, F.** Characterization, toxicity and therapeutic efficacy of adriamycin encapsulated in liposomes. *Eur. J. Cancer Clin. Oncol.* 1982;18:167–176.

403. **Herman, EH., Rahman, A., Ferrans, VJ., Visk, JA. and Schien, PS.** Prevention of chronic doxorubicin cardiotoxicity in beagles by liposome encapsulation. *Cancer Res.* 1983;43:5427–5432.

404. **Van Hoesel, QGCM., and Steerenberg, PA.** Crommelin, DJA. et al. Reduced cardiotoxicity and nephrotoxicity with preservation of antitumor activity of doxorubicin entrapped in stable liposomes in the LOU/M Wsl rat. *Cancer Res.* 1984;44:3698–3705.

405. **Barenholz, Y. and Haran, G.** Loading and controlled-release of amphiphilic pharmaceuticals to and from liposomes. *Eur. Pat. Appl.* EP 361,894 (Cl. A61K9/127) 4 Apr. 1990, *US Appl.* 250, 687, 28 Sep 1988.

406. **Vaage, J., Donovan, D., Uster, P., and Working, P.** Tumor uptake of doxorubicin in polyethylene glycol-coated liposomes and therapeutic effect against a xenografted human pancreatic carcinoma *Br. J. Cancer* 1997;75:482–486.

407. **Goyal, P., Goyal, K., Kumar, SGV., Singh, A., and Katare, OP.** Liposomal drug delivery systems: Clinical applications. *Acta Pharm.* 2005;55:1–25.

408. **Cheung, TW., Remick, SC., Azarnia, N., Proper, JA., Barrueco, JR., and Dezube, BJ.** AIDS-related Kaposi's sarcoma: a phase II study of liposomal doxorubicin. *Clin. Cancer Res.* 1999;5:3432–3437.

409. **Ten Hagen, TL., Van Der Veen, AH., Nooijen, PT., Van Tiel, ST., Seynhaeve, AL., and Eggermont, AM.** Low-dose tumor necrosis factor-alpha augments antitumor activity of stealth liposomal doxorubicin (DoxilTM) in soft tissue sarcoma-bearing rats. *Int. J. Cancer.* 2000;87:829–837.

410. **Yasui, K. and Nakamura, Y.** Positively charged liposomes containing tumor necrosis factor in solid tumors. *Biol. Pharm. Bull.* 2000;23:318–322.

411. **Tseng, YL., Hong, RL., Tao, MH., and Chang, FH.** Sterically stabilized anti-idiotype immunoliposomes improve the therapeutic efficacy of doxorubicin in a murine B-cell lymphoma model. *Int. J. Cancer* 1999;80:723–730.

412. **Lopes de Menezes, DE., Pilarski, LM., and Allen, TM.** In vitro and in vivo targeting of immunoliposomal doxorubicin to human B-cell lymphoma. *Cancer Res.* 1998;58:3320–3330.

413. **Pastorino, F., Brignole, C., Marimpietri, D., et al.** Doxorubicin-loaded Fab' fragments of anti-disialoganglioside mmunoliposomes selectively inhibit the growth and dissemination of human neuroblastoma in nude mice. *Cancer Res.* 2003;63:86–92.

414. **Brignole, C., Marimpietri, D., Gambini, C., Allen, TM., Ponzoni, M., and Pastorino, F.** Development of Fab' fragments of anti-GD(2) immunoliposomes entrapping doxorubicin for experimental therapy of human neuroblastoma. *Cancer Lett.* 2003;197:199–204.

415. **Arndt, D., Zeisig, R., Eue, I., Sternberg B., and Fichtner, I.** Antineoplastic activity of sterically stabilized alkyl phosphocholine liposomes in human breast carcinomas. *Breast Cancer Res. Treat.* 1997;43:237–246.

416. **Wollina, U., Hohaus, K., Schonlebe, J., Haroske, E., and Kostler, E.** Liposomal daunorubicin in tumor stage cutaneous T-cell lymphoma: report of three cases. *J. Cancer Res. Clin. Oncol.* 2003;129:65–69.

417. **Fiorillo, A., Maggi, G., Greco, N., et al.** Second-line chemotherapy with the association of liposomal daunorubicin, carboplatin and etoposide in children with recurrent malignant brain tumors. *J. Neurooncol.* 2004;66:179–185.

418. **Guthlein, F., Burger, AM., Brandl, M., et al.** Pharmacokinetics and antitumor activity of vincristine entrapped in vesicular phospholipid gels. *Anticancer Drugs* 2002;13:797–805.

419. **Kubo, T., Sugita, T., Shimose, S., Nitta, Y., Ikuta, Y., and Murakami, T.** Targeted delivery of anticancer drugs with intravenously administered magnetic liposomes in osteosarcoma-bearing hamsters. *Int. J. Oncol.* 2000;17:309–315.

420. **Matsuoka, F., Shinkai, M., Honda, H., Kubo, T., Sugita T., and Kobayashi, T.** Hyperthermia using magnetite cationic liposomes for hamster osteosarcoma. *Biomagn. Res. Technol.* 2004;2:3.

421. **Chelvi, TP., Jain, SK., and Ralhan, R.** Hyperthermia-mediated targeted delivery of thermosensitive liposome-encapsulated melphalan in murine tumors. *Oncol. Res.* 1995;7:393–398.

422. **Vodovozova, EL., Gayenko, GP., Razinkov, VI., Korchagina, EY., Bovin NV., and Molotkovsky, JG.** Saccharide-assisted delivery of cytotoxic liposomes to human malignant cells. *Biochem. Mol. Biol. Int.* 1998;44:543–553.

423. **Yachi, K., Kikuchi, H., Yamauchi, H., Hirota, S., and Tomikawa, M.** Distribution of liposomes containing mannobiose esters of fatty acid in rats. *J. Microencaps.* 1995;12:377–388.

424. **Gokhale, PC., Pei, J., Zhang, C., Ahmad, I., Rahman, A., and Kasid, U.** Improved safety, pharmacokinetics and therapeutic efficacy profiles of a novel liposomal formulation of mitoxantrone. *Anticancer Res.* 2001;21:3313–3321.

425. **Sengupta, S., Tyagi, P., Chandra, S., Kochupillai, V., and Gupta, SK.** Encapsulation in cationic liposomes enhances antitumor efficacy and reduces the toxicity of etoposide, a topo-isomerase II inhibitor. *Pharmacol* 2001;62:163–171.

426. **Peacock, GF., Ji, B., Wang, CK., and Lu, DR.** Cell culture studies of a carborane cholesteryl ester with conventional and PEG liposomes. *Drug Deliv.* 2003;10:29–34.

427. **Shabbits, JA. and Mayer, LD.** High ceramide content liposomes with *in vivo* antitumor activity. *Anticancer Res.* 2003;23:3663–3669.

428. **Ozpolat, B., Lopez-Berestein, G., Adamson, P., Fu CJ., and Williams, AH.** Pharmacokinetics of intravenously administered liposomal all-trans-retinoic acid (ATRA) and orally administered ATRA in healthy volunteers. *J. Pharm. Pharm. Sci.* 2003;6:292–301.

429. **Pagnan, G., Stuart, DD., Pastorino, F., et al.** Delivery of c-myb antisense oligodeoxynucleotides to human neuroblastoma cells via disialoganglioside GD(2)-targeted immunoliposomes: antitumor effects. *J. Natl. Cancer Inst.* 2000;92:253–261.

430. **Stuart, DD., Kao, GY., and Allen, TM.** A novel, long-circulating and functional liposomal formulation of antisense oligodeoxynucleotides targeted against MDR1. *Cancer Gene Ther.* 2000;7:466–475.

431. **Stuart, DD. and Allen, TM.** A new liposomal formulation for antisense oligodeoxynucleotides with small size, high incorporation efficiency and good stability, *Biochim. Biophys. Acta* 2000;1463:219–229.

432. **Oku, N., Saito, N., Namba, Y., Tsukada, H., Dolphin, D., and Okada, S.** Application of long-circulating liposomes to cancer photodynamic therapy. *Biol. Pharm. Bull.* 1997;20:670–673.

433. **Barrow, WW.** Treatment of mycobacterial infections. *Rev. Sci. Tech.* 2001;20:55–70.

434. **Morgan, JR. and Williams, KE.** Preparation and properties of liposome associated gentamicin. *Antimicrob. Agents Chemother.* 1980;17:544–548.

435. **Cabanes, A., Reig, F., Garcia-Anton, JM., and Arboix, M.** Evaluation of free and liposome-encapsulated gentamycin for intramuscular sustained release in rabbits. *Res. Vet. Sci.* 1998;64:213–217.

436. **Cynamon, MH., Klemens SP., and Swenson, CE.,** TLC G-65 in combination with other agents in the therapy of *Mycobacterium avium* infection in beige mice. *J. Antimicrob. Chemother.* 1992;29:693–699.

437. **Gaspar, MM., Neves, S., Portaels, F., Pedrosa, J., Silva MT., and Cruz, ME.** Therapeutic efficacy of liposomal rifabutin in a *Mycobacterium avium* model of infection. *Antimicrob. Agents Chemother.* 2000;44:2424–2430.

438. **Agarwal, A., Kandpal, H., Gupta, HP., Singh NB., and Gupta, CM.** Tuftsin-bearing liposomes as rifampin vehicles in treatment of tuberculosis in mice. *Antimicrob. Agents Chemother.* 1994;38:588–593.

439. **Onyeji, CO., Nightingale, CH., Nicolau, DP., and Quintiliani, R.** Efficacies of liposome-encapsulated clarithromycin and ofloxacin against *Mycobacterium avium*-M. intracellular complex in human macrophages. *Antimicrob. Agents Chemother.* 1994;38:523–527.

440. **Webb, MS., Boman, NL., Wiseman, DJ., et al.** Antibacterial efficacy against an *in vivo Salmonella typhimurium* infection model and pharmacokinetics of a liposomal ciprofloxacin formulation. *Antimicrob. Agents Chemother.* 1998;42:45–52.

441. **Stevenson, M., Baillie AJ., and Richards, RM.** Enhanced activity of streptomycin and chloramphenicol against intracellular Escherichia coli in the J774 macrophage cell line mediated by liposome delivery. *Antimicrob. Agents Chemother.* 1983;24:742–749.

442. **Gangadharam, PR., Ashtekar, DA., Ghori, N., Goldstein, JA., Debs, RJ., and Duzgunes, N.** Chemotherapeutic potential of free and liposome encapsulated streptomycin against experimental *Mycobacterium avium* complex infections in beige mice. *J. Antimicrob. Chemother.* 1991;28:425–435.

443. **Gangadharam, PR., Ashtekar, DR., Flasher, DL., and Duzgunes, N.** Therapy of *Mycobacterium avium* complex infections in beige mice with streptomycin encapsulated in sterically stabilized liposomes. *Antimicrob. Agents Chemother.* 1995;39:725–730.

444. **Yanagihara, K.** Design of anti-bacterial drug and anti-mycobacterial drug for drug delivery system. *Curr. Pharm. Des.* 2002;8:475–482.

445. **Duzgunes, N., Perumal, VK., Kesavalu, L., Goldstein, JA., and Debs, RJ.** Enhanced effect of liposomes-encapsulated amikacin on *Mycobacterium avium*-M. intracellular complex infection in beige mice. *Antimicrob. Agents Chemother.* 1988;32:1404–1411.

446. **Fielding, RM., Moon-McDermott, L., and Lewis, RO.** Bioavailability of a small unilamellar low-clearance liposomal amikacin formulation after extravascular administration, *J. Drug Targ.* 1999;6:415–426.

447. **Desiderio, JV. and Campbell, SG.** Intraphagocytic killing of *Salmonelle typhimurium* by liposome encapsulated cephalothin. *J. Infect. Dis.* 1983;148:563–570.

448. **Barsoum, IS. and Reich, M.** The effect of liposome-entrapped penicillin G on *Staphylococcus aureus* infection in mice. *Pharmacol* 1982;10:358–363.

449. **Bonventre, P. and Gregoriadis, G.** Killing of intraphagocytic *Staphylococcus aureus* by dihydrostreptomycin entrapped within liposomes. *Antimicrob. Agents Chemother.* 1978;13:1049–1051.

450. **Kerridge, D.** Mode of action of clinically important antifungal drugs. *Adv. Microb. Physiol.* 1986;27:1–72.

451. **Utz, JP.** Amphotericin B toxicity: general side effects. *Ann. Intern. Med.* 1964;61:340–343.

452. **Bodey, G., Bueltmann, B., and Duguid, W.** Fungal infections in cancer patients: an international autopsy survey. *Eur. J. Clin. Microbial Infect. Dis.* 1992;11:99–109.

453. **Michaud, D.** Liposomal amphotericin B for the treatment of severe fungal infection. *Dynamics* 2001;12:17–21.

454. **Dupont, B.** Overview of the lipid formulations of amphotericin B. *J. Antimicrob. Chemother.* 2002;49:31–36.

455. **Adler-Moore, J. and Proffitt, RT.** AmBisome: liposomal formulation, structure, mechanism of action and pre-clinical experience. *J. Antimicrob. Chemother.* 2002;49:21–30.

456. **Chopra, R., Blair, S., Strang, J., Cervi, P., Patterson KG., and Goldstone, AH.** Liposomal amphotericin B (AmBisome) in the treatment of fungal infections in neutropenic patients. *J. Antimicrob. Chemother.* 1991;28:93–104.

457. **Meunier, F., Prentice HG., and Ringden, O.** Liposomal amphotericin B (AmBisome): safety data form and phase-II/III clinical trial. *J. Antimicrob. Chemother.* 1991;28:83–91.

458. **Ringden, O., Meunier, F., Tollemar, J., et al.** Efficacy of amphotericin B encapsulated in liposomes (AmBisome) in the treatment of invasive fungal infections in immunocompromised patients. *J. Antimicrob. Chemother.* 1991;28:73–82.

459. **Moribe, K. and Maruyama, K.** Pharmaceutical design of the liposomal antimicrobial agents for infectious disease. *Curr. Pharm. Des.* 2002;8:441–454.

460 **Moribe, K., Maruyama, K., and Iwatsuru, M.** Encapsulation characteristics of nystatin in liposomes: effects of cholesterol and polyethylene glycol derivatives. *Int. J. Pharm.* 1999;188:193–202.

461. **Moribe, K., Maruyama, K., and Iwatsuru, M.** Spectroscopic investigation of the molecular state of nystatin encapsulated in liposomes. *Int. J. Pharm.* 2000;201:37–49.

462. **Arikan, S. and Rex, JH.** Lipid-based antifungal agents: current status, *Curr. Pharm. Des.* 2001;7:393–415.

463. **Sarin, PS., Gallo, RC., Scheer, DI., Crews, F., and Lippa, AS.** Effects of a novel compound (AL 721) on HTLV-III infectivity *in vitro*. *N. Eng. J. Med.* 1985;313:1289–1290.

464. **Rios, A., Rosenblum, M., Crofoot, G., Lenk, RP., Hayman, A., and Lopez-Berestein, G.** Pharmacokinetics of liposomal nystatin in patients with human immunodeficiency virus infection. *J. Infect. Dis.* 1993;168:253–254.

465. **Sinha, J., Mukhopadhyay, S., Das, N., and Basu, MK.** Targeting of liposomal andrographolide to L. donovani-infected macrophages *in vivo*. *Drug Deliv.* 2000;7:209–213.

466. **Mahato, RI., Rolland, A., and Tomlinson, E.** Cationic lipid-based gene delivery systems: pharmaceutical perspectives. *Pharm. Res.* 1997;14:853–859.

467. **Crystal, RG.** Transfer of genes to humans: early lesions and obstacles to success. *Science*1995;270:404–410.

468. **Felgner, PL., Gadek, TR., Holm, M., et al.** Lipofectin: a highly efficient, lipid mediated DNA transfection procedures. *Proc. Natl. Acad. Sci. USA* 1987;84:7413–7417.

469. **Lasic, D.** Liposomes—an industrial view. *Chem. Ind.* 1996;6:210–213.

470. **Tomlinson, E. and Rolland, AP.** Controllable gene therapy: pharmaceutics of non viral gene delivery systems. *J. Control. Release*1996;39:357–372.

471. **Sharma, A. and Sharma, US.** Liposomes in drug delivery: progress and limitations. *Int. J. Pharm.* 1997;154:123–140.

472. **Zou, Y., Zong, G., Ling YH., and Perez-Soler, R.** Development of cationic liposome formulations for intratracheal gene therapy of early lung cancer. *Cancer Gene Ther.* 2000;7:683–696.

473. **Bandyopadhyay, P., Kren, BT., Ma X., and Steer, CJ.** Enhanced gene transfer into HuH-7 cells and primary rat hepatocytes using targeted liposomes and polyethylenimine. *Biotechniques* 1998;25:282–284.

474. **Shimizu, K., Maitani, Y., Takayama, K., and Nagai, T.** Formulation of liposomes with a soybean-derived sterylglucoside mixture and cholesterol for liver targeting. *Biol. Pharm. Bull.* 1997;20:881–886.

475. **Kawaura, C., Hasegawa, S., Hirashima, N., and Nakanishi, M.** Monosialoganglioside containing cationic liposomes with a cationic cholesterol derivative promote the efficiency of gene transfection in mammalian culture cells. *Biol. Pharm. Bull.* 2000;23:778–780.

476. **Ishiwata, H., Suzuki, N., Ando, S., Kikuchi, H., and Kitagawa, T.** Characteristics and biodistribution of cationic liposomes and their DNA complexes. *J. Control. Release* 2000;69:139–148.

477. **Yoshida, J., Mizuno, M., Fujii, M., et al.** Human gene therapy for malignant gliomas (glioblastoma multiforme and anaplastic astrocytoma) by *in vivo* transduction with human interferon beta gene using cationic liposomes. *Human Gene Ther.* 2004;15:77–86.

478. **Kim, A., Lee, EH., Choi, SH., and Kim, CK.** *In vitro* and *in vivo* transfection efficiency of a novel ultradeformable cationic liposome. *Biomaterials* 2004;25:305–313.

479. **Kawakami, S., Yamashita, F., Nishida, K., Nakamura, J., and Hashida, M.** Glycosylated cationic liposomes for cell-selective gene delivery. *Crit. Rev. Ther. Drug Carrier Syst.* 2002;19:171–190.

480. **Joo, SY. and Kim, JS.** Enhancement of gene transfer to cervical cancer cells using transferrin-conjugated liposome. *Drug Dev. Ind. Pharm.* 2002;28:1023–1031.

481. **Shi, N. and Pardridge, WM.** Noninvasive gene targeting to the brain. *Proc. Natl. Acad. Sci. USA* 2000;97:7567–7572.

482. **Shi, N., Zhang, Y., Zhu, C., Boado, RJ., and Pardridge, WM.** Brain-specific expression of an exogenous gene after i.v. administration. *Proc. Natl. Acad. Sci. USA* 2001;98:12,754–12,759.

483. **Nabel, GJ., Chang, AE., Hersh, EM., et al.** Combined experience from Phase I studies with Allovectin-7, a direct gene transfer immunotherapeutic, 31st Annual Meeting of American Society of Clinical Oncology, May 20–23, 1995, Los Angeles; *Proc. Annu. Meet. Am. Soc. Clin. Oncol.* 1995;14:582A.

484. **Ono, I., Yamashita, T., Jin, HY., et al.** Combination of porous hydroxyapatite and cationic liposomes as a vector for BMP-2 gene therapy. *Biomaterials* 2004;19:4709–4718.

485. **Mathew, E., Hardee, GE., Bennett, CF., and Lee, KD.** Cytosolic delivery antisense oligonucleotides by listeriolysin O-containing liposomes. *Gene Ther.* 2003;10:1105–1115.

486. **Allison, AG. and Gregoriadis, G.** Liposomes as immunological adjuvants. *Nature* 1974;252(5480):252.

487. **Allison, AC. and Gregoriadis, G.** In recent results in cancer research, (Mathe, G., Florintin, I., and Simmler, MC., eds.), Heideberg, Springer Verlag, 1976, 58 p.

488. **Latif, N. and Bachhawat, BK.** The effect of surface charges of liposomes in immunopotentiation. *Biosci. Rep.* 1984;4(2):99–107.

489. **Tyrrell, DA., Heath, TD., Colley, CM., and Ryman, BE.** New aspects of liposomes. *Biochim. Biophys. Acta* 1976;457(3–4):259–302.

490. **van Rooijen, N. and van Nieuwmegen, R.** Liposomes in immunology: the immune response against antigen-containing liposomes. *Immunol. Commun.* 1977;6(5):489–498.

491. **van Rooijen, N. and van Nieuwmegen, R.** Liposomes in immunology: further evidence for the adjuvant activity of liposomes. *Immunol. Commun.* 1978;7(6):635–644.

492. **Hudson, LD., Fiddler, MB., and Desnick, RJ.** Enzyme therapy. X. Immune response induced by enzyme- and buffer-loaded liposomes in C3H/HeJ Gus(h) mice. *J. Pharmacol. Exp. Ther.* 1979;208(3):507–514.

493. **Sanchez, Y., Ionescu-Matiu, I., Dreesman, GR., et al.** Humoral and cellular immunity to hepatitis B virus-derived antigens: comparative activity of Freund complete adjuvant alum, and liposomes. *Infect. Immun.* 1980;30(3):728–733.

494. **Raphael, L. and Tom, BH.** Liposome facilitated xenographic approach for studying human colon cancer immunity: carrier and adjuvant effect of liposomes. *Clin. Exp. Immunol.* 1984;55(1):1–13.

495. **Shek, PN. and Heath, TD.** Immune response mediated by liposome-associated protein antigens. III. Immunogenicity of bovine serum albumin covalently coupled to vesicle surface. *Immunol* 1983;50(1):101–106.

496. **Alving, CR.** In the antigens, (Sela, M., ed.), vol. 4, Academic Press, New York, 1977, 1 p.

497. **Schuster, BG., Neidig, M., Alving, BM., and Alving, CR.** Production of antibodies against phosphocholine, phosphatidylcholine, sphingomyelin, and lipid A by injection of liposomes containing lipid A. *J. Immunol.* 1979;122(3):900–905.

498. **Uemura, K., Nicolotti, RA., Six, HR., and Kinsky, SC.** Antibody formation in response to liposomal model membranes sensitized with N-substituted phosphatidylethanolamine derivatives. *Biochem.* 1974;13(8):1572–1578.

499. **Dancey, GF., Yasuda, T., and Kinsky, SC.** Enhancement of liposomal model membrane immunogenicity by incorporation of lipid A. *J. Immunol.* 1977;119(6):1868–1873.

500. **Hudson, LDS.** Studies in enzyme therapy: Evaluation of enzyme delivery strategies in a mammalian system, Ph.D. Thesis, University of Minnesota, Minnesota, 1977.

501. **Heath, TD., Macher, BA., and Papahadjopoulos, D.** Covalent attachment of immunoglobulins to liposomes via glycosphingolipids. *Biochim. Biophys. Acta.* 1981;640(1):66–81.

502. **Heath, TD., Edwards, DC., and Ryman, BE.** The adjuvant properties of liposomes. *Biochem. Soc. Trans.* 1976;4(1):129–133.

503. **Shek, PN. and Sabiston, BH.** Immune response mediated by liposome-associated protein antigens. I. Potentiation of the plaque-forming cell response. *Immunol* 1982a;45(2):349–356.

504. **Shek, PN. and Sabiston, BH.** Immune response mediated by liposome-associated protein antigens. II. Comparison of the effectiveness of vesicle-entrapped and surface-associated antigen in immunopotentiation. *Immunol* 1982b;47(4):627–632.

505. **Ogmundsdottir, HM. and Weir, DM.** Stimulation of phosphatidylinositol turnover in the macrophage plasma membrane: a possible mechanism for signal transmission. *Immunol* 1979;37(3):689–696.

506. **Ghosh, P. and Bachhawat, BK.** Grafting of different glycosides on the surface of liposomes and its effect on the tissue distribution of 125I-labelled gamma-globulin encapsulated in liposomes. *Biochim. Biophys. Acta.* 1980;632(4):562–572.

507. **Latif, N. and Bachhawat, BK.** The effect of surface sugars on liposomes in immunopotentiation. *Immunol. Lett.* 1984b;8(2):75–78.

508. **Kinsky, SC.** Immunogenicity of liposomal model membranes. *Ann. NY Acad. Sci.* 1978;308:111–123.

509. **Tan, CT., Chan, SW., and Hsia, JC.** Specific anti-thyroxine antisera induced by thyroxine sensitized liposomes. *Immunol. Commun.* 1981;10(1):27–34.

510. **van Houte, AJ., Snippe, H., and Willers, JM.** Characterization of immunogenic properties of haptenated liposomal model membranes in mice. IV. induction of IgM memory. *Immunol* 1981;43(4):627–634.

511. **Wood, C. and Kabat, EA.** Immunochemical studies of conjugates of isomaltosyl oligosaccharides to lipid. I. Antigenicity of the glycolipids and the production of specific antibodies in rabbits. *J. Exp. Med.* 1981;154(2):432–449.

512. **Das, MK., Roy, SK., and Sarkar, DP.** Characterization of anti-N-acetyl-D-glucosamine antibodies elicited through haptenated liposomes. *Carbohydr. Res.* 1984;128(2):335–340.

513. **Das, PK., Ghosh, P., Bachhawat, BK., and Das, MK.** Liposomes as immunological carriers for the preparation of antimannosyl antibodies. *Experientia* 1982;38(5):629–630.

514. **Das, PK., Ghosh, P., Bachhawat, BK., and Das, MK.** Liposomes as carrier for production of sugar specific antibodies: preparation of antigalactosyl antiserum. *Immunol. Commun.* 1982;11(1):17–24.

515. **Latif, N.** Liposomes as tools in biomedicine, Ph.D. Thesis, University of Calcutta, 1984, Calcutta.

516. **Chedid, L., Carelli, C., and Audibert, F.** Recent developments concerning muramyl dipeptide, a synthetic immunoregulating molecule. *J. Reticuloendothel. Soc.* 1979;26:631–641.

517. **Fraser-Smith, EB., Eppstein, DA., Larsen, MA., and Matthews, TR.** Protective effect of a muramyl dipeptide analog encapsulated in or mixed with liposomes against Candida albicans infection. *Infect. Immun.* 1983;39(1):172–178.

518. **Fidler, IJ., Sone, S., Fogler, WE., and Barnes, ZL.** Eradication of spontaneous metastases and activation of alveolar macrophages by intravenous injection of liposomes containing muramyl dipeptide. *Proc. Natl. Acad. Sci. USA* 1981;78(3):1680–1684.

519. **Kleinerman, ES., Schroit, AJ., Fogler, WE., and Fidler, IJ.** Tumoricidal activity of human monocytes activated in vitro by free and liposome-encapsulated human lymphokines. *J. Clin. Invest.* 1983;72(1):304–315.

520. **Vemuri, S. and Rhodes, CT.** Preparation and characterization of liposomes as therapeutic delivery systems: a review. *Pharm. Acta Helv.* 1995;70(2):95–111.

521. **Wagner, A., Platzgummer, M., Kreismayr, G., et al.** GMP production of liposomes-a new industrial approach. *J. Liposome Res.* 2006;16(3):311–319.

522. **Wagner, A., Vorauer-Uhl, K., and Katinger, H.** Liposomes produced in a pilot scale: production, purification and efficiency aspects. *Euro. J. Pharm. Biopharm.* 2002;54(2):213–219.

523. **Schwendener, RA.** The preparation of large volumes of homogeneous, sterile liposomes containing various lipophilic cytostatic drugs by the use of a capillary dialyzer. *Cancer Drug Deliv.* 1986;3(2):123–129.

524. **Barnadas-Rodriguez, R. and Sabes, M.** Factors involved in the production of liposomes with a high-pressure homogenizer. *Int. J. Pharm.* 2001;213(1–2):175–186.

525. **Sorgi, FL. and Huang, L.,** Large scale production of DC-Chol cationic liposomes by microfluidization. *Int. J. Pharm.* 1996;144(2):131–139.

526. **Kikuchi, H., Carlsson, A., Yachi, K., and Hirota, S.** Possibility of heat sterilization of liposomes. *Chem. Pharm. Bull.* 1991;39(4):1018–1022.

527. **Zuidam, NJ., Lee, SS., and Crommelin, DJ.** Sterilization of liposomes by heat treatment. *Pharm. Res.* 1993;10(11):1591–1596.

528. **Zuidam, NJ., Lee, SS., and Crommelin, DJ.** Gamma-irradiation of non-frozen, frozen, and freeze-dried liposomes. *Pharm. Res.* 1995;12(11):1761–1768.

529. **Goldbach, P., Brochart, H., Wehrlé, P., and Stamm, A.** Sterile filtration of liposomes: retention of encapsulated carboxyfluorescein. *Int. J. Pharm.* 1995;117(2):225–230.

2

Niosomes

R.S.R. Murthy, M.PHARM, PhD

CONTENTS

1. INTRODUCTION

Vanlerberghe *et al.* *(1)* in 1972 reported non-ionic surfactant vesicles (NSVs) or niosomes which are formed in aqueous media with or without the presence of cholesterol (CHOL) or other lipids. Like liposomes, niosomes can also entrap both hydrophilic and lipophilic drugs, either in aqueous layer or in lipoidal vesicular membrane. Because of the presence of non-ionic surfactant they possess better intrinsic targeting potential and may prove very useful for targeting drugs for treating cancer, parasitic, viral and other microbial diseases.

Advantages that niosomes offer are as follows:

1. Entrap solute in manner analogous to liposomes.
2. Osmotically active and stable, increase the stability of entrapped drug.
3. Handling and storage of surfactants require no special conditions.
4. Accommodate drug molecules with a wide range of solubility.
5. Exhibit flexibility in their structural characteristics (composition fluidity and size) and can be designed according to the desired situation.
6. Improve oral bioavailability of poorly absorbed drugs and can also enhance skin penetration of drugs.
7. Can be made to reach the site of action by oral, parenteral as well as topical routes.
8. Niosomal surfactants are biodegradable, biocompatible and non-immunogenic and non-toxic.
9. Niosomes improve the therapeutic performance of the drug molecules by delayed clearance from the circulation, protecting the drug form biological environment and restricting the effects to target cells.
10. They can prolong the circulation of the entrapped drugs.

Disadvantages:

Niosomes as such are biocompatible and safe. However in rare cases, nonionic surfactants interacts with other components of the system rendering the formulation turn homogenous or form precipitates.

2. STRUCTURE AND CLASSIFICATION

Vesicles are closed bilayer structures that enclose an aqueous pool and are surrounded by an aqueous solution *(2)*. Vesicles are not only interesting because they mimic biological membranes, they have recently also been used in applications such as drug delivery, nanotechnology *(3)* and two-dimensional (2D)-crystallisation of proteins. On the other hand, micelle-forming surfactants are widely used in enhanced oil recovery, rinse-off preparations and as detergents.

Both micelles and vesicles have amphiphilic molecules as building blocks, and the issue is to tune the structures of these building blocks so that a stable aggregates of the desired morphology and properties are obtained. In case of micelles, the aim is to predict and tune the critical micelle concentration, whereas for vesicles the phase-transition temperature of bilayer is of particular importance.

3. MORPHOLOGY OF SURFACTANT AGGREGATES: THE PACKING PARAMETER

The ability of amphiphiles to form aggregates of a well-defined morphology depends on molecular architecture of surfactant molecule. The packing properties of surfactants depend on the balance between the optimal cross-sectional surface area of the head groups (a_o), the volume (v) of the hydrocarbon chains and the maximum length (l_c) that the chains can attain. The dimensionless packing parameter $P = v/a_o l_c$ characterises the ability of the surfactants to form spherical micelles (cone-shaped surfactant molecules, $P < 1/3$), rod-like micelles (truncated cone, $1/3 < P < 1/2$) or bilayers ($1/2 < P < 1$) *(5)*.

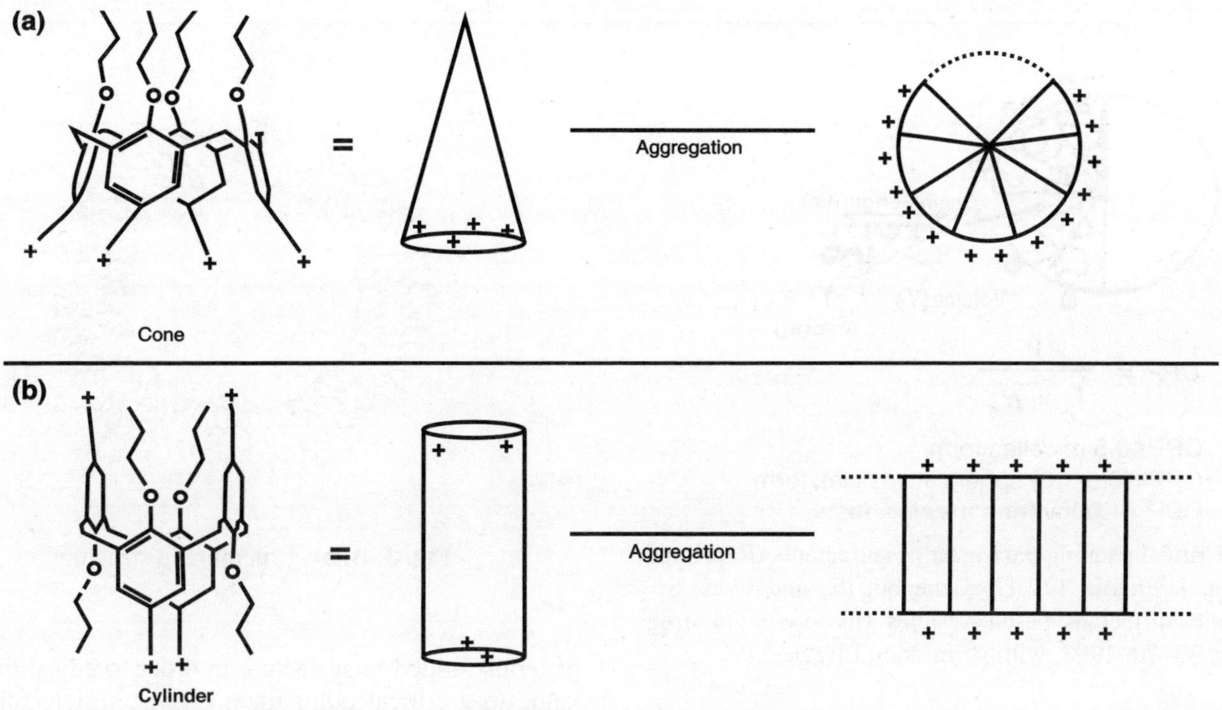

Fig. 1. Expected aggregation modes of **(a)** cone-shaped cone-1 and **(b)** cylindrical 1,3-alternate-1 (or 2 n) (Reprinted from J. Chem. Soc. Perkin. Trans. 2, 2. Arimori, S., Nagasaki, T., and Shinkai, S. Self-assembly of tetracationic amphiphiles bearing a calix [4] arene core correlation between the core structure and the aggeration properties, 679–683, 1995, with permission from Royal society of chemistry) *(8)*.

There are many recent examples of a wide variety of surfactant molecules that obey these geometrical rules. For instance, C12EO3 forms vesicles, whereas C12EO7 having a larger head group, forms rod-like micelles *(6)*. Even polystyrene (PS)-*b*-poly(acrylic acid) (PAA) diblock co-polymers form vesicles (PS-*b*-PAA = 400-*b*-16) or rod-like micelles (200-*b*-15) depending on the hydrophobic chain length (i.e., PS content) at constant head group area (i.e., PAA content) *(7)*. Arimori and co-workers *(8)* synthesized some remarkable tetracationic amphiphiles bearing a calyx *(5)* arene core. The hypothesis proposed was that, the monomer shape, the cone isomer favourably forms micelles, whereas the 1,3-alternate isomer preferably aggregates as 2D lamellae (Fig. 1). The bilayer thickness of lamella; however, is about twice the predicted value *(8)*. Therefore, one could envisage a model in which the cylindrical 1,3-alternate is turned 90° in-plane so that it can form a monolayer characterised by a rectangular head group and four hydrophobic tails per head group. The monolayers can be stuck together at the hydrophobic interface to form a bilayer having twice the thickness of the bilayer originally proposed.

Niosomes may be formed from a diverse array of amphiphiles bearing sugar, polyoxyethylene, polyglycerol, crown ether and amino acid hydrophilic head groups and these amphiphiles typically possess one to two hydrophobic alkyl, perfluoro alkyl or steroidal groups. The self assembly of surfactants into niosomes is governed not only by the nature of the surfactant but by the presence of membrane additives, nature of drug encapsulated and the actual method of preparation *(9)*. Most of the ionic surfactants being toxic have limited applications in designing and are unsuitable for use as drug carriers. NSVs or "niosomes" are prepared using methods similar to liposome preparation *(10)*. These formulations use alternative materials to phospholipids such as Span 60, Span 40 and Span 20, which are inexpensive and widely available permitted food additives *(10–16)*. For example, niosomes has been used to encapsulate colchicine *(17)*, estradiol *(18)*, tretinoin *(19,20)*, dithranol *(21,22)*, enoxacin *(23)* and several other class of drugs such as anti-cancer *(24)*, anti-tubercular, anti-leishmanial, anti-inflammatory, hormonal drugs and oral vaccine.

4. GENERAL CHARACTERISTICS OF NON-IONIC SURFACTANT

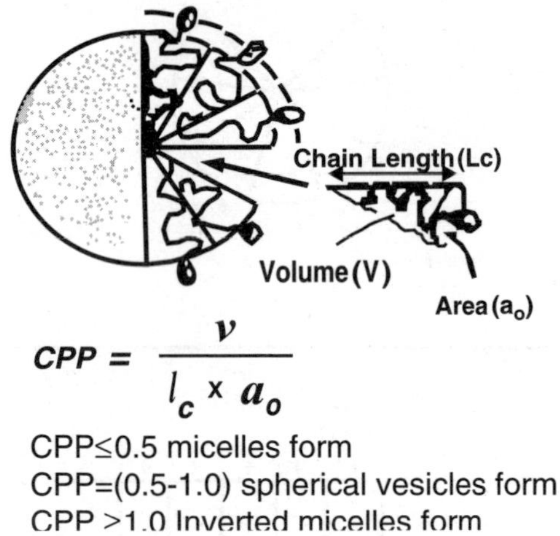

Fig. 2. Critical packing parameter of surfactants (Reprinted from Int. J. Pharm, 172 (2) Uchegbu, IF., and Vyas, Sp. Non-ionic surfactant based vesicles (niosomes) in drug delivery, 33–70, 1998, with permission Elsevier) *(9)*.

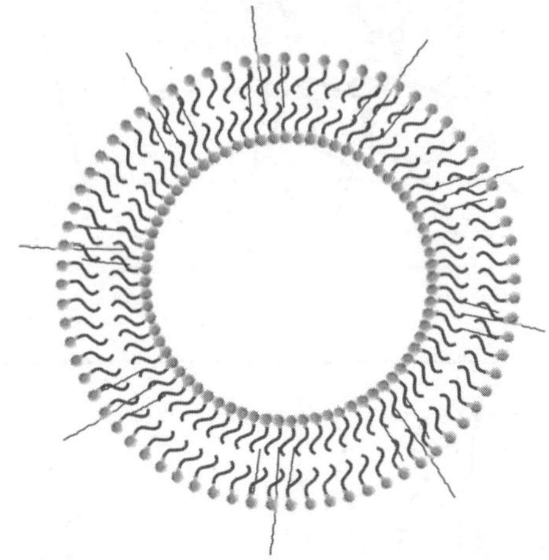

Fig. 3. Bilayer membrane structure.

The ability of non-ionic surfactant to form bilayer vesicles instead of micelles is dependant on hydrophilic–lipophilic balance (HLB) values of the surfactant, the chemical structure of components and the critical packing parameter *(9)*. The relationship between the structure of the surfactant including size of hydrophilic head group, and length of lipophilic alkyl chain in the ability to form vesicles is described in Fig. 2 and the general form of a single bilayer vesicle is shown in Fig. 3

Non-ionic surfactants generally used in the preparation of niosomes are shown in Table 1. Cholesterol is generally added to surfactant in order to adjust the HLB value to a critical point for a bilayer vesicle formation *(12)* and some times, to make vesicles more stable. The addition of CHOL may also enables more hydrophobic surfactants to form vesicles, suppresses tendency of the surfactants to form aggregates and lends greater stability to the bilayer membranes by raising gel–liquid transition temperature of vesicles *(13)*. Below mentioned are the phase-transition temperatures of non-ionic surfactants (Table 2). The transition temperatures of surfactants increases from 46–47°C to 56–58°C as the hydrocarbon length is increased (C9–C15). This stability decreases leakage of the vesicles and stabilises against osmotic gradients *(13)*.

Table 1. Chemical Specifications of Surfactants Used in Niosome Preparation

Chemical specification	*Description*	*Molecular weight (g/mol)*	*Molecular formula*	*HLB[54]*
Sorbitan monolaurate (Span 20)	Clear viscous liquid	346.5	$C_{18}H_{34}O_6$	8.6
Sorbitan monopalmitate (Span 40)	Yellowish powder	402.6	$C_{22}H_{42}O_6$	6.7
Sorbitan monostearate (Span 60)	White powder	430.6	$C_{24}H_{46}O_6$	4.7
CHOL	White powder	386.7	$C_{27}H_{46}O$	N/A
Dicetyl phosphate	White powder	546.9	$C_{32}H_{67}O_4P$	N/A
5(6)-Carboxyfluorescein (CF)	Yellowish powder	376.0	$C_{21}H_{12}O_7$	N/A

Table 2. Phase-Transition Temperature of Span 20, Span 40 and Span 60

Non-ionic surfactant	*Acyl composition*	*Gel transition temperature*
Sorbitan monolaurate (Span 20)	C9	Liquid at room temperature
Sorbitan monopalmitate (Span 40)	C13	46–47°C
Sorbitan monostearate (Span 60)	C15	56–58°C

4.1. Spherulites

Spherulites are liposome like vesicles made of surfactants and, in some rare cases, polymers under shear. They are considered structurally to have lyotropic lamellar phases and are closely packed vesicles made of repeated lamellar units forming onion-like structures. Their size is governed by shear and can vary between 0.1 and 50 lm and have between 10 and 1000 layers. The multi-lamellar vesicles (MLVs), made in this way have properties similar to the lamellar phase, like solubilisation of water or oil, inter-lamellar spacing and bending rigidity. In recent years, a number of studies have explored the prospects of encapsulating sub-micron particles *(25)*, fatty acids, enzymes *(26)* and use of MLVs as chemical microreactors *(27)* and as a pH regulator inside microcapsules *(28)* using so-called spherulite technology. At rest, the lamellar state is the equilibrium structure. When subjected to shear, the phase experiences a series of transformations that modify the topology of lamellae in space relative to the direction of shear field *(29,30)*.

5. METHODS OF PREPARATION

Niosomes are prepared by methods similar to that used for liposome preparation and these methods are described in detail under liposome chapter.

The traditional method for producing niosomes involves drying the surfactant and lipid mixture to a thin film from organic solvent, and then hydrating this film with the aqueous solvent of choice *(32)*. The resulting MLVs can be further processed by sonication, extrusion or other treatments to optimise drug entrapment *(33)*. Other methods includes injection of surfactant and lipid mixture in water-miscible or water-immiscible solvents into an aqueous solution, detergent dialysis or reverse-phase evaporation. *(33)*. All of these methods are time consuming and many involve specialised equipment. The thin film approach allows only for a pre-determined lot size, so material is often wasted if smaller quantities are required for a particular application or dose.

The influence of formulation factors on niosome stability is examined as methods to optimise drug loading. Physical properties like particle size, shape and charge are also to be optimised for their *in vivo* performance as these systems have been used as immunological adjuvant, carriers for various class of drugs for target delivery. Niosomes have also been used in diagnostic imaging. Efforts to achieve transdermal and ophthalmic drug delivery with some formulations are also reported *(9)*.

Large polyhedral niosomes of size 2–10 μm were prepared from mixtures of a hexadecyl diglycerol ether (C16G2), a cholesteryl poly-24-oxyethylene ether (Solulan C24) and a low level of CHOL. They are investigated as slow-release systems for ophthalmic, sub-cutaneous or intra-muscular administration. The phase-diagram constructed of this three-component system showed that these polyhedral vesicles are found to be in gel (L-β) phase. The complex morphology of these vesicles was confirmed by confocal laser-scanning microscopy *(9)*.

Nasseri and Florence prepared the same niosome formulation by extrusion through micro-capillaries under pressure to form multi-lamellar tubules up to about 80 μm in length *(15)*. The diameter of the extruded tubules depends on the exit diameter of the capillaries used (around 1 μm). Under some circumstances, instead of linear tubules, the tubules form as concentric whorls, which can be unraveled into their constituent tubules, indicating the strength of the systems. They also reported that these microtubules formed under the pressure, lead to the fusion of many vesicles giving rise to the formation of three distinctive structures, namely tubules, vesicle within tubule and concentric ("whorl") morphologies *(34)*. The entrapment efficiency of the tubules was influenced by shear stress and the compaction pressure on release of the entrapped solute. Deformation of the structures affects their ability to retain entrapped solute. Tubular structures heated above their transition temperatures reversibly transform into discrete vesicular structures *(35)*. They are described as early prototype of a pulsatile delivery system for drug containing NSVs (niosomes). The pulsatile release profile of luteinising hormone releasing hormone (LHRH) from such a system was found to be due to pulsatile expulsion of groups of niosomes from them.

Membrane composition of the niosomes determined their size and shape. Spherical or polyhedral niosomes were formed when polyoxyethylene alkyl ethers (CnEOm) was used with and without CHOL, respectively. Niosomes with diameters larger than exit diameter of the capillary did not retain their membrane integrity on extrusion and were sheared to form new ultrastructures. However, tetradecyl-β-D-maltoside niosomes with sizes smaller than the exit diameter were also achieved readily.

Arunothayanun and co-workers *(36)*, studied the effects of processing variables, particularly temperature and sonication, on the physical characteristics and phase-transitional behaviour of two niosomal systems based on a hexadecyl diglycerol ether (C[16]G[2]). Systems containing C(16)G(2), CHOL and poly-24-oxyethylene cholesteryl ether (solulan C24) in the molar ratios 91:0:9 and 49:49:2 were prepared by aqueous dispersion of films, followed by examination of 5(6)-CF entrapment, particle size and morphology. The thermal behaviour examined using high-sensitivity differential scanning calorimetry and hot stage microscopy, showed the polyhedral vesicles to convert to spherical structures at approximately 48°C, while on cooling the spherical vesicles split into smaller structures and reverted to the polyhedral shape at approximately 49°C. Sonication resulted in the polyhedral vesicles forming spherical structures, which underwent a particle size increase on storage at room temperature but not at 60°C *(35)*.

Ketoconazole niosome were prepared by ether injection technique using surfactant (Tween-40 or -80), CHOL and drug in five different ratios by weight, 1:1:1, 1.5:1:1, 2:1:1, 2.5:1:1 and 3:1:1 and were characterised for size, shape, entrapment efficiency and *in vitro* drug release (by exhaustive dialysis). The formulations when tested for *in vitro* (cup-plate method) and *in vivo* anti-fungal activity (in rabbits) in comparison to free ketoconazole, indicated that niosomes have the potential to reduce the therapeutic dose of ketoconazole by improving its performance *(37)*.

Tretinoin-loaded niosomes were prepared from polyoxyethylene lauryl ether, sorbitan esters and a commercial mixture of octyl decyl polyglucosides, in the presence of CHOL and dicetyl phosphate. Liposomes made of hydrogenated and non-hydrogenated phosphatidylcholine were also prepared as a comparison reference. A study made to assess the influence of vesicle composition and preparation method on the vesicle structure (MLV, large unilamellar vesicles [LUVs] and small unilamellar vesicles [SUVs]), size distribution, entrapment efficiency and *in vitro* release of incorporated tretinoin showed that (a) vesicle sizes were dependent on the preparation method, bilayer composition and drug load, (b) drug-loaded vesicles were generally smaller than empty ones, (c) entrapment efficiencies of tretinoin were always very high especially for multi-lamellar (91–99%) and extruded (88–98%) vesicles, (d) the rate of drug release through a Silastic membrane from niosomal tretinoin dispersion was generally faster than from a tretinoin solution and (e) tretinoin delivery is mainly affected by the vesicular structure and that tretinoin delivery increased from MLVs to LUVs to small unilamellar vesicles (SUVs) *(19)*.

Van Hal *et al.* (1996) prepared NSVs from CnEOm and sugar ester surfactants to establish the relationship between the HLB, gel–liquid transition temperature (T_c) of the surfactants and vesicle formation. Results indicated that for spontaneous vesicle formation both an HLB between 7.5 and 10.5 and a T_c below the experimental temperature were necessary. However, surfactants with a suitable HLB, but with a high T_c, were also able to form vesicles upon sonication. CHOL encapsulation facilitated vesicle formation and the minimum amount of CHOL necessary to form vesicles and the maximum amount that could be encapsulated were related to the HLB and T_c. Addition of CHOL and dicetylphosphate decreased the size of NSVs while CHOL alone decreased the floating and increased the sedimentation behaviour of vesicles. Dicetylphosphate stabilised the suspensions and minimised the aggregation behaviour of sugar ester vesicles *(6)*.

6. PRO-NIOSOMES

All the traditional methods generally adopted for producing niosomes or liposomes like thin film hydration, sonication and extrusion, lipid injection and detergent dialysis, or reverse-phase evaporation methods are complicated and need downstream processing to remove certain components following liposome formation *(32,33)*. In addition, these methods are time consuming, difficult to scale up and many involve specialised equipment. Pro-niosomes *(38)* and pro-liposomes *(39)* circumvent all of these complications. These are dry formulations of surfactant-coated carrier, which can be measured out as needed and re-hydrated by brief agitation in hot water. Pro-niosomes (and pro-liposomes) are normally made by spraying surfactant in organic solvent onto sorbitol powder and then evaporating the solvent. Because the sorbitol carrier is soluble in organic solvent, it is necessary to repeat process until the desired surfactant loading has been achieved. The surfactant coating on the carrier is very thin and hydration of this coating allows MLVs to form as the carrier dissolves *(11,32)*. The resulting niosomes are very similar to those produced by conventional methods and the size distribution is more uniform. It was suggested that this formulation could provide a suitable method for formulating hydrophobic drugs in a lipid suspension without concerns over instability of the suspension or susceptibility of active ingredient to hydrolysis *(38)*.

7. PROPERTIES

In addition to common spherical niosomes, disc-like, tubular and polyhedral niosomes have also been reported. The permeability and osmotic activity of niosomes are important in determining their use as controlled-release drug delivery systems. These properties have been compared for polyhedral niosomes prepared by hydrating a mixture of hexadecyl diglycerol ether (C16G2), a poly(24) oxyethylene cholesteryl ether (solulan C24), 91:9 or 98:2, and conventional spherical niosomes prepared from the same surfactants but with CHOL. When subjected to osmotic gradients, polyhedral niosomes, the membranes of which are in gel phase, swell and shrink less than their spherical counterparts and they are more permeable to hydrophilic solute, 5(6)-CF. In 2 *M* NaCl solution, the rate of release of CF from polyhedral niosomes (both containing 9% solulan C24) into either a hypotonic medium (water) or 2 *M* NaCl solution was low. This contrasted with similarly loaded spherical niosomes and polyhedral niosomes containing 2% solulan C24, from which release was high in hypotonic media (e.g., water) but less in 2 *M* NaCl. For both polyhedral and spherical niosomes encapsulating CF (pK_a = 6.4), release rates were higher at pH 8.0 than at pH 5.0. Polyhedral niosomes are thus, in general, less osmotically active than spherical niosomes because of their rigid but highly permeable membranes. The unusual polyhedral membrane impermeability to CF co-entrapped with salt in hypotonic media is a function of solulan C24 content, and is possibly a result of salting out of polyoxyethylene chains; this is, therefore, a property that might be manipulated in the design of a drug delivery system *(40)*.

8. RELEASE BEHAVIOUR

The thermo-responsive nature of release of CF and nicotinamide adenine dinucleotide entrapped in polyhedral niosome prepared from mixtures of a hexadecyl diglycerol ether (C16G2), a cholesteryl poly-24-oxyethylene ether (solulan C24) and a low level of CHOL has been studied by Uchegbu *et al. (1)*. The release was found to increase with increase in temperature (37°C). However, even then the polyhedral shape of vesicles still maintained at this temperature. This result indicates that the thermo-responsive features of the niosomes are a result of reversible changes in bilayer permeability caused by temperature-mediated alteration in the membrane packing characteristics of polyethoxylated CHOL ether.

9. CHARACTERISATION

Niosomes are required to be characterised for structural and transformational properties, rheological behaviour, bilayer thickness and molecular interfacial area in addition to general characteristics like particle size, shape, entrapment and charge by methods which are similar to those for liposomes.

9.1. Structural and Transformational Properties

Niosomes formed by a hexadecyl diglycerol ether (C16G2) and a series of CnEoM exhibit a variety of shapes dependent on their membrane composition. These surfactants form with an equimolar amount of CHOL a mixture of largely spherical and tubular niosomes while in the absence of CHOL, they form faceted polyhedral structures. The physicochemical and biological differences between polyhedral and spherical/tubular niosomes as described above. Polyhedral niosomes undergo a reversible shape transformation into spherical structures on heating above their phase-transition temperature (T_c) and are determined by differential scanning calorimetric studies (DSC).

9.2. Rheological Behaviour

The viscosity of polyhedral niosomes at room temperature is higher than their spherical counterparts due to their faceted and relatively rigid shape and is more dependent on temperature due to shape transformation. At room temperature, polyhedral niosomes possess more rigid gel phase membranes and are less osmotically sensitive; however, they are more permeable because of a lack of or low levels of CHOL in their membranes. Polyhedral niosomes loaded with LHRH, nonetheless, slow the release of drug compared with solution, albeit to a small extent *(41)*.

9.3. Bilayer Thickness and Molecular Interfacial Area

Small-angle neutron-scattering (SANS) studies are used extensively in conjugation with SANS data fitting software to determine bilayer thickness and molecular interfacial area. Drug delivery vesicles formed from 1,2-di-*O*-octadecyl- and 1,2-di-*O*-hexadecyl-rac-glycerol-3-(ω-methoxydode-caethylene glycol) (2C18-E12 and 2C16E12, respectively) were subjected to SANS showed the 2C18E12 vesicles to be delimited by single bilayers 55 Å thick, while the 2C16E12 vesicles are more likely delimited by twin bilayers (with lamellae thicknesses of 104 Å). For both types of surfactants, the molecular interfacial areas occupied in the vesicle bilayers are calculated to be approximately 100 Å. Through model fitting of the SANS data, approximating the vesicle lamellae as infinite sheets, it is shown that the lamellae have undulating (rather than perfectly flat) surfaces, with a small proportion of the surfactant's polyoxyethylene chains inter-mixed with the hydrocarbon chains, and a rather low level of headgroup hydration (of the order of 1 H_2O per oxyethylene unit). In the presence of 0.15 *M* NaCl (used as a crude approximation to human blood plasma), the 2C18E12 vesicle lamellae are completely unaffected, while the 2C16E12 vesicles have mean lamellae thicknesses that are reduced by approximately 20%, possibly because the salt causes changes in the relative proportions of unilamellar and bilamellar vesicles in samples *(42)*.

10. PHARMACOKINETIC AND *IN VIVO* EVALUATION

Niosomes are vesicles formed by the self-assembly of non-ionic surfactants in aqueous dispersions. They can entrap drugs and have been used experimentally as sustained drug delivery systems. Apart from conventional spherical niosomes, various types of vesicle ultrastructures (polyhedral, spherical, tubular, etc.) can be formed by varying the composition of vesicle membrane. The properties of two forms of niosomes were studied using LHRH as a model peptide demonstrated high entrapment of LHRH acetate in polyhedral niosomes when prepared by remote loading methods using pH or $(NH_4)_2SO_4$ gradients; in contrast, only low entrapment was achieved by passive loading methods (direct hydration at pH 7.4 or pH 3.0, dehydration–re-hydration and reversed-phase evaporation). *In vitro* studies demonstrated that both polyhedral and spherical/tubular niosomes were more stable in 5% rat skeletal muscle homogenate than in rat plasma. Also, LHRH than spherical/tubular niosomes in both muscle homogenate and plasma. In clearance experiments in rat, following intra-muscular injection, both polyhedral and spherical/-tubular niosomes gradually released ^{125}I LHRH into the blood, but some radioactivity remained at the injection site for 25 and 49 h, respectively. In contrast, ^{125}I LHRH in phosphate buffered saline was completely cleared from the injection site at 2 h. The release of drug is sustained by both niosome formulations, but spherical/tubular niosomes possess more stable membranes than polyhedral niosomes due to presence of CHOL *(43)*.

NSVs (niosomes) have potential applications in targeted drug delivery and imaging because of their ability to encapsulate therapeutic agents and their enhanced uptake by physiological membranes. Ultrasound may be used to mediate delivery non-invasively by altering the niosome membrane structure. Niosomes made up of polyoxyethylene sorbitan monostearate (Tween-61), CHOL and dicetyl phosphate was encapsulated with a fluorescing dye, CF as a drug model. The amount of dye in niosomes, the concentration of the vesicles and their mean particle size after each 5 min incremental exposure to ultrasound were monitored. Dye concentration encapsulated by the niosomes in the samples decreased while the population and size distribution of niosome remained largely unchanged. The conclusion is that ultrasound enhances the rate of dye diffusion across the niosome membrane non-destructively *(44)*.

A series of novel niosomes with amphiphilic co-polymer of poly(methoxy-polyethyleneglycol cyanoacrylate-*co*-n-hexadecylcyanoacrylate) (PEG-PHDCA) acted as surface modification materials were prepared and hydroxycamptothecin (HCPT) was used as a model drug. This work was concentrated on the effects of PEG chain length and particle sizes on niosomes surface properties, *in vitro* drug release, phagocytic uptake, *in vivo* pharmacokinetics and anti-tumour activity. Within the range of PEG molecular weight from 2000 to 10,000, the increasing ζ-potential (from 16.08 to 5.25 mV) and thicker fixed aqueous layer (3.82–5.78 nm) would facilitate the niosomes stealth effects, while the reduced PEG chain density (from 0.53 to 0.17 PEG/nm^2) and the quickened speed of drug release would diminish the effects. As a result, the PEG 5000-PHDCA niosomes had the least phagocytic uptake, the longest half-life of 11.46 h and the best tumour inhibition rate of 97.1%.

In the groups different in particle size (PEG 5000-PHDCA niosomes from 92.5 to 204.6 nm), the bigger particles could be taken up by macrophages more quickly, regardless of changes of other physicochemical parameters. Correspondingly, PEG 5000-PHDCA niosomes with particle sizes of 92.5, 144.2 and 204.6 nm could extend the half-life of HCPT to 11.46, 6.33 and 4.46 h, respectively. The tumour inhibition rate of PEG 5000-PHDCA niosomes (92.5 nm) at a dose of 2 mg/kg was five times that of HCPT injection at 4 mg/kg. The stealth effects of the PEG-PHDCA niosomes and the enhanced stability of lactone form of HCPT were accountable for the powerful anti-tumour effects of niosomes *(45)*.

11. APPLICATIONS

The concept of carriers to deliver drugs to target organs and modify drug disposition has been widely discussed. The majority of such reports have concerned the use of phospholipid vesicles of liposomes, which exhibit certain disadvantages, such as chemical instability, high cost and variable purity of lipids used, which militates against their adoption as drug delivery vehicle. Alternatives to phospholipids are thus of interest from the technical viewpoint and could also allow a wider study of influence of chemical composition on biological fate of vesicles *(47)*.

Non-ionic surfactant vesicles (niosomes) were prepared and appended with a polysaccharide cap using hydrophobic anchors *(46)*. Hydrophobised polysaccharides, O-palmitoyl pullulan (OPPu) and cholesteroyl pullulan (CHPu) were anchored onto propranolol:HCL containing preformed niosomes. The coated niosomes showed no significant difference in percentage encapsulation in comparison to uncoated vesicles. However, a significant lowering ($P < 0.01$) of drug release for the coated systems in simulated gastric and intestinal fluids with a biphasic release profile was reported.

The influence of the hydrophobised polysaccharide cap on niosomal membrane integrity and stabilisation against harsh bio-environment conditions was investigated using parameters like detergent and bile challenge, freeze–thaw cycling, osmotic stress, and long term and shelf stability studies. Uncoated niosomes underwent bilayer solubilisation into intermediate micellar structures, whereas coated niosomes were able to maintain their structural integrity. Similarly, freeze–thaw cycling could not bring any fusion or collapse of the niosomal membrane in coated niosomes unlike the uncoated ones. Furthermore, the exceptional shelf stability of the coated vesicles both at 37 ± 1°C and at 4 ± 1°C establishes the potential of polysaccharide coated niosomes as an oral delivery system for water-soluble agents *(46)*.

Jain and Vyas *(48)* developed mannosylated niosomes as a topical vaccine delivery carrier and adjuvant for the induction of both humoral and cellular immunity. Bovine serum albumin (BSA)-loaded niosomes composed of sorbitan monostearate/sorbitan trioleate (Span 60/Span 85), cholesterol and stearylamine as constitutive lipids were prepared by the reverse-phase evaporation method. The niosomes were coated with a modified polysaccharide *O*-palmitoyl mannan (OPM) to target them to Langerhan's cells, the major antigen presenting cells found in abundance beneath the stratum corneum. The immune stimulating activity studied by measuring serum IgG titre and its subclasses (IgG2a/IgG1 ratio) following topical application in albino rats showed that niosomal formulations elicited a significantly higher serum IgG titre as compared with topically applied alum adsorbed BSA ($P < 0.05$). The serum IgG levels were significantly higher for the mannosylated niosomes as compared with plain uncoated niosomes ($P < 0.05$). All formulations displayed a combined serum IgG2a/IgG1 response, which suggested that the formulations were capable of eliciting both humoral and cellular responses. The proposed system would be simple, stable, and cost effective and might be clinically acceptable *(48)*.

Christine *et al. (49)* evaluated glucose-bearing niosomes as a brain targeted delivery system for the vasoactive intestinal peptide (VIP) in mice. Brain uptake was determined by measuring the radioactivity of ^{125}I-labeled VIP using γ-counting, after intravenous administration of VIP in solution or encapsulated in glucose-bearing niosomes or in control niosomes. HPLC analysis confirmed the presence of intact VIP in brain after administration of VIP-loaded niosomes, but not after administration of VIP solution. Encapsulation within glucose-bearing niosomes mainly allowed a significantly higher VIP brain uptake compared to control niosomes particularly in posterior and anterior parts of the brain as assessed by radioactive study.

Niosome vaginal delivery system for systemic treatment of insulin was studied using two kinds of vesicles prepared with Span 40 and Span 60 by lipid phase evaporation methods with sonication *(50)*. The particle sizes of Span 40 niosomes and Span 60 niosomes were 242.5 ± 20.5 nm and 259.7 ± 33.8 nm, respectively. The hypoglycemic effects, and insulin concentrations after vaginal administration of insulin vesicles to rats were compared with subcutaneous administration of insulin solution.The relative pharmacological bioavailability and relative bioavailability of Span 60 and Span 40 niosomes were both higher than blank Span 40, Span 60 vesicles, and free insulin physical mixture groups ($p < 0.05$) indicating an enhancing effect of insulin-Span 60, Span 40 niosomes on vaginal delivery of insulin.

Niosomes containing salbutamol sulphate were prepared *(51)* using different non-ionic surfactants like Tween-20, -40, -60 and -80, Span 20, 40, 60 and 80 and Brij 35 by transmembrane pH gradient method. The drug encapsulation efficiency varied from 28% to 79%. *In vitro* drug release studies carried out in phosphate buffer, pH 7.4 exhibited retarded release for 24 h and Span 60 was found to be the most satisfactory surfactant which released 78.4% of drug in 24 h. Tissue distribution studies carried out on rabbits showed maximum concentration in lungs.

An alternative formulation for the vaginal administration of clotrimazole to provide sustained and controlled release of the drug for local vaginal therapy was prepared as liposome/niosomes and were evaluated as delivery vehicles *(52)*. The ability of the systems to deliver clotrimazole into and through the mucosa was evaluated *in vitro* using rabbit vaginal mucosa with vertical Franz diffusion cell. The *in vitro* permeation data showed that the liposomes/niosomes system increased the clotrimazole total penetration through the vaginal mucosa by 1.6/1.5-fold, the accumulation of clotrimazole into the mucosa was increased by 3.1, 2.3-fold, respectively, as compared with control during 24 h.

11.1. Anti-Cancer Niosomes

The success achieved with liposomal systems stimulated the search for other vesicle forming amphiphiles for anti-cancer drug delivery. Non-ionic surfactants were among the first alternative materials studied *(53)* and a large number of surfactants capable of self assemble into closed bilayer vesicles *(54)* are used to develop anti-cancer drug delivery. Suitably designed anti-cancer niosomes are expected to accumulate within tumours in a similar manner to that of liposomes. The niosomal encapsulation of methotrexate *(55)* and doxorubicin *(56,57)* increased drug delivery to the tumour and tumouricidal activity. Unlike non-stealth liposomes, 800 nm doxorubicin niosomes, possessing a triglycerol *(56,58)* or 200 nm doxorubicin niosomes possessing a muramic acid *(59)* surface are not taken up significantly by the liver. As such, these triglycerol niosomes accumulate in the tumour *(56)*. However, muramic acid vesicles are found to accumulate in the spleen *(59)*. On the other hand, 200 nm doxorubicin niosomes with a polyoxyethylene (molecular weight 1000) surface are rapidly taken up by the liver *(57)* and accumulate to a lesser extent in tumour while, a polyoxyethylene coating with a molecular weight of 2000 was found to be optimal for stealth liposomes. It is obvious that, like liposomes and presumably any parenterally administered colloidal particulates, body disposition may be controlled by alterations in particulate surface chemistry.

The accumulation of certain niosomes within the liver may be exploited; however, doxorubicin polymer conjugates *(61)* are prepared by conjugating the anti-cancer drug to a polymeric backbone through an enzymatically cleavable spacer. The encapsulation of these polymeric prodrugs within 200 nm niosomes *(62)* provides a depot system within the liver from which free drug is gradually cleaved off and liver levels of drug are seen to rise over a 24 h period *(62)*. This technology may prove advantageous for treatment of hepatic neoplasms. The activity of other anti-cancer drugs, such as vincristine *(63)*, bleomycin *(64)* and plumbagin, a plant derived anti-cancer agent *(65)*, are also improved on niosomal encapsulation.

Uptake by liver and spleen *(54)* make niosomes ideal for targeting diseases manifesting in these organs. One such condition is leishmaniasis and a number of studies *(66–68)* have shown that niosomal formulations of sodium Stilbogluconate improve parasite suppression in liver *(66,67)*, spleen and bone marrow *(69)* Niosomes may also be used as depot systems for short acting peptide drugs on intra-muscular administration *(43)*.

11.2. Niosomes as Vaccine Adjuvants

Niosomal antigens are potent stimulators of cellular and humoral immune response *(70,71)*. The formulation of antigens as a niosome in water-in-oil emulsion further increases the activity of antigens *(72)*. The controlled release property of emulsion formulation is responsible for enhancing the immunological response.

11.3. Niosomes in Imaging

NSVs are considered as carriers of iobitridol, a diagnostic agent used for X-ray imaging. The niosomes, with a diameter between 150 and 175 nm, are prepared using the film-hydration method followed by sonication. These vesicles were obtained with appropriate mixtures of D-α tocopheryl polyethylene glycol 1000 succinate, polyoxyethylene glycol 4000 stearate, sorbitan monostearate, CHOL and dicetylphosphate. Methods allowing increase of the rate of encapsulation and the stability of vesicles were carried out. In addition to study of formulation of the vesicles, the physicochemical and morphological properties of vesicles have been studied *(73)*.

11.4. Other Vesicles

Vesicles for use in drug delivery have also been prepared from amphiphilic carbohydrate and amino acid based polymers *(74,75)* and also from aged red blood cells *(76)*. The latter increase intra-cellular drug delivery to virus infected cells. Non-ionic surfactants and other amphiphiles may be used to prepare a number of different drug carriers with varied surfaces. This should provide the basis for the development of drug delivery vesicles with different biodistribution profiles *(60)*.

12. TOXICITY

Two different toxicity models were used to assess the relationship between physicochemical properties of NSVs, and safety of these vesicles for topical drug administration. The vesicles used in this study consisted of C*n*EO*m* in which the number of C atoms (*n*) varied between 12 and 18 and the number of oxyethylene units (*m*) between 3 and 7. The first toxicity model, comprising the measurement of ciliary beat frequency, is a tool to assess the safety of intra-nasally applied formulations. Studies using this ciliotoxicity model revealed that by increasing the length of the alkyl chain of surfactant, a decrease in toxicity was observed. The opposite correlation was found if the length of the polyoxyethylene headgroup was increased. Furthermore, it was observed that gel-state vesicles produce less of an effect on the ciliary beat frequency than liquid state vesicles. The second toxicity model, comprising the determination of cell proliferation of human keratinocytes, is a method to assess skin irritancy. In contrast to the ciliotoxicity model the length of polyoxyethylene headgroup and of the alkyl chains did not seem to have an effect on the safety of the vesicles *(77)*.

13. REFERENCES

1. **Uchegbu, IF., Schatzlein, A., Vanlerberghe, G., and Morgatini, N., Florence, AT.** Polyhedral non-ionic surfactant vesicles. *J. Pharm. Pharmacol.* 1997;49(6):606–610.
2. **Engberts, JBFN. and Hoekstra, D.** Vesicle-forming synthetic amphiphiles. *Biochim. Biophys. Acta* 1996;1241:323–340.
3. **Engberts, JBFN. and Kevelam, J.** Formation and stability of micelles and vesicles. *Curr. Opin. Colloid Interf. Sci.* 1996;1:779–789.
4. **Singh, A., Chow, GM., Chang, EL., and Markowitz, MA.** Making stable nanospheres and tubules. *Chem. Tech.* 1995;25:38–43.
5. **Israelachvili, JN.** Inter-molecular and surface forces, ed. 4, London, Academic Press, 1994.
6. **Van Hal, DA., Bouwstra, JA., Van Rensen, A., Jeremiasse, E., De Vringer, T., and Junginger, HE.** Preparation and characterization of non-ionic surfactant vesicles. *J. Colloid Interf. Sci.* 1996;178:263–273.
7. **Zhang, LF. and Eisenberg, A.** Multiple morphologies and characteristics of crew-cut micelle-like aggregates of polystyrene-b-poly (acrylic acid) diblock copolymers in aqueous solutions. *J. Am. Chem. Soc.* 1996;118:3168–3181.
8. **Arimori, S., Nagasaki, T., and Shinkai, S.** Self-assambly of tetracationic amphiphiles bearing a calix[4]arene core. Correlation between the core structure and the aggregation properties. *J. Chem. Soc. Perkin. Trans.* 1995;2:679–683.
9. **Uchegbu, IF. and Vyas, SP.** Non-ionic surfactant based vesicles (niosomes) in drug delivery. *Int. J. pharm.* 1998;172(2):33–70.
10. **Uchegbu, IF. and Florence, AT.** Non-ionic surfactant vesicles (niosomes): physical and pharmaceutical chemistry. *Adv. Colloid Interf. Sci.* 1995;58:1–55.
11. **Yoshioka, T., Sternberg, B., and Florence, AT.** Preparation of vesicles (niosomes) of sorbitan monoesters (Span 20, 40, 60 and 80) and a sorbitan trimester (Span 85). *Int. J. Pharm.* 1994;105:1–6.
12. **Lawrence, MJ.** The formation, characterization and stability of non-ionic surfactant vesicles. *STP Pharma. Sci.* 1996;1:49–60.
13. **Bouwstra, JA., van Hal, DA., and Hofland, HE.** Preparation and characterization of non-ionic surfactant vesicles. *Colloids surf. A: Physiochem. Eng. Aspects* 1997;123–124:71–80.
14. **Manosroi, A., Wongtrakul, P., Manosroi, J., et al.** Characterization of vesicles prepared with various non-ionic surfactants mixed with cholesterol. *Colloids Surf. B: Biointerf.* 2003;30:129–138.
15. **Nasseri, B. and Florence, AT.** Microtubules formed by capillary extrusion and fusion of surfactant vesicles. *Int. J. Pharm.* 2003;266:91–98.
16. **Nasseri, B. and Florence, AT.** A vesicular shuttle: transport of a vesicle within a flexible microtube. *J. Control. Release* 2003;92:233–240.
17. **Hao, Y., Zhao, F., Li, N., Yang, Y., and Li, K.** Studies on a high encapsulation of colchicine by a niosome system. *Int. J. Pharm.* 2002; 244:73–80.
18. **Fang, JY., Yu, SY., Wu, PC., Huang, YB., and Tsai, YH.** *In vitro* skin permeation of estradiol from various proniosome formulations. *Int. J. Pharm.* 2001;215:91–99.
19. **Manconi, M., Sinico, C., Valenti, D., Loy, G., and Fadda, AM.** Niosomes as carriers for tretinoin I. Preparation and properties. *Int. J. Pharm.* 2002;234:237–248.
20. **Manconi, M., Valenti, D., Sinico, C., Lai, F., Loy, G., and Fadda, AM.** Niosomes as carriers for tretinoin II. Influence of vesicular incorporation on tretinoin photostability. *Int. J. Pharm.* 2003;260:261–272.
21. **Touitou, E., Junginger, HE., Weiner, ND., Nagai, T., and Mezei, M.** Liposomes as carriers for topical and transdermal delivery. *J. Pharm. Sci.* 1994;83:1189–1203.
22. **Agarwal, R., Katare, OP., and Vyas, SP.** Preparation and *in vitro* evaluation of liposomal/niosomal delivery systems for antipsoriatic drug dithranol. *Int. J. Pharm.* 2001;228:43–52.
23. **Fang, JY., Hong, CT., Chiu, WT., and Wang, YY.** Effect of liposomes and niosomes on skin permeation of enoxacin. *Int. J. Pharm.* 2001;219:61–72.
24. **Udupa, N., Chandraprakash, KS., Umadevi, P., and Pillai, GK.** Formulation and evaluation of methotrexate niosomes. *Drug Dev. Industr. Pharm.* 1993;19:1331–1342.
25. **Arrault, J., Grand, C., Poon, *WCK.*, and Cates, ME.** Stuffed onions: Particles in multilamellar vesicles, *Europhys. Lett.* 1997;38:625.
26. **Bernheim-Grosswasser, A., Ugazio, S., Gauffre, F., Viratelle, O., Mahy, P., and Roux, D.** Spherulites: A new vesicular system with promising applications. An example: Enzyme microencapsulation, *J. Chem. Phys.* 2000;112:3424.
27. **Gauffre, F. and Roux, D.** Studying a new type of surfactant aggregate ("Spherulites") as chemical microreactors. A first example: copper ion entrapping and particle synthesis. *Langmuir* 1999;15(11):3738.
28. **Gauffre, F. and Roux, D.** Evidence for a pH difference controlled by thermodynamics between the interior and the exterior of a new type of vesicles in suspension. *Langmuir* 1999;15(9):3070.
29. **Diat, O., Roux, D., and Nallet, F.** Effect of shear on a lyotropic lamellar phase olivier diat, didier roux and frédéric nallet**.** *J. Phys. II (France)* 1993;3:1427–1452.
30. **Le, TD., Olssona, U., and Mortensen, K.** Packing states of multilamellar vesicles in a non ionic surfactant system. *Phys. Chem. Chem. Phys.* 2001;3:1310–1316.
31. **Almira, I., Blazek-Welsh., and David, G.** Rhodes maltodextrin-based proniosomes. *AAPS Pharmsci.* 2001;3(1):*article 1.*
32. **Bangham, AD., Standish, MM., and Watkins, JC.** Diffusion of univalent ions across the lamellae of swollen phospholipids. *J. Mol. Biol.* 1965;13:238–252.
33. **Van Winden, ECA., Zuidam, NJ., and Crommelin, DJA.** Strategies for large scale production and optimized stability of pharmaceutical liposomes developed for parenteral use, (Lasic, DD. and Papahadjopoulos, D., eds.), Amsterdam, Elsevier, *Med. Appl. Liposomes* 1998;567–604.
34. **Nasseri, B. and Florence, AT.** Some properties of extruded non-ionic surfactant micro-tubes. *Int. J. Pharm.* 2003;254(1):11–16.
35. **Arunothayanun, P., Sooksawate, T., and Florence, AT.** Extrusion of niosomes from capillaries: approaches to a pulsed delivery device. *J. Control. Release* 1999;60(2–3):391–397.

36. **Arunothayanun, P., Bernard, MS., Craig, DQ., Uchegbu, IF., and Florence, AT.** The effect of processing variables on the physical characteristics of non-ionic surfactant vesicles (niosomes) formed from a hexadecyl diglycerol ether. *Int. J. Pharm.* 2000;201(1):7–14.

37. **Satturwar, PM., Fulzele, SV., Nande, VS., and Khandare, JN.** Formulation and evaluation of ketoconazole niosomes. *Ind. J. Pharm. Sci.* 2002;64(2):155–158.

38. **Hu, C. and Rhodes, DG.** Proniosomes: a novel drug carrier preparation. *Int. J. Pharm.* 1999;185(1):23–35.

39. **Payne, NI., Timmins, P., Ambrose, CV., Ward, MD., and Ridgway, F.** Proliposomes: a novel solution to an old problem. *J. Pharm. Sci.* 1986;75(4):325–329.

40. **Arunothayanun, P., Uchegbu, IF., and Florence, AT.** Osmotic behaviour of polyhedral non-ionic surfactant vesicles (niosomes). *J. Pharm. Pharmacol.* 1999;51(6):651–657.

41. **Arunothayanun, P., Uchegbu, IF., Craig, DQ., Turton, JA., and Florence, AT.** *In vitro/in vivo* characterisation of polyhedral niosomes. *Int. J. Pharm.* 1999;183(1):57–61.

42. **Ma, G., Barlow, DJ., Lawrence, MJ., Heenan, RK., and Timmins, P.** Small-angle neutron-scattering studies of non ionic surfactant vesicles. *J. Phys. Chem. B.* 2000;104(39):9081–9085.

43. **Arunothayanun, P., Turton, JA., Uchegbu, IF., and Florence, AT.** Preparation and *in vitro/in vivo* evaluation of luteinizing hormone releasing hormone (LHRH)-loaded polyhedral and spherical/tubular niosomes. *J. Pharm. Sci.* 1999;88(1):34–38.

44. **Hood, E., Gonzalez, M., Strom, J., and Vanauker, M.** Ultrasound enhancement of drug release across non ionic surfactant vesicle membranes. *Conf. Proc. IEEE Eng. Med. Biol. Soc.* 2004;5:3527–3530.

45. **Shi, B., Fang, C., and Pei, Y.** Stealth PEG-PHDCA niosomes: effects of chain length of PEG and particle size on niosomes surface properties, in vitro drug release, phagocytic uptake, in vivo pharmacokinetics and anti-tumor activity. *J. Pharm. Sci.* 2006;95(9):1873–1887.

46. **Sihorkar, V. and Vyas, SP.** Polysaccharide coated niosomes for oral drug delivery: formulation and in vitro stability studies. *Pharmazie.* 2000;55(2):107–113.

47. **Namdeo, A. and Jain, NK.** Niosomes as drug carriers. *Ind. J. Pharm. Sci.* 1996;58(2):41–46.

48. **Jain, S. and Vyas, SP.** Mannosylated niosomes as carrier adjuvant system for topical immunization. *J. Pharm. Pharmacol.* 2005;57(9):1177.

49. **Dufes, C., Gaillard, F., Uchegbu, IF., Schhtzlein, AG., Olivier, JC., and Muller JM.** Glucose-targeted niosomes deliver vasoactive intestinal peptide (VIP) to the brain. *Int. J. Pharm.* 2004;285(1–2):77–85.

50. **Ning, M., Guo,Y., Pan, H., Yu, H., and Gu, Z.** Niosomes with sorbitan monoester as a carrier for vaginal delivery of insulin: studies in rats. *Drug Deliv.* 2005;12(6):399–407.

51. **Bhaskaran, S. and Panigrahi, L.** Formulation and evaluation of niosomes using different non-ionic surfactants *Ind. J. Pharm. Sci.* 2002;64(1):63–65.

52. **Ning, M., Gu, Z., Pan, H., Yu, H., and Xiao, K.** Preparation and in vitro evaluation of liposomal/niosomal delivery systems for antifungal drug clotrimazole. *Ind. J. Expt. Biol.* 2005;43: 158–162.

53. **Iga, K., Ohkouchi, K., Ogawa, Y., and Toguchi, H.** Membrane modification by negatively charged stearylpolyoxyethylene derivatives for thermosensitive liposomes: reduced liposomal aggregation and avoidance of reticuloendothelial system uptake. *J. Drug Target* 1994;2:259–267.

54. **Ahl, PL., Bhatia, SK., Meers, P., et al.** Enhancement of the in vivo circulation lifetime of L-alpha-distearoylphosphatidylcholine liposomes: importance of liposomal aggregation versus complement opsonization. *Biochim. Biophys. Acta.* 1997;1329:370–382.

55. **Chandraprakash, KS., Udupa, N., Devi, PU., and Pillai, GK.** Effect of niosome encapsulation of methotrexate, macrophage activation on tissue distribution of methotrexate and tumour size. *Drug Deliv.* 1993;1:133–137.

56. **Rogerson, A., Cummings, J., Willmott, N., and Florence, AT.** The distribution of doxorubicin in mice following administration in niosomes. *J. Pharm. Pharmacol.* 1988;40:337–342.

57. **Uchegbu, IF., Double, JA., Turton, JA., and Florence, AT.** Distribution, metabolism and tumoricidal activity of doxorubicin administered in sorbitan monostearate (Span 60) niosomes in the mouse. *Pharm. Res.* 1995;12:1019–1024.

58. **Cable, C.** An examination of the effects of surface modifications on the physicochemical and biological properties of non-ionic surfactant vesicles (PhD thesis), Glasgow, University of Strathclyde, 1989.

59. **Uchegbu, IF.** The biodistribution of novel 200 nm palmitoyl muramic acid vesicles. *Int. J. Pharm.* 1998;162:19–27.

60. **Uchegbu, IF.** Science in pharmacy, parenteral drug delivery: 1. *Pharm. J.* 1999; 263(7060):309–318.

61. **Duncan, R.** Drug polymer conjugates—potential for improved chemotherapy. *Anti-Cancer Drugs* 1992;3:175–210.

62. **Uchegbu, IF. and Duncan, R.** Niosomes containing N-(2-hydroxypropyl) methacrylamide copolymer-doxorubicin (PK1): effect of method of preparation and choice of surfactant on niosome characteristics and a preliminary study of body distribution. *Int. J. Pharm.* 1997;155:7–17.

63. **Parthasarathi, G., Udupa, N., Umadevi, P., and Pillai, GK.** Niosome encapsulated of vincristine sulfate: improved anticancer activity with reduced toxicity in mice. *J. Drug Target* 1994;2:173–182.

64. **Naresh, RAR. and Udupa, N.** Niosome encapsulated bleomycin. *STP Pharm. Sci.* 1996;6:61–71.

65. **Naresh, RAR., Udupa, N., and Devi, PU.** Niosomal plumbagin with reduced toxicity and improved anticancer activity in Balb/C mice. *J. Pharm. Pharmacol.* 1996;48:1128–1132.

66. **Baillie, AJ., Coombs, GH., Dolan, TF., and Laurie, J.** Non-ionic surfactant vesicles, niosomes, as a delivery system for the anti-leishmanial drug, sodium stibogluconate. *J. Pharm. Pharmacol.* 1986;38:502–505.

67. **Carter, KC., Baillie, AJ., Alexander, J., and Dolan, TF.** The therapeutic effect of sodium stibogluconate in Balb/C mice infected with *Leishmania donovani* is organ dependent. *J. Pharm. Pharmacol.* 1988;40:370–373.

68. **Hunter, CA., Dolan, TF., Coombs, GH., and Baillie, AJ.** Vesicular systems (niosomes and liposomes) for delivery of sodium

stibogluconate in experimental murine visceral leishmaniasis. *J. Pharm. Pharmacol.* 1988;40:161–165.

69. **Williams, DM., Carter, KC., and Baillie, AJ.** Visceral leishmaniasis in the Balb/C mouse—a comparison of the in-vivo activity of 5 non-ionic surfactant vesicle preparations of sodium stibogluconate. *J. Drug Target* 1995;3:1–7.

70. **Brewer, JM. and Alexander, J.** The adjuvant activity of non ionic surfactant vesicles (niosomes) on the Balb/C humoral response to bovine serum albumin. 1992;75:570–575.

71. **Hassan, Y., Brewer, JM., Alexander, J., and Jennings, R.** Immune responses in mice induced by HSV-1 glycoproteins presented with ISCOMs or NISV delivery systems. *Vaccine* 1996;14:1581–1589.

72. **Yoshioka, T., Skalko, N., Gursel, M., Gregoriadis, G., and Florence, AT.** A non-ionic surfactant vesicle-in-water-in-oil (V/W/O) system—potential uses in drug and vaccine delivery. *J. Drug Target* 1995;2:533–539.

73. **Muller, D., Foulon, M., Bonnemain, B., and Vandamme, TF.** Niosomes as carriers of radiopaque contrast agents for X-ray imaging. *J. Microencapsul.* 2000;17(2):227–243.

74. **Uchegbu, IF., Schätzlein, AG., Tetley, L., et al.** Polymeric chitosan based vesicles for drug delivery. *J. Pharm. Pharmacol.* 1998;50:453–458.

75. **Uchegbu, IF., Schätzlein, AG., Tetley, L., Brown, M., Siddique, S., and Jack, V.** Polymeric vesicles from amino acid homopolymers. *Proc. Int. Symp. Control. Rel. Bioact. Mater.* 1998;25:186–187.

76. **Grimaldi, S., Lisi, A., Pozzi, D., and Santoro, N.** Attempts to use liposomes and RBC ghosts as vectors in drug and antisense therapy of virus infection. *Res. Virol.* 1997;148: 177–180.

77. **Hofland, HE., Bouwstra, JA., Verhoef, JC., et al.** Safety aspects of non-ionic surfactant vesicles: a toxicity study related to the physicochemical characteristics of non-ionic surfactants. *J. Pharm. Pharmacol.* 1992;44(4):287–294.

3

Microemulsion

Dr. P. K. Ghosh, M.PHARM, PhD
Dr. Gour Mukherji, M.PHARM, PhD

CONTENTS

1. INTRODUCTION

Schulman and co-workers (1959) coined the term microemulsion to describe the clear, fluid system of an ordinary milky emulsion (macroemulsion) obtained by titration with medium-chain alcohol, such as pentanol or hexanol, to the point of clarity *(1–3)*. Microemulsions were probably discovered well before the studies of Schulman. Since the beginning of last century, Australian housewives have used water–eucalyptus oil–soap flake white spirit mixtures to wash wool. The first commercial microemulsions were probably the liquid waxes discovered by Rodawald in 1928. Interest in microemulsions really took off in late 1970s and early 1980s, when it was recognised that such systems could improve oil recovery, when oil prices reached levels where such tertiary recovery methods became profit earning *(6)*. However, microemulsion applications have been discovered; in pharmaceutical preparations, catalysis, preparation of sub-micron particles, solar energy conversion and liquid–liquid extraction (minerals, proteins, etc.). Together with classical applications in detergency and lubrication, the field remains sufficiently important to continue to attract a number of scientists. From fundamental research point of view, a great deal of progress has been made in the last 20 yr in understanding microemulsion properties.

In 1981, Danielsson and Lindman provided the definition of microemulsion, which was used as a point of reference for aqueous systems with or without electrolyte, oil and non-ionic surfactants that are single isotropic and thermodynamically stable liquid solutions *(4)*.

Microemulsion is thus defined as a thermodynamically stable, translucent dispersions of oil and water stabilised by an interfacial film of surfactant molecules *(5)*. These homogenous systems, which can be prepared over a wide range of surfactant concentrations and oil-to-water ratios, are all fluids of low viscosity.

1.1. Composition of Microemulsion

1.1.1. Surfactants

The surfactants are conveniently classified on an empirical scale known as hydrophilic–lipophilic balance (HLB), which runs from 1 to 20. In general, water dispersed in oil (W/O) microemulsions are formed using surfactants, which have HLBs in the range of about 3–6, whereas oil dispersed in water (O/W) microemulsions are formed using surfactants, which have HLB values in the range of about 8–18.

If the surfactant is ionic and contains a single hydrocarbon chain (e.g., sodium dodecyl sulphate [SDS]) microemulsions are only formed if a co-surfactant (e.g., usually a 4–8 carbon chain aliphatic alcohol, such as pentanol) is present in the system. The most fundamental property for the formation of microemulsions is an ultra-low interfacial tension between oil and water phases, ($\gamma_{O/W}$). The main role of a surfactant is to lower the oil–water interfacial tension by way of their interfacial adsorption. This helps to minimise the relative positive free energy change of dispersion associated with surface formation—so that spontaneous dispersion of water or oil droplets occurs and the system becomes thermodynamically stable. As a result, they are dynamic, and able to rearrange structure in response to changing environmental conditions. Surfactants used in these formulations are also known to improve bioavailability by various mechanisms, including the following:

1. Improved drug dissolution.
2. Increased intestinal epithelial permeability.
3. Increased tight junction permeability.
4. Inhibition of p-glycoprotein efflux.

1.1.2. Co-surfactants

The role of co-surfactant, usually a short-chain alcohol, is to increase the interfacial fluidity by penetrating into the surfactant film. Consequently, it creates a disordered film within the void spaces among surfactant molecules and lowers the interfacial tension *(6)*. This causes easier surface bending to energetically favoured dispersion. A surfactant mixed with a co-surfactant in a certain proportion is most often convenient.

1.2. Microemulsion as a Drug Carrier System

In recent years, considerable emphasis has been given to the development of a microemulsion (O/W or W/O) as a drug carrier system, because of its improved drug solubilisation, long shelf life, ease of preparation, modified drug release characteristic and improvement of bioavailability *(7)*. Microemulsions allow incorporation of hydrophilic, as well as lipophilic compounds, depending on their internal structure. These aggregates have been described as reservoir systems, which allow slow release of drugs, thus providing prolonged effects and avoiding high concentrations in blood. Since microemulsion contains a surfactant among

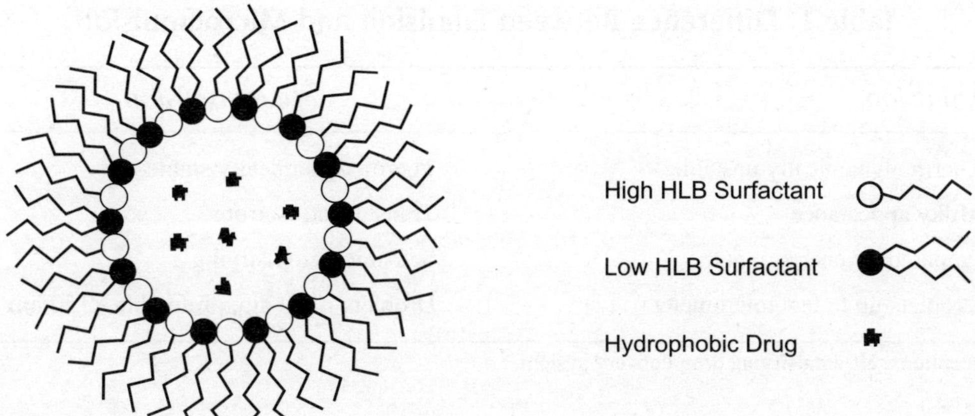

Fig. 1. Common structure of a microemulsion.

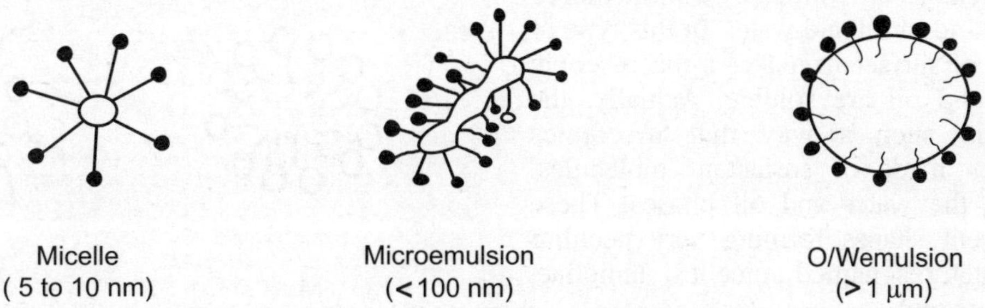

Fig. 2. Structural diagram of different types of emulsions and their dimensions.

its components, application to skin surface usually produces an increase in membrane permeability thus facilitating transdermic transport *(8)*. The common structure of a microemulsion is shown in Fig. 1.

1.3. Emulsion Vs Microemulsion—A Comparison

Microemulsion embraces a number of different microstructures, most of which have little in common with classical two-phase emulsions and are readily distinguished from normal emulsions by their particle size, transparency, low viscosity and more fundamentally, their thermodynamic stability. In addition microemulsions have very flexible, near zero curvature structures whose thermodynamic stability depicts an ultra-low interfacial tension leading to easy interfacial deformation. In other words, a microemulsion can be said to be as not an emulsion with small droplets, but some kind of a weaved complex fabric with oil and water in interconnected domains. The structural diagram of different types of emulsions and their dimensions are shown in Fig.2.

Although systems containing low concentrations of dispersed phases (<25%) may, like emulsions, be composed of droplets of either O/W or W/O, they are essentially stable, single-phase swollen micellar solutions rather than unstable two-phase dispersions. In addition, there are distinct differences in their methods of preparation, since emulsions require a large input of energy while microemulsions do not. A mixture of the right composition of water, amphiphile and oil, may spontaneously homogenise, forming a microemulsion. This has obvious implications when considering the relative cost of commercial production of two types of systems. Table 1 summarises basic differences of an emulsion from a microemulsion.

Table 1. Difference Between Emulsion and Microemulsion

Emulsion	*Microemulsion*
Thermodynamically unstable	Thermodynamically stable
Milky appearance	Translucent, isotropic
Prepared by energy input[a]	Self-microemulsifying
Droplets up to few micrometer	Droplets <200 nm, preferable <150 nm

[a]Exception: self-emulsifying drug delivery system.

2. STRUCTURE OF MICROEMULSIONS

The interfaces observed in a microemulsion, which are of microscopic dimensions, are formed by a surfactant or co-surfactant, some kind of oil and water. In this type of system, the addition of surfactant makes a macroscopic illusion that water and oil are soluble. Actually, the system organises in such a way that it creates microscopic surfaces made of surfactant molecules, whereby, separating the water and oil phases. These surfaces have different shapes forming very peculiar supra-molecular structures named micelles, lamellae, bi-continuous structure, etc.

A *micelle* (plural micellae) is an aggregate of surfactant molecules dispersed in a liquid colloid. A typical micelle in aqueous solution forms a roughly spherical or globular aggregate with hydrophilic "head" regions in contact with surrounding solvent, sequestering the hydrophobic tail regions in the micelle centre. Micelles are often globular and roughly spherical in shape, but ellipsoids, cylinders and bi-layers, are also possible. The shape of a micelle is a function of molecular geometry of its surfactant molecules and solution conditions such as surfactant concentration, temperature, pH and p*I*s. The difference in micelles and reverse micelles in microemulsion is shown in Fig. 3, and the different shapes of micelles and vesicles are shown in Fig. 4. The process of forming micelles is known as micellisation.

Micelles form only when the surfactant concentration is greater than the critical micellar concentration (CMC), and the temperature of system is greater than the critical micellar temperature, or Krafft temperature. The formation of micelles can be understood using thermodynamics. It can form spontaneously because of a balance between entropy and enthalpy. In water, the

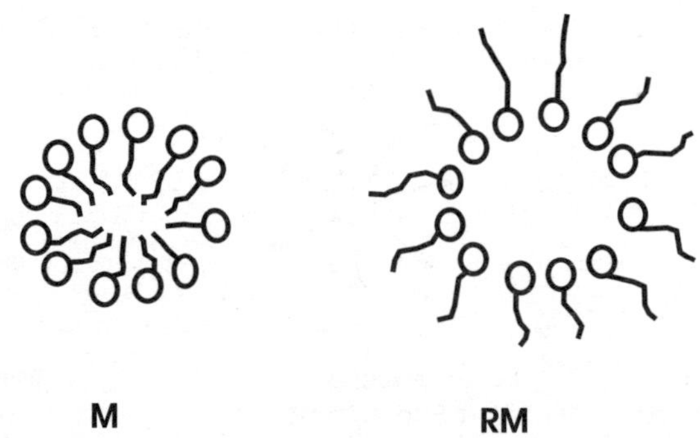

Fig. 3. Difference in micelles and reverse micelles in microemulsion. M, micelles for O/W microemulsion; RM, reverse micelles for W/O microemulsion.

hydrophobic effect is the driving force for micellar formation, despite the fact that assembling surfactant molecules together reduce their entropy. The fact is that, above CMC, the entropic penalty of assembling the surfactant molecules is less than the entropic penalty of caging water molecules, and also that they can act as emulsifiers that will solubilise a compound normally insoluble in solvent being used. This occurs because the insoluble species can be incorporated into the micelle core, which is itself solubilised in bulk solvent by virtue of the head groups favourable interactions with solvent species. The emulsifying ability of surfactants is also the basis for emulsion polymerisation. Enthalpic considerations, such as the electrostatic interactions that occur between charged (or ionic) surfactants, are important factors too.

A reverse micelle is topologically similar to a water–oil microemulsion, wherein the polar heads of amphiphile are oriented inwards and non-polar tails orient towards the oil phase. Their description rests

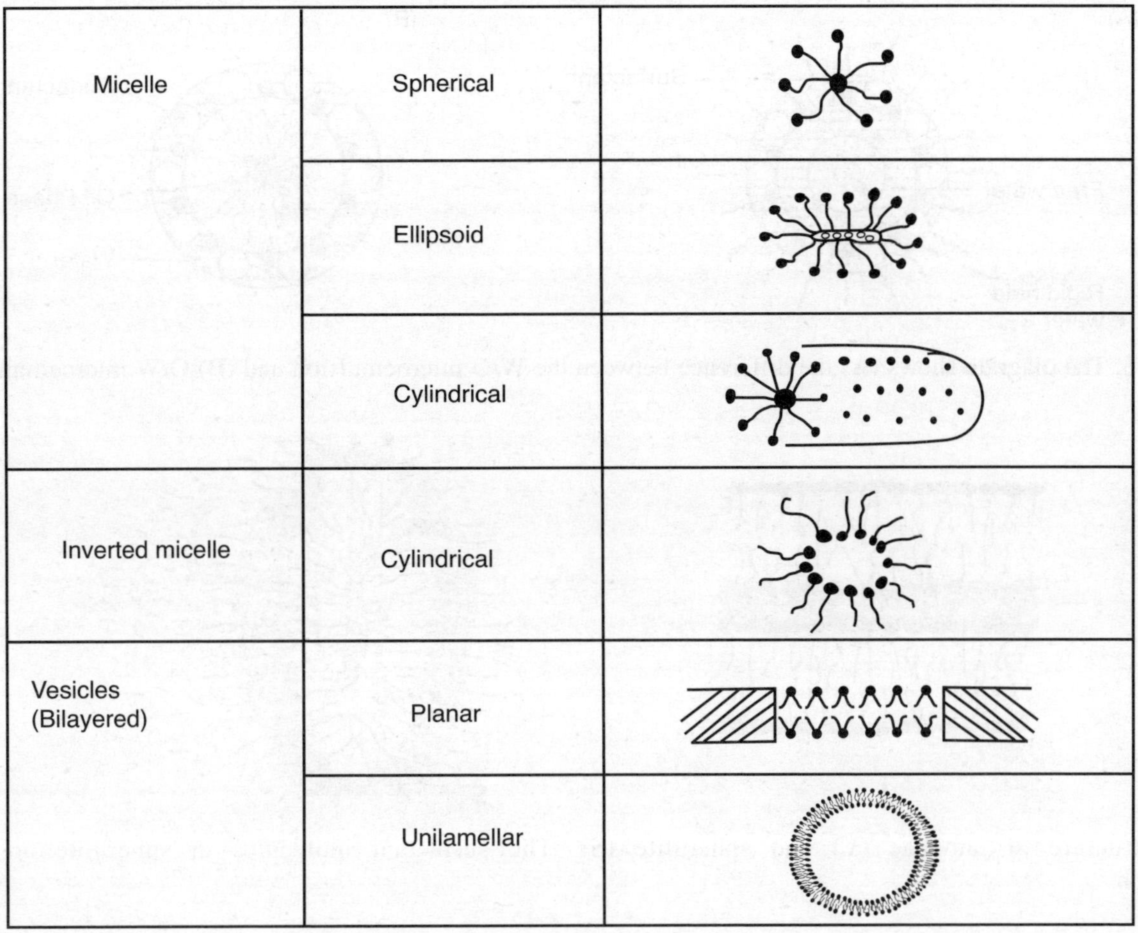

Fig. 4. Different shapes of micelles and vesicles.

on the availability of free water in the core called "micro-pool".

The composition of reverse micelles yields a rigid interior core by immobilisation of water present, by way of hydration of polar, ionic heads of the amphiphile and the counter-ions, when present. These reverse micelles are extremely difficult to form from surfactants with charged head groups, since hydrophilic sequestration would create highly unfavourable electrostatic interactions. The compositions having mobile or free water in the core after satisfying the hydration requirements of amphiphile head groups and counter-ions are called "microemulsions" *(2)*. The diagrammatic figure of such a water in oil microemulsion is compared with oil in water microemulsion as shown as Fig. 5.

Another microemulsion structure is *lamellae*: water and oil consecutive layers separated by surfactant layers conveniently oriented. The lamellae structure is similar to the smectic thermotropic phase; it presents birefringence and maintains the order even at diluted concentrations. This structure is related with spherulite structure (onion-like structure). It is possible that spherulites are only out-of-equilibrium transient lamellar phases induced by mechanical work (yet to be proved) or by any other stimulus. The thermodynamic stability of spherulites is not defined yet and still under study. The structures are shown in Fig. 6.

The *bi-continuous structure* or sponge phase is quite a complicated structure. As its name indicates, in this structure water and oil are continuous phases. The sponge has a continuous structure, but it is possible to "fill" the sponge with a liquid. The liquid forms a continuous phase and the material of sponge also forms a continuous phase. Thinking that the sponge surface is surfactant, a diagrammatic illustration of a bi-continuous structure can be presented as shown in Fig. 7.

Other possible microemulsion structures are inter-connected rod-like micelles (B), onions with a different inner structure like vesicles (A), etc. The principal factors involved in microemulsion structural changes are

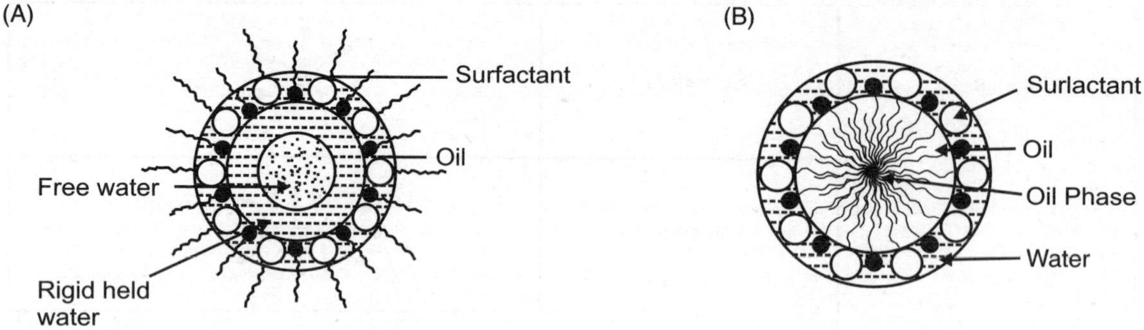

Fig. 5. The diagram shows **(A)** the difference between the W/O microemulsion and **(B)** O/W microemulsion.

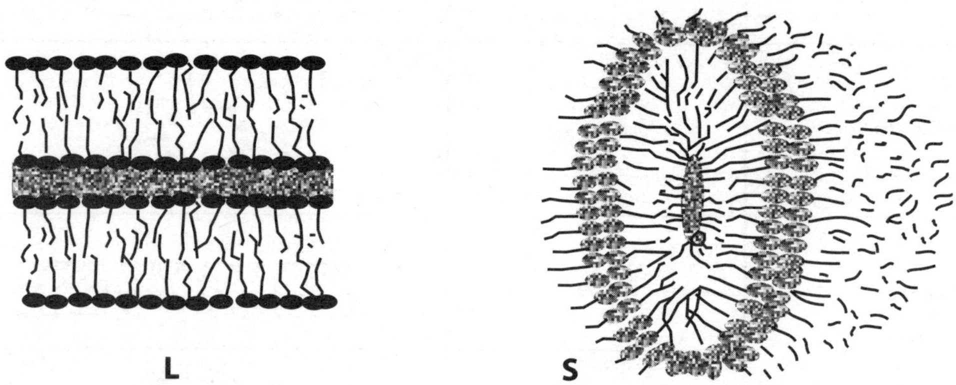

Fig. 6. Structure of lamellae **(L)** and spherulite **(S)**. The surfactant molecules in spherulite are arranged like an onion.

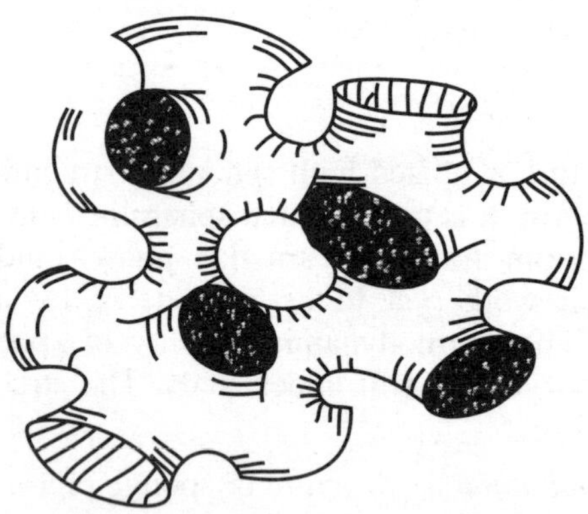

Fig. 7. Bi-continuous structure. The "pipeline" forms an oil-continuous phase and the exterior forms a water-continuous phase *(9)*.

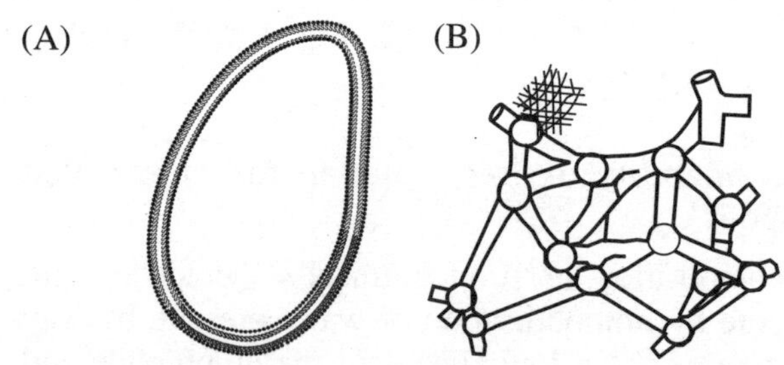

Fig. 8. Possible microemulsion structures: **(A)** vesicles **(B)** inter-connected rod-like micelles *(9)*.

surfactant shape, entropic energy terms, as well as, solvent properties such as ionic force and pH are shown in Fig. 8.

The internal structure of a microemulsion may be complex and varied *(10–16)*. It is physicochemically conceived that when concentration of water is on lower side, the surfactant requirement to boost dispersion is low, and on an average, spherical dispersion of surfactant-coated water nanodroplets exist in oil-continuous phase. The situation is reverse for compositions with a low percentage of oil and high percentage of water. The increasing dispersant concentration ends up with increased droplet dimension together with distortion of spherical shape; at comparable proportions of water and oil, irregular dispersions of both oil and water may simultaneously exist. This is called the "bi-continuous state", which is considered to be a sponge-like random network *(17)*.

Lagues *et al. (18)* have considered in their work oil and water globules, which are hard and have a relatively

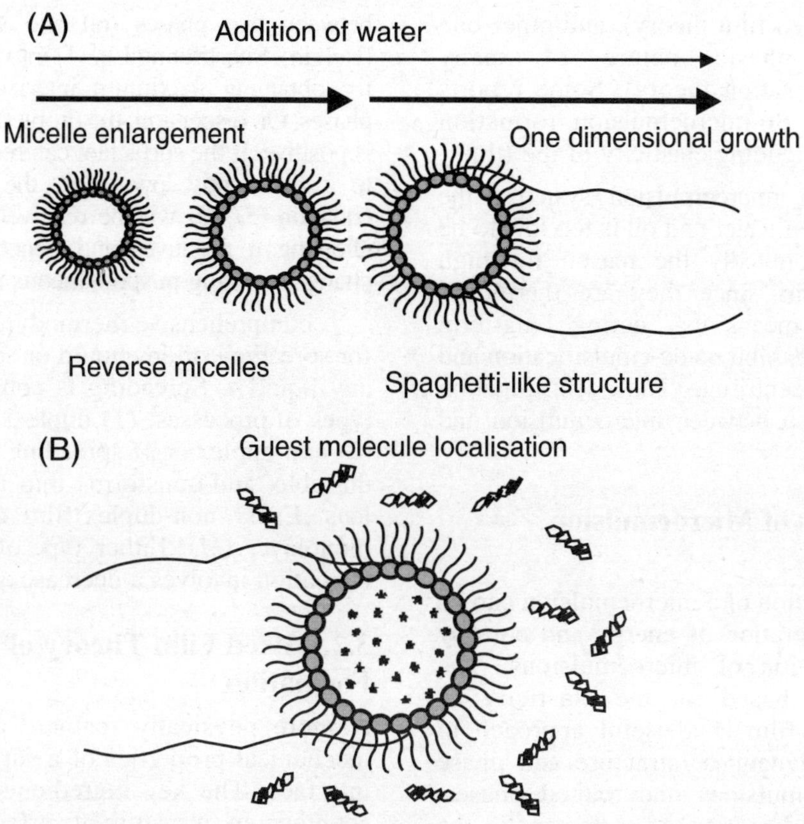

Fig. 9. Microemulsion-based lecithin gels. **(A)** Schematic representation of formation of lecithin gels upon addition of water to small phosphatidylcholine reverse micelles in polar solvent. **(B)** Localisation of solubilised "guest" molecules within lecithin gels. Lipophilic drug (stripped bar), hydrophilic drug (black circle) and amphiphilic drug (shaded head with attached tail).

sharp transition between them. Alternative layers of water, amphiphile and hydrocarbon in the form of a lamellar structure have been considered by Shinoda *et al.* *(19)*, whereas Tamlon and Prager have proposed randomly arranged hard hydrophobic and hydrophilic polyhedra *(20)*. According to Scriven, the internal structure is a complex three-dimensional network with both hydrocarbon and water continuity *(21)*. A random structure with varying curvatures has been proposed by Friberg *et al.* *(22)*. Lindman *et al.* *(23)* have proposed a hard and well-defined interface as in lamellar liquid crystals or micelles. A typical microemulsion has a polydispersity in aggregate size and shape; the size and shape of the aggregates changes, very rapidly and the hydrophilic–hydrophobic interface maintains a relatively low order. Other workers *(24–26)* also bear similar ideas about internal structures of microemulsions. The amphiphiles at lower state of concentration reside in the interfacial region between oil and water domains; on incorporation of macroscopic amount of surfactant, the system may become anisotropic and liquid crystalline, generating globular or tubular structures *(27)*.

The micellar structure changes on addition of water, as well as, enlargement of micelles (Fig. 9) in presence of guest molecules.

3. THEORIES OF MICROEMULSION FORMATION

The formation of a microemulsion involves creation of a situation in which the oil–water interfacial tension approaches zero *(28)*. They are colloidally dispersed systems and hence show an essential distinction from molecular solutions of hydrocarbons and water *(29)*. There are different theories involved in formation of microemulsions; among those, one which emphasises on the formation of an interfacial film and production of interfacial tensions (mixed film theory), and other one describes the mono-phasic nature of many microemulsions (solubilisation theory). Some reports considered free energy of microemulsion formation (thermodynamics) and blending elasticity of the film.

Studies show that in microemulsion systems, the interfacial tension between water and oil is too low to be measured. This is undoubtedly the reason for high stability of such systems since they are thermodynamically stable. This means that during long-term storage, microemulsions exhibit no de-emulsification and cannot be stratified by a centrifuge. Thus, centrifugation can be used to distinguish between microemulsion and emulsion.

3.1. Thermodynamics of Microemulsion Formulation

A thermodynamic definition of a microemulsion can be obtained from a consideration of energy and entropy involved in the formation of microemulsions. The interfacial description based on the elasticity of curvature of surfactant film is a useful approach to understand the thermodynamics (structure and phase equilibrium) of microemulsions and related phases. The driving force for adsorption of surfactant is the lowering of free energy (interfacial free energy per unit area is the amount of work required to expand the interface) of the phase boundary in a two-phase system. This interfacial free energy, referred to as surface or interfacial tension (g), is given in mJ/m^2 or mN/m. Adsorption of surfactant molecules at the interface lowers g, and higher the adsorption of surfactant (i.e., denser the layer) larger the reduction in g. The degree of surfactant adsorption at interface depends on surfactant structure and the nature of two phases that meet at the interface *(30)*.

A microemulsion formation involves sub-division of dispersed phase into very small droplets. Then, the resultant configurational entropy change (S^{conf}), can be approximately expressed as (Eq. 1)

$$S^{conf} = -nk^b\,[1n\phi + \{(1-\phi)/\phi\}1n(1-\phi)] \qquad (1)$$

where n is the number of droplets of dispersed phase, k^b the Boltzmann constant and ϕ^b the dispersed phase volume fraction. The associated free energy change can be expressed as a sum of the free energy for creating new area of interface, $\Delta A \cdot \gamma^{12}$, and configurational entropy (ΔG^{form}) in the form (Eq. 2)

$$\Delta G^{form} = \Delta A \cdot \gamma^{12} - T\,\Delta S^{conf} \qquad (2)$$

where A is the change in interfacial area, which is equal to $4\pi r^2$ per droplet of radius (r) and γ^{12} the interfacial tension between two phases (oil and water) at temperature (T) (Kelvin). Substituting Eq. (1) into Eq. (2) gives an expression for obtaining maximum interfacial tension between two phases. On dispersion, the droplet number increases and S^{conf} is positive. If the surfactant can reduce the interfacial tension to a sufficiently low value, the energy term ($\Delta A \cdot \gamma^{12}$) in equation *(31,32)* will be relatively small and positive, thus allowing a negative (and hence favourable) free energy change resulting in spontaneous microemulsion formation.

A comprehensive thermodynamic theory is developed for spreading of any liquid or solid b over the surface of any liquid a. Spreading is considered to occur by two types of processes: (1) duplex film or D spreading and (2) non-duplex or M spreading. A duplex film is always unstable, and transforms into a non-duplex film and a lens. Every non-duplex film of known structure is a monolayer (M). Either type of film may spread if its formation involves a decrease of free energy.

3.2. Mixed Film Theory of Microemulsion Formation

A more physically realistic approach is to consider mechanical properties of a surfactant film at oil–water interface. The key ingredients in this description are spontaneous curvature of surfactant film and two elastic moduli, the bending rigidity, which is a stiffness parameter and the saddle splay modulus, which tells about preferred topology of surfactant film. Many efforts have been made to measure these quantities but it is difficult, and different approaches or methods often give significantly different results. Particularly difficult is to measure the saddle splay modulus *(33)*. It is important to understand how these parameters relate to interfacial stability since surfactant films determine the static and dynamic properties of microemulsions. These include phase behaviour and stability, structure and solubilisation capacity.

Formation of microemulsion is accompanied by ultra-low interfacial oil–water tensions ($\gamma_{O/W}$), typically 10^{-2}–10^{-4} mN/m. They are affected by the presence of a co-surfactant, as well as, electrolyte and/or temperature, pressure and oil chain length.

Some surfactants (double-chain ionics and some non-ionics) can produce extremely low interfacial tensions—typically 10^{-2}–10^{-4} mN/m—but in most cases, such low values cannot be achieved by a single surfactant because CMC is reached before a low value of $\gamma_{O/W}$ is attained *[34,35,36]*. An effective way to further decrease $\gamma_{O/W}$ is to include a second surface-active species, for example, either a surfactant or medium-chain alcohol (a co-surfactant). This can be understood in terms of the Gibb's equation extended to multi-component systems. It enables the extent of adsorption at a liquid surface to be estimated from surface tension data. Typical low interfacial tensions are found in microemulsions, in this case spanning about 1–10^{-3} mN/m. In the absence of a co-surfactant, such as a medium-chain alcohol, the surfactant mixture exists in the form of a precipitate or tends to form a lamellar liquid crystal, instead of isotropic microemulsions, due to strong interaction between oppositely charged head groups *(37)*.

Adam and Harkins obtained the duplex film with following assumptions: (1) the momentum of each entire molecule contributes to monolayer gas pressure, (2) the interaction potential between the "liquid ends" of molecules is equivalent to an "intrinsic pressure", which has effect of increasing the surface tension at interface between parent liquid and monolayer, (3) this intrinsic pressure is derivable from a Lennard-Jones type of interaction potential depending on mean molecular area: $W = W_0 + \alpha/A^{4.5} - \beta/A^3$ and (4) the tails of molecules can form clusters, thus forming micelles in the duplex film, in which there are six bonds per molecule, each with interaction energy $\notin = -8.8 \times 10^{-14}$ erg per molecule. The field constants α and β seem to depend slightly on the nature of parent liquid, but the energy $\notin$ is independent of this. The duplex film therefore appears to have its liquid layer in contact with parent liquid, the free tails forming the gas layer. More data on different parent liquids are needed before a definite decision on this point can be made *(38)*.

3.3. Solubilisation Theory of Microemulsion Formation

In a system formed by a solvent, an association *colloid* and at least one other component (solubilisate), the incorporation of one additional component into or on the *micelles* is called micellar solubilisation, or, briefly, solubilisation. Surface-active agents also aggregate in solution-forming micelles. The driving force for micelle formation (or micellisation) is the reduction of contact between hydrocarbon chain and water, thereby reducing the free energy of system. In micelle, the surfactant hydrophobic groups are directed towards the interior of aggregate and the polar head groups are directed towards solvent. These micelles are in dynamic equilibrium and the rate of exchange between a surfactant molecule and the micelle may vary by orders of magnitude, depending on the structure of surfactant molecule. Although the molecules are intertwined, they are in constant motion like those of a liquid. Thus, the interior of a micelle can be thought of as a separate phase and a miceller solution can be thought of as a microdispersion of that phase in water. If the micelle is considered to be a separate phase, it is then convenient to evaluate the solubilisation capacity (k) in terms of partition between micelle and water. The micellar partition coefficient (K^m), is defined as the ratio of solute concentration in micelle (C^m), to that of water, C^w (Eq. 3)

$$K^m = C^m/C^w \tag{3}$$

The micelle/water partition coefficient for many solutes has been shown to correlate with the octanol/water partition coefficient. Finally, miceller solubilisation for both semi-polar and non-polar surfactants can be obtained. Due to the limitation on surfactant quantity that can be practically used, due to biological constraints micellar solubilisation is typically more advantageous for low dose formulations.

4. FORMULATION CONSIDERATIONS

Microemulsions require minimal effort for their formation, and once formed they have exceptional long-term thermodynamic stability. Furthermore, they are capable of solubilizing significant amounts of water-soluble and oil-soluble compounds (guest molecules or solubilisates) *(39,40)*. However, isotropic systems are usually more difficult to formulate than ordinary emulsions because their formulation is a highly specific process involving spontaneous interaction. Pharmaceutical acceptability of excipients, and the toxicity issues of components used, make the formulation of microemulsion really critical.

The formation of microemulsions usually involves a combination of three to five components, namely, oil, water, surfactant, co-surfactant and electrolyte. The micro-structural state of a microemulsion may be affected by the presence of additives. The tendency towards a W/O or an O/W microemulsion is dependent on the properties of oil, surfactant, water-to-oil ratio and temperature. The type of associated structures formed from these components at a particular temperature depends not only on the chemical nature of each component but also on their relative concentration.

Early studies revealed that the self-microemulsifying process is specific to:

- Nature of oil.
- Surfactant.

- Concentration of surfactant.
- Oil/surfactant ratio.
- Concentration and nature of the co-surfactant.
- Surfactant/co-surfactant ratio.
- Temperature at which microemulsion forms.

Although there is no strict rule for choosing appropriate microemulsion components, there are some general guidelines based on empirical observations. The important parameter is to choose a suitable surfactant and co-surfactant for particular oil.

4.1. Choice of Various Components

The choice of components for pharmaceutical microemulsions is often a balance between compounds which are able to form microemulsions, are non-toxic and are able to fulfil the requirements of a good vehicle for optimal absorption, i.e., high solubility of drug of interest and a high thermodynamic activity of drug. As the level of surfactant and oil in microemulsion is fairly high, it is important to consider the irritancy of these compounds *(41)*. A crucial step lies in the choice of a surfactant and a co-surfactant for particular oil.

4.1.1. Surfactant

The desirable properties of a surfactant to form a microemulsion are *(42)*:

- Lower interfacial tension to a very low value to aid dispersion processes during the preparation of microemulsion.
- With appropriate hydrophilic–lipophilic character to provide correct curvature at the interfacial region for desired microemulsion type—O/W, W/O or bi-continuous.
- Provide a flexible film that can readily deform around small droplets.
- Be adsorbed quickly around the dispersed drops as a condensed, non-adherent film, which will prevent coalescence.
- Impart to the droplets an adequate electric potential so that mutual repulsion occurs.
- Increase the viscosity of emulsion.
- Be effective in a reasonably low concentration.

Pharmaceutically acceptable surfactant must also:

- Be stable.
- Be compatible with other ingredients.
- Be non-toxic.
- Possess little odour, taste or colour.
- Not interfere with stability or efficacy of a drug.

The surfactant used to stabilise a microemulsion may be:

- Cationic.
- Anionic.
- Zwitterionic.

In general, for aqueous solutions of polyoxyethylenated non-ionic surfactants, the extent of solubilisation of aliphatic hydrocarbons at a given temperature appears to increase as length of hydrophobic group increases and as length of polyoxyethylene chain decreases. This reflects increase in aggregation number of micelles produced by these conditions. It is also of importance to note that as the degree of branching in hydrocarbon tail of a non-ionic surfactant increases, a significant result in solubilisation is evident. As the amount of branching to hydrocarbon tail increases, the net solubilisation decreases.

Non-ionic surfactants, which have low CMCs, are better solubilising agents than ionic surfactants in dilute systems. The experimental order for solubilising ability of hydrocarbons and polar compounds, which are solubilised in inner core, appears to be: anionics < cationics < non-ionics (for surfactants with comparable hydrophobic chain lengths). The greater solubilising capacity of cationics, when compared with anionics of same hydrophobic chain length, is probably due to looser packing of surfactant molecules in the micelles of anionics.

Although it is possible to form a microemulsion using a single surfactant as emulsifier, there are several criteria for this to be plausible. The surfactant must have a good affinity for bulk phases present. It must also have right geometry for packing at the interface. Finally, it must be able to reduce the interfacial tension between bulk phases to low values.

The extent to which a substance can be solubilised into a particular micelle depends on the portion of micelle that is locus for solubilisation. The volume of that portion depends on the shape of micelle that is formed. The particular shape of micelle is directly related to the volume occupied by hydrophobic groups in micellar core, the length of hydrophobic groups in core and the cross-sectional area occupied by hydrophilic groups at micelle/solution interface. As the ratio of volume occupied by hydrophobic group to volume of hydrophilic group increases, the micelle becomes increasingly asymmetrical.

The selection of a surfactant for formation of a microemulsion is also based upon the route of administration and the type of microemulsion. The selection of surfactant additionally depends upon HLB of surfactant, phase inversion temperature (PIT), presence of other additives or electrolytes, among others.

4.1.1.1. HLB Concept

HLB takes into account the relative contribution of hydrophilic and hydrophobic fragments of surfactant molecule. Since a surfactant contains both hydrophobic and hydrophilic groups, and phase in which the surfactant is more soluble is generally the continuous phase. The type of emulsion produced (i.e., O/W or W/O) can be predicted on basis of relative hydrophilic–lipophilic properties of the emulsifier. According to HLB concept, each of the surfactants can be assigned a numerical value representing its HLB. Experimental determination of HLB number for a given emulsifier is a tedious process. However, this value may be calculated with satisfactory accuracy based on easily determined characteristics of emulsifier. Griffin suggested the following equation for polyhydric alcohol and fatty acid esters:

$$HLB = 20(1 - S/A) \quad (4)$$

where S is the saponification number of ester and A is acid number of acid.

In certain cases, where accurate determination of saponification number is difficult, the relationship $HLB = (E + P)/5$ is used.

Where E is the weight percent of oxyethylene and P the weight percent of polyhydric alcohol. When ethylene oxide is the only hydrophilic group present the equation is reduced to $HLB = E/5$. HLB numbers for some common surfactants are listed in Table 2.

It is generally accepted that low HLB surfactants are favoured for formulation of W/O microemulsion, whereas surfactants having high HLB (>12) are preferred for formation of O/W microemulsion *(43–44)*. Ionic surfactants having HLB >20 often require presence of co-surfactants to reduce their effective HLB to a value within the range required for microemulsion formation.

Combination of (1) an anionic or a cationic surfactant of high HLB with a co-surfactant of lower HLB, (2) a double-chained surfactant of appropriate molecular composition or (3) a single-chained non-ionic surfactant of polyethylene glycol alkyl ether type at appropriate temperature are generally used for the formulation of microemulsion. Such combinations, particularly ionic and non-ionic surfactant, can be very effective in increasing extent of microemulsion region. An example of non-ionic surfactant includes sorbitan monooleate (Span 80) or polyoxyethylene surfactant such as Brij® 35 ($C_{12}H_{23}$) (Atlas Chemicals Co., USA)

Table 2. HLB Value of Some Commonly Used Surfactants

Surfactants	*HLB value*
Glycerol monostearate	3.8
Diglycerol monostearate	5.5
Tetraglycerol monostearate	9.1
Succinic acid ester of monoglycerides	5.3
Diacetyl tartaric acid ester of monoglycerides	9.2
Sodium stearoyl-2-lactylate	21.0
Sorbitan tristerate	2.1
Sorbitan monostearate	4.7
Sorbitan monooleate	4.3
Poloxyethylene sorbitan monostearate	14.9
Propylene glycol monostearate	3.4
Polyoxyethylene sorbitan monooleate	15

Many non-ionic surfactants can produce microemulsions without addition of a co-surfactant. Systems that have been reported, are generally produced from combinations of hydrocarbon, water and a polyoxyethylene glycol alkyl ether non-ionic surfactant (C_mE_n, where m is hydrocarbon chain length and n is number of oxyethylene units). There are several research papers available using $C_{12}E_5$ for microemulsion formation *(45,46)*.

Sometimes, microemulsions form with double-chained surfactants, such as anionic surfactants (e.g., aerosol-OT [AOT]), and cationic surfactants (e.g., didodecyldimethylammonium bromide [DDAB]), in absence of co-surfactants. Because of bulky hydrophobic groups they have required HLB to form W/O microemulsion spontaneously. Unfortunately, they are too toxic for general pharmaceutical and biotechnological application. Lecithin is a double-chained phospholipid

Table 3. Factors Affecting Spontaneous Curvature of Monolayers

Variable	*Curvature effect*	*Cause*
Increase oil chain length	More positive	Less penetration of surfactant tail region
Addition of shorter-chain co-surfactant	More positive	Alcohol swells head region more than tail region
Addition of longer-chain co-surfactant	More negative	Alcohol swells surfactant chain region more than head region
Addition of salt (ionic surfactant)	More negative	Screened repulsion between polar head groups
Addition of salt (non-ionic surfactant)	More negative	Head group size reduced by dehydration
Branched or double-chained surfactant	More negative	Increased tail group area
Reduced surfactant head group size	More negative	—
Increased temperature (non-ionic surfactant)	More negative	Head group size reduced by dehydration
Increased temperature (ionic surfactant)	More positive	Increased surfactant counter-ion dissociation

From *ref. 50.*

surfactant, which forms pharmaceutically acceptable microemulsion *(47)*. The characteristic properties of lecithin that must be taken into account while formulating microemulsion include:

- A strong non-polar portion due to two long hydrocarbon chains.
- A strong polar portion due to zwitterionic polar head groups, which are strongly hydrated.
- A close balance between polar and non-polar regions although slightly towards lipophilic side.
- A strong tendency to form lamellar liquid crystals.

Alteration of HLB can be achieved by adding short-chain alcohols, which make the polar solvent less hydrophilic. In addition, incorporation of these weakly amphiphilic co-solvents in polar parts of lipid layers increase area of lipid polar head to produce required spontaneous curvature of lipid layers. It also decreases the stability of lamellar liquid crystalline phase.

HLB also determines the type of microemulsion; for example, O/W, W/O or bi-continuous, through its influence on molecular packing and film curvature. The analysis of film curvature for surfactant association leading to microemulsion formation has been explained in terms of packing ratio (P), defined as V/al, where V is the partial molar volume of surfactant, a is cross-sectional area (i.e., size) of surfactant head group and l is maximum length of surfactant chain *(48)*. The packing ratio provides a direct measure of HLB and is influenced by same factors. O/W microemulsions are favoured if the effective polar part of surfactant is more bulky than hydrophobic part; that is, P varies from 0 to 1, and the interface curves spontaneously towards water (positive curvature). W/O microemulsions form when the interface curves in opposite direction; that is, when $P > 1$ (negative curvature). At zero curvature, when the HLB is balanced and $P = 0$, either bi-continuous or lamellar structures may form according to the rigidity of film. The critical packing parameter (P), is based purely on geometric considerations. Hydration of surfactant head group and penetration of oil and co-surfactant into the surfactant film also affect the packing and film curvature, as summarised in Table 3, which also illustrates how formulation variables may be manipulated to produce a microemulsion of desired type *(49)*.

4.1.1.2. PIT Concept

Another important factor for surfactant selection is PIT. It employs a characteristic property of emulsion rather than the properties of surfactants in isolation *(51)*. The method uses the fact that stabilities of O/W emulsions containing non-ionic surfactants are closely related to the degree of hydration of interfacial films. Emulsion stability is reduced by increase in temperature or added salts because these decrease the extent of interfacial film hydration. Phase inversion, due to a change from preferential water solubility of emulsifier film at low temperature to preferential oil solubility at high temperature, will occur at a specific temperature unique to particular emulsion and this can be determined experimentally. As a general rule, relatively stable O/W emulsions are obtained when their temperatures during storage and use are between 20 and 65°C below PIT, presumably because the films are sufficiently hydrated. Mixtures of emulsifiers with identical HLBs produce emulsions with quite different PITs because additives and interactions between the components affect PIT but not HLB.

Shinoda *et al. (52)* defined this critical point of PIT:

- If T < PIT, an O/W microemulsion forms.
- If T > PIT, a W/O microemulsion forms.
- At T = PIT, a middle-phase microemulsion exists with a spontaneous curvature equal to zero, and a HLB number approximately equal to 10.

The HLB number and PIT are inter-related; hence the term HLB temperature is sometimes employed *(53)*.

4.1.2. Co-Surfactant

An essential requirement for formation and stability of a microemulsion is attainment of a very low interfacial tension, γ. Since microemulsions have a very large interface between oil and water because of small droplet size, they can only be thermodynamically stable if the interfacial tension is so low that the positive interfacial energy (given, γA, where A is the interfacial area) can be compensated by negative free energy of mixing ΔGm. We can calculate a rough measure of limiting γ value required as follows: ΔGm is given by $-T \cdot \Delta S$m (where T is the temperature), and the entropy of mixing ΔSm is of the order of Boltzmann constant K_B.

Hence the equation can be written as

$$K_B T = 4\pi r^2 \gamma$$

Thus, for a droplet radius (r) of about 10 nm, an interfacial tension of 0.03 mN/m would be required. The role of surfactants in system is thus to reduce the interfacial tension between oil and water (typically about 50 mN/m) to this low level.

With the possible exception of double alkyl chain surfactants and a few non-ionic surfactants, it is generally not possible to achieve required interfacial area with the use of a single surfactant. If, co-surfactant is added to system, the effects of two surfactants can be additive, provided, the adsorption of one does not adversely affect that of the other and that mixed micelle formation does not reduce the available concentration of surfactant molecule.

Surfactants having single chain are not able to form microemulsion, as they are not able to decrease interfacial tension sufficiently, as well as, they are not having the correct molecular structure (e.g., HLB). For further reduction of interfacial tension between oil and water phases, as well as, to fluidise the hydrocarbon region of interfacial film and it's curvature, the co-surfactant is necessary. Although free energy associated with formation of microemulsion is negative, it is small, and therefore the order of mixing plays an important role in time taken to reach equilibrium *(54)*. For example, the equilibrium is established faster if the surfactant is injected into the oil phase, as its greater solubility in this phase hinders its diffusion into aqueous phase. Thus, the most appropriate co-surfactant is generally a small molecule, typically an alcohol of short- to medium-chain length (C3–C8), which can diffuse rapidly between bulk oil and water phases and the interface. Co-surfactant of short- to medium-chain-length alcohols also ensures that the interfacial film is flexible enough to deform readily around droplets, as the inter-calation between primary and surfactant molecules decreases both the polar head group interactions and the hydrocarbon chain interactions. Lamellar liquid crystalline phases rather than microemulsion phase often form with longer-chain-length co-surfactant or in absence of co-surfactant due to rigidity of interfacial film *(55)*.

Overbeek illustrates the importance of co-surfactant in the following example taken from a review *(56)*. The interfacial tension between cyclohexane and water is about 42 mN/m in absence of any added surfactant. The addition of ionic surfactant sodium lauryl sulphate (SLS) in increasing amounts cause a gradual reduction of γ to a value of about 2 mN/m at a SLS concentration of 10^{-4} g/mL. Further reduction of interfacial tension does not occur, because the cyclohexane/water interface is now saturated with SLS and any further increase of SLS concentration forms micelles in aqueous solution. Addition of 20% pentanol to cyclohexane/water system in the absence of SLS reduces interfacial tension to 10 mN/m. It is then theoretically possible by the addition of SLS to achieve a negative interfacial tension at SLS concentration below the level at which it forms micelles (CMC). Although pentanol is not generally regarded as a surfactant, it has the ability to reduce interfacial tension by virtue of its amphiphile nature (a short hydrophilic chain and a terminal hydrophilic hydroxyl group) and functions as a co-surfactant in this system. Its presence in this system means that the SLS is now required to produce a much smaller lowering of interfacial tension (10 mN/m rather than 42 mN/m in its absence) in order to produce a microemulsion *(57)*.

A lot of characterisation studies of microemulsions have been done with medium-chain alcohols as co-surfactants *(58–60)* as they are considered to form microemulsions with many surfactants and oil. Fletcher *et al.* reported that the length of alcohol co-surfactant influences curvature, with long-chain alcohols swelling the oil group region (negative curvature) more than those of shorter-chain length *(49)*. Although most researchers use medium-chain alcohols, like pentanol and hexanol, because of their effectiveness for microemulsion, they are not suitable for pharmaceutical use due to their high irritant potential. Furthermore, the evaporation of alcohol could destabilise the system. Administration of 6–9% propanol or 32% ethanol in water was shown to produce elongated mitochondria in rat liver after 1 mo and mega-mitochondria after 2 mo. Beside this ethanol, fatty acid esters of propylene glycol, oleic esters of polyglycerol, ethyldiglycol and polyethylene glycol were also evaluated as co-surfactants for microemulsion formulation*(61)*.

Due to problem with medium-chain alcohols, many researchers investigated less-irritant non-ionic surfactants (polyoxyethylene alcohol esters) for use as co-surfactant during microemulsion formulation *(62)*. Polyethylene glycol (PEG)-liquid (PEG derivative of distearoyl phosphatidyl ethanolamine [PEG-DSPE] mean molecular weight of PEG: 2000) was used as co-surfactant for preparation of vincristine microemulsion *(63)*. Alternative co-surfactants with better tolerability, for example, Plurol Isostearique, have recently been introduced into topical microemulsion formulations. Alany *et al.* have shown the effect of eight different co-surfactants on phase behaviour of pseudoternary system water: ethyl oleate:non-ionic surfactant blends (sorbitan monolaurate/polyoxy-ethylene-20-sorbitan monooleate) *(64)*. Four aliphatic alcohols (1-propanolol, 1-butanol, 1-hexanol and 1-octanol) and four 1,2-alkanediols (1,2-propanediol, 1,2-pentadiol, 1,2-hexanediol and 1,2-octanediol) were used as co-surfactant. They showed how the zone of microemulsion changes in presence of different co-surfactant in comparison to co-surfactant-free system.

In short, the functions of co-surfactants in micro-emulsion formulations are as follows:

1. They provide very low interfacial tensions (near zero) required for the formation of microemulsions with their thermodynamic stability.
2. They can modify the curvature of interface based on relative importance of their polar groups.
3. They act on fluidity of interfacial film. If the film is too rigid, it prevents formation of microemulsion and results in a more viscous and birefringent phase. The existence of unsaturated bonds on hydrocarbon chain of surfactants equally increases the fluidity of film.

4.1.3. Oil

The third and most important component of microemulsion formulation is the oil phase. If drug of interest is lipophilic, the solvent properties of oil should be compatible with drug. Larger oil molecules are generally able to dissolve lipophilic compounds of multiple sizes *(65)*. However, to enable the formation of microemulsions, the importance of penetration and association of molecules of oil phase with the interfacial surfactant film, which is governed by smaller oil molecules, must be recalled. A balance between these two properties in choice of oil phase must therefore be found.

Non-modified edible oils provide the most "natural" basis for lipid vehicles, but their poor ability to dissolve large amounts of hydrophobic drugs and their relative difficulty in efficient self-emulsification, makes them unsuitable for frequent uses. In contrast, modified or hydrolysed vegetable oils have contributed widely in the formation of microemulsions since they exhibit formulative and physiological advantages *(65,66)*.

Oils with excessively long hydrocarbon chains do not result in microemulsions. Short-chain oils penetrate tail group region more than long-chain alkanes, and hence swell this region to a greater extent, resulting in an increased negative curvature (reduced effective HLB value). Shorter the chain, deeper the penetration of organic phase into the interfacial film. On contrary, capacity of solubilisation by organic phase increases with the length of chain. Therefore, the choice of oil is dependent on the solubility of drug.

Polar oils, such as triglycerides with medium or long chains (MCT, LCT) are also preferred instead of non-polar oils, based on better solubility of drugs. In addition, the organic phases should not be too polar because they prevent the formation of microemulsion. The most often used external phases consist of vegetable oils, like soya oil, castor oil *(67)*, triglycerides for which 95% of fatty acids are made of 8–10 carbon atoms, Myglyol 812® (triesters of glycerol, capric and caprylic acids: Dynamit. Nobel, Witten/Ruhr, FRG), isopropyl myristate, fatty acids, such as oleic acid, and esters of saccharose, such as mono-, di- or tripalmitates of saccharose *(68)*.

The preparation of microemulsions with mineral oils, synthetic surfactants, either ionic or non-ionic and, if necessary, alkanols as co-solvents, have become a well-established practice *(69)*. Because mineral oils and synthetic amphiphiles, as well as, alkanols, in general, are harmful, there is some problem in preparing microemulsions with suitable components for possible applications in pharmaceutical industry *(70)*.

Unfortunately, most work till date on microemulsions has utilised oils, surfactants and co-surfactants, which are unacceptable for pharmaceutical purposes. In order to make these systems pharmaceutically acceptable, it is necessary to prepare such systems by using non-toxic and safe components *(71)*. Oils from natural sources and their derivatives, for example, triglycerides and fatty acid methyl esters, are easily degraded by micro-organisms and are considered to be harmless to the environment. The formation of bi-continuous micro-emulsions with mineral oils has been investigated in model experiments and for application in industrial products *(72)*; but such systems with natural oils and esters are infrequently published in literature *(73)*.

An acceptable lipophilic phase for pharmaceutical use would be vegetable oils *(74)*. The extension of a microemulsion region is generally dependent on the nature of oil. This is due to differences in oil penetration into the surfactant layer *(75)*. Relatively few studies have been done using triglycerides as the lipophilic phase in a microemulsion of soybean oil, polyoxyethylene(40), sorbitan-hexaoleate and water–ethanol. They found that the extension of W/O microemulsion regions were significantly dependent on temperature. Moreover, water–ethanol ratios also affected the phase behaviour. In these systems, large amounts of surfactant had to be used to form a microemulsion with equal amounts of triglyceride and aqueous phase. Owing to their high molecular weight, triglycerides form bi-continuous microemulsions only at relatively high temperatures with a high amount of hydrophobic surfactants. Esters of fatty acids, however, show suitable phase behaviour forming three phases at appropriate temperature and moderate surfactant content *(76)*. Alander and Warnheim observed that microemulsion phase diagrams for high-molecular weight triglycerides exhibit smaller homogeneous regions than low-molecular weight esters and hydrocarbons *(73)*. This effect has been attributed to better penetration of interfacial film by small oil molecules, which aids in obtaining optimal curvature of W/O or O/W droplets *(77)*. Triglycerides, in particular, large triglycerides, like peanut oil, are significantly more difficult to solubilise into microemulsions than hydrocarbons or alkyl esters. El-Nokaly *et al.* explained following reasons that present difficulties concerning formation of triglyceride microemulsions *(78)*:

- Triglycerides are semi-polar as compared with hydrocarbons.
- A surfactant of higher HLB is needed to favour a W/O system, with lower solubility in bulk and increased adsorption at interface.
- In case of triglycerides, the ratio of surfactant/water is high.
- The surfactant efficiency is decreased if it is lost to the bulk and is unavailable at the interface.

Edible triglycerides, such as soybean, rapeseed or sunflower oils, contain long alkyl chains mainly of C_{16}, C_{18}, C_{20} and C_{22}. The oil may be very bulky to penetrate interfacial layer to assist the formation of an optimum curvature. Reports of oil being solubilised in aggregates palisade layer may be due to shortness of alkyl chains in triglycerides used *(79)*. To increase the triglyceride microemulsion regions, a different strategy was applied. By using a suitable hydrotrope to destabilise liquid crystalline phase of triglycerides, surfactant and water led preferentially to the formation of microemulsion *(80)*. The preparation of triglyceride microemulsions can be achieved by incorporating sucrose and short-chain alcohols, such as ethanol. The alcohol acts synergistically with sucrose to destabilise the liquid crystalline mesophase *(81)*. Sucrose enhanced the formation of O/W microemulsion phase while destroying the W/O microemulsion phase. Triglycerides containing unsaturated or short-chain fatty acids have improved solubility in O/W microemulsions compared with triglycerides with saturated or long-chain fatty acids *(81)*.

In case of parenteral, ocular delivery, and like, the oil selected should be well tolerated by eye and their degree of purity must be high in order to prevent any contamination with potentially irritating substances.

4.1.4. Temperature

Temperature is mainly involved in formation of microemulsion when a non-ionic surfactant is used. At low temperature, non-ionic surfactants are hydrophilic and produce O/W microemulsion; but at high temperature, they behave as lipophilic moiety and produce W/O microemulsion. At an intermediate temperature (HLB temperature), hydrophilic–lipophilic interactions balance each other and microemulsions may have bi-continuous structure *(82)*.

Temperature usually also exerts an effect on formation and region of existence of microemulsions, as the HLB of surfactants can change with temperature and destabilise surfactant interface. Therefore, the stability of final microemulsion formulation should always be examined within the temperature ranges of storage and application.

4.1.5. Surfactant to Co-Surfactant Ratio

It plays a main role in influencing phase properties. Some researchers studied that when an ionic surfactant, such as SDS or dodecyl trimethylammonium bromide (DTAB), is used to prepare a microemulsion, alcohol and salt, generally, should be introduced in the system to form a fish-like phase diagram similar to that shown for non-ionic surfactants. As surfactant and alcohol are mixed, addition of salt always induces the surfactant, including alcohol, to adsorb at water–oil interface. The structure of microemulsion at the three-phase point of fish-type phase diagram is a bi-continuous microemulsion, in equilibrium with aqueous and oil phases. Within bi-continuous microemulsion, an ionic surfactant such as SDS is supposed to be adsorbed at interface, while alcohol can be either dissolved in oil micro-domain or adsorbed at interface. The solubilisation of water and oil increases with increasing cationic surfactant weight fraction due to formation of a surfactant interface with a decreased mean curvature *(82–84)*.

Zhong-Gao *et al.* prepared microemulsions with varying weight ratio of compositions such as oil, surfactant–co-surfactant mixture and cyclosporin A *(85)*. In addition, the effect of composition on physicochemical characteristics of each microemulsion system was investigated for the optimisation of microemulsion system. They observed that surfactant to co-surfactant ratio of S_{mix} greatly affected the physicochemical characteristics of resultant microemulsion systems obtained using Cremophor EL as a surfactant, Transcutol as a co-surfactant and Captex 355 as oil. The stable microemulsion with its high solubility of cyclosporin A, small droplet size and fast dispersion rate was obtained from a mixture composed of 10:5:4 ratio of the above, respectively.

4.1.6. Aqueous Phase

In the formulation of microemulsions, water served as aqueous phase. It has been recently reported that certain mixtures of non-ionic surfactants can provide enhancement of solubilisation of water in W/O microemulsions. Gradual changes in micro-structure occur with the addition of water phase into mixture of oil and surfactants during the preparation of microemulsions *(86)*.

The knowledge of hydration and the environmental aqueous fluidity in water droplets in W/O microemulsions is essential in understanding the dynamics of physicochemical processes studied in interface.

The structures of interfacial water of both O/W and W/O microemulsion systems are different from bulk water. According to reports by various physical and thermodynamic methods, the amphiphile, like AOT, can attach six water molecules per SO_3^- group; the counter Na^+ ion also acquires its share *(87–93)*. A similar physical state may also arise with SDS as amphiphile.

The existence of three types of water (bound, aggregated and free) in various proportions has been realised. The relative extents of the states depend on volume, pressure and temperature. The solubilisation of water and rotational isomerism of AOT are significantly influenced by the addition of salts.

5. ADVANTAGE OF MICROEMULSIONS

5.1. Enhancement in Oral Bioavailability

For poorly water-soluble drugs, the rate-limiting step for absorption and subsequent bioavailability, is dependent upon availability of soluble drug at the absorption site, which is further dependent on the dissolution rate. Microemulsion is a novel approach to improve the water solubility, and ultimately, bioavailability of poorly water-soluble drugs and/or for lipophilic drugs. Microemulsion presents the drug to gastrointestinal tract (GIT) in a solubilised and microemulsified form. Subsequent increase in specific surface area enables more efficient drug transport through intestinal aqueous boundary layer and through the absorptive brush border membrane leading to improved bioavailability *(94,95)*.

5.2. Reduction of Inter-Subject and Intra-Subject Variation

There are several drugs, like peptide group of drugs, which show large inter- and intra-subject variation in absorption, leading to decreased therapeutic performance of drugs and also patient non-compliance. Micro-emulsion drug delivery system is a proven approach to overcome inter- and intra-subject variation *(94,95)*.

5.3. Reduction of Food Effects

Food is a major factor affecting therapeutic performance of a drug in body. Several researchers have found that there was no food effect on plasma profiles when drugs were given as microemulsion formulations *(94)*.

5.4. Ease of Manufacturing and Scale Up

The unique quality of microemulsion is its simplicity of method of preparation, which makes it more popular when compared with others, like solid dispersions, liposomes and nanoparticles, among others. Micro-emulsion requires very simple and economical manufacturing facilities, like simple mixers with agitators and volumetric liquid-filling equipments, for large-scale manufacturing. This explains the interest of industry for microemulsion-based drug delivery systems.

5.5. Ability to Deliver Peptides that are Prone to Enzymatic Hydrolysis in GIT

One unique property of a microemulsion is its ability to deliver macromolecules, like peptides, hormones, enzyme substrates and inhibitors, and the ability to offer protection from enzymatic hydrolysis.

5.6. No Influence of Lipid Digestion Process

Unlike other lipid-based drug delivery systems, the performance of a microemulsion is not influenced by lipolysis, emulsification by bile salts, action of pancreatic lipases and mixed micellar formations. Microemulsions are not necessarily digested before the drug is absorbed. Since they present drug in a microemulsified form, they can easily penetrate the mucin and unstirred-water layer.

5.7. Useful for Topical Application

The nanometric size of micelles, improved solubilisation capacity for lipophilic drugs, transparency etc., makes the system more suitable for transdermal application. It was also proved by several researches that there was an improvement in bioavailability for anti-fungal and anti-inflammatory drugs when the system was compared against solution.

6. FACTORS INFLUENCING FORMATION OF MICROEMULSIONS

6.1. Effect of Surfactants

The formation of a microemulsion is strongly dependent on the chemical nature of both the surfactants and the oil *(96,97)*. Li and Wang studied solubilisation of W/O microemulsions formed with mixed surfactants and they have concluded that such a formation is due to synergistic effect resulting from the strong Coulombic interactions between cationic and anionic surfactants.

6.2. Effect of Co-Surfactants

Addition of co-surfactants can reduce surfactant concentration in a microemulsion preparation. Normally, low molecular weight alcohols, such as *n*-butanol, can be used for this purpose. The amphiphilic nature of co-surfactants could also enable them to distribute between aqueous and oil phases *(98)*. In doing so, it substantially changes the composition of oil so that its interfacial tension with water is reduced. Binding of alcohol molecules to surfactant aggregates decreases their interfacial free energy and enhances solubility of water and oil in W/O and O/W microemulsions, respectively *(99)*.

Nave *et al.* observed that some microemulsion systems could be formulated without presence of a co-surfactant *(100)*. They investigated 11 AOT-related surfactants, which are efficient for forming microemulsions. These surfactants were from two homogenous series, with either linear or branched hydrocarbon tails.

With linear di-chain compounds, W/O micro-emulsion phase could be formed in presence of a short-chain alcohol, while all the branched surfactants form microemulsions even in absence of a co-surfactant.

6.3. Effect of Oil Type

It appears that stability of W/O microemulsions is dependent on the molecular weight of oil *(101)*. When oil chain length is increased, the water solubility is decreased, and the chain length is compatible when the system contains a medium-chain alcohol. The oil phase containing LCTs or MCTs and mono-/di-glycerides or sorbiton esters (low HLB values) and Polysorbate 80 (high HLB value) were used for stable self-emulsifying W/O microemulsions of extremely small particle size (5–30 nm) *(102)*.

6.4. Effect of Alcohol Chain Length

Alcohol is essential in promoting interfacial fluidity for formation of microemulsions. It was found that decreasing the alcohol chain length in a microemulsion system leads to decrease in the radius of droplets and an increase in interfacial fluidity. In contrast, increasing the alcohol chain length may lead to increase in droplet size and a rigid interface. It appears that a small change in alcohol chain length can strongly influence the interfacial elasticity and, hence, the phase behaviour of a microemulsion. In addition, alcohol (co-surfactant) can increase the total interfacial area at low concentration, thus increasing solubilisation property. Increasing the alcohol concentration can increase the alcohol partitioning at interface, and consequently increase total interfacial area available for solubilisation. However, at sufficiently high concentrations, the fluidity of interface increases, and hence solubilisation decreases.

6.5. Effect of Salt Concentration

In general, increasing the concentration of salt causes a reduction in total aqueous phase solubilised. Leung and Shah studied that decreasing brine solubi-lisation with increasing salinity is due to an increase in the interfacial rigidity with increasing salinity *(103)*. A decreasing alcohol partitioning at interface with increasing salinity may also contribute to decrease in brine solubilisation.

Watt *et al.* studied that with increased salt concentration, formation of W/O microemulsions is favoured. This is due to electrostatic interactions of surfactant head groups which are suppressed, causing packing ratio to increase and inducing formation of a W/O microemulsion. However, the excessive salt concentration tends to drive the alcohol into oil phase *(104)*.

Leung and Shah observed that the optimal salinity addition tends to reduce the attractive interaction of fluid interfaces and, hence, increase the maximum solubilisation of W/O microemulsions. For salinity lower than optimal salinity, these effects, together with salting-out effect, tend to increase the solubilisation. However, for salinity higher than optimal salinity, they increase interfacial rigidity and curvature, thus decrease the solubilisation *(103)*.

6.6. Effect of HLB

Huibers and Shah studied that there are two different approaches to be considered in order to achieve a high level of water solubilisation in W/O microemulsions *(105)*. First, maximise the amount of surfactant in the HLB 9–13 region, where it intermediates between high oil solubility and high water solubility. Second, use mixtures of highly oil-soluble surfactants and high water-soluble surfactants.

7. PHASE DIAGRAMS

When oil, water and surfactant (presence or absence of a co-surfactant) are mixed, microemulsions are only one of a number of association structures (including emulsion, micelles, lamellar, hexagonal and cubic and various gels and oily dispersion) that can form, depending on the chemical composition and concentration of each component. A phase diagram is a graphical repre-sentation of the combinations of oil, surfactant, water or other variables for which specific phases exist at equilibrium. Several types of phase diagram can be identified depending on the number of variables involved. In using an adequate mode of representation, it is possible to describe not only the limits of existence of single and multi-phase regions, but also to characterise equilibrium between phases (tie-lines, tie-triangles, critical points, etc.). At constant temperature and pressure, the ternary phase diagram of a simple three-component microemulsion is divided into two or four regions. In each case, every composition point within single-phase region above the de-mixing line corresponds to a microemulsion. Composition points below this line correspond to multi-phase regions comprising in general microemulsion in equilibrium with either an aqueous or an organic phase or both systems. Although quaternary phase diagram is a good approach to describe the different association structures of oil, water, surfactant and co-surfactants (four-component system), it is very time consuming and difficult to interpret. Therefore, pseudotertiary phase diagram is often constructed to find different zones, including, microemulsion zone, in which each corner of the diagram represents 100% of particular component. Figure 10 shows a hypothetical phase diagram with representation of microemulsion structures.

At high water concentrations, microemulsions consist of small oil droplets dispersed in water (O/W microemulsion), while at lower water concentrations the situation is reversed and the system consists of water droplets dispersed in oil (W/O microemulsions). In each phase, a surfactant-rich film separates oil and water droplets. In systems containing comparable amounts of oil and water, equilibrium bi-continuous structures in which the oil and the water domains interpenetrate in a more complicated manner are formed. In this region, infinite curved channels of both oil and water domains extend over macroscopic distances and the surfactant forms an interface of rapidly fluctuating curvature, but in which the net curvature is near zero.

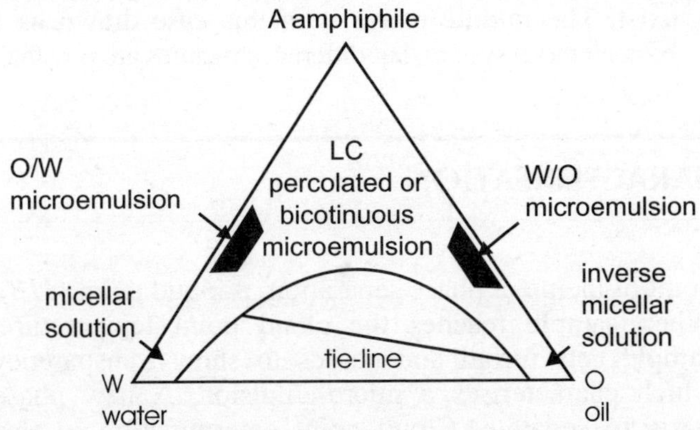

Fig. 10. Ternary phase diagram of oil, water and surfactant showing microemulsion formation zone.

Surfactants are surface-active molecules that can form interfaces between immiscible fluids (such as oil and water). A large number of structurally different phases can be formed, such as droplet, rod-like and bi-continuous microemulsions, along with hexagonal, lamellar and cubic liquid crystalline phases. Ternary phase diagram shows compositional ranges for different phases.

Interesting things happen in region where a surfactant transitions from being water soluble to oil soluble. At the incipient point of transition, the surfactant repels both the water and the oil phases and prefers to be at interface, but there is insufficient room at interface to accommodate all of surfactant. New phase forms, which is called a middle-phase microemulsion *(106)*. The middle-phase microemulsion combines virtually all of surfactant with portions of the oil and water phases, giving it an intermediate density, and exists in equilibrium with virtually surfactant-free oil and water phases. Middle-phase microemulsions appear at intermediate salt concentrations, unlike oil–water emulsion which break if given sufficient time. A middle-phase microemulsion system is thermodynamically stable and does not break with time (given that system conditions remain constant). Winsor referred to this middle phase as a Type III microemulsion, as opposed to Type I (micelles) and Type II (inverse micelle) microemulsions. Middle-phase microemulsions have several highly desirable properties, including ultra-low interfacial tensions with water or oil phases, potentially $<10^{-4}$ mN/m, and ultra-high solubilisation potentials for oil or water, potentially two to three orders of magnitude higher than in simple micellar systems. To illustrate the remarkable ability for oil and water to co-exist in a middle-phase microemulsion, a few weight percent surfactants can cause equal amounts of oil and water to be contained in the microemulsion.

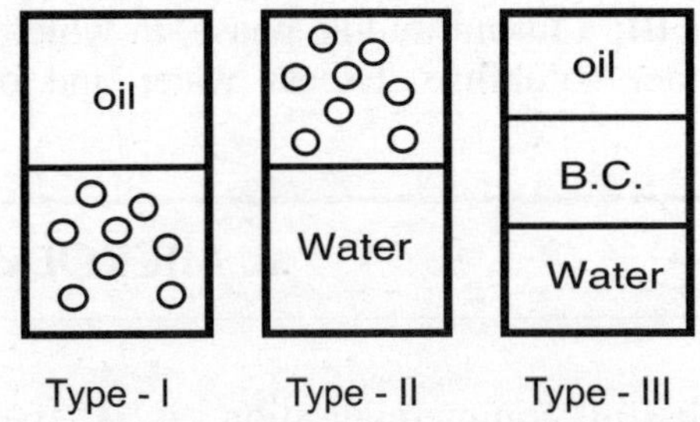

Fig. 11. Types of microemulsion.

While the middle-phase microemulsion appears at a discrete point in temperature or salinity scan, system properties change continuously through the scan. The interfacial tension decreases continuously as the system transitions through Type I region towards the Type III boundary, and it will decrease by orders of magnitude prior to appearance of a middle-phase microemulsion. Likewise, the solubilisation potential will increase by an order of magnitude or more prior to the appearance of a middle phase. We refer to the Type I microemulsion region just before a Type III microemulsion forms as super-solubilisation region.

As surfactant concentration increases, there is more surfactant in the middle-phase region. Because the surfactant is accumulating at oil–water layers within the middle-phase, as the surfactant concentration increases, the volume of middle phase must increase to accommodate additional surfactant. Eventually, at elevated surfactant concentrations, the volume of middle phase grows sufficiently to consume all of the oil and water phases, and this results in a single-phase microemulsion. As a microemulsion transitions from a Type I towards a Type III system, micelles become swollen, and eventually, a bi-continuous structure forms with a monomolecular surfactant film separating regions of oil from regions of water. Hence, water and oil are continuous; this bi-continuous structure is present, not only in middle-phase microemulsions containing approximately equal volumes of oil and water, but also as we approach Type I or II microemulsion boundaries within the middle-phase region.

1. Winsor I: oil is emulsified in water phase (lower phase) and the water phase appears turbid and contains solubilised oil. The upper excess oil phase is clear.
2. Winsor II: water is emulsified in oil phase (upper phase) and this phase appears turbid and contains solubilised water in reverse micelles. The lower excess water phase is clear.

3. Winsor III: a turbid middle phase, in which both oil and water solubilise. Excess water and oil phase exist. The middle phase is in this case drawn as a bi-continuous system, but different structures are possible.

8. MICROEMULSION CHARACTERISATION

For successful commercialisation, it is essential to characterise the system in detail, even though it is very difficult to determine. Different techniques are used to characterise the microemulsion system macroscopically, as well as, microscopically. Visual assessment may provide important information about self-emulsifying properties of mixture and about the resulting dispersion system, although more objective criteria are required for microemulsion characterisation and comparison *(109–111)*.

8.1. Macroscopic Study

At macroscopic level, viscosity, conductivity, refractive index and dielectric measurements provide useful information for characterisation of a micro-emulsion system. Viscosity measurements not only provide information about the pourability of system but it also provides information about the presence of rod-like or worm-like reverse micelles *(112,113)*. Using any commercial viscometer, such as Brookfield viscometer, Cannon-Manning semi-microviscometer, etc., the viscosity of microemulsion system can be measured. It is advisable to calibrate the instrument before measurement of viscosity.

Conductivity measurements provide a means of determining whether a microemulsion is oil-continuous or water-continuous, as well as, providing means of monitoring percolation or phase inversion phenomena *(112,114,115)*. The conducting properties of micro-emulsions are given mainly by surfactant or by addition of a supporting electrolyte. Due to the small interfacial tension, usually <0.001 dyne/cm, these systems are able to dissolve a large number of substances. *(116,117)*. Conductivity is measured using conductivity meter equipped with a platinum electrode. Traces of sodium chloride can be added to water to a concentration sufficient to ensure a well defined p*I*. This small amount of sodium chloride does not influence the phase behaviour to any significant degree.

A stable homogeneous mixture is transparent, whereas an unstable non-homogeneous mixture is turbid unless the components of mixture have identical refractive index. Transition from transparent to turbid state can be brought about by variations of temperature, pressure or composition of mixture. This transition point, within the point of incipient phase separation, is cloud point *(118)*. When sample reaches the cloud point temperature, sample gets turbid and ceases to show transparency which characterises a micro-emulsion. A new phase starts to separate. Cloud point determination is also useful tool for determination of microemulsion stability. Cloud point is determined using a spectrophotometer, by measuring transmitted light through solution at a wavelength of 600 nm and at increasing temperature, at constant rate.

Electro-analytical techniques may provide valuable information concerning the structural evolution, inter-particle interaction and transport data *(119–121)*. Yet there are very few studies employing electro-analytical methods in microemulsion.

8.2. Particle Size Analysis

The size range of microemulsion droplets and the inability to dilute many microemulsions to infinite dilution makes size determination difficult. Various techniques have been employed with varying successes in size analysis of microemulsions. It is generally true to say that, because of the limitation of technique, it is preferable to employ a combination of techniques to determine the particle size.

The micro-structure of microemulsion has been elucidated by various techniques, as for example, static and dynamic light scattering (DLS), dielectric relaxation, time-resolved fluorescence or phosphore-scence quenching, electric field or temperature jump, small-angle neutron scattering (SANS) and small-angle X-ray scattering (SAXS). These techniques can afford fruitful information about core and surface monolayer structures, particle size distribution, polydispersity, droplet clustering and diffusion dynamics, inter-droplet exchange rate and fluidity of monolayer.

8.3. Electron Microscopy

The size of droplets in microemulsion can be measured using transmission electron microscopy (TEM) and freeze-fracture transmission electron microscopy (FFTEM). In TEM technique, freezing of microemulsion must be achieved sufficiently rapidly to avoid phase separation or crystallisation.

This objective can be achieved either by plunging the specimen into a liquid cryogen, or by propane jetting, or by spray freezing. The sample is subsequently fractured and its visibility is enhanced by deposition of platinum–carbon layer in vacuum. The microemulsion sample, mounted on a support film and grid, is replicated by breaking apart the film and grid. The replica is then viewed by TEM and assumed to be representative of bulk microemulsion. Recent developments in the cryo-fixation technique have overcome many of problems associated with artefact formation in earlier studies, which were due to slow cooling rates.

Recent FFTEM studies utilising rapid cooling rate and adequate environmental control of samples before freezing (to prevent loss of volatile components) has been investigated in microemulsion structures of pentaethylene glycol dodecyl ether, water and *n*-octane *(122)*. This one of the earliest methods, is not currently used because of limitations of this technique.

Another method involves direct imaging, in which thin portions of specimen are directly investigated in frozen hydrated state by using a cryostage in TEM. The development of glass-forming microemulsions that do not break down during cooling process has provided a way for direct studies of microemulsion structures. The first types of such systems reported were O/W microemulsions with a non-crystallising aqueous matrix obtained by adding propylene glycol to water in the ratio 1:3. It was thought that propylene glycol functioned as co-surfactant since the usual addition of an alcohol was not necessary. The fact that neither phase crystallised on cooling below 273 K meant that possible modifications of microemulsion structure by crystal growth were avoided. This approach was extended to W/O microemulsion by Greek, who used glycerol/water mixture as dispersed phase, a glass-forming oil (ethyl-cyclohexane) as continuous phase and DDAB as surfactant *(123)*. Direct electron microscope imaging of vitrified microemulsion using freeze fracture technique revealed clearly separated droplets of 20 nm diameter.

8.4. Scattering Technique

The capacity of measuring very small particle size (<10 nm) makes this technique ideal for determining particle size in microemulsions. Various scattering methods, which were employed for determining particle sizes in microemulsions, include SAXS *(124–130)*, SANS *(131–134)* and SLS and DLS. Particles as low as 2 nm in size and up to 100 nm in size, can be measured using SANS and SAXS (up to few microns by light scattering).

In scattering techniques, the waves scattered at a given angle by all points in sample interfere with each other to produce one point in an interference pattern, which is then transformed to reconstruct an image of all correlations within sample. For structural information, experiments must be designed which can measure distances on a scale comparable with the dimensions of aggregates. For micelles and microemulsions, this can be profitably achieved by the use of neutron and X-ray radiations (wavelength <1 nm) where measurements at low angles produce enough interference to derive information about scattering species. In small-angle scattering method, the measured intensity is correlated with number density of scatterers, the inter-particle form factor and inter-particle structure factor to derive information on the particle size and structural correlation.

In case of monodisperse spheres interacting through hard spheres repulsion, the general expression for scattering intensity $I(Q)$ is

$$I(Q) = nP(Q)S(Q) \quad (5)$$

where n is the number density of aggregates and the form factor,

$$Q = 4\pi \sin \theta/\lambda \quad (6)$$

where θ is the scattering angle and λ is wavelength. $P(Q)$ describes the aggregate's size, shape and scattering properties, while $S(Q)$ is structure factor for scattering particles, which is a Fourier transform of the radial distribution function. The radial distribution function describes the probability of finding centre of a particle at a particular distance from another particle. For dilute or non-interacting particles, $S(Q) = 1$ (a uniform probability). If there are interactions between particles $S(Q)$ will have a peak shape, indicating liquid-like ordering. Analytical expression may be used to calculate both $P(Q)$ and $S(Q)$ under favourable circumstances.

8.4.1. Static Light Scattering

Static light scattering is a well-established technique for determining size, shape and structure by measuring the intensity, $I(Q)$, as a function of scattering wave vector, Q. In some cases, when there is independent information about sample, the interpretation of $I(Q)$ is straightforward; however, when little is known about sample, the analysis can be more difficult. Measurement of $I(Q)$ provides an ensemble average over the entire illumination volume, making the interpretation of scattering from highly heterogeneous samples particularly challenging.

In contrast to DLS, time-averaged scattering intensities are detected in SLS and observed at one specific

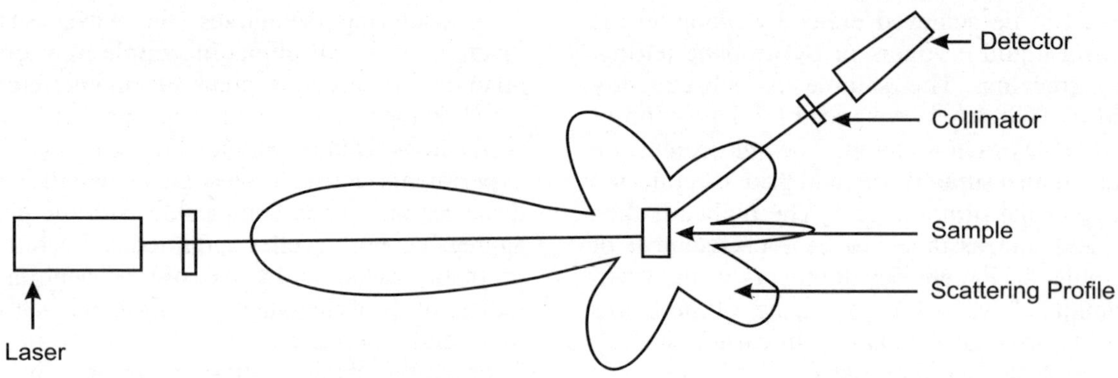

Fig. 12. Basic principle and set up of static light scattering measurements.

scattering angle. One has to consider that colloids, from which the incident laser beam is scattered, are no point scatterer. Their scattering pattern depends on their shape and size. If primary light waves are scattered on several scattering centres the resulting secondary waves differ in their path lengths. This difference of path lengths results into a phase-factor difference of the scattered light waves. Because of a strong relation between the phases of scattered waves, there is interference. Up to a specific size having same range as scattered light wavelength, colloids are not point scatterer anymore. So one has to consider the interference of scattered light resulting from scattering centres of different colloids, as well as, scattered intensities for a single large particle in presence of intra-particle interference. From there the scattering ability of a colloid depends on scattering angle where scattering light is detected. This leads to particle form factor *P*(*Q*). With increasing concentration of colloidal dispersion, one can obtain information about the static structure factor *S*(*Q*) from time-averaged intensities. The structure factor represents the structural arrangement of particles and is determined by particle interactions.

In static light scattering technique, the angular dependency of time-mean-intensity of laser light scattered by the particles is measured. The course of scattered intensity as a function of detector angle depends on size and structure of particles (Fig. 12).

Rayleigh developed a theory that predicts the angular intensity distribution of light scattered by particles much smaller than the wavelength of light (R < λ/20). In this case, the intensity of scattered light depends only on the size of particles and not on their structure or concentration. If the intensity of scattered light is measured in a plane orthogonal to the polarisation plane of incident light, there will be no angular distribution of scattered light.

$$R_\theta = \frac{16\pi^4 R^6 \left(\frac{n^2-1}{n^2+2}\right)^2}{\lambda^4} \qquad (7)$$

In this expression, R_θ is the Rayleigh ratio, *R* the particle size, *n* the relative refractive index of solute and λ the wavelength of incident light.

8.4.2. Dynamic Light Scattering

DLS (also known as *quasi*-elastic light scattering) can be used to determine the size of dispersed colloidal droplets *(135)*. Very dilute emulsions are illuminated by a polarised light source. Droplets in sample will scatter the incident light beam, if there is a difference in refractive indices of droplets and emulsifying medium.

A schematic representation of dynamic light scattering is shown in Fig. 13. For simplicity, two droplets are considered represented with two dots. Incident light is scattered by both droplets to the detector at point *P* at an angle θ. The two droplets move with respect to each other due to temperature fluctuations (Brownian motion). Therefore, δ, the path difference in scattered beams changes continuously. As a result, there is a time-dependent phase difference between two scattered waves arriving at *P*. This time dependence causes interference.

The detector measures a fluctuating intensity over a period of time. An example of this intensity vs time diagram is plotted in Fig. 14. The intensity $I(s,t)$ fluctuates over an average. $I(s,t)$ stands for the intensity, *I*, in time, *t*, where *s* stands for scattering vector *(136)*. The fluctuations around the average have to be correlated to a time interval. Therefore, intensities in time I_k and time I_{k+1} are summed. The time interval between I_k and I_{k+1} is called Δt or delay time t_d, named that way since it represents the delay in time between two signals $i(s,k\Delta t)$

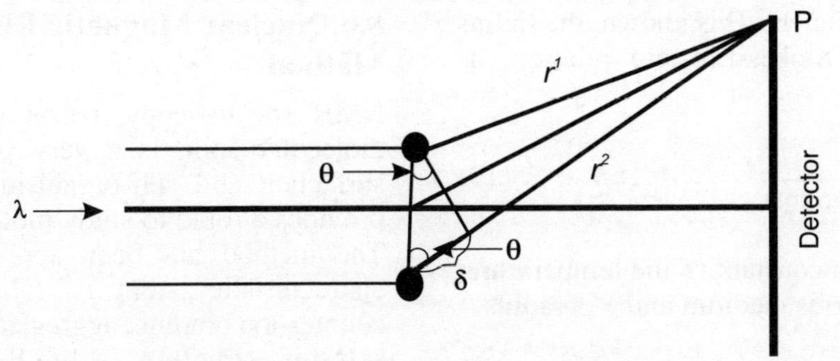

Fig. 13. Scattering of radiation in emulsion.

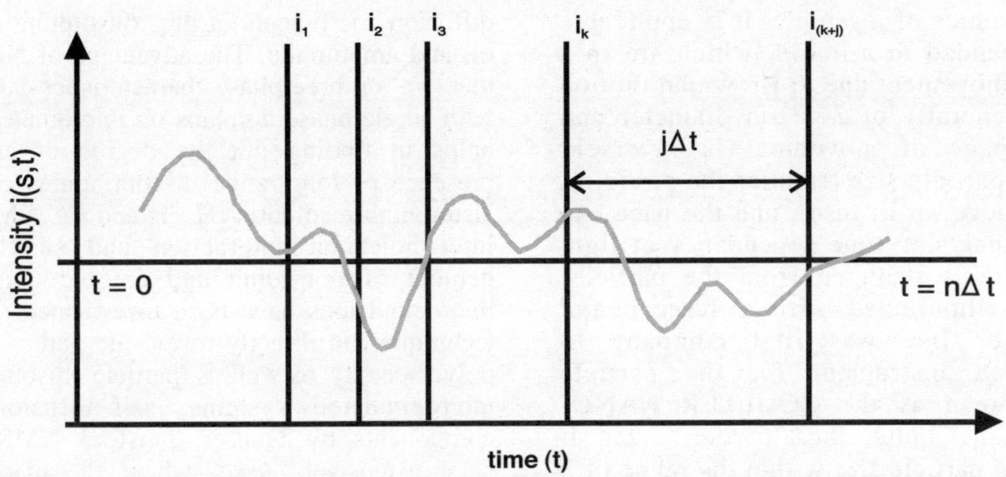

Fig. 14. Intensity fluctuations in time as a result of light scattering by dissolved particles. (Reprinted from Int. J. Pharm, 244 Paollino, D., Ventura, CA., Nistico, S., Puglisi, G., and Fresta, M. Lecithin microemulsion for the topical administration of ketoprofen percutaneous adsorption through human skin tolerability, 21–23, 2002 with permission from Elsevier) *(154)*.

and $i[s,(k+j)\Delta t]$ and is equal to $j\Delta t$ *(136)*. The intensities then are summed over larger intervals, such as $2\Delta t$, $3\Delta t$, $4\Delta t$, and so on.

To obtain a particle size from the intensity measurements, time dependence of fluctuations is of interest. Therefore, the fluctuations are transformed to the auto-correlation function.

$$C(s,t_d) = \lim_{n\to\infty}\frac{1}{n}\sum_{k=0}^{n} i(s,k\Delta t)i[s,(k+j)\Delta t] \tag{8}$$

The auto-correlation function has its largest value at $t_d = 0$. If $t_d \to \alpha$, then $I(s,t)$ becomes uncorrelated. The ratio of the auto-correlation function to its asymptotic value $[I(s,t)]$ can be read from Eq. (9).

$$\frac{C(s,t_d)}{[\bar{i}(s,t)]^2} = 1 + \xi\left|g_1(s,t_d)\right|^2 \tag{9}$$

This is also known as Siegert relation *(135)*. In this equation, ξ, stands for an instrument constant. The decay in $g_1(s, t_d)$ is given by

$$g_1(s, t_d) = e^{-2Dq^2 t_d} \tag{10}$$

where t_d is delay time and d the diffusion coefficient. The scattering vector (q) is given by

$$q = \frac{4\pi n}{\lambda}\sin\left(\frac{\theta}{2}\right) \tag{11}$$

where θ the angle, λ the wavelength and n the refractive index of solvent.

To calculate a radius from auto-correlation function, Eq. (10) is transformed to

$$\ln g_1(s,t_d) = \ln\left[g_1(s,t_d)\right]^{1/2} - \frac{1}{2}\ln\xi \tag{12}$$

A plot of ln $g_1(s,t_d)$ vs s,t_d should yield a straight line. The slope is equal to the negative diffusion coefficient,

D. If t_d and diffusion coefficient, D is known, the radius can be calculated from Stokes-Einstein relation, as given by

$$r = \frac{k_b T}{6\pi\eta D} \tag{13}$$

where k_b is the Boltzmann constant, T the temperature, η the viscosity of continuous medium and r is radius.

8.5. Photon Correlation Spectroscopy

Photon correlation spectroscopy is a powerful way to study the dynamics of a sample. It is applicable to particles suspended in a liquid, which are in a state of random movement due to Brownian motion (i.e., particles generally of 2–3 µm diameter and smaller). The pace of movement is inversely propor-tional to particle size (smaller the particles, the faster they move, or diffuse), and the pace can be detected by analysing time dependency of light intensity fluctuations scattered from the particles when they are illuminated with a laser beam. Beckman Coulter Inc. was first company to commercialise an instrument for the particle technologist, known as the COULTER NANO-SIZER® (Beckman Coulter Inc.) particle sizer. It presented average particle size within the range of 3 µm down to 40 nm, and also gave an indication of width of size distribution.

8.6. Nuclear Magnetic Resonance (NMR) Method

NMR spectroscopy, based on physical properties of molecular spin, is a very powerful method to study surfactant and self-organising systems in solution. It provides a route to study molecular degrees of freedom. The method has been applied to determine micellar characteristics, that is, CMC, aggregation number, counter-ion binding, aggregate shape, size and hydration, solution structure, solubilisation equilibria, among others. The reverse micelles and microemulsions can be understood by the possibilities of determination of self-diffusion coefficients of the constituting species, water, oil and amphiphile. The advantage of NMR method is that two- or three-phase characteristics can be monitored with single-phase domains on micrometer scale. It also helps in finding out the degree of anisotropy and presence of long-range discontinuities or continuities. Using high-resolution ^{1}H, ^{2}H and ^{13}C NMR techniques, inter-molecular interaction and structural rearran-gement of non-ionic and anionic amphiphile-aided microemulsions have been investigated *(137,138)*. The technique can directly reveal the nature of mono- and polydispersity, as well as, particle anisotropy *(139)*. For microemulsion systems, self-diffusion studies of components by Fourier transform-NMR method has been extensively used, where the macroscopic self-diffusion of constituents confined to droplets will be that of droplets and will be low *(140)*.

9. STABILITY OF MICROEMULSION

There are many thermodynamic properties that can be involved when considering the dynamic stability of a microemulsion formation. Among these are solubility parameters, chemical potentials, concentrations of species present, interfacial entropy and enthalpy, interfacial free energy, interfacial compressibility, stress gradients, osmotic pressure and Laplace pressure differences across curved interfaces.

All of these properties have one factor in common; the interface is treated as an oriented monolayer. The concept of a thermodynamically stable microemulsion evolved via the perceived need for a transient negative interfacial tension to spontaneously form these systems.

A correlation of solubilisation rate, interfacial tension and size of the surfactant aggregate can accu-rately approximate the micellar size for a given emul-sion. The lowering of interfacial tension between oil–surfactant solution interface is a function of rate of solubilisation of oil. This rate of solubilisation (*DS/Dt*) is a function of effective volume for solubilisation and can be shown as:

$$DS/Dt = \mathrm{k} n V_{\mathrm{eff}}$$

In this equation, k is the constant, n the number of aggregates in unit volume of surfactant solution and V_{eff} the effective volume for solubilisation by an aggregate. V_{eff} is impacted by the actual accessible volume of hydrocarbon core of an O/W mycelia, the chemical nature of surfactant molecule(s) and that of oil.

It should also be noted that the effective volume for solubilisation may or may not be proportional to the geometrical size of aggregate. It depends on pac-king of molecules in the aggregate and mutual compatibility of surfactant and oil molecules. In most cases, V_{eff} is proportional to size of the micelle. When aggregate size is too large and the packing becomes too tight, V_{eff} may decrease with aggregate size.

For hydrocarbons and long-chain polar compounds that are solubilised in the interior of micelle or deep in the palisade layer, the amount of material solubilised generally increases with an increase in size of micelles. Therefore, any factor that causes an increase in either the diameter of micelle or its aggregation number can be expected to produce an increase in solubilisation capacity for this type of material.

Since aggregation numbers increase with an increase in degree of dissimilarity between solvent and surfactant, an increase in chain length of hydrophobic portion of surfactant generally results in increased solubilisation capacity for hydrocarbons in the interior of micelle in an aqueous media.

10. APPLICATION OF MICROEMULSION IN DRUG DELIVERY

The advantages of microemulsions as drug delivery systems essentially include the improvement of drug solubilisation and protection against enzymatic hydrolysis, as well as, the potential for enhanced absorption due to surfactant-induced permeability changes.

Microemulsions are used as drug delivery systems because of their solubilisation capacity for poorly water-soluble compounds and enhancement of topical and systemic drug availability. In recent times up to 50% of new chemical entities are poorly water-soluble and, therefore, largely show poor bioavailability. Lipid-based formulations, such as microemulsions, are increasingly recommended for such candidates.

Beside the obvious advantages of microemulsions, including physical stability and ease of preparation, these systems may offer additional benefits for periodontal uses. These include an increased drug release rate due to smaller particle size compared with emulsions, and improved handling due to transparency of formulation. Particularly interesting microemulsion systems for pharmaceutical applications are those based on non-ionic surfactants, since these require no additional surfactant or co-surfactant to form a microemulsion.

One of the most important properties of a colloidal drug delivery system is the release profile, which describes how the drug diffuses out of the colloidal carrier after administration. Many methods have been described to measure the release rate of a drug from colloidal particles *(141,142)*. The measurement of drug release from emulsions is a particularly troublesome process. Since these systems have a liquid-dispersed phase and the solute diffuses rapidly through the droplet, it becomes impossible to separate the drug released from particles within the timescale of release process.

Washington and Evans recently described a method widely applicable to study of drugs with weak acidic or basic properties *(143)*. This method highlights rapid release of drugs from sub-micron emulsions by monitoring the change in pH of an acceptor phase as the release system is diluted into it. Release rates from triglyceride emulsions were rapid, but consistent with an interfacial barrier being the rate-limiting step for solute release.

10.1. Topical Delivery

Transdermal drug delivery system exhibits several advantages over other routes, notably oral route, by avoiding systemic side effects. But the main limiting factor for this delivery system is penetration of drug through stratum corneum, the outermost layer of the skin, which comprises keratin-rich dead cells embedded in a lipid matrix. Considering the solubilising capacity of microemulsion, these are expected to significantly affect the structure of stratum corneum lipid self-assemblies, with obvious consequences for drug penetration. There have been several studies regarding penetration enhancement by microemulsion drug carriers, for example, lecithin containing W/O microemulsion for transdermal administration of scopolamine and broxaterol. It was found that the transport rate obtained with a lecithin microemulsion gel was much higher than that obtained with an aqueous solution at same concentration *(144)*.

Microemulsions are appropriate vehicles for administration of drugs and this may enhance transdermal penetration by various mechanisms *(145–147)*. Many molecules have been solubilised in microemulsions. In addition, microemulsions induce a change in thermodynamic activity of drugs they contain, modifying their partition coefficient, and thus favour penetration through the stratum corneum.

Many studies have shown that microemulsion formulations possessed improved transdermal and dermal delivery properties, mostly *in vitro (148–151)*, and several *in vivo (152,153)*. As demonstrated by two recent publications, the intra-dermal permeation rates of a lipophilic drug were significantly increased from microemulsions as compared with commercial macro-emulsions *(151,153)*.

In vitro release of piroxicam from microemulsion provides a reservoir effect for piroxicam release. Retardation of piroxicam release was obtained on incorporation of microemulsion into carboxyvinilic gel and *in vitro* studies showed significant inhibition of inflammation process. Paolino *et al.* showed four to five times improvement in ketoprofen percutaneous penetration using two microemulsions as compared with a conventional formulation, which is due to small particle size of internal phase droplets of microemulsions *(154)*. Improvement of permeation was also due to the solubilising effect of drug elicited by the microemulsion lecithin matrix, having high affinity for epidermal tissue, and is able to mix with skin lipid components. Permeation-enhancer effect was also mediated by lecithin component. Similar studies also suggested that the percutaneous absorption of tyrosine from O/W microemulsion was superior in comparison to liquid–crystal system and an emulsion *(155)*.

Enhanced delivery rate in a hairless mouse model was found in O/W microemulsion as compared with W/O microemulsions for delivery of prostaglandin E1. The microemulsions were based on oleic acid or Gellucire 44/14® as oil phase and were stabilised by a mixture of Labrasol (C8 and C1 polyglycolised glycerides) and Plurol Olique CC 497 as surfactants *(156)*. The transdermal delivery from W/O microemulsion of diphenhydramine HCl into excised human skin was evaluated. The microemulsions were based on combination of Tween-80 and Span 20 with isopropyl myristate. Skin permeation of felodipine, a calcium antagonist, from O/W microemulsions based on mixture containing Tween-20 and taurodeoxycholate (as surfactant), isopropyl myristate (as oil phase) and benzyl alcohol (as co-surfactant) was evaluated *(157)*. The transdermal penetration of glyceryl trinitrate through mouse skin was found as enhanced about 10 times by formulating the drug in AOT micelles, reverse micelles and W/O microemulsions. Irritation studies showed that AOT reverse micellar solutions show little or no erythema whereas normal micelles caused moderate irritation *(158)*. The use of lecithin, isopropyl myristate and water microemulsion for transdermal transport of indomethacin and diclofenac was reported. Improvement of skin permeation of diazepam from "visosised" O/W microemulsions prepared using egg lecithin, polysorbate 20, benzyl alcohol, isopropyl myristate and water/propylene glycol mixture was also reported *(159)*. Gasco *et al.* studied the gel-like system obtained by adding the polymer Carbopol 934® to a microemulsion of decanol, dodecanol, Tween-20 and propylene glycol containing solubilised azelaic acid *(160)*. The diffusion studies on hairless mouse skin implied that microemulsion gel was more efficient than the gel alone or cream. Comparative studies done by El-Faham *et al.* in 1992 have shown that an O/W microemulsion gel containing analgesic anti-inflammatory agent, flufenamic acid and stabilised by polyethylene glycol-7glyceryl coccoate (Cetiol HE) was having higher bioavailability after topical administration as compared against macro-emulsion, hydrogel and cream.

Sintov studied microemulsion systems possessing a potentially improved skin bioavailability of lidocaine and explored for some characteristic features *(161)*. The percutaneous penetration studies using rat skin *in vitro* showed that the transdermal flux of lidocaine was significantly improved by microemulsion composed of glyceryl oleate–PEG-40 stearate combination rather than glyceryl oleate–PEG-40 hydroxylated castor oil. Two principal factors were found to govern the transdermal penetration of lidocaine from microemulsion, viz., water content and co-surfactant–surfactant ratio. By analysing skin layers (epidermis and dermis) for lidocaine content, significantly higher concentrations were found after rats were treated *in vivo* with liquid microemulsions (when co-surfactant and surfactant ratio was 1.8, water content 30% w/w) or patches compared with those measured after application of EMLA cream (reference product from Astra AB containing 25 mg/g of lidocaine and prilocaine respectively) (Fig. 15).

Lu and Jun studied that methotrexate (MTX) is a folic acid antagonist with anti-neoplastic activity but it is also effective for the treatment of psoriasis when administered by oral or parenteral route over long periods of time *(162)*. However, the systemic use of this drug may provoke any of numerous side effects, notably hepatotoxic effects *(163,164)*. To reduce such effects, it would be preferable to administer MTX topically in the form of microemulsion or hydrogel and this may enhance transdermal delivery of this drug *(165)*.

10.2. Influence on Drug Release Characteristics

Drug incorporated in microemulsions will partition between the hydrophilic and hydrophobic phases depending on their lipophilicity. Trotta *et al.* reported the usefulness of partition coefficient of a drug on its release characteristics *(166)*.

Garcia-Celma has reviewed microemulsions as drug delivery systems for different types of drugs, viz., anti-

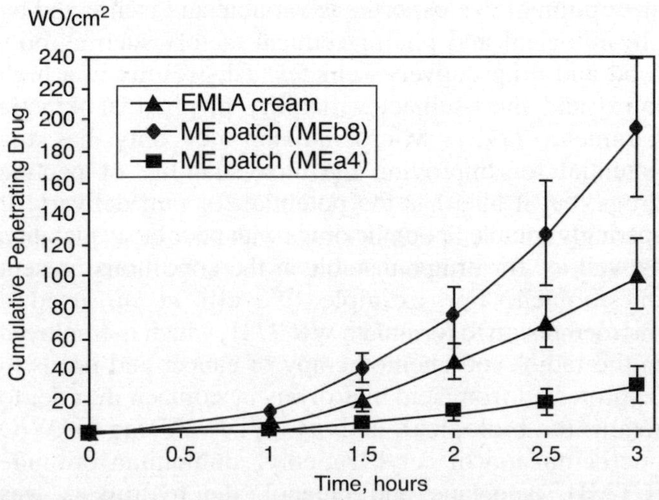

Fig. 15. Percutaneous penetration of lidocaine from microemulsion patches of system b (MEb8, $n = 6$) and system a (MEa4, $n = 12$) through rat skin *in vitro* during 3 h. The penetration profiles (diamonds for MEb8 and squares for MEa4) are compared with the transport kinetics of lidocaine from EMLA cream (triangles). (Reprinted from Int. J. Pharm., 62, Gasco, MR., Pattarino, F., and Lattanzi, F. Longacting delivery system for peptides: reduced plasma testosterone levels in male rats after a single injection, 119–123, 1990, with permission from Elsevier.) *(183)*

neoplastics/anti-tumour agents (doxorubicin, idarubicin and tetrabenzamidine derivative), peptide drugs (cyclosporine, insulin and vassopressin), sympatholytics (bupranolol, timolol, levobunolol and propanolol), local anaesthetics (lidocaine, benzocaine, tetracaine and heptacaine), steroids (testosterone, testosterone -1- propionate, testosterone enanthate, progesterone and medroxyprogestorane acetate), anxiolytics (benzodiazepines), anti-infective drugs (cloitrimazole, ciclopirox olamine, econazole nitrate and tetracycline hydrochloride), vitamins (menadione and ascorbic acid) and dermatological products (tyrocine, azelaic acid, octyl dimethyl para aminobenzoic acid and 2-ethyl hexyl *p*-methoxy cinnamate) *(167)*.

The release of five drugs with different lipophilicity from O/W microemulsions composed of isopropyl myristate, butanol, AOT and buffer (pH 7.0) was studied by determining the mass transfer constants of drugs through a hydrophilic membrane separating the microemulsion from receiving aqueous phase. A linear relationship between the release rate of drug and its isopropyl myristate/water partition coefficient was noted. The rate of drug release from microemulsified drug delivery system was modified by the nature of phase structure *(168)*, interaction between drug and surfactant *(169)* and concentration of co-surfactant. Gasco *et al.* achieved prolonged release of propranolol by increasing the partitioning of drug using administration of octanoic acid into dispersed oil phase *(170)*. As a result, release rate through a hydrophilic membrane was decreased due to its decreased concentration in continuous phase, providing a prolonged release of drug.

The release of piroxicam–β-cyclodextrin complex in microemulsions can be modified by inclusion of Carbopol 940® (Noveon, Inc.) as reported by Dalmora *et al. (66)*. Incorporation of an inert polymer gelled matrix into a self-microemulsifying system, which forms a microemulsion, continuous and uniform release of microemulsified active agent occurs after ingestion (on contrast with physiological fluid) *(171)*.

Panayiotis Constantinides *et al.* developed stable self-emulsifying W/O microemulsions having particle sizes of 5–30 nm using water-soluble molecules/peptides of different molecular sizes and charges *(113)*. They tried with various long-chain glycerides and/or sorbitan esters and medium-chain glycerides (mono-/di-/triglycerides) and these systems are discussed in terms of their drug delivery potential. The formulas, which they developed is given below.

Table 4: For medium-chain glycerides:

S.No.	*Ingredients*	*Percentage (w/w)*
1	Captex 355	65
2	Capmul MCM	22
3	Tween-80	10
4	Saline	03

Table 5:
For LCTs and long-chain monoglycerides:

S.No.	*Ingredients*	*Percentage (w/w)*
1	Soybean oil	65
2	Arlacel 186	22
3	Tween-80	10
4	Saline	03

10.3. Oral Delivery

Microemulsion formulations offer several benefits over conventional formulation for oral administration including increased absorption, improved clinical potency and decreased drug toxicity. Therefore, microemulsions have been reported to be ideal delivery systems for drugs, such as steroids, hormones, diuretic and antibiotics. Pharmaceutical drugs of peptides and proteins are highly potent and specific in their physiological functions. However, most are difficult to administer orally. With an oral bioavailability in conventional (i.e., non-microemulsion based) formulation of <10%, they are usually not therapeutically active by oral administration. Because of their low oral bioavailability, most protein drugs are only available as parenteral formulations. However, peptide drugs have an extremely short biological half-life when administered parenterally, so require multiple dosing.

A microemulsion formulation of cyclosporine named Neoral® has been introduced to replace Sandimmune®, a crude O/W emulsion of cyclosporine formulation. Neoral® is formulated with a finer dispersion, giving it a more rapid and predictable absorption and less inter- and intra-patient variability.

Apart from those involving penetration enhancement in topical administration, the most interesting drug delivery application lie in oral administration of peptide and protein drugs. Despite the many promising features of peptides in drug delivery, many of them are difficult to administer orally without a loss in activity. The general low bioavailability of peptides administered orally means that the intra- and inter-subject variability is magnified and a major reason for maximising the oral peptide bioavailability is ability to control *in vivo* drug (Arg-Gly-Asp) concentration. For example, SK & F-106760 and SK & F-110679, both water-soluble RGD fibrinogen-receptor antagonists, were formulated in microemulsion at pharmaceutically relevant levels and their uptake after intra-duodenal administration was investigated. It was found that the presence of SK & F-110679 peptide in varying concentration did not influence the structure of W/O microemulsion studied. Furthermore, bioavailability of SK & F-106760 was increased dramatically for microemulsion formulations compared with that of aqueous solution *(172)*.

The oral bioavailability of peptide drugs, for example, cyclosporine, a potent immunosuppressive agent, when given orally, the absorption of cyclosporine is incomplete, amounting to about 30% or less. Furthermore, the absorption of cyclosporine is variable and is affected by physiological and pharmaceutical factors such as bile, food and drug delivery vehicles. This results in a high intra- and inter-subject variability in pharmacokinetic parameter *(173)*. Microemulsion not only has the potential for improving the bioavailability of peptide drugs, but it also has the potential for oral delivery of sparingly soluble lipophilic drugs with poor bioavailability, as well as, for drugs unstable at the conditions present in stomach. For example, Novelli *et al.* used a microemulsion to formulate WR 2721, which is employed in the radio- and chemotherapy of cancer and needs to be protected from acid hydrolysis in stomach in order to retain its biological activity *(174)*. Using a W/O microemulsion of cetyl trimethyl ammonium bromide (CTAB), isooctane and butanol, the hydrolysis was slowed down considerably in microemulsion compared with aqueous solution. A two fold increase in bioavailability of CoQ10 was observed when compared with powder formulation in an *in vivo* rat model. The microemulsion formulation used for bioavailability studies contained Myvacet 9-45® (Eastman Chemical Company) (40%), Labrasol (50%) and Lauroglycol® (Gattefosse) (10%) *(175)*. An oral microemulsion formulation was reported for N-4472 (N-2-[3,5-di-tert-butyl-4-hydroxyphenethyl]-4,6-difluorophenyl)-N-(4-[*n*-benzyl piperidyl]) urea, which is a poorly water-soluble drug having a lipid-lowering effect, using microemulsion technique *(176)*. The above microemulsion formulation was prepared using L-ascorbic acid, Gellucire 44/14, hydrogenated castor oil (e.g., HCO-60®, Nikko Chemical K.K.) and SDS.

Nitrendipine, a poorly soluble drug, has shown a remarkable enhancement of bioavailability when HCO-60 microemulsion formulation of nitrendipine was compared against a suspension or an oily solution in rat model *(177)*. The bioavailability of several drugs, including peptides, using microemulsion delivery system depends not only on the nanometric particle size and thermodynamic stability but also on the composition of microemulsion including type of oil phase, ionic nature of surfactant, etc. Recently, reported data shows that incorporation of water-soluble cellulosic polymer such as hydroxypropyl methyl-cellulose improves concentration time profile, as well as, bioavailability of thiazolidinedione analogue PNU-91325, which is a poorly soluble drug and used as insulin action-enhancing agent, in comparison to the microemulsion having same formulation without hydroxyl propyl methyl cellulose (HPMC). This is due to generation and maintenance of high free drug concentration during the absorption phase via generation of a super-saturated state that is stabilised by precipitation inhibitors such as HPMC.

As a result, the dynamic equilibrium between micro-emulsion micelles and free drug, the resulting super-saturated solution dictates drug transport and absorption kinetics *(178)*. A five fold increase in bioavailability of biphenyl dimethyl dicaroboxylate, a drug used for treatment of liver diseases, was observed from a pre-microemulsion concentrate composed of Tween-80 and Neobee M-5® (Stepan Company) at the ratio of 2:1 and 35% of triacetin, which not only increases the solubility and immediate dispersion of drug in GIT but also increases its bioavailability *(179)*.

Khoo *et al.* showed improvement of oral bioavailability of halofantrine, an anti-malarial drug, using microemulsion drug delivery system (52–67%) as compared with commercially available tablet formulation (8.6 ± 5.3%) and crystalline halofantrine base alone in a hard gelatin capsule *(180)*. The increase in oral bioavailability was a consequence of delivering the drug in a solubilised and rapidly dispersed manner. They also showed the difference in bioavailability when microemulsion formulation was composed of different triglycerides (medium- vs long-chain length) in oil phase, along with Cremophor EL as surfactant and absolute alcohol as co-surfactant. Commercially available drugs that are formulated as self-microemulsifying systems include cyclosporine (Sandimmune Neoral®, Novartis Pharmaceuticals UK Ltd)), ritonavir (Norvir®, Abbot) and saquinavir (Fortovase®, Hoffmann-La Roche Inc) *(181,182)*.

Zhong-Gao *et al.* reported cyclosporin A-loaded O/W microemulsion systems to improve solubility and enhance bioavailability. Varying weight ratios of surfactant to co-surfactant were prepared using caprylic:capric triglyceride (Captex 355) as an oil, polyoxyethylated castor oil (Cremophor EL) as a surfactant, Transcutol as a co-surfactant and saline. The solubility of cyclosporin A in microemulsion systems reached the maximum with 2:1 mixture of Cremophor EL and Trancutol. They concluded that the absolute bioavailability of cyclosporin A loaded in this microemulsion system was increased about 3.3- and 1.25-fold compared with Sandimmune and Sandimmune Neoral® (marketed formulation). The enhanced bioavailability of cyclosporin A loaded in this microemulsion system might be due to the reduced droplet size of microemulsion systems. The formula developed by them is given below:

Table 6:

Formula	*Ingredients*	*I*	*II*	*III*	*IV*	*V*
Captex-355	Oil	4	4	4	4	4
Cremorphor	EL Surfactant	5	7.5	10	11.25	12
Transcutol	Co-surfactant	10	7.5	5	3.75	3

Compositions (% [w:w]) of the oil–surfactant–co-surfactant systems for preparing cyclosporin A microemulsions.

10.4. Parenteral, Pulmonary and Ocular Delivery

Gasco and his group found that prolonged action and protection of biodegradable molecules might be achieved by administering W/O microemulsion parenterally. By using microemulsion, plasma concentration of testosterone was similar compared with other sustained release formulation *(183)*. The area under curve (AUC) of vincristine, an anti-tumour agent, was much higher when given as a microemulsion formulation as compared with solution of free drug. The microemulsion formulation was composed of surfactant as polyethylene glycol–lipid and cholesterol, oil phase as vitamin E solution of oleic acid. A non-aqueous microemulsion formulation composed of lecithin/glycerol/-soybean oil and contained octyl ester of Ibuprofen. Microemulsion formulation was modified by the addition of poloxamer, which altered the absorption process resulting in drug being targeted to reticulo-endothelial system-rich organs *(184)*. Lecithin-stabilised microemulsion formulation has been designed for pulmonary delivery of salbutamol, a bronchodialating agent, as pressurised aerosol system *(185)*. A potential ophthalmic microemulsion formulation of indomethacin, diclofenac and chloramphenicol was prepared by using triacetin, castor oil, water and propylene glycol and stabilised by poloxamer, and *in vitro* permeation study was evaluated *(186)*. Later on, an ocular microemulsion formulation of pilocarpine was also evaluated which was stabilised by sucrose fatty acid ester surfactants *(187)*.

Table 7: Established Microemulsion Technology in Pharmaceutical Formulation

Technology	*Company*	*Details*
ISP-microemulsion technology	International specialty products (ISP)	Utilises unique properties of AgsolEx® solvents and Agrimer® co-polymers from ISP, offer new levels of performance to water-based formulations containing water-insoluble active ingredients
NanoDerma microemulsion technology	NanoDerma Ltd.	The technology offers a dispersion system of nanosized droplets (10–100 nm) that forms viscous semi-solid or homogeneous liquid gel, with transparent or translucent appearance
Non-flammable aerosol propellant microemulsion system	U.S. Patent. No. 3,207,386 to Presant *et al.*	This invention relates to a propellant composition for aerosol dispensers, which is in the form of an O/W microemulsion to suppress the flammability of gaseous propellants for aerosol dispensers by dissolving the propellant in a continuous liquid aqueous phase

REFERENCES

1. **Becher, P.** Encyclopedia of emulsion technology, Marcel Dekker, New York, 1983.
2. **Schulman, JH., Stoeckenius, W., and Prince, M.** Mechanism of formation and structure of micro-emulsions by eletron microscopy. *J. Phy. Chem.* 1959;63:1677–1680.
3. **Kaahiwelt, M., Lessner, E., and Stery, R.** Influence of the properties of the oil and the surfactant on the phase behavior of systems of the type H[2]O-oil-nonionic surfactant. *J. Phy. Chem.* 1983;87:5032–5040.
4. **Danielson, I. and Lindman, B.** The definition of microemulsion. *Colloids Surf.* 1981;3:392–393.
5. **Shinoda, K. and Lindman, B.** Organized surfactant systems: microemulsions. *Langmuir* 1987;3:135–149.
6. **Leung, R. and Shah, DO.** Microemulsions: an evolving technology for pharmaceutical applications, (Rossof, M. ed.), VCH, New York, *Control. Release Drugs: Pol. Aggregate Syst.* 1989, pp. 85–215.
7. **Lawrence, MJ. and Rees, GD.** Microemulsion based media as novel drug delivery system. *Adv. Drug Deliv. Rev.* 2000;45:89–121.
8. **Bagwe, RP., Kanicky, JR., Palla, BJ., Patanjali, PK., and Shah, DO.** Improved drug delivery using microemulsion: rationale, recent progress and new horizons. *Crit. Rev. Ther. Drug Carrier Syst.* 2001;18:77–140.
9. **Daoud, M. and Williams, CE. (eds.)** Soft matter physics, Springer-Verlag, Berlin, Germany, 1999.
10. **Frontell, K., Hernqvist, L., Larsson, K., and Sjoblom.** On structural relations between lipid mesophases and isotropic reversed micellar (L2) solutions. J. *J. Colloid Interf. Sci.* 1983;93:453.
11. **Luisi, PL., Scartazzini, R., Haering, G., and Schurtenbarger, P.** Organogels from water-in-oil microemulsions. *Colloid Polym. Sci.* 1990;268:356.
12. **Shioi, A., Harada, M., and Matsumoto, K.** Phase equilibrium of sodium bis(2-ethylhexyl) phosphate/water/ n-heptaneisodium chloride microemulsion. *J. Phy. Chem.* 1991;95:7495.
13. **Kern, F., Zana, R., and Candau, SJ.** Rheological properties of semidilute and concentrated aqueous solutions of cetyltrimethylammonium in the presence of sodium salicylate and sodium chloride. *Langmuir* 1991;7:1344.

14. **Kahlweit, M., Strey, R., and Schomaker, R.** Reactions in compartmentallized liquids, (Knoche, W. and Schomarker R., eds.), Springer Verlag, New York, 1989, 1 p.

15. **Sjoblom, E. and Friberg, S.** Light-scattering and electron microscopy determinations of association structures in W/O microemulsions. *J. Colloid Interf. Sci.* 1978;67:16.

16. **Koper, GJM., Sager, WFC., Smeets, J., and Bedeaux, D.** Aggregation in oil-continuous water/sodium bis(2-ethylhexyl)sulfosuccinate/oil microemulsions. *J. Phy. Chem.* 1995;99:13,291.

17. **Eicke, HF., Borkovec, H., and Dasgupta, B.** Conductivity of a water-in-oil microemulsion: a quantitative charge fluctuation model. *J. Phy. Chem.* 1989;93:314.

18. **Lagues, M., Ober, R., and Taupin, C.** Study of structure and electrical conductivity in microemulsions: evidence for percolation mechanism. *J. Phy. Lett.* 1978;39:487.

19. **Shinoda, K. and Saito, H.** The effect of temperature on the phase equilibria and the types of dispersions of the ternary system composed of water, cyclohexane, and nonionic surfactant. *J. Colloid Interf. Sci.* 1968;26:70.

20. **Tamlon, Y. and Prager, S.** Statistical thermodynamics of phase equilibria in microemulsions. *J. Chem. Phy.* 1978;69(7): 2984–2991.

21. **Scriven, LE.** Micellization, solubilization, and micro-emulsions, (Mittal, KL. ed.), vol. 2, Plenum Press, New York, 1977, 877 p.

22. **Friberg, S., Lapczynska, I., and Gillberg, G.** Microemulsions containing nonionic surfactants—the importance of the pit value. *J. Colloid Interf. Sci.* 1976;56:19.

23. **Lindman, B., Kamenka, N., Brun, B., and Nilsson, PG.** Microemulsions, (Robb, ID. ed.), Plenum Press, New York, 1982, 115p.

24. **Zulauf, M. and Eicke, HF.** Inverted micelles and microemulsions in the ternary system water/aerosol-OT/isooctane as studied by photon correlation spectroscopy. *J. Phy. Chem.* 1979;83:480.

25. **Eicke, HF.** Aggregation in surfactant solutions: formation and properties of micelles and microemulsions. *J. Pure Appl. Chem.* 1980;52:1349.

26. **Zana, R. and Lang, J.** Solution chemistry of surfactants, (Fendler, EJ. and Mittal KL., eds.), Plenum Press, New York, 1984.

27. **Borkovec, M., Eicke, HF., Hammerich, H., and Dasgupta, B.** Two percolation processes in microemulsions. *J. Phy. Chem.* 1988;92:206.

28. **Ruckenstein, Eli.** Thermodynamic approaches to microemulsions. *J. Colloid Interf. Sci.* 1998;204:143–150.

29. **da Graca Miguel., Burrows, HD., Pereira, MAE., and Varela, AP.** Probing solute distribution and acid-base behaviour in water-in-oil microemulsions by fluorescence techniques. *Colloid surf.* 2001; 176:85–99.

30. **Overbeek, J. and Th, G.** The first rideal lecture. Micro-emulsions, a field at the border between lyophobic and lyophilic colloids. *Faraday Discuss. Chem. Soc.* 1978;65:72.

31. **Tadros, TF., Vincent, B., and Becher, P (eds.).** Encyclopaedia of emulsion technology, Marcel Dekker, New York, 1980.

32. **Harkins, WD.** A general thermodynamic theory of the spreading of liquids to form duplex films and of liquids or solids to form monolayers. *J. Chem. Phy.* 1941;9(7):552–568.

33. **Olsson, ULF.** Physical chemistry 1: surfactant self-assembly, Research projects, Lund University, Lund, Sweden, 2006, http://www.fkem1.lu.se/research_projects/surfactant.asp., Last accessed date: July, 26th, 2007.

34. **Kunieda, H. and Shinoda.** Solution behavior and hydrophile-lipophile balance temperature in the aerosol OT-isooctane-brine system: correlation between microemulsions and ultralow interfacial tensions, K. *J. Colloid Interf. Sci.* 1980;75:601.

35. **Chen, SJ., Evans, FD., and Ninham, BW.** Properties and structure of three-component ionic microemulsions. *J. Phy. Chem.* 1984;88:1631.

36. **Kahlweit, M., Strey, R., and Busse, G.** Microemulsions: a qualitative thermodynamic approach. *J. Phy. Chem.* 1990;94:3881–3894.

37. **Li, X. and Kunieda, H.** Catanionic surfactants: microemulsion formation and solubilization. *Curr. Opin. Colloid Interf. Sci.* 2003;8:327–336.

38. **Feng, LSK. and Band, W.** Statistical theory of duplex films. *J. Chem. Phy.* 1940;8:977–980.

39. **Garti, N., Yaghmur, A., Aserin, A., Spernath, A., Elfakess, R., and Ezrahi, S.** Solubilization of active molecules in microemulsions for improved environmental protection. *Colloids Surf. A Physicochem. Eng. Asp.* 2004;230:183.

40. **Lawrence, MJ.** Microemulsions as drug delivery vehicles. *Curr. Opin. Colloid Interf. Sci.* 1996;1:826.

41. **Kreilgaard, M.** Influence of microemulsions on cutaneous drug delivery. *Adv. Drug Deliv. Rev.* 2002;54(1):S77–S98.

42. **Goodwin, JW.** Colloids and interfaces with surfactants and polymers-An Introduction, John Wiley and sons Ltd, England, 2004.

43. **Danielsson, I. and Lindman, B.** The definition of micro-emulsion. Colloids and surfaces. *Colloids Surf.* 1992;3:391–392.

44. **Sachdeva, A., Guati, R., Gupta, U., and Bapna, JS.** Comparative bioavailability of two brands of cyclosporine. *Ind. J. Pharmacol.* 1997;29:135–137.

45. **John, W. and Strey, R.** Microstructure of microemulsions by freeze fracture electron microscopy. *J. Phy. Chem.* 1988;92:2294.

46. **Vinson, PK., Sheeban, JG., Mille, WG., Scriven, LE., and Davis, HT.** Viewing microemulsions with freeze-fracture transmission electron microscopy. *J. Phy. Chem.* 1991;95:2546.

47. **Eccleston, GM., Swarbrick, J., and Boylan, JC.** Microemulsions, encyclopedia of pharmaceutical technology, 1st ed, vol. 9, Marcel Dekker Inc., New York, 1995, pp. 375–421.

48. **Mitchell, DJ. and Ninham, B.** Micelles vesicles and microemulsions. *J. Chem. Soc. Faraday Trans.* 1981;2(677): 601–629.

49. **Fletcher, DI., Parrott, D., and Pileni, MP.** Protein partitioning between microemulsion phases and conjugate aqueous phases, structure and reactivity in reverse micelles, Elsevier, New York, 1988, pp. 303–322.

50. **Kupferman, A., Ryan, WJ., and Leibowitz, HM.** Prolongation of anti-inflammatory effect of prednisolone acetate. *Arch. Ophthalmol.* 1981;99:2028–2029.

51. **Shinoda, K. and Saito, H.** The stability of O/W type emulsions as functions of temperature and the HLB of emulsifiers: the emulsification by PIT method. *J. Colloid Int. Sci.* 1969;30: 258–263.

52. **Shinoda, K. and Saito, H.** The effect of temperature on the phase equilibria and the types of dispersions of the ternary system composed of water, cyclohexane, and nonionic surfactant. *J. Colloid Interf. Sci.* 1968;26:70–74.

53. **Shinoda, K., Kunieda, H., and Becher, P.** Encyclopaedia of emulsion technology, Marcel Dekker, New York, 1983, 1 p.

54. **Rosano, HL., Cavello, JL., Chang, DL., and Whittam, JH.** Microemulsions: a commentary on their preparation. *J. Soc. Cosmet. Chem.* 1988;39:201–209.

55. **Shinoda, K., Kunieda, H., Arai, T., and Saijo, H.** Principles of attaining very large solubilization (microemulsion): inclusive understanding of the solubilization of oil and water in aqueous and hydrocarbon media. *J. Phy. Chem.* 1984;88:5126.

56. **Overbeek. J. The First Rideal Lecture.** Microemulsions, a field at the border between lyophobic and lyophilic colloids. *Faraday Discuss.* 1978;65:7–19.

57. **Wakabayashi, T., Horiuchi, M., Sakaguchi, M., Onda, H., and Iljima, M.** Induction of megamitochondria in the rat liver by N-propyl alcohol and N-butyl alcohol. *Acta Patho. Jpn.* 1984;4:471.

58. **Hoar, TP. and Schulman, JH.** Transparent water in oil dispersions: oleopathic hydromicelle. *Nature* 1943;102:152.

59. **Attwood, D., Mallon, C., and Taylor, CJ.** Phase studies on oil-in-water phospholipid microemulsions. *Int. J. Pharm.* 1992;84:5–8.

60. **Aboofazeli, R., Patel, M., Thomas, M., and Lawrence, MJ.** Investigations into the formation and characterization of phospholipid microemulsions. IV. Pseudo-ternary phase diagrams of systems containing water-lecithin-alcohol and oil; the influence of oil. *Int. J. Pharm.* 1995;125:107–116.

61. **Dalmora, ME., Dalmora, SL., and Oliveira, AG.** Inclusion complex of piroxicam with b-cyclodextrin and incorporation in cationic microemulsion. *Int. J. Pharm.* 2001;222:45–55.

62. **Johnson, KA. and Shah, DO.** Effect of oil chain length and electrolytes on water solubilization in alcohol-free pharmaceutical microemulsions. *J. Colloid Int. Sci.* 1985;107: 269–271.

63. **Junping, W., Takayama, K., Nagai, T., and Maitani, Y.** Pharmacokinetics and antitumor effects of vincristine carried by microemulsions composed of PEG-lipid, oleic acid, vitamin E and cholesterol. *Int. J. Pharm.* 2003;251:13–21.

64. **Lawrence, J.** Surfactant systems: microemulsions and vesicles as vehicles for drug delivery. *Eur. J. Drug Metab. Pharmacokinet.* 1994;3:257–269.

65. **Constantinides, PP.** Lipid microemulsions for improving drug dissolution and oral absorption: physical and biopharmaceutical aspects. *Pharm. Res.* 1995;12:1561–1572.

66. **Hauss, DJ., Fogal, SE., Ficorilli, JV., *et al.*** Lipid-based delivery systems for improving the bioavailability and lymphatic transport of a poorly water-soluble LTB4 inhibitor. *J. Pharm. Sci.* 1998;87:164–169.

67. **Evitts, DP., Olejnik, O., Musson, DG., and Bilgood, AM.** Aqueous ophtalmic microemulsions of tepoxalin. European patent application 0 480 690 A1, 1991.

68. **Vandamme, TF.** Microemulsions as ocular drug delivery systems: recent developments and future challenges. *Prog. Reti. Eye Res.* 2002;21:15–34.

69. **Kahlweit, M.** How to prepare microemulsions at prescribed temperature, oil, and brine. *J. Phy. Chem.* 1995;99:1281–1284.

70. **Kahlweit, M., Lessner, E., and Strey, R.** Phase behavior of quaternary systems of the type H_2O-oil-nonionic surfactant-inorganic electrolyte. *J. Phy. Chem.* 1984;88:1937–1944.

71. **Aboofazeli, R. and Lawrence, MJ.** Investigations into the formation and characterization of phospholipid microemulsions, II: pseudoternary phase diagrams of systems containing water-lecithin-isopropyl myristate and alcohol: influence of purity of lecithin. *Int. J. Pharm.* 1994;106:51–61.

72. **Schwuger, MJ. and Stickdorn, K.** Microemulsions in technical processes. *Chem. Rev.* 1995;95(4):849.

73. **Alander, J. and Warnheim, W.** Model microemulsions containing vegetable oils. Part 1: nonionic surfactant systems. *J. Amer. Oil Chem. Soc.* 1989;66(11):1656–1660.

74. **Von Corswant, C., Engstrom, S., and Soderman, O.** Microemulsions based on soybean phosphatidylcholine and triglycerides. Phase behavior and microstructure. *Langmuir* 1997;13:5061–5070.

75. **Caboi, F., Capuzzi, G., Baglioni, P., and Monduzzi, M.** Microstructure of Ca-AOT/water/decane w/o microemulsions. *J. Phy. Chem.* 1997;B101:10,205.

76. **Monig, K., Haegel., and Schwuger, MJ.** Microemulsions with plant oils. *Tenside Surf. Det.* 1996;33(3):228–232.

77. **Dreher, F., Walde, P., Walther, P., and Wehrli, E.** Interaction of a lecithin microemulsion gel with human stratum corneum and its effect on transdermal transport. *J. Control. Release* 1997;45:131–140.

78. **El-Nokaly, M., Hiler, G., and McGrady, J.** Microemulsionsand emulsions in foods, (El-Nokaly, M. and Cornell, D., eds.), *Am. Chem. Soc.* Washington DC, 1991, pp. 26–43.

79. **Kunieda, H., Asaoka, H., and Shinoda, K.** Two types of surfactant phases and four co-existing liquid phases in a water/ non-ionic surfactant. *J. Phy. Chem.* 1988;92:185.

80. **Joubran, RF., Cornell, DG., and Parris, N.** Microemulsions of triglyceride and non-ionic surfactant—effect of temperature and aqueous phase composition. *Colloid Surf. A Physicochem. Eng. Asp.* 1993;80:153–160.

81. **Parris, N., Joubran, RF., and Lu, DP.** Triglyceride microemulsions—effect of nonionic surfactants and the nature of the oil. *J. Agri. Food Chem.* 1994;42(6):1295–1299.

82. **Bourrel, M. and Schechter, RS.** Microemulsions and related systems: formation solvency and physical properties, Academic Press, New York, 1988, pp. 30, 152, 315, 343 (Chapters 4 and 5).

83. **Li, X., Ueda, K., and Kunieda, H.** Solubilization and phase behavior of microemulsions with mixed anionic–cationic surfactants and hexanol. *Langmuir* 1999;15:7973–7979.

84. **Kunieda, H. and Aoki, R.** Effect of added salt on the maximum solubilization in an ionic surfactant microemulsion. *Langmuir* 1996;12:5796–5799.

85. **Gao, KH. Oh, and Kim, CK.** Physicochemical characterization and evaluation of a microemulsion system for oral delivery of cyclosporin A. *Int. J. Pharm.* 1998;161:75–86.

86. **Djordjevic, L., Primorac, M., Stupar, M., and Krajisnik, D.** Characterization of caprylocaproyl macrogolglycerides based microemulsion drug delivery vehicles for an amphiphilic drug. *Int. J. Pharm.* 2004;271:11–19.

87. **Hauser, H., Haering, G., Pande, A., and Luisi, PL.** Interaction of water with sodium bis(2-ethyl-1-hexyl) sulfosuccinate in reversed micelles. *J. Phy. Chem.* 1989;93:7869.

88. **Quist, PQ. and Halle, B.** Water dynamics and aggregate structure in reversed micelles at sub-zero temperatures. A deuteron spin relaxation study. *J. Chem. Soc. Faraday Trans.* 1988;1:1038.

89. **Haandrikman, G., Daane, GJR., Kerkhof, FJM., Van Os, NM., and Rupert, LAM.** A microcalorimetric investigation of the solubilization of water in reversed micelles and water-in-oil microemulsions. *J. Phy. Chem.* 1992;96:9061.

90. **Wong, M., Thomas, JK., and Nowak, T.** Structure and state of water in reversed micelles. *J. Am. Chem. Soc.* 1977;79:4730.

91. **Moran, PD., Bowmaker, GA., Cooney, RP., Bartlett, JR., and Woolfrey, JL.** Vibrational spectroscopic study of the structure of sodium bis(2-ethylhexyl)sulfosuccinate reverse micelles and water-in-oil microemulsions. *Langmuir* 1995;11:738.

92. **Giammona, G., Gofferedi, F., Liveri, VT., and Vassallo, G.** Water structure in water/AOT/n-heptane microemulsions by FT-IR spectroscopy. *J. Colloid Interf. Sci.* 1992;154:411.

93. **Ikushima, Y., Saito, N., and Arai, M.** The nature and structure of water/AOT/ethane (w/o) microemulsion under supercritical conditions studied by high-pressure FT-IR spectroscopy. *J. Colloid Interf. Sci.* 1997;186:254.

94. **Nazzal, S., Smalykh, II., Lavrentovich, OD., and Khan, MA.** Preparation and *in vitro* characterization of a eutectic based semisolid self-nanoemulsified drug delivery system (SNEDDS) of ubiquinone: mechanism and progress of emulsion formation. *Int. J. Pharm.* 2002;235:47–65.

95. **Cortesi, R. and Nastruzzi, C.** Liposomes, micelles and microemulsions as new delivery systems for cytotoxic alkaloids. *Pharm. Sci. Tech. Today* 1999;2(7):288–298.

96. **Bastogne, F. and David, C.** Quaternary N-alkylaldonamide–brine–decane–alcohol systems. Part I: phase behaviour and microemulsions. *Colloid Surf. A: Physicochem. Eng. Asp.* 139;1998:311–320.

97. **Li, X. and Wang, J.** Effects of mixed anionic-cationic surfactants and alcohol on solubilization of water-in-oil microemulsions. *J. Disp. Sci. Tech.* 1999;20:993–1007.

98. **Alany, RG., Rades, T., Agatonovic-Kustrin, S., Davies, NM., and Tucker, IG.** Effects of alcohols and diols on the phase behaviour of quaternary systems. *Int. J. Pharm.* 2000; 196:141–145.

99. **Yao, JY. and Romsted, LR.** Effects of hydrocarbon and triglyceride oils on butanol distribution in water-in-oil cationic microemulsions. *Colloid Surf. A: Physicochem. Eng. Asp.* 1997;123–124:89–105.

100. **Nave, S., Eastoe, J., Heenan, RK., Steytler, D., and Grillo, I.** What is so special about aerosol-OT? 2. Microemulsion systems. *Langmuir* 2000;16:8741–8748.

101. **Warisnoicharoen, W., Lansley, AB., and Lawrence, M.** Nonionic oil-in-water microemulsions: the effect of oil type on phase behaviour. *Int. J. Pharm.* 2000;198:7–27.

102. **Panayiotis, PC. and Scalart, JP.** Formulation and physical characterization of water-in-oil microemulsions containing long- versus medium-chain glycerides. *Int. J. Pharm.* 1997; 158:57–68.

103. **Leung, R. and Shah, DO.** Solubilization and phase equilibria of water-in-oil microemulsions : II. Effects of alcohols, oils, and salinity on single-chain surfactant systems. *J. Colloid Int. Sci.* 1987;120:330–344.

104. **Watt, SL., Tunaley, D., and Biggs, S.** The formation of water-in-oil microemulsions using a concentrated saline aqueous phase. *Colloid Surf. A: Physicochem. Eng. Asp.* 1998;137:25–33.

105. **Huibers, PD. and Shah, DO.** Evidence for synergism in nonionic surfactant mixtures: enhancement of solubilization in water-in-oil microemulsions. *Langmuir* 1997;13:5762–5765.

106. **Mittal, KL.** Micellization, solubilization, and microemulsions, vol 2, Plenum, New York, 1977, pp. 1–2.

107. **Mittal, KL. and Kumar, P.** Handbook of microemulsion science and technology, Marcel Dekker, New York, 1999, pp. 50–53.

108. **Overbeek, GT., Verhoeckx, GJ., Bruyn De, PL., and Lekkerkerker, HNW.** On understanding microemulsions. II thermodynamics of droplet-type microemulsions. *J. Colloid Interf. Sci.* 1987;119:2.

109. **Craig, DQM., Barker, SA., Banning, D., and Booth, SW.** An investigation into the mechanisms of self-emulsification using particle size analysis and low frequency dielectric spectroscopy. *Int. J. Pharm.* 1995;114:103–110.

110. **Pouton, CW.** Self-emulsifying drug delivery systems: assessment of the efficiency of emulsification. *Int. J. Pharm.* 1985;27:335–348.

111. **Gershanik, T. and Benita, S.** Positively charged self-emulsifying oil formulation for improving oral bioavailability of progesterone. *Pharm. Dev. Technol.* 1996;1:147–157.

112. **Yu, ZJ. and Neuman, RD.** Reversed micellar solution-to-bicontinuous microemulsion transition in sodium bis(2-ethylhexyl) phosphate/n-heptane/water system. *Langmuir* 1995;11:101–108.

113. **Angelico, R., Palazzo, G., Colafemmina, G., Cirkel, PA., Giustini, M., and Ceglie, A.** Water diffusion and headgroup mobility in polymer-like reverse micelles: evidence of a sphere-to-rod-to-sphere transition. *J. Phy. Chem.* 1998;B102:2883–2889.

114. **D'Angelo, M., Fiorette, D., Onori, G., Palmieri, L., and Sntneci, A.** Dynamics of water-containing sodium bis(2-ethylhexyl) sulfosuccinate (AOT) reverse micelles: a high-frequency dielectric study. *Phy. Rev. E.* 1996;E54:993–996.

115. **Mehta, SK., Kavaljit, XX., and Bala, K.** Phase behavior, structural effects, and volumetric and transport properties in nonaqueous microemulsions. *Phy. Rev. E.* 1999; E59:4317–4325.

116. **Klier, J., Tucker, CJ., Kalantar, TH., and Green, DP.** Properties and applications of microemulsions. *Adv. Mater.* 2000; 12:1751.

117. **Gradzielski, M. and Hoffmann, H.** Influence of charges on structure and dynamics of an O/W microemulsion. Effect of admixing ionic surfactants. *J. Phy. Chem.* 1994;98:2613.

118. **Olabisi, O., Robeson, LM., and Shaw, MT.** Polymer-polymer miscibility, Academic Press, New York, 1979.

119. **Charlton, ID. and Doherty, AP.** Simultaneous observation of attractive interaction, depletion forces, and "Sticky" encounters between AOT reverse micelles in isooctane using microelectrode voltammetry. *J. Phy. Chem. B* 2000;104:8061.

120. **Myers, SA., Mackay, RA., and Btajter-Toth, A.** Solution microstructure and electrochemical reactivity. Effect of probe partitioning on electrochemical formal potentials in microheterogeneous solutions. *Anal. Chem.* 1993;65:34.

121. **Mackay, RA., Myers, SA., Bodalbhai, L., and Btajter-Toth, A.** Microemulsion structure and its effect on electrochemical reactions. *Anal. Chem.* 1990;62:1084.

122. **Bodet, JF., Bellare, JR., Davies, HT., Scriven, LE., and Miller, WG.** Fluid microstructure transition from globular to bicontinuous in mid rang microemulsions. *J. Phy. Chem.* 1988;92:1898.

123. **Greek, JL.** Electron microscopy study of a glass-forming water/oil psudo-three-component microemulsion system. *J. Phy. Chem.* 1990;94:5647.

124. **Barnes, IS., Hyde, ST., Ninham, BW., Derian, P. J., Drifford, M., Warr, GG., and Zemb, TN.** The dissordered open connected model of microemulsions. *Progr. Colloid Polym. Sci.* 1988;76:90–95.

125. **Regev, O., Ezrahi, S., Aserin, A., Garti, N., Wachtel, E. and Talmon, Y.** A Study of the microstructure of a four-component nonionic microemulsion by cryo-TEM, NMR, SAXS, and SANS. *Langmuir* 1996;12:668–674.

126. **Kahlweit, M., Strey, R., Hasse, D., *et al.*** How to study microemulsions. *J. Colloid Interf. Sci.* 1987;118:436–453.

127. **Nakamura, N., Yamaguchi, Y., Hakansson, B., Olsson, U., Tagawa, T., and Kunieda, H.** Formation of microemulsion and liquid crystal in biocompatible sucrose alkanoate systems. *J. Disp. Sci. Technol.* 1999;20:535–557.

128. **Hirai, M., Hirai, RK., Jwase, H., *et al.*** Dynamics of w/o AOT microemulsions studied by neutron spin echo. *J. Phy. Chem. Solids* 1999;60:1359–1361.

129. **Auvray, L., Cotton, JP., Ober, R., and Taupin, C.** Evidence for zero mean curvature microemulsions. *J. Phy. Chem.* 1984;88:4586–4589.

130. **Zemb, TN., Barnes, IS., Derian, PJ., and Ninham, BW.** Scattering as a critical test of microemulsion structure models. *Progr. Colloid Polym. Sci.* 1990;81:20–29.

131. **Bergenholtz, J., Romagnoli, AA., and Wagner, NJ.** Viscosity, mi-crostructure, and interparticle potential of AOT/H2O/n-Decane inverse microemulsions. *Langmuir* 1995;11:1559–1570.

132. **Bolzinger, MA., Thevenin, MA., Grossiord, JL., and Poelman, MC.** Characterization of a sucrose ester microemulsion by freeze fracture electron micrograph and small angle neutron scattering experiments. *Langmuir* 1999;15:2307–2315.

133. **Tabony, J.** Occurrence of liquid-crystalline mesophases in microemulsion dispersions. *J. Nature* 1986;320:338–340.

134. **Tabony, J.** Formation of cubic structures in microemulsions containing equal volumes of oil and water. *J. Nature* 1986;319:400.

135. **Pecora, R.** (ed.) Dynamic light scattering, Plenum Press, New York, 1985, 15 p.

136. **Hiemens, PC. and Rajagopalan, R.** Principles of colloid and surface chemistry, 3rd ed., Marcel Dekker, New York, 1997.

137. **Vesetova, OV., Nikolaev, BP., and Shlyakov, AM.** *Kollid Zh.* 1985;47:1027.

138. **Mesa, CL., Coppola, L., Raniera, GA., Terenzi, M., and Chidichimo, G.** Phase diagram and phase properties of the system water-hexane-aerosol OT. *Langmuir* 1992;8:26.

139. **Garti, N., Feldenkriez, R., Aserin, A., Ezrahi, S., and Shapira, D.** Hydraulic fluid based on water in oil microemulsions, STLE. *Lubracation Engg.* 1993;49:404.

140. **Lindman, B., Stilbs, P., Friberg, S., and Bothorel, P (eds.).** Microemulsions, CRC Press, Boca Raton Florida, 1986, 295 p.

141. **Washington, C.** Drug release from microdisperse systems. *Int. J. Pharm.* 1990;58:1–12.

142. **Illum, L., Khan, MA., Mak, E., and Davis, SS.** Evaluation of carrier capacity and release characteristics for poly(butyl-2-cyanoacrylate) nanoparticles. *Int. J. Pharm.* 1986;30:17–28.

143. **Washington, C. and Evans, K.** Release rate measurements of model hydrophobic solutes from submicron triglyceride emulsions. *J. Control. Release* 33;1995:383–390.

144. **Williman, H., Walde, P., Luisi, PL., Gazzaniga, A., and Stroppolo, F.** Lecithin organogel as matrix for transdermal transport of drugs. *J. Pharm. Sci.* 1992;81:871–874.

145. **Osborne, DW., Ward, JL., and O'Neill, KJ.** Microemulsions as topical drug delivery vehicles: in-vitro transdermal studies of a model hydrophilic drug. *J. Pharm. Pharmacol.* 1991;43:451–454.

146. **Swarbrink, J. and Boylan, JC (eds.).** Encyclopedia of pharmaceutical technology, Marcel Dekker, Inc., USA, 1994; 9:375–421.

147. **Thacharodi, D. and Rao, KP.** Transdermal absortion of nifedipine from microemulsions of lipophilic skin penetrations enhancers. *Int. J. Pharm.* 1994;111:235–240.

148. **Delgado-Charro, MB., Iglesias-Vilas, G., Blanco-Mendez, J., Lopez-Quintela, MA., Marty, J-P., and Guy, RH.** Delivery of a hydrophilic solute through the skin from novel microemulsion systems. *Eur. J. Pharm. Biopharm.* 1997;43:37–42.

149. **Parra, JL., Coderch, L., Yuste, I., and De La Maza, A.** Incorporation of non-steroidal anti-inflammatory drugs into specific monophasic formulations. *Colloids Surf. A: Physicochem. Eng. Asp.* 1997;123–124:115–123.

150. **Schmalfuss, U., Neubert, R., and Wohlrab, W.** Modification of drug penetration into human skin using microemulsions. *J. Control. Release* 1997;46:279–285.

151. **Kreilgaard, M., Pedersen, EJ., and Jaroszewski, JW.** NMR characterization and transdermal drug delivery potential of microemulsion systems. *J. Control. Release* 2000; 69:421–433.

152. **Kemken, J., Ziegler, A., and Mueller, BW.** Influence of super saturation on the pharmacodynamic effect of bupranolol after dermal administration using microemulsions as vehicle. *Pharm. Res.* 1992;9:554–558.

153. **Kreilgaard, M., Kemme, MJB., Burggraaf, J., Schoemaker, RC., and Cohen, AF.** Influence of a microemulsion vehicle on cutaneous bioequivalence of a lipophilic model drug assessed by microdialysis and pharmacodynamics. *Pharm. Res.* 2001;18:593–599.

154. **Paollino, D., Ventura, CA., Nistico, S., Puglisi, G., and Fresta, M.** Lecithin microemulsions for the topical administration of ketoprofen: percutaneous adsorption through human skin and in vivo human skin tolerability. *Int. J. Pharm.* 2002;244:21–23.

155. **Fevrier, F., Bobin, MF., Lafforgue, C., and Martini, MC.** Advances in microemulsions and transepidermal penetration of tyrosine. *S. T. P. Pharm. Sci.* 1991;1:60.

156. **Ho, HO., Huang, MC., Chen, LC., *et al.*** *J. Chin. Pharm.* 1998;50:257–266.

157. **Trotta, M., Morel, S., and Gasco, MR.** Effect of oil phase composition on the skin permeation of felodipine from o/w microemulsions. *Pharmazie* 1997;52:50–53.

158. **Varshney, M., Khanna, T., and Changez, M.** Effects of AOT micellar systems on the transdermal permeation of glyceryl trinitrate. *Colloids Surf. B Biointerf.* 1999;13:1–11; Bolonga, Italy, 1991, 388p.

159. **Trotta, M., Gasco, MR., and Pattarino, F.** Diffusion of steroid hormones from o/w microemulsions: influence of the cosurfactant. *Acta Pharm. Technol.* 1990;36:226–231.

160. **Gasco, MR., Morel, S., and Mazoni, R.** *Il Farmaco Ed. Pr.* 1988;43:373.

161. **Sintov, AC. and Shapiro, L.** New microemulsion vehicle facilitates percutaneous penetration in vitro and cutaneous drug bioavailability *in vivo*. *J. Control. Release* 2004;95:173–183.

162. **Lu, G. and Jun, HW.** Diffusion studies of methotrexate in carbopol and poloxamer gels. *Int. J. Pharm.* 1998;160:1–9.

163. **Bookbinder, SA., Espinoza, LR., Fenske, NA., Germain, BF., and Vasey, FB.** Methotrexate: its use in the rheumatic diseases. *Clin. Exp. Dermatol.* 1984;2:185–193.

164. **Van Dooren-Greebe, RJ., Kuijpers, ALA., Mulder, J., De Boo, T., Van der., and Kerkhof, PCM.** Methotrexate revisited: effects of long-term treatment in psoriasis. *Br. J. Dermatol.* 1994;130:204–210.

165. **Hwang, GC., Lin, AY., Chen, W., and Sharpe, RJ.** Development and optimization of a methotrexate topical formulation. *Drug Dev. Ind. Pharm.* 1995;21(17):1941–1952.

166. **Trotta, M., Gasco, MR., and Morel, S.** Release of drugs from oil-water microemulsions. *J. Control. Release* 1989;10:237.

167. **Von Conxita Solans, Infante, MR., and Garcia-Celma, MJ.** Trends in colloid and interface science X, Steinkopff Verlag, 1996, pp. 123–145.

168. **Kriwet, K. and Müller-Goymann, CC.** Diclofenac release from ármacoipids drug systems and permeation through excised human stratum corneum. *Int. J. Pharm.* 1995;125:231–242.

169. **Pattarino, F., Gasco, MR., and Trotta, M.** Accumulation of anthracycline, a W/O microemulsion. *Il Farmaco.* 1989;44:339.

170. **Gasco, MR., Pattarino, F., and Voltani, I.** Behavior of doxorubicin in o/w microemulsions. *Il Farmaco Ed. Pr.* 1988;43:3.

171. **Benameur, H. and Bartheelemy, P.** Composition with sustained release of active principle, capable of forming a microemulsion US patent no. 6309665.

172. **Constantinides, PP., Scalart, JP., Lancaster, C., *et al.*** Formulation and intestinal absorption enhancement evaluation of water-in-oil microemulsions incorporating medium-chain glycerides. *Pharm. Res.* 1994;11:385.

173. **Drewe, J., Fricker, G., Vonderscher, J., and Beglinger, C.** Enteral absorption of octreotide: absorption enhancement by polyoxyethylene-24-cholesterol ether. *Br. J. Pharmacol.* 1993;108:247–265;298–303.

174. **Novelli, A., Rico, I., and Lattes, A.** Novel microemulsion formulation reduces acid hydrolysis of radioprotector WR 2721. *New J. Chem.* 1992;16:395.

175. **Kommuru, TR., Gurley, B., Khan, MA., and Reddy, IK.** Self-emulsifying drug delivery systems (SEDDS) of coenzyme Q10: formulation development and bioavailability assessment. *Int. J. Pharm.* 2001;212:233–246.

176. **Itoh, K., Tozuka, Y., Oguchi, T., and Yamamoto, K.** Improvement of physicochemical properties of N-4472 part I formulation design by using self-microemulsifying system. *Int. J. Pharm.* 2002;238:153–160.

177. **Kawakami, K., Yoshikawa, T., Hayashi, T., Nishihara, Y., and Masuda, K.** Microemulsion formulation for enhanced absorption of poorly soluble drugs: II. In vivo study. *J. Control. Release* 2003;81:75–82.

178. **Gao, P., Guyton, ME., Huang, T., Bauer, JM., Stefanski, KJ., and Lu, Q.** Enhanced oral bioavailability of a poorly water soluble drug PNU-91325 by supersaturatable formulations. *Drug Dev. Ind. Pharm.* 2004;30(2):221–229.

179. **Kim, CK., Cho, Ju, Y., and Gao, ZG.** Preparation and evaluation of biphenyl dimethyl dicarboxylate microemulsions for oral delivery. *J. Control. Release* 2001;70:149–155.

180. **Khoo, SM., Humberstone, AJ., Porter, CJH., Edwards, GA., and Charman, WN.** Formulation design and bioavailability assessment of lipidic self-emulsifying formulations of halofantrine. *Int. J. Pharm.* 1998;167:155–164.

181. **Cooney, GF., Jeevananandan, V., Choudhury, S., Feutren, G., Muller, EA., and Eisen, H.** Comparative bioavailability of Neoral and Sandimmune in cardiac transplant recipients over one year. *J. Transplant.* 1998;30:1892–1894.

182. **Porter, CJH. and Charman, WN.** Uptake of drugs into the intestinal lymphatics after oral administration. *Adv. Drug Deliv. Rev.* 2001;25:47–58.

183. **Gasco, MR., Pattarino, F., and Lattanzi, F.** Long-acting delivery systems for peptides: reduced plasma testosterone levels in male rats after a single injection. *Int. J. Pharm.* 1990;62:119–123.

184. **Li, MJ., Lee, MH., and Shin, CK.** Inverse targeting of drugs to reticuloendothelial system-rich organs by lipid microemulsion emulsified with poloxamer 338. *Int. J. Pharm.* 1995;113: 175–187.

185. **Evans, RM. and Farr, SJ.** The development of novel, pressurised aerosols formulated as solutions. *J. Biopharm. Sci.* 1992;3:33–40.

186. **Siebenbrodt, I. and Keipert, S.** Poloxamer-systems as potential ophthalmics. II. Microemulsions. *Eur. J. Pharm. Biopharm.* 1993;39:25–30.

187. **Keipert, S. and Schulz, G.** Microemulsions with sucrose fatty ester surfactants. I: In vitro characterization. *Pharmazie* 1994;49:195–197.

4

Multiple Emulsion

Prof. (Mrs)K. K. Sawant, M.PHARM, PhD
Prof. K. S. Rajesh, M.PHARM, PhD

CONTENTS

1. INTRODUCTION

Multiple emulsions are novel development in the field of emulsion technology and more complex type of dispersed systems. Multiple emulsions were first described by Seiferiz in 1925 as double or complex emulsions during an inversion of oil-in-water (O/W) olive oil emulsion into water-in-oil (W/O) emulsion *(1)*, but it is only in the last 30 yr that they have been extensively studied and investigated in such diverse fields as separation of hydrocarbons, treatment of waste water, immobilisation of enzymes, prolongation of drug release, treatment of overdose, etc. Their applications in the pharmaceutical and cosmetological field include taste masking, adjuvant vaccines, enzyme immobilisation, absorption or permeation enhancement, protection and stabilisation of entrapped active, sustained and prolonged release, etc. *(2)*.

Multiple emulsions may also be called as "emulsion of emulsions", "double or triple emulsions" because the internal phase itself contains dispersed globules, which are miscible with the continuous phase. This leads to two types, viz. water-in-oil-in-water (W/O/W) and oil-in-water-in-oil (O/W/O) wherein the two miscible phases are separated by an immiscible phase. This phase is sometimes called a "liquid membrane" which acts as semi-permeable membrane through which a solute may diffuse from one phase to another. Hence multiple emulsions are also called "Liquid membrane systems" *(3)*. Schematic representation of a W/O/W double emulsion droplet is shown in Fig. 1. The internal droplets that usually contain the therapeutic agent are dispersed in the oil phase (primary W/O emulsification stage), which in turn is dispersed in external aqueous phase (secondary emulsification stage). To prepare multiple emulsions, two types of surfactants are used. In primary W/O emulsification stage, lipophilic surfactants are used while in secondary emulsification stage, hydrophilic surfactant is used.

A typical W/O/W double emulsion stabilised by monomeric emulsifiers will consist of inner W/O droplets of 0.5–2 μm in size and double W/O/W droplets (outer phase) of 10–60 μm (4). Because of the presence of a reservoir phase inside droplets of another phase, multiple emulsions find many applications in pharmaceutical and cosmetic fields.

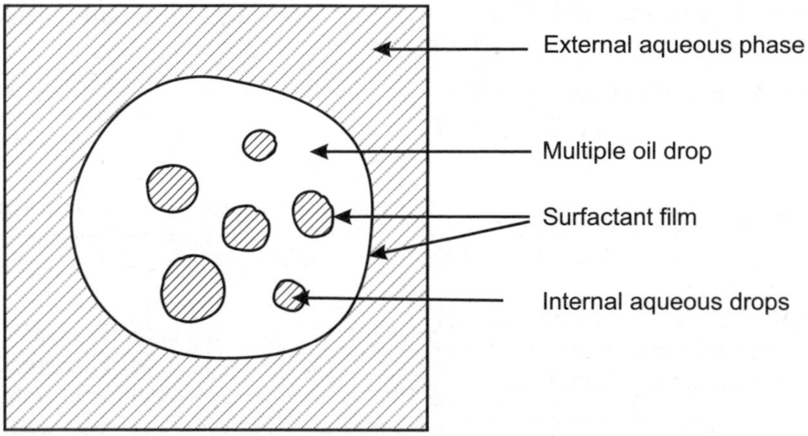

Fig. 1. Schematic representation of a W/O/W double emulsion droplet.

2. ADVANTAGES AND DRAWBACKS OF MULTIPLE EMULSIONS AS DRUG DELIVERY SYSTEM

2.1. Advantages

1. They protect bioactives from degradation.
2. They are easy to administer via oral, nasal, ocular, parenteral or any other route.
3. They offer encapsulating compartments for both hydrophilic and lipophilic compounds with very high encapsulation efficiency; the drug may be encapsulated as a solution or suspension.
4. They may be targeted by both passive and active means by surface modification.
5. The drug release pattern may be prolonged or controlled.

6. They utilise pharmaceutically acceptable components, which are non-toxic, non-immunogenic and biocompatible/biodegradable.
7. The components of formulation are economical and manufacturing equipments are easily accessible.
8. They are easy to produce and scale-up.

2.2. Drawbacks

1. They have low thermodynamic stability.
2. They are bulkier systems.
3. They have disagreeable taste in some cases *(5)*.

In practice, double emulsions are thermodynamically unstable systems with a strong tendency for coalescence, flocculation and creaming. Most double emulsions consist of relatively large droplets, cannot withstand storage regime and have a strong tendency to release the entrapped matter in an uncontrolled manner *(6,7)*.

3. THEORETICAL ASPECT OF MULTIPLE EMULSION FORMATION

In order to specify the location of formation region of multiple emulsions, one of the generalised phase diagram for a mixture of water–oil emulsifier was proposed by Florence, AT. and Whitehill, D.1982 *(8)*. The phase diagram is shown in Fig. 2.

The micellar phase of surfactant solution solubilises a small amount of oil, while a large part of oil remains immiscible with solution. This area can be specified by location for providing O/W microemulsions, when one makes disruption of the interface between two separate phases. On the other hand, a variety of hydrophilic emulsifiers dissolved in oil phase presumably as reverse micelles, solubilises a small quantity of water. A large amount of residual water remains separated from reversed micellar solution. This zone is featured by the area for preparing W/O microemulsions due to disruption of two separated phases.

Some emulsifiers can neither be dissolved in water nor in oil, but they form the continuous phase that consists of D-phase and contains a certain amount of water and/or oil among lamellar structure of D-phase. Such a phase can be provided by increasing temperature of non-ionic emulsifier or by mixing different types of emulsifiers. The region for obtaining W/O/W and O/W/O emulsions should be located very closely to either sides of D-phase.

A typical W/O/W double emulsion stabilised by monomeric emulsifiers will consist of inner W/O droplets of 0.5–2 μm in size and double W/O/W droplets (outer phase) of 10–60 μm. It was found that there is a significant correlation between the droplet size, number of compartments of inner W/O emulsion and the stability of W/O/W emulsion, with 'weighted hydrophilic–lipophilic balance (HLB) value of emulsion *(9–11)*. Simple calculations based on the required oil HLB are not relevant since migration of surfactant from inner to outer phase, and *vice versa*, takes place. The weighted HLB serves as a good approximation for evaluating best mixture of emulsifiers to be selected for the formation of optimal droplet size and maximum yield of formation of double emulsion droplets.

$$\text{Weighted HLB} = \frac{\text{HLB}_{(I)} \times \Phi_{(w/o/w)} \times C_{(I)} + \text{HLB}_{(II)} \times C_{(II)}}{\Phi_{(w/o/w)} \times C_{(I)} + C_{(II)}} \quad (1)$$

where $\text{HLB}_{(I)}$ is HLB value of hydrophobic emulsifier used for first step procedure, Φ is fraction of inner W/O emulsion in final W/O/W emulsion, $C_{(I)}$ is weight percent of hydrophobic emulsifier in starting W/O emulsion, $\text{HLB}_{(II)}$ is HLB value hydrophobic emulsifier used in second step procedure and $C_{(II)}$ is weight percent of the hydrophilic emulsifier in W/O/W emulsion.

There is a significant correlation between droplet size of W/O/W emulsion and the 'weighted HLB' value, and W/O/W emulsion may inverse into an O/W emulsion when 'weighted HLB' approaches 10 or lower values. At the correct 'weighted HLB' the droplet size can be about 5 μm.

Kita *et al.* found that the weight ratio of hydrophobic to hydrophilic emulsifiers in system should be between 2 and 20 in order to obtain best yields *(12)*. It is, therefore, common practice to use 10-fold ratios of Span 80 (sorbitan-monooleate, the hydrophobic emulsifier) over the hydrophilic non-ionic emulsifiers to obtain minimum size of double emulsion droplets with high yields.

It was also clearly demonstrated that hydrophilic emulsifier had a negative effect on the flux of water molecules from inner phase to outer dispersion phase. In addition, there is a significant influence of emulsifier concentration on the flux of water. At higher

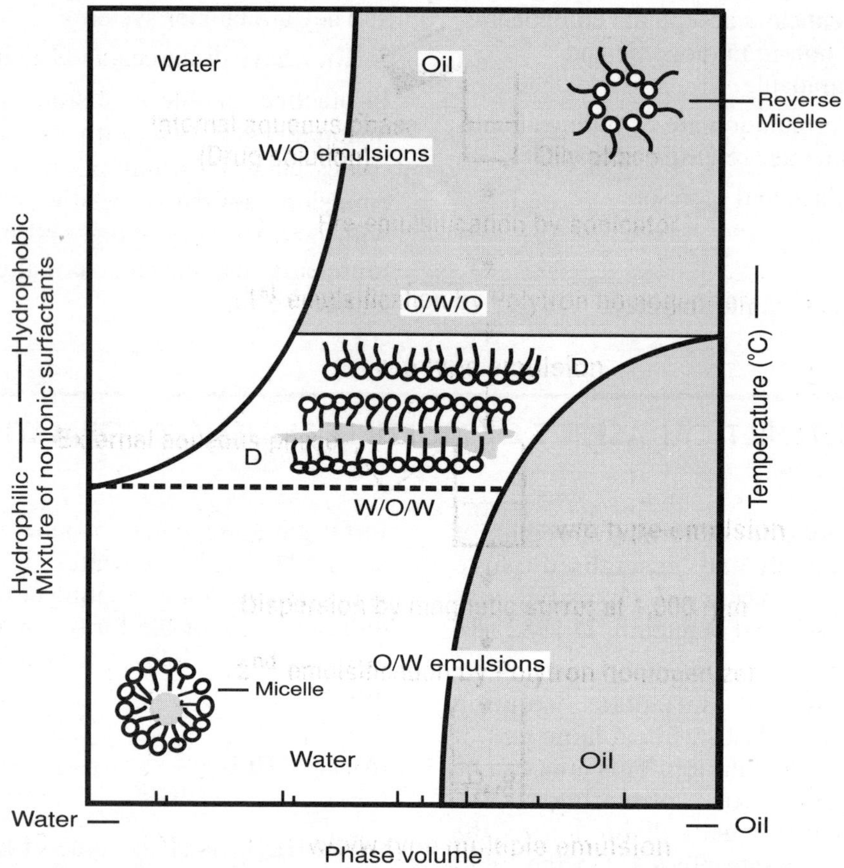

Fig. 2. Schematic phase diagram of the phase volume of oil, water and hydrophobicity of a mixture of non-ionic emulsifiers.

emulsifier concentrations more water is solubilised by the emulsifier and its transport 'in' and 'out' (controlled by osmotic pressure gradient) is enhanced. This is an additional reason to keep the concentration of hydrophilic emulsifier as low as possible. However, at concentrations lower than 0.5 g/100 g, hydrophilic emulsifier of double emulsion will invert into an O/W emulsion.

4. FORMULATION AND MANUFACTURE OF MULTIPLE EMULSIONS

A multiple phase system can be obtained by mainly four methods:

1. Two-step emulsification/double emulsification.
2. One-step emulsification/phase inversion.
3. Use of phase diagram of water–emulsifier–oil.
4. Membrane emulsification.

4.1. Double Emulsification/Two-Step Emulsification

Two-step emulsification methods involve re-emulsification of primary W/O or O/W emulsion using suitable emulsifier agent *(13)*.

1. The first step involves preparation of an ordinary W/O or O/W primary emulsion wherein an appropriate emulsifier system is utilised.
2. In second step, freshly prepared W/O or O/W primary emulsion is re-emulsified with an excess of aqueous phase or oil phase.

The primary emulsion is prepared in usual manner; i.e., with a laboratory mixer, by ultrasonication, etc. To prepare W/O/W emulsion, a lipophilic surfactant is used to promote formation of a W/O emulsion. The emulsion is poured into a solution or dispersion of secondary surfactant in water. The secondary surfactant is hydrophilic to promote O/W emulsification in which the 'oil' phase is W/O emulsion. *(11)*.

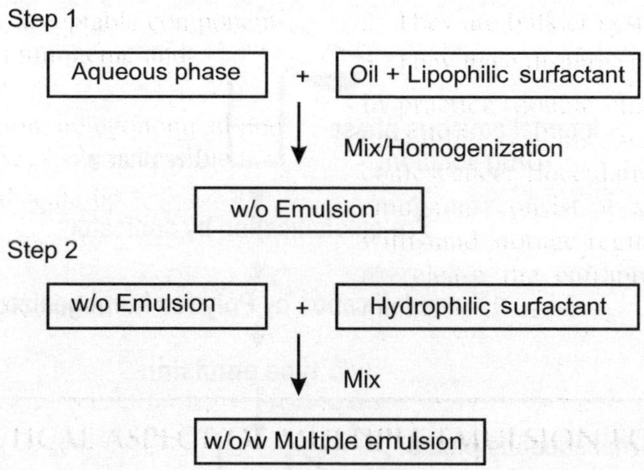

Fig. 3. Schematic representation of two-step emulsification of a W/O/W double emulsion.

The second emulsification step is crucial as it can lead to fracture of internal droplets forming simple emulsion of either W/O or O/W type depending upon number of factors. The finally prepared emulsion could be W/O/W or O/W/O, respectively. The method is schematically illustrated in Fig. 3.

In two-step emulsification, it was observed that the physicochemical characteristics of multiple emulsions are directly related to ratio of amount of Span 80 to that of a series of hydrophilic emulsifiers existing in entire system *(14)*.

A typical formulation might be as follows:

The primary emulsion (W/O) could be formed from isopropyl myristate (47.5%), sorbitan monooleate (Span 80)-lipophilic surfactant (2.5%), and distilled water upto 100%.

The multiple emulsion (W/O/W) may be prepared by adding primary (W/O) emulsion (50%) into a polyoxyethylene sorbitan monooleate (Tween-80)-hydrophilic surfactant (2% [w/v]) solution in water.

By this technique, one can set different requirements for each emulsion, such as droplet size and viscosity. The primary emulsion can be prepared by high shear equipment to get very fine size (<1 μm) while second step may be prepared by a low shear homogeniser, forming larger droplets *(15)*.

Law *et al.* prepared a stable multiple emulsion with 10% (w/w) Span-80, 0–0.5% (w/w) bovine serum albumin (BSA) as inner emulsifying agent and 2% NaCl by weight in inner aqueous phase. The outer interface was stabilised with 5% of Tween-80 by weight. Using this procedure, multiple emulsions may be prepared with high reproducibility *(16)*.

O/W/O multiple emulsion using soyabean oil as oil phase was prepared and camphor/cyclodextrin complexation was used for stability of multiple emulsion *(17)*. They stirred primary emulsion at 3000 rpm for 20 min and secondary emulsification at 2000 rpm for 1 min.

Matsumoto *et al.* prepared W/O/W multiple emulsion using Triester F-1801, viz., medium chain triglyceride (MCT) as oil phase *(10)*. The lipophilic and hydrophilic surfactants used were hexaglyceryl-condensed (poly)ricinolate (Hexaglyn PR-15; HLB-3.2) and polyoxyethylene hydrogenated castor oil-60 (HCO-60, HLB-14.0), respectively.

A W/O/W multiple emulsion was prepared composed of MCTs containing insulin with aprotinin, a protease inhibitor, and/or sodium taurocholate, an absorption enhancer, by a two-step emulsification method at 15°C *(18)*.

A modified two-step emulsification technique for preparation of W/O/W emulsion was reported (Fig. 4). This method is different from the conventional two-step technique in two points. Firstly, sonication and stirring are used to obtain fine, homogeneous and stable W/O emulsion. Secondly, a continuous phase is poured into a dispersed phase for preparing W/O/W emulsion (in contrast to conventional method in which a dispersed phase is poured into a continuous phase). Moreover, the ratio of internal aqueous phase to oil phase (external phase) is fixed at 1:45, which produces most stable formulation.

Okochi and Nakano prepared W/O/W multiple emulsions of vancomycin (VCM) using lipiodol as oil phase *(19)*. They used 5% HCO-40 as emulsifier in oil phase and Pluronic F-68 emulsifier in external phase. They prepared stable W/O/W emulsions with a particle size of about 3 μm and an entrapment efficiency of VCM of about 70% and showed that when this emulsion was administered intravenously to rats, plasma concentrations of VCM were prolonged compared to VCM solution alone.

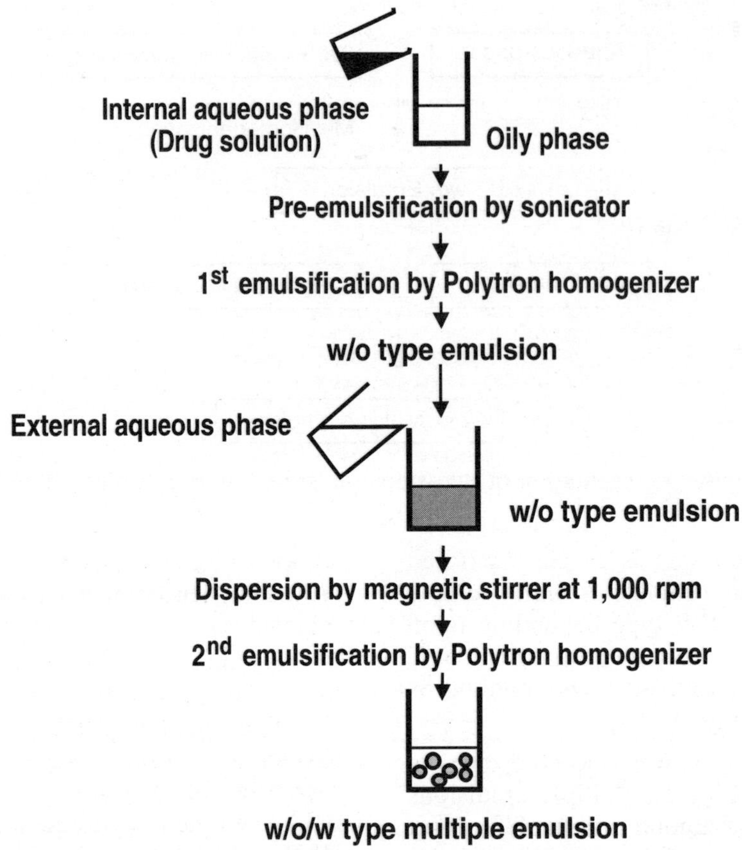

Fig. 4. A modified two-step emulsification technique for preparation of W/O/W emulsion. (Reprinted from Adv. Drug Deliv Rev, 45(1), Okochi, H., Nokano, M., Preparation and evaluation of W/O/W type emulsion containing vancomycin, 5–26, 2000, with permission from Elsevier) *(19)*.

W/O/W multiple emulsion using semi-crystalline oil phase was prepared by Weiss *et al.* using 5% gelatin as additive in inner aqueous phase and 2–8% polyglycerol polyricinoleate (PGPR), a lipophilic surfactant and 1% whey protein isolate (WPI) as hydrophilic surfactants *(20)*.

W/O/W multiple emulsions of chlorhexidine digluconate and benzalkonium chloride was prepared for local vaginal therapy. Abil EM 90® (cetyl dimethicone copolyol) was used as the lipophilic surfactant, Synperonic PE/F127® (ethylene and propylene oxide copolymer) was used as hydrophilic surfactant which was introduced in external aqueous phase. Sodium chloride was used as swelling–breakdown marker *(21)*. Preparation of a stable multiple emulsion using Pluronic (Poloxamer) and polyacrylic acid complexes was also reported by Cole and Whateley *(22)*.

Sugiura *et al.* described a micro-channel (MC) emulsification as a novel two-step technique for preparing monodispersed emulsions using triolein as oil phase *(23)*. The mild action of droplet formation based on spontaneous transformation led to a high entrapment yield during MC emulsification.

4.2. Phase Inversion Technique/One-Step emulsification Technique

Spontaneous formation of multiple emulsions was first reported during phase inversion of a simple emulsion *(24)*. When aqueous solution of hydrophilic emulsifier is introduced into oil containing lipophilic surfactant, W/O/W emulsion is obtained due to phase inversion of W/O emulsion, which occurs due to migration of the emulsifier between phases *(25)*.

The phase inversion of emulsion also occurs when the concentration of dispersed globules in dispersion medium is quite high, i.e., globules are packed very closely in suspending fluid.

It is possible to obtain multiple emulsions by this technique using an emulsifier with a HLB value that does not favour a certain type of emulsion, for example, sorbitan monopalmitate *(26)* or concentrated O/W emulsion is thermally induced to produce W/O/W emulsion, mainly with ethoxylated emulsifiers, near their phase inversion temperature *(27)*.

Gohla *et al.* proposed a new one-step procedure to produce a stable W/O/W emulsion *(28)*. The process involves a partial solubilisation—inversion technology based on controlled salting out of hydrophilic emulsifier during droplet formation. Phase inversion technique can be exploited to produce emulsions characterised by their fine droplet size.

Devani *et al.* described the formation of multiple emulsion droplets from two oil systems (Labrafil M 1944 CS and Labrafac Lipophile WL 1349) via a one-step process involving minimal agitation in aqueous media and investigated it in terms of multiple character of droplets, particle size distribution, stability and lipolysis profile in presence of pancreatic lipase *(29)*.

4.3. Use of Phase Diagrams of Water–Emulsifier–Oil

It has been shown that multiple emulsions can be produced with use of only one surfactant to stabilise both primary and secondary emulsion. But the incorporation of liquid crystalline mesophase in external phase of either primary or secondary emulsion is important. This is evident in three-phase region for such system where an aqueous micellar solution of emulsifier and oil rich solution of emulsifier are in equilibrium with each other with a mesomorphous phase. The presence of a liquid crystalline phase in ternary system consisting of water emulsifier oil has been shown to greatly improve the stability of emulsion.

Phase diagram was prepared by Kim *et al.* to identify the range of heat-denatured WPI (HD-WPI) and pectin concentrations where phase separation occurred *(30)*. Under certain conditions, the biopolymers formed a two-phase system consisting of a HD-WPI-enriched lower phase (W_1) and a pectin-enriched upper phase (W_2), which was attributed to thermodynamic incompatibility to two biopolymers. Water-in-water emulsions (W_1/W_2 or W_2/W_1) could be formed by blending incompatible upper and lower phases together at different ratios. Then they showed that whey protein stabilised oil droplets preferentialy partition into HD-WPI rich phase of two-phase biopolymer systems. This enabled them to prepare multiple emulsions by mixing a whey protein stabilised O/W emulsion with incompatible upper and lower phases. These multiple emulsions were either of oil-in-water-in-water ($O/W_1/W_2$) type or the mixed oil-in-water/water-in-water (O/W_1–W_2/W_1) type depending on initial biopolymer composition of system.

4.4. Membrane Emulsification Technique

Recently, a membrane emulsification technique has been developed as a novel emulsification method. In this method, a W/O emulsion (a dispersed phase) is extruded into an external aqueous phase (a continuous phase) with a constant pressure through a porous glass membrane. The particle size of resulting emulsion can be controlled with proper selection of porous glass membrane as droplet size depends upon the pore size of membrane.

Multiple W/O/W emulsions for drug delivery systems were produced by extruding a coarse W/O/W emulsion five times under pressure of 70–150 kPa through Shirasu porous glass (SPG) (SPG Technology, Miyazaki, Japan) membrane with a mean pore size of 5.4, 7.6, 10.7, 14.8 and 20.3 μm *(31)*.

Scherze *et al.* reported that membrane emulsification resulted in multiple emulsions with a yield of the W_1-phase close to 100% and in a tailored particle size range *(32)*.

4.5. Parameters Affecting Multiple Emulsion Preparation

4.5.1. Composition

Nature of oil is of great importance since it controls the permeability of liquid membrane, which in turn controls release of solute across it. The stability of oily layer against leakage of entrapped material depends upon nature of oil. Besides the concentration of oil phase, physiochemical characteristics of oil used such as density and viscosity influence the behaviour of system. Refined hydrocarbon oils such as mineral oil and squalene have been used extensively. Esters of long chain fatty acids including isopropyl myristate or oleate and vegetable oils such as peanut oil, olive oil, sesame oil, maize/corn oil, jojoba oil and arachis oil have also been used to vary the physiochemical properties of multiple emulsions *(3)*.

The yield of multiple emulsion droplets depends upon nature of oil. Optimal stabilities of multiple emulsions can be obtained when there is a similarity between hydrophobic part of emulsifier and oil phase. This suggests that stability of multiple emulsions depends on adsorption of emulsifiers at oil–water interface and on the properties of adsorbed layer. The nature of oil phase affects the nature of interfacial film and together these are of crucial importance in determining globule size and stability *(13)*.

Benichou *et al.* concluded that the differentiation between two types of oils, O_1 (inner) and O_2 (outer), in O/W/O emulsions enabled high entrapment capacity of drug in inner oil phase. In addition, when inner oil phase (O_1) was a 1:1 (w/w) mixture of MCT/triacetin and external oil phase (O_2) was silicone oil, it was possible to slow the release of entrapped matter while the solubility of inner phase in external oil phase remained constant *(33)*.

4.5.2. Surfactants

Formation of multiple emulsions requires at least two surfactants of different nature, i.e., one hydrophilic and other lipophilic as primary and secondary surfactants depending on the type of emulsion (O/W/O or W/O/W) required. In a W/O/W emulsion, the optimal HLB value of primary surfactant is usually in range of 2–7 while it is 6–16 for secondary surfactant. The concentration of secondary emulsifier is generally less than 1/5th of primary emulsifier. It is beneficial to use hydrophobic emulsifier in excess, i.e., about 10–30% (w/w) of oil phase or primary emulsion whereas hydrophilic emulsifier is used in low concentration, i.e., about 0.5–5% (w/w) of external phase.

Non-ionic surfactants are reported to give better yields of multiple drops than ionic surfactants. Also, non-ionic emulsifiers are preferred because of their lower toxicity and also they are less to likely to interact with other compounds *(7)*. Examples include sorbitan esters, polysorbates, Cetearth 12, and poly oxyethylene (POE) docosyl ethers. A correlation between oil–water interfacial tension and emulsifier has been reported.

The concentration and type of emulsifier is reported to be optimised on basis of concentration v/s. interfacial relationship for various emulsifiers. Two types of curves are generally observed. The suitable surfactant is shown by a steep lowering curve with a sharp break at its optimum concentration. Other surfactants show relatively flat curve without a sharp break but with a slow change. There will be an optimal concentration of surfactant required to stabilise system; low concentrations may not be sufficient to stabilise emulsion and may result in rapid degradation of emulsion. High concentration may serve to increase viscosity of system but may be objectionable from the point of view of toxicity.

The lipophilic surfactant should be at least 10 times greater than the hydrophilic surfactant to obtain a yield of more than 90% *(9)*.

Florence and Whitehill *(28)* observed that the nature of multiple emulsion depends on surfactant used to prepare secondary emulsion in case of isopropyl myristate and Span 80 based primary emulsions.

- Type A droplets contained one large internal droplet when Brij 30 (2%) was used.
- Type B droplets contained several small internal droplets when 2% Triton X-165 was used.
- Type C droplets entrapped large number of small internal droplets and were prepared using Span 80:Tween-80 (3:1) mixture.

In another study, they further reported that the character of each multiple emulsion was significantly different.

1. Type A—composed of small multiple emulsion drops (mean diameter 8.6 μm) 82% of this contained only one internal aqueous droplet (mean diameter 3.3 μm).
2. Type B—composed of large multiple drops (mean diameter 19 μm) containing smaller, but more numerous internal aqueous droplets (mean diameter 2.2 μm).
3. Type C—composed of very large multiple drops (mean diameter 25 μm), which contained very large numbers of internal droplets, which were difficult to resolve.

They suggested that the concentrations of more than 30% by weight of Span 80 in oil phase are required to obtain yields of more than 90% of multiple drops. They also found out that yields of primary emulsion fell markedly when concentration of secondary emulsifier in external phase was increased. This is thought to be due to solubilisation of molecules of primary (lipophilic) surfactant in outer aqueous phase when the concentration of secondary (hydrophilic) surfactant exceeds critical micellar concentration. As concentration of secondary surfactant increases, more of the primary surfactant may be incorporated into secondary surfactant micelles, reducing the concentration of primary surfactant in oil phase able to stabilise W/O system. This would lead, if the primary surfactant at the interface falls, to rupture of oil layer resulting in loss of internal aqueous drops.

Ohwaki *et al.* studied influence of addition of hydrophilic surfactants into the internal aqueous compartment of emulsion, on breakdown of suspending vesicular globules of W/O/W *(34)*. Only addition of hydrophilic surfactant into internal aqueous compartments was demonstrated to inhibit both coalescence of internal aqueous compartments and influx of water to internal aqueous compartment from the external aqueous phase.

The structure of multiple drops probably depends on efficiency of second emulsification step.

Vasiljevic reported that the concentration of lipophilic primary emulsifier markedly affected rheological behaviour as well as droplet size and *in vitro* drug release kinetics of investigated systems *(35)*. The multiple emulsion systems with highest concentration (2.4% [w/w]) of the primary emulsifier had lowest droplet size, highest apparent viscosity and highest elastic characteristics.

4.5.3. Phase Volume

Over a range of low volume fractions, the secondary phase volume influences yield of multiple emulsions. The multiple emulsions can be prepared using internal phase volume W/O in an optimal range 25–50% and phase volume ratio of as large as 70–90% can produce a stable multiple emulsion. The order of addition of phases becomes important for required type of multiple emulsions. Internal phase volume influences the stability and release of solute from multiple emulsions. Usually slow addition of dispersed phase into continuous phase during emulsification is always advantageous and beneficial to multiple emulsion preparation.

It was suggested that internal phase volume influenced the release of material from internal aqueous phase and that the secondary phase volume influences the yield of multiple drops over a range of low volume fractions *(36)*.

4.5.4. Shear/Agitation

The choice of modes of emulsification is very important because multiple emulsions systems are rather fragile systems. The high shear disrupts large percentage of multiple drops and thus results in instability of system. Therefore, the yield of system falls rapidly as homogenisation time is decreased.

Pin mixers and micro-vortex stirrers are usually preferred to high shear producing Ultra-Turrax and ultrasonication. Ultra-Turrax causes incorporation of air and excessive frothing resulting in loss of surfactant at air–water interface. Thus, shear combined with air bubbles may lead to instability. Even if formation of high yield emulsion is achieved, the use of high energy like sonication leads to complete loss of multiple drops on storage. The rule of thumb is that high agitation speed for primary and lower speed for secondary emulsification are necessary for manufacture of multiple emulsions. The minimum requirements seem to be 800 rpm for primary and 200 rpm for secondary emulsification, below which the multiple emulsions will tend to coalesce or cream.

4.5.5. Temperature

Temperature plays a significant role in emulsion formation. It is advised to dissolve surfactant in respective phases completely, with aid of heat, only if required. The hydrophilic emulsifier becomes more lipophilic as it tends to precipitate upon increasing temperature from its solution (cloud point). Therefore temperature must be precisely controlled during preparation of primary emulsion.

5. CHARACTERISATION OF MULTIPLE EMULSIONS

For multiple emulsions, there is at present no general agreement on design of evaluation tests. Various tests employed differ from laboratory to laboratory. The important ones are discussed below:

5.1. Macroscopic Examination

Colour, consistency and homogeneity are first investigated subjectively in order to ensure formation of an emulsion. The idea of type (W/O/W or O/W/O) is obtained by dilution with external phase.

Yield: The estimation of yield is based on the quantitative measurement of release of marker compounds such as electrolytes (NaCl or ephedrine HCl) *(37–38)*, water-soluble additives (glucose) using fluorescent probes, specific electrodes *(40)*, micro-analysis *(10)*, electrical conductivity *(37,39,41)* or fluorescent measurements *(37–39)*.

The yield is given by:

$$Y = (M_{in}/M_{in} + M_{out}) \times 100 \quad (2)$$

where M_{in} and M_{out} are the amounts of marker in internal and external phases, respectively.

The determination of release of marker could be studied directly or by dialysis or after filtration.

The yield of multiple droplets in emulsions made from mineral oils (liquid paraffin and squalane) and vegetable oils (sesame oil, maize oil and arachis oil) has been followed using a tracer method based on 6-carboxyfluorescein *(39)*.

The W/O/W emulsion entrapment yield was measured fluorometrically and found to be 91% by Sugiura *et al.* *(23)*. Nuclear magnetic resonance (NMR) technique has also been suggested as a direct technique for measuring yield *(42)*.

5.2. Microscopic Examination

The multiplicity of multiple emulsions is verified by light microscopy and/or electron microscopic technique. The optical microscopy method using calibrated ocular and stage micrometer can be utilised for globule size determinations of both multiple emulsion droplets as well as droplets of internal dispersed phase. Freeze-etching electron microscopy has also been reported for studying both internal and external droplet size distribution *(43)*.

Three types of multiple emulsions are classified based on size, namely:

1. Coarse multiple emulsions of >3 μm diameter.
2. Fine multiple emulsions of about 1–3 μm diameter.
3. Micro-multiple emulsions with <1 μm diameter.

Very small multiple emulsion diameters are measured using Laser diffraction Granulometer or Coulter-counter (Beckman, UK) and their multiple nature is proved by calculating yield using a suitable marker. The droplet size distribution of freshly made emulsion can be measured by light scattering using a Malvern Mastersizer and surface mean droplet diameter and the specific surface area can also be derived. The number of globules per unit volume can also be measured using Haemocytometer cell *(44)*.

Eads *et al.* demonstrated increased resolution in proton (^{1}H) magic angle spinning (MAS) NMR spectra of emulsions *(42)*. Relative volumes of internal and external water phases of W/O/W type multiple emulsions were estimated by integration of water resonances separated by use of a shift reagent, while broadening due to magnetic susceptibility mismatch among phases was removed by magic angle sample spinning. Internal water may also be uniquely detected in Carr-Purcell-Meiboom-Gill (CPMG) spin-echo spectrum of a sample containing added $MnCl_2$ as a relaxation reagent.

Scherze *et al.* measured particle size distribution by laser diffraction microscopy and developed image processing automated image analysis of $W_1/O/W_2$ emulsions for visualising oil droplet size as well as distribution of inner aqueous W_1-phase *(32)*.

5.3. Entrapment Efficiency

Entrapment efficiency of drug or active moiety in multiple emulsions is generally determined using dialysis, centrifugation, filtration or conductivity measurements. However, recently an internal marker was used to evaluate entrapment of an impermeable marker molecule contained in inner phase of W/O/W emulsion. The unentrapped marker is calculated and the amount entrapped can be thus calculated by deducting unentrapped amount from initially added amount *(45)*. The entrapment (%) can be calculated using the following equation:

$$C = \frac{100}{\left[1 - n_1 V^* / (n_0 - n_1) V_1\right]} \tag{3}$$

$$V^* = \frac{V_d (V_1 + V_2 + V_0)}{V_2} + V_s \tag{4}$$

where, n_0 is initial concentration of drug in inner aqueous phase, n_1 is concentration of drug in dialysate, V_1, V_2 and V_0 represents drug volume of inner, middle and outer phase respectively, and V_s and V_d represent volume of dialysing media and dialysed emulsion, respectively, V^* is a constant.

The encapsulation efficiency of a marker ($CaNa_2$-EDTA) was determined by inductively coupled plasma emission spectrophotometer by Vladisavljević *et al. (31)*.

5.4. ζ-Potential

The ζ-potential measurements are pivotal in designing of surface modified or ligand anchored multiple emulsions systems. The ζ-potential and surface charge can be calculated using Smouchowski's equation from mobility and electrophoretic velocity of dispersed globules using the ζ-potentiometer. A cylindrically bored micro-electrophoresis cell equipped with platinum–iridium electrodes was used to measure electrophoretic mobility of diluted W/O/W emulsion and ζ-potential was calculated *(46)*.

$$\zeta = \frac{4\pi\eta\mu}{\varepsilon \cdot E} \times 10^3 \tag{5}$$

where, ζ is zeta potential (mv), η is viscosity of dispersion medium (poise), μ is migration velocity (cm/s), ε is dielectric constant of dispersion medium and E is potential gradient (voltage applied/distance between globules).

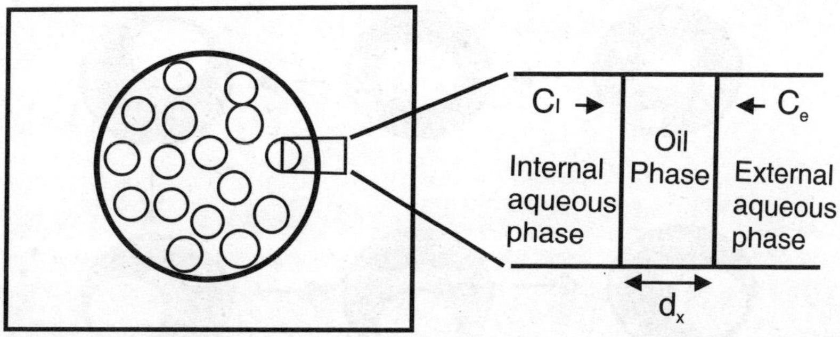

Fig. 5. Two-dimensional model for diffusion controlled transport of unionised materials. From the external aqueous phase to internal aqueous droplets in a W/O/W system. (Reprinted from J. Colloid Int. Sci., 144, Zheng, S., Beissinger, R.L., and Wasan, D.T. The stabilization of hemoglobin multiple emulsion for use as a red blood cell substitute, 72–85, 1991, with permission from Elsevier) *(15)*.

5.5. Rheological Analysis

The viscosity of multiple emulsions can be measured by Brookfield rotational viscometer (Brookfield Engineering Laboratory, USA) or a rheometer. Oil phase viscosity can be determined by stress viscometry using a Bohlin controlled rheometer.

Interfacial film strength can be evaluated by interfacial rheology measurements, using a tensiometer, i.e., elasticity of (W/O) and (O/W) components of (W/O/W) multiple emulsions and these data may relate to emulsion stability. Interfacial rheology (i.e., interfacial elasticity at oil–aqueous interface) can be investigated at mineral O/W interface using an oscillatory surface rheometer.

5.6. Drug Release Mechanisms and Models

There are several possible mechanisms by which the active compound may be transferred across the oil layer in a W/O/W system. Some of the mechanisms include:

- Diffusion of unionised drug (hydrophobic species) through oil layer.
- Carrier mediated transport.
- Micellar transport.
- Rupture of oil membrane.
- Thinning of oil membrane.

5.6.1. Diffusion Rate Model (Diffusion of Unionised Drug Through Oil Layer)

The most obvious release mechanism is by diffusion of unionised drug (hydrophobic species) through oil layer (semi-permeable liquid membrane), especially in stable multiple emulsion system *(15)*. Hence, the drug transport *in vitro* has been found to follow first order kinetics and obeyed Fick's law (Fig. 5).

$$\frac{\mathrm{d}C_o}{\mathrm{d}t} = \frac{-DA\Delta C}{\mathrm{d}x} = \frac{-DA}{\mathrm{d}x} \times (C_o - C_i) \qquad (6)$$

Because $C_e = C_o/P$

$$\frac{\mathrm{d}C_e}{\mathrm{d}t} = \frac{P(\mathrm{d}t)}{\mathrm{d}x} = \frac{-DA}{P\mathrm{d}x} \times \mathrm{P}(C_o - C_i) \qquad (7)$$

where, C_o is the concentration of drug in oil phase, C_i is concentration of drug in internal aqueous phase, C_e is concentration of drug in external aqueous phase, D is diffusion coefficient of drug in oil phase, dx is diffusion layer thickness, P is partition coefficient of drug between oil and external phase and t is time.

When a trapping agent is used in internal aqueous phase, the material becomes ionised and C_i turns to be negligible; equation can be written as

$$\frac{\mathrm{d}C_e}{\mathrm{d}t} = \frac{-DAC_e}{\mathrm{d}x} = -\mathrm{K}C_e \qquad (8)$$

The rate constant K is a function of diffusion coefficient of drug, the area between external phase and liquid membrane and membrane thickness.

Both water soluble and ionisable compounds can migrate through the oil membrane.

5.6.2. Planar-Sheet Model

The uniform planar-sheet model of multiple emulsion droplets for release mechanism was also suggested *(47)*. The model is schematically represented in Fig. 6. It is generally based on assumption that the thickness of oil phase is negligible compared to the droplet average radius (r). The area for mass transfer can be considered to be constant and a uniform planar

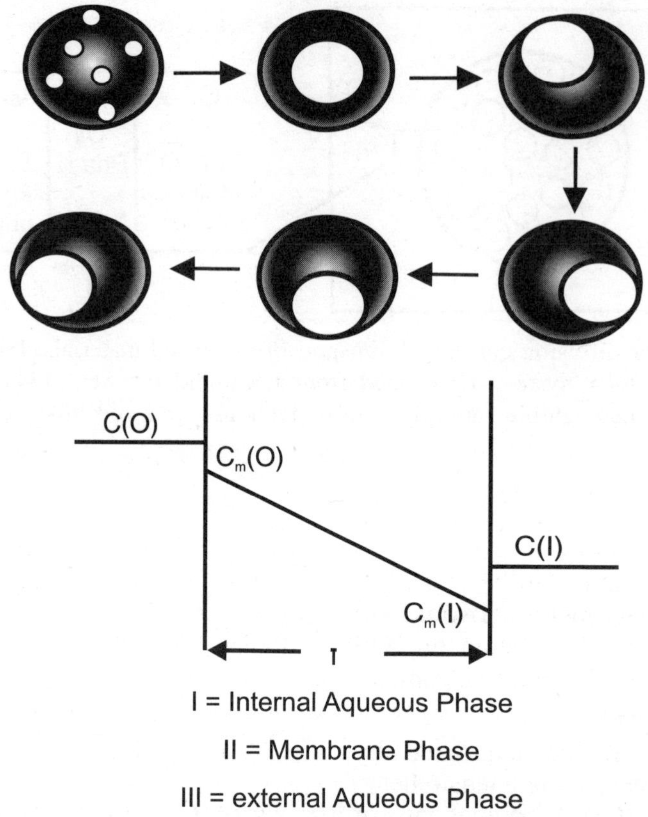

Fig. 6. Uniform planer-sheet model of multiple emulsion droplets. (Reprinted from J. Control Release, 45, Jager-Lezer, N., Terrisse, I., Bruneou, F., Tokgoz, S., Ferreira, L., Clausse, D., Seiller, M., and Grossiord, J.L. Influence of lipophilic surfactant on the release kinetics of water soluble molecules entraped in a W/O/W multiple emulsion, 1–13, 1997, with permission from Elsevier) *(47)*.

membrane of thickness (*L*). The equation governing the release from a slab with a non-constant source has the form:

$$M_t = \frac{M_{\text{infinite}}\left\{V_2 \exp\left[-ADK\left(V_1+V_2\right)t / LV_1 \cdot V_2\right]+V_1\right\}}{V_1+V_2} \quad (9)$$

where, M_t is the amount of drug in internal drops at time (*t*), M_{infinite} is initial amount of drug, *A* is surface area of multiple drops, *K* is partition-coefficient of solute in oil phase, *L* is thickness of oil layer, V_1 is internal volume, V_2 is sink solution volume and *D* is diffusion coefficient.

Suppose $V_2 >> V_1$, then, equation simplifies to

$$M_t = M_{\text{infinite}} \exp\left(-ADKt/L \cdot V_1\right) \quad (10)$$

The permeability coefficient (*P*) is given by $P = DK/L$ and substituting (*P*) in previous equation.

$$\text{Log } M_t = -\left(APt/2.303\ V_1\right) + \log M_{\text{infinite}} \quad (11)$$

This equation is first order expression and permits the evaluation of *P* from plots of log M_t against *t*.

5.6.3. Swelling–Breakdown Phenomenon

This model is based on process wherein the drug release is caused by water flow from external aqueous phase to internal aqueous phase, which leads to progressive swelling and finally breakdown of internal phase globules.

This is dependent on concentration of lipophilic surfactant, which increases swelling of oil globules and delays the release *(48)*.

5.6.4. Micelle Formation Model/Oil Thinning or Rupture Model

Kita *et al.* suggested two possible mechanisms forpermeation of water and water soluble materials through oil phases in W/O/W emulsions *(48)*.

They are micelle formation model and oil rupture model. The presence of both lipophilic and hydrophilic

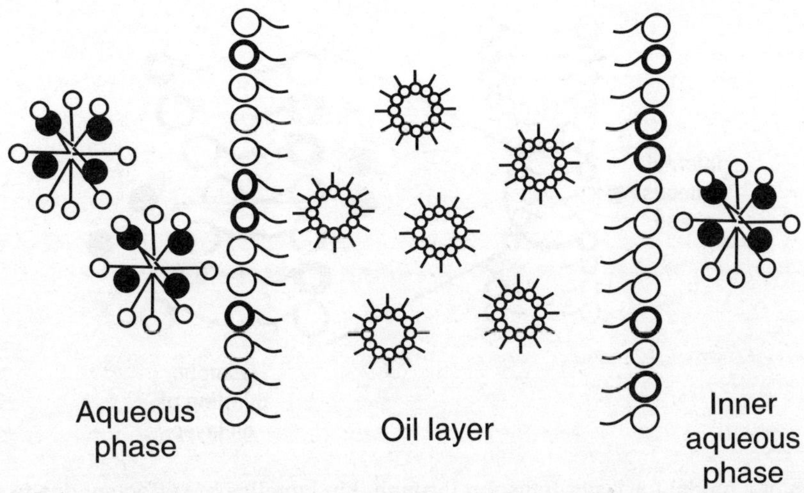

Fig. 7. Schematic illustration of a model for micellar transport of water from outer aqueous phase to inner aqueous phase through the oil layer in W/O/W emulsions. (Reprinted from J. colloid Int. Sci., 62, Kita, Y., Matsumoto, S., and Yonezawo, D. Viscometric method for estimating the stablity of W/O/W type multiple-phase emulsions, 87–94, 1977, with permission from Elsevier) *(48)*.

surfactants in oil phase facilitates the formation of water swollen inverse micelles, which may act as a mobile carrier for both ionised and unionised drugs (Fig. 7).

Electrolytes are mainly transported through a reverse micellar mechanism, controlled by viscosity and nature of oil membrane.

A modified diffusion controlled equation was used to calculate the release factor *B*

$$B = 3/2\,[1 - (1 - F)^{2/3}] - F \qquad (12)$$

or

$$B = 3D_e t/r_o 2C_o \qquad (13)$$

where *F* is the release fraction of soluble marker in inner phase, D_e is effective diffusion coefficient, r_o is radius of droplet, 't' is time of release and C_o is initial concentration of marker.

Osmotic pressure gradient between two aqueous phases may also act as a driving force for migration of drug and water (Fig. 8) *(49)*.

Release rates of methotrexate loaded multiple emulsions were found to be via diffusion from inverse micelles and were increased by surfactants with high HLB values *(50)*.

Avendano-Gomez *et al.* reported that the mechanism of mass transfer of tetradecane through aqueous membrane of $O_1/W/O_2$ emulsion is a solution-diffusion enhanced by micelles of surfactant Tween-20 *(51)*. The model of mass transfer confirms that osmotic pressure difference controls the kinetics of tetradecane transfer.

Another possibility is that water molecules may diffuse across thin lamellae of surfactants formed where the oil layer is very thin.

It was also suggested that the drug release could be due to rupture of oil membrane as illustrated in Fig. 9 and this will lead to release of drug in external aqueous medium *(52)*.

The drug released by rupture is transported through the cellulose membrane into the acceptor phase according to Fick's law:

$$V_3 dC_3/dt = D{\cdot}S\,(C_2 - C_3)/h \qquad (14)$$

where *D, S* and *h* are diffusion coefficient, effective cross sectional area and thickness respectively, while C_2, C_3 and V_3 are the concentrations in the outer and inner aqueous phases and volume of acceptor phases respectively *(53)*.

Hino *et al.* reported that the release of theophylline from W/O/W emulsions was satisfactorily explained by oil membrane rupture model *(54)*.

The mechanism of release of two fluorescent markers, fluorescein isothiocyanate–BSA (FITC– BSA) and fluorescein, from W/O/W emulsions was investigated using a rapid and sensitive method based on fluorescence-activated cell sorting (FACS). The release of FITC–BSA from a W/O/W emulsion was controlled by diffusion rather than by simple breakdown of multiple droplets or by formation of reverse micelles in oil phase. In contrast, the release of fluorescein from a double emulsion was controlled by formation of reverse micelles rather than by diffusion or simple breakdown of multiple droplets *(55)*.

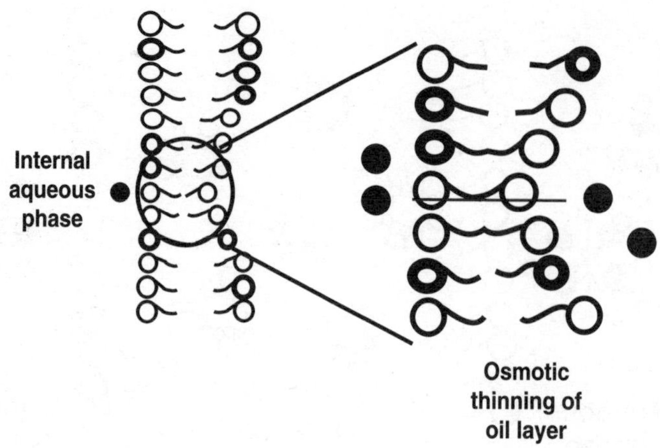

Fig. 8. Schematic illustration of a model for water transport through thin lamellae of surfactant due to fluctuation in the thickness of oil layer.

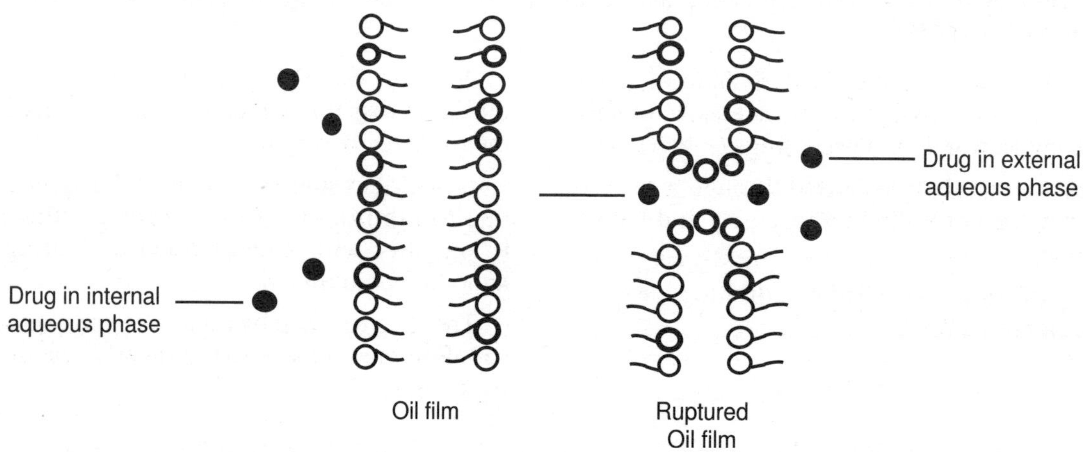

Fig. 9. Schematic illustration of a model for release of drug on rupturing of oil layer.

Silicone based surfactants were used as stabilisers for W/O/W double emulsions with unusual mechanical stability. W/O/W multiple emulsions containing several markers were prepared. The entrapped markers were: (1) halide salts, (2) a typical drug, ephedrine hydrochloride, and (3) KNO_3 (water-soluble fertiliser) *(56)*. They concluded that the release seems to be composed of three separate stages: lag time, fast release and "no release". The release mechanism seems to comply, in part, with a transport mechanism involving "reverse micelles" and is also dependent on hydrophobicity of marker. The more hydrophobic markers (drug and iodide) seem to be released also by "direct diffusion of molecule through oil" in addition to their release through reverse micelles.

5.6.5. Carrier Oriented Transport

Another possible transport mechanism, which possibly operates for release of drug, is carrier-oriented transport (Fig. 10). This involves either incorporation of some material into internal aqueous phase of membrane phase, which reacts with permeating compound to render it liposoluble. The carrier compounds effectively pump permeating compound across the membrane, for example, stearic acid facilitated diffusion of Cu^{2+} ions *(7)*.

The mechanism is especially effective for transport of highly hydrophilic compounds, which explains rapid partitioning of lipophilic molecules into oil phase and subsequently into external medium.

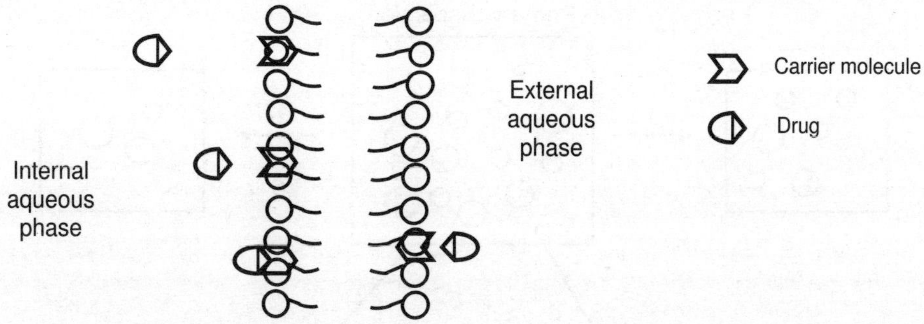

Fig. 10. Schematic illustration of a model for carrier oriented transport.

The last and probably much less important transport mechanism is solubilisation of small amounts of internal phase in membrane phase resulting into generation of diffusive passages of very small quantities of materials.

The release kinetics of molecules across the liquid membrane system are affected by various factors such as:

- Internal and multiple droplet size.
- pH of internal and external aqueous phases.
- Phase volume ratios ($\Phi_{W/O}$ and $\Phi_{W/O/W}$).
- Viscosity.
- Nature of entrapped material.
- Nature and concentration of primary and secondary emulsifiers *(7)*.

Most commonly, drug release from multiple emulsions can be measured by dialysis technique using cellophane tubing. The drug coming out of inner aqueous phase to outer aqueous phase through the intermediary liquid membrane (oil phase) will pass through dialysis tube. Drug released are thus separated and estimated by suitable analytical technique.

Avendano *et al. (52)* characterised and measured time-dependent changes within emulsion. In particular, interest was focused to quantify the concentration changes in internal and external phases of $O_1/W/O_2$ multiple emulsion. In order to accomplish the objective, the measurement and analysis was carried out by differential scanning calorimeter based on crystallisation behaviour of emulsion.

6. STABILITY OF MULTIPLE EMULSIONS

Multiple emulsions are thermodynamically unstable and their stability depends upon equilibrium between water, oil and surfactant. Mechanisms of instability are complex and may include *(6)*:

1. Coalescence of internal droplets and/or leakage of contents from inner aqueous phase.
2. Coalescence of multiple emulsion droplets.
3. Rupture of oil layer on surface of internal droplets, i.e., expulsion of internal droplet in external phase.
4. Shrinkage and swelling of internal drops due to osmotic gradient across oil membrane.
5. Phase separation.

Some of the breakdown pathways that may be involved in W/O/W destabilisation are summarised in Fig. 11.

1. Some breakdown pathways involve rupture of oil layer and consequent loss of internal aqueous drop. This results when the concentration of the primary emulsifier is depleted via transfer through oil layer to aqueous compartment.
2. Emulsifier migration is responsible for a decrease in effective HLB of second emulsifier, i.e., an increase in optimal HLB is proportional to the concentration of primary emulsifier. At a fixed concentration of primary emulsifier, the HLB shift is inversely proportional to the concentration of secondary emulsifier.

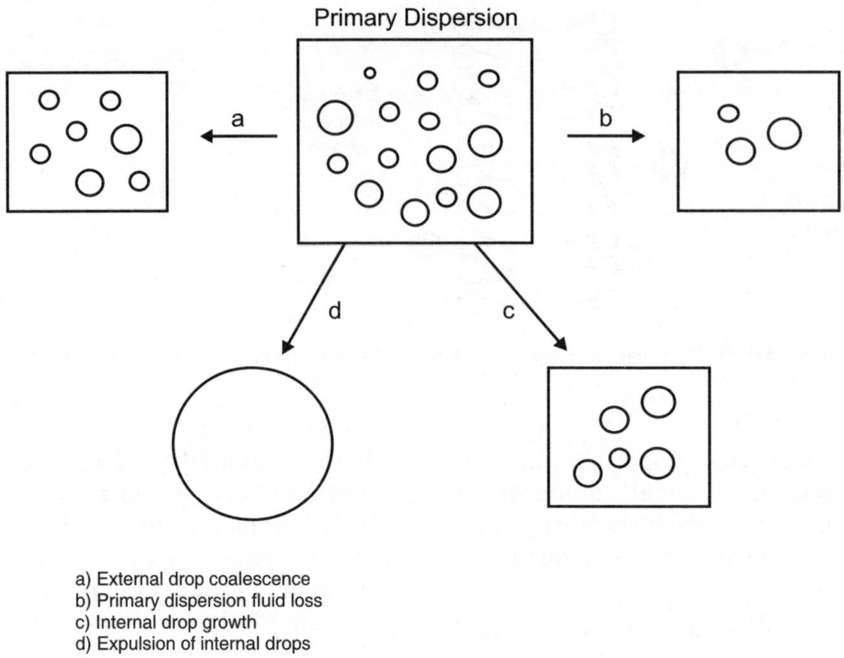

Fig. 11. Breakdown pathways that occur in a W/O/W emulsion.

3. Inversion of W/O/W emulsions to O/W emulsion occurs if HLB of total emulsifiers approaches the required HLB of oil or if droplet size, as a result of increasing secondary emulsifier concentration, becomes too small to obtain desired internal droplet size.
4. Coalescence of multiple drops produces a large decrease in oil/water interfacial area, whereas coalescence of small internal droplets would not contribute significantly to breakdown pathways.
5. The reduction in diameter of a multiple emulsion droplet as a result of expulsion of internal droplet by rupture of oil membrane leads to a significant diminution of the van der Waals forces of attraction between multiple emulsion droplets.

A photodensitometric method to follow breakdown of multiple emulsions has been suggested. The method is based on the change in optical density of multiple emulsion due to it's breakdown. A cinemicrography technique to evaluate water transfer rates from single drops in a W/O/W system is reported. The lives of single drops in an osmotic gradient were recorded on film so that changes in drop size could be measured by frame to frame on a film analyser.

6.1. Factors Affecting Stability of Multiple Emulsions

Influence of ripening and interfacial interaction on W/O/W emulsion was studied by Rosano *et al. (57).* They described three possible factors influencing the stability of $W_1/O/W_2$:

1. Laplace and osmotic effects between two aqueous phases.
2. The interactions between the low and high HLB emulsifiers at the O/W_2 interface.
3. Polymeric thickener like carboxy methyl cellulose (CMC), hydroxy propyl methyl cellulose (HPMC) and their interaction with hydrophilic emulsifier in the outer phase.

They explained how a small quantity of salt in W/O droplets is able to balance the excess pressure due to differences in Laplace pressure between droplets of W_1 in oil and droplets of first W_1/O emulsion by osmotic opposition. Thus, multiple emulsions can be stabilised by addition of right salt concentration necessary to balance osmotic pressure between two water phases.

The effect of surfactant and electrolyte concentration on emulsion bulk rheological properties was investigated by Jiao *et al. (58).* Salt added to inner aqueous phase exerted an osmotic pressure that caused diffusion of water into inner aqueous phase and increased W/O/W emulsion viscosity through an increase in volume fraction of primary W/O emulsion. This type of viscosity increase imposed a destabilising effect because of likelihood of rupture of the inner and multiple droplets.

Kanouni *et al.* reported that the long-term stability of double emulsion requires a balance between

Laplace and osmotic pressures (between W_1 droplets in O and between W_1 droplets and the external aqueous phase W_2) *(59)*. The presence of a thickener in outer phase is necessary in order to reach a viscosity ratio (preferably ~1) between W_1/O and W_2 phases, allowing dispersion of viscous primary emulsion into W_2 aqueous phase. The thickener, which also serves as a dispersant and consequently prevents phase separation due to its thixotropic properties, must be compatible with the surfactants. Finally, the interactions between low and high HLB emulsifiers at O/W_2 interface should not destabilise the films. It was observed that such destructive interaction for system could be prevented by use of two high HLB surfactants in outer aqueous phase: an amphoteric surfactant, betaine, and an anionic surfactant, sodium lauryl ether sulfate. The combination of such pairs of surfactants was found to contribute to the films stability.

The nature of oil phase of W/O/W multiple emulsions stabilised by interfacial complexation between Span 80 and albumin was studied by Omotosho *et al. (60)*. They suggested that diffusion of unionised species of 5-fluorouracil (FU) across oil phase or through localised thin oil lamellae is the primary transport mechanism. In presence of surface active agents, water is solublilised in inverse micelles, which would possess the ability to solubilise other water-soluble components, such as NaCl and 5-FU. The mixed micellar units of Span 80 and polysorbate (Tween-80) therefore acts as solute carriers across liquid hydrocarbon membrane separating two aqueous phases of emulsions. The main factor determining the differences in rates of release from hydrocarbon emulsions appears to be droplet size of internal aqueous phase.

A study on the effect of addition of surfactants in internal aqueous phase of emulsions on water flux showed that only addition of hydrophilic surfactant into internal aqueous compartments demonstrated both coalescence of internal aqueous compartments and influx of water to internal from external aqueous phase *(34)*. The formation percentage of multiple emulsions was improved by increasing the concentration of additives, viz., sorbitol and sodium chloride due to a decrease in interfacial tension between internal aqueous phase of W/O/W emulsion and oily phase of emulsion.

Lezer *et al. (47)* suggested that stability can be improved by increasing the lipophilic surfactant concentration which could strengthen interfacial film whereas an excess of hydrophilic surfactant destabilises the emulsion.

Three main mechanisms of stabilisation with polymeric amphiphiles as reviewed by Garti *(61)* include:

1. Depletion of stabilisation by non-adsorbing macromolecules that prevent collision between particles (droplets) and provide elasticity to the system.
2. Electrostatic repulsions between two droplets carrying same charge.
3. Steric stabilisation resulting from hydrophobic interactions between adsorbed polymers.

The main contribution to the stability of macromolecular stabilised emulsions is related to droplets approaching a distance where compression due to polymer–polymer interactions occurs (without interpenetration).

Cyclodextrins (α, β and γ) were shown to be potential stabilisers for O/W/O emulsions. The advantages of cyclodextrins are their ability to complex with certain oil components at oil/water interface without additional surfactant. It appears that the stabiliser efficacy depends on nature of oil and type of cyclodextrin (α/β/γ). The presence of any active matter in inner phase (such as benzophenone) destabilised the emulsion. Only the α-cyclodextrin yielded stable emulsions. The reason is that interfacial interactions between the components at interface change HLB and cause destabilisation effect *(17)*.

6.2. Approaches to Improve Stability

Various methods have been described to stabilise multiple emulsions.

6.2.1. Gelation of Phases

The earlier approaches were to increase viscosity either by gelating (viscofying) the internal or external water phase or by gelating (viscofying) the oil phase.

It is possible to stabilise multiple emulsions by forming a polymeric gel in either internal or external aqueous phase using gelatin or a non-ionic surfactant like poloxamer that can be polymerised *in situ*, with the consequence that multiple globules become established in a network of cross-linked surfactant molecules. Polyacrylamide and a series of acryloyl derivatives of poloxamer surfactants can also be used. Polymerisation in external aqueous phase increases its viscosity, increases stability by reducing the close approach of particles *(62–64)*.

Ozer *et al. (18)* reported improved stability of emulsions wherein viscofying agents like magnesium silicate, veegum, aerosil, hydroxy propyl cellulose (HPC), HPMC, hydroxy ethyl cellulose (HEC), guar gum, carbopol, etc. were used in outer aqueous phase.

A stable W/O/W thermo-reversible multiple emulsion was obtained by Olivieri *et al.* based on high molecular weight graft-copolymers of poly(acrylic acid) and Pluronic F127 as stabilising agents *(65)*.

6.2.2. Formation of Interfacial Complex Films

A very strong interfacial film will help to stabilise multiple emulsion either by *in situ* polymerisation at the interface or by interfacial interaction between a polymer and surfactants.

This mode of stabilisation can be executed through formation of stable complex interfacial films between polymeric surfactant and monomeric lipophilic surfactant. The film is thick, viscous, gel-like and imparts elasticity and resistance to rupture *(59)*.

Use of amphiphilic proteins such as BSA and casein along with monomeric emulsifiers or synthetic block copolymers based on silicon backbones and polyethylene oxide side-chains have also been studied *(66)*. The stability of W/O/W emulsions has been significantly improved by using a blend of non-ionic surfactant (Span 80) and BSA as an interfacial complex in inner phase. Improved stability was obtained by replacing common non-ionic hydrophilic monomeric emulsifier by BSA in outer phase *(67)*.

The formation of multiple W/O/W emulsions containing chloroquine phosphate with improved stability due to formation of interfacial complex films between acacia, gelatin, polyvinylpyrrolidone (PVP) and sorbitan monooleate is described by Omotosho *(68)*.

Sela *et al.* reported that multiple emulsions based on silicone surfactants with unusual mechanical stability can be used as slow release systems for agricultural applications *(56)*.

Another approach of formation of stable interfacial membrane is by interfacial interaction between a macromolecule like albumin, acacia, gelatin or a polyanion such as polyacrylic acid in internal aqueous phase and a lipophilic surfactant in oil phase. The increased stability allows the film to withstand thinning and also delay the release of entrapped solutes *(69)*.

Benichou, A., Aserin, A., and Garti, N. (69) reported that formation of amphiphilic biopolymer adducts between protein (WPI) and polysaccharide (xanthan gum and fenugreek gum) gave very high yield of addendum entrapment (>95%). WPI/xanthan gum adducts served as thick and efficient barriers against release of flumethrin® (a veterinary drug model) entrapped in core of O/W/O multiple globules.

6.2.3. Modulating Surfactant Concentration

The classical approach of choosing the best combination of emulsifers by HLB approach or the newer Liquid–crystal stabilisation approach can also be employed for improving emulsion stability.

In many stable and commercially available emulsions, the emulsifier, water and oil molecules contribute to regular structure of multi-molecular layers, which are known as "liquid crystal layers". The liquid crystalline phase around droplets acts as a rheological barrier to shear. In addition, some liquid crystalline phases have a tendency to form a network similar to semi-solid phase extending through continuous phase. This network impedes the movement of droplets and adds to the stability of emulsion *(70)*.

6.2.4. Additives in Internal Aqueous Phase

Soluble material like electrolytes (ascorbic acid, sodium chloride, sodium citrate and acetic acid), when used as additives in internal aqueous phase can influence the stability and release profile. Glucose and sucrose could increase viscosity and as a result stability of emulsion system. Adeyeye and Price studied the effect of dextrose in internal phase and its effect on improving the stability of multiple emulsions by controlling osmolarity *(71)*. Yazan *et al.* reported addition of PVP into multiple emulsions containing vitamin A for improved stability *(41)* whereas Zheng *et al.* stabilised Hb-containing multiple emulsions by adding human serum albumin into both aqueous phases and dextran into outer water phase *(15)*.

The addition of lysozyme to aqueous phase or stearylamine and oleic acid to oil phase can effectively improve the stability of oil layer. Biopolymers like BSA, HEC, CMC and sodium alginate have also been reported to improve stability and control release of active agent *(72)*.

6.2.5. Stabilisation by Additive in Oily Phase

Colloidal silica has been reported to have stabilised the oil film in a urea-containing multiple emulsion *(73)*.

6.2.6. Steric Stabilisation

Steric stabilisation can be achieved using either adsorption or grafting of natural polymers or by using polymeric surfactants or lipid grafted polymers. The steric cloud may help in preventing their instability due to environmental changes.

Oza and Frank have suggested the use of colloidal CMC and monomeric surfactants for mechanical stabilisation of double emulsions *(74)*.

Multiple emulsions can be stabilised by coating them with hydrophobised polysaccharides like cholesteroyl pullulan, mannan and amylopectin. Similar potential of poloxamer or Pluronic coated systems can also be elucidated.

Lawson and Papadopoulos incorporated activated form of *N*-glutaryl-phosphatidylethanolamine into $W_1/O/W_2$ double-emulsion globules and observed that external coalescence of internal droplets was prolonged in globules containing this co-surfactant as compared to globules containing only Span 80 *(75)*.

6.2.7. Micellar Solution

A W/O emulsion whose inner phase is composed of a micellar solution of inverse type, will form a new multiple emulsion, the micellar solution-in-oil-in-water, when emulsified in water *(76)*.

6.3. Estimation of Stability

The stability of a pharmaceutical emulsion is characterised by the absence of coalescence of internal phase, absence of creaming and maintenance of elegance with respect to appearance, odour, colour and other physical properties.

Basic studies performed on multiple emulsion prepared freshly, and/or stored for different time periods for estimation of stability are:

1. Droplet size and polydispersity of internal and multiple droplets: The precise method for determining stability involves a size frequency analysis of internal and multiple droplets from time to time as the product ages.

   Geiger *et al.* proposed a novel micro-pipette aspiration technique to study globule deformability on a microscopic scale *(77)*. The method consists of aspirating, step-by-step, individual globules into a cylindrical glass tube under well-controlled conditions and studying its deformability by micromanipulation technique.

   Values of shear elastic modulus (μ) can be determined using the equation,

$$Rp \cdot \Delta P = \mu[(2Lp/Rp) - 1 + \log(2Lp/Rp)] \qquad (15)$$

where *Rp* is the internal radius of micro-pipette, ΔP is pressure required to aspirate and *Lp* is length of globule.

2. Creaming: Creaming of multiple emulsions can be studied to determine the stability of multiple emulsions. Creaming results from flocculation and concentration of globules of internal phase, which represents potential step towards complete coalescence of internal phase. Furthermore, creaming results in a lack of uniformity of drug distribution and, unless the preparation is thoroughly shaken before administration, leads to variable dosage.

   If the dispersed phase is less dense than continuous phase, which is in case of W/O/W multiple emulsions, the velocity of sedimentation becomes negative, that is, an upward creaming results. If the internal phase is heavier than external phase, which is in case of O/W/O multiple emulsions, the globules settle and this effect is referred to as creaming in downward direction. Greater the difference between the density of the two phases, larger the oil globules and less viscous the external phase, greater is rate of creaming. By adjusting the densities of two phases, rate of creaming can be reduced down.

   To test flocculation in multiple emulsions, sodium dodecyl sulphate (10%) is added and then the particle size analysis is repeated and degree of flocculation is assessed.

3. Coalescence and breaking: During stability study, breaking of multiple emulsions into simple emulsion has to be studied to evaluate stability of multiple emulsions. Breaking of multiple emulsion can be judged macroscopically by observing phase separation of multiple emulsion.

   The volume of aqueous phase separated is measured from time to time and percent phase separation is calculated:

$$B(\%) = 100(V_{sep}/20)/[(V_1 + V_2)/V_1 + V_2 + V_0] \qquad (16)$$

   where, V_1, V_2 and V_0 are volumes of internal, external and middle phases, respectively.

   Globule size, viscosity, phase-volume ratio and ζ-potential of system can be adjusted to retard the breaking of multiple emulsions.

4. Viscosity measurements: To characterise the stability of multiple emulsions, viscosity of the multiple emulsions can be studied time to time as system ages. Decrease in viscosity of multiple emulsion indicates the diffusion of water from internal phase to external phase and hence the instability of multiple emulsions.

   Kita *et al.* made an attempt to establish method for estimating the stability of W/O/W-type multiple-phase emulsions in light of correlation between viscosity and disperse phase concentration using Mooney's theory, as in

$$\eta_{rel} = \Phi W_i + \Phi_o \approx 1 - \lambda(\Phi W_i + \Phi_o)\sim, \quad (17)$$

where η_{rel} is relative viscosity of W/O/W emulsion, ΦW_i and Φ_o are the volume fractions of inner aqueous phase and oil phase, and α and λ are constants *(48)*. As a result of rupture of oil layer on the surface of dispersed inner aqueous-phase globules, the volume fraction ΦW_i should decrease following the mixing of inner aqueous-phase component with outer aqueous phase *(78)*. This may reduce the viscosity of W/O/W emulsion according to relationship

$$\Phi W_i = \alpha[\log \eta_{rel} \approx (2.303/\alpha) - (2.303\lambda\Phi_o/\alpha) - \Phi_o] (\alpha + 2.303\lambda \log \eta_{rel}). \quad (18)$$

The experimental results obtained suggest that it is possible to estimate stability of W/O/W emulsions by measuring the time dependence of viscosity in a range of relatively low disperse phase concentrations, although the presence of ingredients, such as protein, electrolytes, saccharides, in both aqueous phases affects the rheological properties of W/O/W emulsions.

5. Turbidometry: Turbidometric measurements can be made using a Turbiscan wherein the optical properties of dispersion is monitored from top to bottom at periodic time intervals *(79)*.
6. Drug leakage: Drug leakage is one of the important parameters to study stability of multiple emulsions as the system ages. Drug leakage in multiple emulsion indicates the diffusion of drug from internal phase to external phase and hence the instability of multiple emulsions.
7. Conductometry: Conductivity measurements correspond to release of entrapped electrolyte in the innermost phase, which can be correlated to emulsion stability.
8. Osmotic pressure: Osmotic pressure measurement or osmolarity calculations can also be used for assessing the stability of multiple emulsions.

A method to study the stability of W/O/W multiple drops by an ion selective membrane electrode, using a marker compound, ephedrine HCl was suggested. The effect of 1st emulsifier concentration and influence of W/O emulsion ratio on stability was studied by a power function relationship to characterise the multiple emulsion breakdown during storage. Lesser the W/O emulsion ratio and higher the first emulsifier concentration, slower the multiple drop number decrease rate *(79)*.

For accelerated stability testing, tests to be performed include, osmotic fragility test, turbulence shock tests, ortho-kinetic stress test, dilution test, centrifugal test, electro-kinetic test, thermal test and freeze–thaw cycle test.

7. APPLICATIONS OF MULTIPLE EMULSION

Multiple emulsions are unique in that a true liquid phase is maintained separate from an external aqueous phase. This may be especially important for bio-active molecule that cannot be appropriately stabilised in solid state. In addition, the separation of aqueous phase enables highly specialised environment, conducive to maintain protein activity.

7.1. Multiple Emulsions in Controlled Drug Delivery

Multiple emulsions show a high potential for prolonged delivery of drugs. Curcumin extract was nanoencapsulated in chitosan cross-linked with tripolyphosphate (TPP) via multiple emulsion/solvent evaporation technique as a potential controlled release system and the resulting nanocapsules were characterised. The nanocapsules in emulsion were essentially spherical with particle size of 253.8–415.2 nm. Fourier transform-infra red analysis confirmed that TPP cross-linked with ammonium groups of chitosan in nanocapsules. The yield of nanoencapsulated curcumin ranged from 18.56 to 96.28% (w/w) *(80)*.

The ratio of hydrophilic and lipophilic surfactants is important in achieving stable multiple emulsions. Of the W/O/W and O/W/O types of emulsions, W/O/W has more areas of application. Favourable drug release mechanisms with modified rate and *in vivo* profiles make multiple emulsions versatile carriers in controlled, sustained release and targeted delivery systems. It can also be used for taste masking, bioavailability enhancement, immobilisation of enzymes, etc. Multiple emulsions can also be used as an intermediate step in process of micro-encapsulation, which are used in oral delivery of hydrophilic drugs that are unstable in gastrointestinal tract like proteins and peptides *(81)*.

Stealth multiple emulsions of small size, containing 6-mercaptopurine, were prepared by incorporation of sphingomyelins (SM) and monosialogangliosides

(GM1) in oily phase and by coating with lipid-grafted polyethylene glycol (PEG-PC) and were characterised for size distribution, ζ-potential, viscosity, encapsulation efficiency, drug release and stability. The tissue distribution studies carried out with PEG grafted multiple emulsion showed that PEG-PC-coated multiple emulsions are superior as prolonged release and extended blood circulating carriers compared to uncoated multiple emulsions bearing either SM or GM1 *(82)*.

A novel method of genetic library construction on magnetic micro-beads based on solid-phase single-molecule polymerase chain reaction (PCR) in a fine and robust water-phase compartment formed in W/O emulsions was developed and critically diluted DNA fragments were distributed over the emulsion as templates, where beads cross-linked with multiple primers and other PCR components were encapsulated to form multiple reaction compartments. This was useful in constructing GLOBE (genetic library on beads), which can be readily applicable to a genomewide global scanning of genetic elements recognised by a defined DNA-binding protein *(83)*.

Multiple emulsions can be used in addition of anti-aging enzymes to cosmetic and beauty products. A multiple emulsion of aqueous oxygen carrying material in oil in outer aqueous phase is suitable for provision of oxygen for oxygen transfer processes. A haemoglobin multiple emulsion in physiologically compatible oil in an outer aqueous saline solution is provided in sufficiently small droplet size to provide oxygen flow through blood vessels to desired body tissues or organs thereby providing a blood substitute. A process is provided wherein haemoglobin, a fragile material, is formulated into high haemoglobin content W/O/W multiple emulsions while maintaining high yields and high oxygen exchange activity *(84)*.

Laugel *et al.* assessed suitability of O/W/O emulsions as prolonged release topical formulations of hydrocortisone *(85)*. A multiple emulsion as well as a simple emulsion were prepared with exactly same composition and the percutaneous absorption of hydrocortisone from these two emulsion types was studied and compared. At a finite dose, the percentage of hydrocortisone absorbed from simple emulsion was 1.5-fold greater than that observed from the multiple emulsion, while the drug was retained for a longer time in epidermis and dermis following application of multiple emulsion.

Caffeine was used as a water soluble model and was found to be transported out by molecular diffusion and through a reverse micellar mechanism controlled by the viscosity of system using multiple emulsions for topical purposes *(86)*.

W/O/W multiple emulsion destined for vaginal application, containing lactic acid in internal aqueous phase, octadecylamine (ODA) in oily phase and CBZ in external aqueous phase was prepared and evaluated against three microbial strains: *Escherichia coli*, *Staphylococcus aureus* and *Candida albicans*. The results were different depending on the procedure used. Interpretable results were obtained if only a gentle agitation was used just after the introduction of microbial suspension to the product due to release of a variable fraction of CBZ or ODA entrapped in micelles of ethylene and propylene oxide copolymer *(21)*.

7.2. Multiple Emulsion in Protein Delivery

Peptides and proteins are growing in importance and attracting increased interest, as they are specifically effective at a comparably low dose. A number of peptide and protein products are now available in market, and numerous studies investigating them have been published in literature. There are various peptide/protein delivery systems and one of methods popularly used is in the form of multiple emulsions *(87)*.

Two W/O emulsions when forced successively through a pre-fabricated scaffold creates coatings, each containing a different protein and has different release characteristics. The model system designed with model proteins (myoglobin and lysozyme) with poly(ether-ester) multi-block co-polymers chosen as polymer matrix showed independent release of two proteins. The myoglobin release was tailored from a burst to a linear release even after 60 days, while the lysozyme release rate was kept constant. This approach could be of value for tissue engineering applications *(88)*.

Small poly(lactic-co-glycolic acid) microspheres (mean size lower than 10 μm) containing small peptides were prepared by a W/O/W emulsion solvent evaporation technique. These microspheres were shown to encapsulate very efficiently a 33 amino acid peptide (V3 BRU) and *in vitro* release kinetics studies showed that such microspheres could be employed for both oral vaccination and controlled release. However, the encapsulation of a seven amino acid peptide (pBC 264) showed very low encapsulation efficiency which could be increased by (1) maintaining basic pH in inner aqueous phase where the peptide was soluble, while the external aqueous phase was acidic; (2) ovalbumin was added to stabilise inner emulsion. *In vitro* release kinetics of peptide were strongly influenced by presence of ovalbumin which seems to form pores in microsphere structure *(89)*.

7.2.1. Insulin Delivery

The effects of eicosapentaenoic acid (EPA) and docosahexanoic acid (DHA) on insulin absorption from rat intestinal loops *in situ* was studied by Suzuki *et al. (90)* using a W/O/W multiple emulsion. The emulsion (insulin dose, 50 U/kg) was administered directly into colonic and rectal loops. Both EPA and DHA strongly enhanced insulin absorption and induced hypoglycemia after colonic and rectal dosing. The results also indicated that a W/O/W multiple emulsion incorporating DHA is a possible means of facilitating the intestinal absorption of insulin without inducing any serious damage to the epithelial cells.

7.3. Lipid Emulsions

Lipid emulsions (LEs) are heterogenous dispersions of two immiscible liquids (O/W or W/O). However, the physical stability of LE can substantially be improved with help of suitable emulsifiers that are capable of forming a mono- or multi-layer coating film around dispersed liquid droplets in such a way to reduce interfacial tension or to increase droplet–droplet repulsion. Depending on the concentrations of these three components (oil–water–emulsifier) and the efficiency of emulsification equipments used to reduce droplet size, the final LE may be in the form of O/W, W/O, micron, submicron and double or multiple emulsions (O/W/O and W/O/W). The O/W type LEs are colloidal drug carriers, which have various therapeutic applications. As an intravenous delivery system, it incorporates lipophilic water non-soluble drugs, stabilise drugs that tend to undergo hydrolysis and reduce side effects of various potent drugs. LE can also be used as ocular delivery system to increase local bioavailability, to sustain the pharmacological effect of drugs and decrease systemic side effects of drugs *(91)*.

7.4. Multiple Emulsions to Deliver Blood Substitutes

Multiple emulsions can be used for delivering blood substitutes, fluorocarbon for treatment of acute respiratory failure by liquid ventilation or also fluorocarbon-based or stabilised gas bubbles. Reverse water-in-fluorocarbon emulsions, oil-in-fluorocarbon emulsions, multiple emulsions, micro-emulsions, fluorocarbon gels, fluorinated liposomes, fluorinated tubules and other novel supra-molecular systems can be used to deliver pulmonary, topical and ophthalmological drug delivery agents and even skin protection barriers though commercialisation is still distant as this is in investigational stages *(92,93)*.

7.5. Multiple Emulsion in Stabilisation of Drugs

Incorporation of triterpene derivatives within an O/W/O multiple emulsion may protect them against oxidation. This is particularly useful for unsaturated derivatives and lead to a modified release after topical application. These triterpene derivatives stimulate total collagen synthesis of skin fibroblasts. Study of influence of incorporation of madecassic acid, asiaticoside and asiatic acid on viscosity and stability of a multiple O/W/O emulsion and the rheological analysis carried out by flow experiments was assessed with 6 month storage at room temperature and at 40°C. These did not affect the stability of emulsions. *In vitro* percutaneous absorption of triterpenc derivatives when investigated by Franz diffusion cells in hairless rats showed O/W/O emulsions as an effective vehicle to preserve these active substances and to control their distribution in skin *(94)*.

7.6. Multiple Emulsion in Micro-Encapsulation

Complex dispersions prepared by dispersing Spherulites within an oily medium, and then emulsifying this oily dispersion of Spherulites within an aqueous solvent are being explored for encapsulation applications. An advantage of complex dispersions over Spherulites is to present an additional oily barrier. Indeed, this barrier retarded the release of encapsulated ions. These new systems of Spherulites known as complex dispersions showed great potential for pharmaceutical applications such as controlled release and protection of encapsulated substances *(95)*.

7.7. Thermo-Reversible Multiple Emulsion

The fabrication of thermo-reversible W/O/W multiple emulsion combined with complete release under shear at body temperature and superior emulsion stability suggest numerous applications in controlled release of drugs.

Thermo-reversible W/O/W multiple emulsion with increased emulsion stability and higher fraction of drug release under shear was prepared by Olivieri *et al (65)*. The formulation employed high molecular weight graft-co-polymers of poly(acrylic acid) and Pluronic F127 as stabilising agents. The product when assessed for thermo-reversible behaviour and the fragmentation-release characteristics, exhibited a 10^3 fold increase in viscosity over a range of temperatures from 20 to 40°C. At moderate shearing, a complete release of marker encapsulated in internal aqueous phase was observed (99.6%) at 35°C, whereas only 30% was released at 20°C.

7.8. Multiple Emulsion in Food Processing

Multiple emulsions have potential applications forformulation and processing of foods, as each dispersed globule in this type of emulsion consists of single or multiple aqueous compartments separated from aqueous suspending fluid by a layer of oil phase components *(96)*. Multiple emulsions are also used in preparation of food emulsion with improved physicochemical properties and also for development of novel delivery systems *(30)*.

REFERENCES

1. **Serifriz, W.** Studies in emulsions. III-V. *J. phy. Chem.* 1925;29(6):738.
2. **Attwood, D. and Florence, AT.** Surfactant systems: their chemistry, pharmacy and biology, Chapman and Hall, Florence, 1983, pp. 509–518.
3. **Florence, AT., Omotosho, JA., and Whateley, TL.** Multiple W/O/W emulsions as drug vehicles in controlled release of drugs: polymers and aggregate systems, (Rosoff, M. ed.), VCH Publishers, 1997, pp. 163–184.
4. **Davis, SS., Hadgraft, J., and Palin, KJ.** Marcel, Encyclopedia of emulsion technology, vol. 2, Dekker,1985, 159 p.
5. **Cunha, S., Cheron, M., Grossiord, JL., Puisieux, F., and Seiller, M.** Multiple emulsions: pharmaceutical potentiality in multiple emulsions: structure, properties and applications, (Grossiord, JL. and Seiller, M. eds.), 1999, pp. 279–312.
6. **Garti, N.** Double emulsions—scope, limitations and new achievements. *Colloid Surf. A: Physicochem. Engg. Asp.* 1997;233:123–124.
7. **Smith, AL. (ed.)** Theory and practice of emulsion technology, Academic Press, London, 1976, 519 p.
8. **Florence, AT. and Whitehill, D.** The formulation and stability of multiple emulsions. *Int. J. Pharm.* 1982;11:277–308.
9. **Matsumoto, S. and Kang, WW.** Formation and applications of multiple emulsions. *J. Dispersion Sci. Technol.* 1989;10: 455–482.
10. **Matsumoto, S., Kita, Y., and Yonezawa, D.** An attempt at preparing water-in-oil -in-water multiple phase emulsions. *J. Colloid Interface Sci.* 1976;57:353–361.
11. **Frenkel, M., Shwartz, R., and Garti, N.** Multiple emulsions: I. stability: inversion, apparent and weighted HLB. *J. Colloid Interface Sci.* 1983;94:174–178.
12. **Kita, Y., Matsumoto, S., and Yonezawa, D.** Permeation of water through oil layer in W/O/W type multiple-phase emulsions. *Nippon Kagaku Kaishi* 1978;1:11–14.
13. **Vyas, SP. and Khar, RK. (eds.)** Multiple emulsions as drug delivery systems in targeted and controlled drug delivery, Novel Carrier Systems (ed.), CBS Publications, 2002, pp. 323–380.
14. **Khopade, AJ. and Jain, NK.** Advances in controlled and novel drug delivery systems, (Jain, NK., ed.), 1st edn., CBS Publications, New Delhi, 2001, pp. 381–393.
15. **Zheng, S., Beissinger, RL., and Wasan, T.** The stabilization of hemoglobin multiple emulsion for use as a red blood cell substitute. *J. Colloid Interface Sci.* 1991;144(1):72–85.
16. **Law, TK., Florence, AT., and Whateley, T.** Release from multiple emulsions (W/O/W) stabilized by interfacial complexation. *J. Pharm. Pharmacol.* 1983;36:50.
17. **Duchene, D., Bochot, A., Yu, SC., Pépin, C., and Seiller, M.** Cyclodextrins and emulsions. *Int. J. Pharm.* 2003;266:85–90.
18. **Ozer, O., Muguet, V., Roy, E., Grossiord, JL., and Seiller, M.** Stability study of W/O/W viscosified multiple emulsions. *Drug Dev. Ind. Pharm.* 2000;26(11):1185–1189.
19. **Okochi, H. and Nakano, M.** Preparation and evaluation of w/o/w type emulsions containing vancomycin. *Adv. Drug Deliv. Rev.* 2000;45:5–26.
20. **Weiss, J., Scherze, I., and Muschiolik, G.** Polysaccharide gel with multiple emulsions. *Food Hydrocolloids* 2005;19:605–615.
21. **Tedajo, GM., Bouttier, S., Grossiord, JL., Marty, JP., Seiller, M., and Fourniat, J.** In vitro microbicidal activity of W/O/W multiple emulsion for vaginal administration. *Int. J. Antimicrobial Agents* 2002;20:50–56.
22. **Cole, ML. and Whateley, TA.** Preparation of stable multiple W/O/W emulsions using pluronic (poloxamer): poly(acrylic acid) complexes. *J. Colloid Interface Sci.* 1995;175:281–288.
23. **Sugiura, S., Nakajima, M., Yamamoto, K., et al.** Preparation characteristics of W/O/W multiple emulsions using microchannel emulsification. *J. Colloid Interface Sci.* 2004;270(1):221–228.
24. **Matsumoto, S., Koh, Y., and Michura, A.** Preparation of w/o/w emulsions in an edible form on the basis of phase inversion technique. *J. Dispersion Sci. Tech.* 1985;6(5):507–521.
25. **Lin, TJ.** Effect of initial surfactant location on the viscosity of emulsions. *J. Soc. Cosmet. Chem.* 1968;19:683–697.
26. **Becher, P.** The effect of the nature of the emulsifying agent on emulsion inversion. *J. Soc. Cosmet. Chem.* 1958;9:141–145.
27. **Sherman, P. and Parkinson, C.** Measurement of phase inversion temperature above 100°C. *Prog. Colloid Polymer. Sci.* 1978;63:10.
28. **Gohla, SH. and Nielson, J.** Partial phase solu-inversion technology (PPSIT): a novel process to manufacture long term stable multiple emulsions by an in situ one step procedure. *SOFW J.* 1995;121:707–713.

29. **Devani, MJ., Ashford, M., and Craig, DQM.** The development and characterization of triglyceride-based 'spontaneous' multiple emulsions. *Int. J. Pharm.* 2005;300(1–2):76–88.

30. **Kim, HJ., Decker, EA., and McClements, DJ.** Preparation of multiple emulsions based on thermodynamic incompatibility of heat-denatured whey protein and pectin solutions. *Food Hydrocolloids* 2006;20(5):586–595.

31. **Vladisavljević, GT., Shimizu, M., and Nakashima, T.** Production of multiple emulsions for drug delivery systems by repeated SPG membrane homogenization: influence of mean pore size, interfacial tension and continuous phase viscosity. *J. Membr. Sci.* 2006;284(1–2):373–383.

32. **Scherze, I., Knöfel, R., and Muschiolik, G.** Automated image analysis as a control tool for multiple emulsions. *Food Hydrocolloids* 2005;193:617–624.

33. **Benichou, A., Aserin, A., and Garti, N.** W/O/W double emulsions stabilized with WPI -polysaccharide complexes. *Colloids Surf. A: Physicochem. Engg. Asp.* 2007;297(1–3):211.

34. **Ohwaki, T., Machida, R., Ozawa, H., et al.** Improvement of the stability of water-in-oil-in-water multiple emulsions by the addition of surfactants in the internal aqueous phase of the emulsions. *Int. J. Pharm.* 1993;93(1–3):61–74.

35. **Vasiljevic, D., Parojcic, J., Primorac, M., and Vuleta, G.** An investigation into the characteristics and drug release properties of multiple W/O/W emulsion systems containing low concentration of lipophilic polymeric emulsifier. *Int. J. Pharm.* 2006;309(1–2):171–177.

36. **Florence, AT. and Whitehill, D.** Some features of breakdown in water-in-oil-in water multiple emulsions. *J. Colloid Interface Sci.* 1981;79:243–256.

37. **Magdassi, S., Frenkel, M., Garti, N., and Kazan, K.** Multiple emulsions II: HLB shift caused by emulsifier migration to external interface. *J. Colloid Interface Sci.* 1984;97:374–379.

38. **Magdassi, S. and Garti, N.** A kinetic model for release of electrolytes from w/o/w multiple emulsions. *J. Control. Release* 1986;3:273–277.

39. **Takahashi, K., Ohtsubo, F., and Takenchi, H.** Study of the stability of (w/o)w-type emulsions using a tracer technique. *J. Chem. Engg. Jpn.* 1981;14(5):416–418.

40. **Davis, SS. and Walker, I.** Measurement of the yield of multiple emulsion droplets by a fluorescent tracer technique. *Int. J. Pharm.* 1983;17:203–213.

41. **Yazan, Y., Arapl, U., Scieller, M., and Grossiord, JL.,** PVP in multiple emulsions. *Cosmet. toilet* 1995;110:53–56.

42. **Eads, TM., Weiler, RK., and Gaonkar, AG.** Detection of water in the internal aqueous phase of W/O/W multiple emulsions using magic angle spinning proton NMR. *J. Colloid Interface Sci.* 1991;145:466–477.

43. **Davis, SS. and Burbage, AG.** Electron micrography of water-in-oil-in-water emulsions. *J. Colloid Interface Sci.* 1977;62: 361–363.

44. **Lonnqvist, I. and Hakansson, B.** NMR self-diffusion studies of the water and the oil components in a W/O/W emulsion. *J. Colloid Interface Sci.* 1997;192:66–73.

45. **Nakhare, S. and Vyas, SP.** Prolonged release multiple emulsion based system bearing rifampicin: in vitro characterization. *Drug Dev. Ind. Pharm.* 1995;21(7):869–878.

46. **Baker, RW. and Lonsdale, HK.** In: controlled release of biologically active agents, (Tonquary, AO. and Lecoy, RE. eds.), Plenum Press, New York, 1974, pp. 15–71.

47. **Jager-Lezer, N., Terrisse, I., Bruneau, F., et al.** Influence of lipophilic surfactant on the release kinetics of water-soluble molecules entrapped in a W/O/W multiple emulsion. *J. Control. Release* 1997;45:1–13.

48. **Kita, Y., Matsumoto, S., and Yonezawa, D.** Viscometric method for estimating the stability of W/O/W-type multiple-phase emulsions. *J. Colloid Interface Sci.* 1977; 62(1):87–94.

49. **Chiang, C., Fuller, GC., Frankenfeld, JW., and Rhodes, CT.** Potential of liquid membranes for drug overdose treatment. *J. Pharm. Sci.* 1978;67:63–66.

50. **Omotosho, JA., Whateley, TL., and Florence, AT.** Methotrexate transport from internal phase of multiple w/o/w emulsion. *J. Microencap.* 1989;6:183–192.

51. **Avendano-Gomez, JR., Grossiord, JL., and Clausse, D.** Study of mass transfer in oil–water–oil multiple emulsions by differential scanning calorimetry. *J. Colloid Interface Sci.* 2005;290(2):533–545.

52. **Magdassi, S., Frenkel, M., and Garti, N.** Correlation between nature of emulsifier and multiple emulsion stability. *Drug Dev. Ind. Pharm.* 1985;11:791–798.

53. **Kawashima, Y., Hino, T., Takeuchi, H., and Niwa, T.** Stabilization of water/oil/water multiple emulsion with hypertonic inner aqueous phase. *Chem. Pharm. Bull.* 1992; 40:1240–1246.

54. **Hino, T., Takeuchi, H., Niwa, T., Kitagawa, M., and Kawashima, Y.** The analysis of drug release from diluted water/oil/water emulsions by a model of the rupture of oil membrane. *J. Pharm. Pharmacol.* 1995;47:1–7.

55. **Hai, M. and Magdassi, S.** Investigation on the release of fluorescent markers from w/o/w emulsions by fluorescence-activated cell sorter. *J. Control. Release* 2004;96(3): 393–402.

56. **Sela, Y., Magdassi, S., and Garti, N.** Release of markers from the inner water phase of W/O/W emulsions stabilized by silicone based polymeric surfactants. *J. Control. Release* 1995;33(1): 1–12.

57. **Rosano, HL. François G, Gandolfo FG and Hidrot JDP.** Stability of $W_1/O/W_2$ multiple emulsions: Influence of ripening and interfacial interactions. *Colloids Surf. A: Physicochem. Engg. Asp.* 1998;138:109.

58. **Jiao, J., Rhodes, DG., and Burgess, DJ.** Multiple emulsion stability: pressure balance and interfacial film strength. *J. Colloid Interface Sci.* 2002;250(2):444–450.

59. **Kanouni, M., Rosano, HL., and Naouli, N.** Preparation of a stable double emulsion (W1/O/W2): role of the interfacial films on the stability of the system. *Adv. Colloid Interface Sci.* 2002;99(3);229–254.

60. **Omotosho, JA., Florence, AT., and Whateley, TLJA.** Absorption and lymphatic uptake of 5-fluorouracil in the rat following oral administration of w/o/w multiple emulsions. *Int. J. Pharm.* 1989;61:51–56.

61. **Garti, N.** Progress in stabilization and transport phenomena of double emulsions in food applications. *Lebensm.-Wiss. u.-Technol.* 1997;30:222–235.

62. **Takahashi, T., Kono, K., and Yamaguchi, T.** Enhancement of the cancer chemotherapeutic effect by anticancer agents in the form of fat emulsion. *Tohoku J. Exp. Med.* 1977;123:235–246.

63. **Florence, AT. and Whitehill, D.** Stabilization of water/oil/water multiple emulsions by polymerization of aqueous phase. *J. Pharm. Pharmacol.* 1982;34:687.

64. **Law, TK., Florence, AT., and Whateley, TL.** Stabilisation of emulsions by interfacial polymerisation of poloxamer surfactant derivatives. *Colloid Polym. Sci.* 1986;264:167–170.

65. **Olivieri, L., Seiller, M., Bromberg, L., Besnard, M., Duong, T-N-L., and Grossiord, J-L.** Optimization of a thermally reversible W/O/W multiple emulsion for shear induced drug release. *J. Control. Release* 2003;88(3):401–412.

66. **Garti, N. and Aserin, A.** Double emulsions stabilized by macromolecular surfactants. *Adv. Colloid Interface Sci.* 1996; 65:37–69.

67. **Garti, N., Aserin, A., and Cohen, Y.** Mechanistic considerations on the release of electrolytes from multiple emulsions stabilized by BSA and nonionic surfactants. *J. Control. Release* 1994;29(1–2):41–51.

68. **Omotosho, JA.** The effect of acacia, gelatin and polyvinylpyrrolidone on chloroquine transport from multiple w/o/w emulsions. *Int. J. Pharm.* 1990;62(1):81–84.

69. **Benichou, A., Aserin, A., and Garti, N.** O/W/O double emulsions stabilized with WPI–polysaccharide conjugates. *Colloids Surf. A: Physicochem. Engg. Asp.* 2007;297(1–3):211–220.

70. **Bevacqua, AJ., Lahanas, KM., Cohen, ID., and Cloca, G.** Liquid crystals in multiple emulsions. *Cosmet. Toilet* 1991;106(55): 53–56.

71. **Adeyeye, CM. and Price, JC.** Effect of nonionic surfactant concentration and type on the formation and stability of multiple emulsions: microscopic and conductometric evaluation. *Drug Dev. Ind. Pharm.* 1990;16:1053–1078.

72. **Pays, K., Geirmanska-Khan, J., Pouligny, B., Bibette, J., and Leal-Calderon, F.** Double emulsions: how does release occur? *J. Control. Release* 2002;79:193–205.

73. **Dupuis, L.** Multiple emulsion and urea on pig skin: a moisturization and penetration study. *SOFW* 1996;122(10): 658–663.

74. **Oza, KP. and Frank, SG.** Drug release from emulsions stabilized by colloidal microcrystalline cellulose. *J. Disp. Sci. Tech.* 1989;10:187–210.

75. **Lawson, LB. and Papadopoulos, KD.** Effects of a phospholipid cosurfactant on external coalescence in water-in-oil-in-water double-emulsion globules. *Colloids Surf. A: Physicochem. Engg. Asp.* 2004;250(1–3):337–342.

76. **Pilman, E., Larsson, K., and Torhberg, E.** Inverse micellar phases in ternary systems of polar lipids/fat/water and protein emulsification of such phases to w/o/w-microemulsion-emulsions. *J. Disp. Sci. Technol.* 1980;1:267–281.

77. **Geiger, S., Tokgoz, S., Fructus, A., et al.** Kinetics of swelling–breakdown of a W/O/W multiple emulsion: possible mechanisms for the lipophilic surfactant effect. *J. Control. Release* 1998;52:99–107.

78. **Cournarie, F., Savelli, M-P., Rosilio, V., et al.** Insulin-loaded W/O/W multiple emulsions: comparison of the performances of systems prepared with medium-chain-triglycerides and fish oil. *Eur. J. Pharm. Biopharm.* 2004;58:477–482.

79. **Csóka, I. and Erős, I.** Stability of multiple emulsions: I. Determination of factors influencing multiple drop breakdown. *Int. J. Pharm.* 1997;156(1):119–123.

80. **Sowasod, N., Charinpanitkul, T., and Tanthapanichakoon, W.** Nanoencapsulation of curcumin in biodegradable chitosan via multiple emulsion/solvent evaporation, N08, Fourth Thailand material science technology conference. 31st March to 1st April, 2006, Thailand.

81. **Khan, AY., Talegaonkar, S., Iqbal, Z., Ahmed, FJ., and Khar, RK.** Multiple emulsions: an overview. *Curr. Drug Deliv.* 2006; 3(4):429–443.

82. **Khopade, AJ. and Jain, NK.** Long-circulating multiple-emulsion system for improved delivery of an anticancer agent. *Drug Deliv.* 1999;6(2):107–110.

83. **Kojima, T., Takei, Y., Ohtsuka, M., Kawarasaki, Y., Yamane, T., and Nakano, H.** PCR amplification from single DNA molecules on magnetic beads in emulsion: application for high-throughput screening of transcription factor targets. *Nucleic Acids Res.* 2005;33(17):e150.

84 **Beissinger, RL, Rosen, AL, Wasan, DT., and Sehgal, LR.**, Hemoglobin multiple emulsion, CA 1330937, 1994.

85. **Laugel, CA., Baillet, MP., Piemi, Y., Marty, JP., and Ferrier, D.** Oil–water–oil multiple emulsions for prolonged delivery of hydrocortisone after topical application: comparison with simple emulsions. *Int. J. Pharm.* 1998;160(1):109–117.

86. **Tirnaksiz, F. and Kalsin, O.** A topical w/o/w multiple emulsions prepared with Tetronic 908 as a hydrophilic surfactant: formulation, characterization and release study. *J. Pharm. Pharm. Sci.* 2005;8(2):299–315.

87. **Degim, IT. and Celebi, N.** Controlled delivery of peptides and proteins. *Curr. Pharm. Des.* 2007;13(1):99–117.

88. **Sohier, J., Vlugt, TJ., Cabrol, N., Van Blitterswijk, C., de Groot, K., and Bezemer, JM.** Dual release of proteins from porous polymeric scaffolds. *J. Control. Release* 2006;111(1–2):95–106.

89. **Couvreur, P., Blanco-Prieto, MJ., Puisieux, F., Roques, B., and Fattal, E.** Multiple emulsion technology for the design of microspheres containing peptides and oligopeptides. *Adv. Drug Deliv. Rev.* 1997;28(1):85–96.

90. **Suzuki, A., Morishita, M., Kajita, M., et al.** Enhanced colonic and rectal absorption of insulin using a multiple emulsion containing eicosapentaenoic acid and docosahexaenoic acid. *J. Pharm. Sci.* 1998;87(10):1196–1202.

91. **Tamilvanan, S.** Oil-in-water lipid emulsions: implications for parenteral and ocular delivering systems. *Prog. Lipid Res.* 2004;43(6):489–533.

92. **Riess, JG. and Krafft, MP.** Advanced fluorocarbon-based systems for oxygen and drug delivery, and diagnosis. *Artif. Cells Blood Substit. Immobil. Biotechnol.* 1997;25(1–2):43–52.

93. **Riess, JG. and Krafft, MP.** Fluorinated materials for in vivo oxygen transport (blood substitutes), diagnosis and drug delivery. *Biomaterials* 1998;19(16):1529–1539.

94. **Laugel, C., Baillet, A., Ferrier, D., Grossiord, JL., and Marty, JP.** Incorporation of triterpenic derivatives within an o/w/o multiple emulsion: structure and release studies. *J. Cosmet. Sci.* 1998;20(3):183–191.

95. **Genty, M., Couarraze, G., Laversanne, R., Degert, C., Maccario, J., and Grossiord, JL.** Complex dispersions of multilamellar vesicles: a promising new carrier for controlled release and protection of encapsulated molecules. *J. Control. Release* 2003;90(1):119–133.

96. **Matsumoto, S.** w/o/w-type multiple emulsions with a view to possible food applications. *J. Texture Stud.* 1986;17(2): 141–159.

5

Vesicular System: Summary, Conclusions and Future Perspectives

Colloidal drug carrier systems have gained much importance due to it's ability for administration by parenteral route covering sub-dermal to intravenous. Encapsulation of drugs in vesicular structures have been proved to possess several advantages like prolongation of systemic half-life, toxicity reduction, selective uptake, drug protection from very fast degradation/metabolism, etc. Consequently a number of vesicular drug delivery systems such as liposome, niosome, transfersome, and pharmacosome were developed. In addition, related drug delivery systems like microemulsion, micellar systems, and dendrimers have also evolved and developed with potentiality to tackle highly complex problems of particularly toxic bioactives. Advances made in the area of vesicular drug delivery paved way to design targeted delivery systems involving highly potent anti-cancer drugs, antibiotics, immunosuppressants, cardiovascular agents, etc. Development of biotechnological products especially in area of immunologicals as vesicular delivery systems revolutionalised the commercial introduction of long acting immunological products. Vesicular delivery has also been considered useful for gene delivery with high transfection especially with cationic liposomes.

Non-ionic surfactant vesicles or niosomes are similar to liposomes and are formed in aqueous media from non-ionic surfactants with or without presence of cholesterol or other lipids. Like liposomes, niosomes can also entrap both hydrophilic and lipophilic drugs, either in aqueous layer or in vesicular membrane which is lipoidal in nature. Because of presence of non-ionic surfactant they possess better intrinsic targeting potential and may prove very useful for targeting drugs for treating cancer, parasitic, viral and other microbial diseases more effectively.

Micellar delivery systems are such systems which can be exploited to deliver such complex and sophisticated molecules. Polymeric micelles formed in this method can also be used for solubilisation, stabilisation, and delivery of challenging agents. It is also useful in encapsulation and delivery of hydrophobic drugs. Microemulsion is thus defined as a system of nanometric sized droplets of an immiscible liquid within another liquid and amphiphile, which is a single optically isotropic and thermodynamically stable liquid solution. In other words, microemulsions are thermodynamically stable, transparent dispersions of oil and water stabilizsed by an interfacial film of surfactant molecules. These homogenous systems, which can be prepared over a wide range of surfactant concentrations and oil to water (O/W) ratios, are all fluids of low viscosity.

Multiple emulsions are novel development in field of emulsion technology and more complex type of dispersed systems. Multiple emulsions were first described by Seiferiz in 1925 as double or complex emulsions during an inversion of O/W olive oil emulsion into W/O emulsion, but it is only in the last 30 yrs that they have been extensively studied and investigated in such diverse fields as separation of hydrocarbons, treatment of waste water, immobilizsation of enzymes, prolongation of drug release, treatment of overdose, etc. Their applications in pharmaceutical and cosmetological field include taste masking, adjuvant vaccines, enzyme immobilisation, absorption or permeation enhancement, protection and stabilisation of entrapped active, sustained and prolonged release, etc.

The initial teething problems encountered with most of the vesicular delivery systems like scale up and commercial production have been solved with development of newer technologies for large scale production, new concepts like pre-liposomes and niosomes manufacturable by freeze drying/spray drying. Recognition of exceptional *in vivo* qualities for non-conventional systems like micellar systems, dendrimers have given new dimensions for research to overcome problems difficult to solve by conventional vesicular systems.

6

Micro Particles in Drug Delivery

Prof. R.S.R Murthy, M.PHARM, PhD
Dr. Rakesh Sharma, M.PHARM, PhD
Prof. K.S Rajesh, M.PHARM, PhD
Prof. (Mrs) K.K. Sawant, M.PHARM, PhD

CONTENTS

1. INTRODUCTION

Micro-particulate systems refer to the technology of re-arranging and processing of atom/molecules to fabricate material of micrometer specifications. The availability of the spheres of different size allows flexibility regarding specific *in vivo* applications and forms of administration. In general, these systems consist of polymeric materials in which the drug is dispersed, entrapped, dissolved or adsorbed *(1–7)*. This relatively young branch of science draws expertise from chemical sciences, polymer science, physical sciences, biomedical sciences, pharmaceutical sciences, engineering and biotechnology, etc., in a truly inter-disciplinary manner *(8,9)*.

Carrier is one of the most important entities essentially required for successful transportation of loaded drugs overcoming challenges posed in drug delivery as shown in Fig. 1.

The function of drug carriers is not only confined as guiding devices but to protect and retain the bioactivity of drugs including enzymes, proteins, peptides, etc., from different physiological environments against inactivation or excretion, to prevent them from eliciting adverse immune reactions or to store them in a reservoir for their release in a gradual fashion *(8–10)*.

An ideal drug carrier designed as a targeting device should possess the following essential features:

- It should be biocompatible, biodegradable, non-toxic and non-immunogenic.
- It must be able to cross anatomical or physiological barriers.
- The target cells must recognise it specifically and selectively.
- The linkage of drug and targeting moiety should be stable in different physiological fluids and environments.

Different kinds of drug carriers used in drug delivery research are summarised in Table 1.

1.1. Nomenclature

Micro-particulate drug delivery systems include micro/nanoparticles, modified or tailor made systems such as magnetic particles and surface modified or coated particles. The term 'microparticle' refers to polymeric drug delivery systems with the particle in size range of 1–1000 μm diameter irrespective of the precise interior or exterior structure, whereas the 'nanoparticles' are in the size range of 10–1000 nm *(1–4)*. Depending upon the morphology, micro-particles can be subcategorised into two categories—microspheres and microcapsules. Despite the specific and logical sub-categories, many authors use the terms interchangeably often to the confusion of the reader.

Microspheres are monolithic or matrix-type spherical micro-particles.

Microcapsules are microspheres having a core surrounded by a material, which is distinctly different from that of the core. Microcapsules are assumed to have one or more discrete domain of active agent(s). As domains and sub-domains of active agent within microcapsules become increasingly smaller, the microcapsules become microspheres. All these devices differ not only in the structure (Fig. 2) but also in their biopharmaceutical properties and therapeutic uses *(3)*.

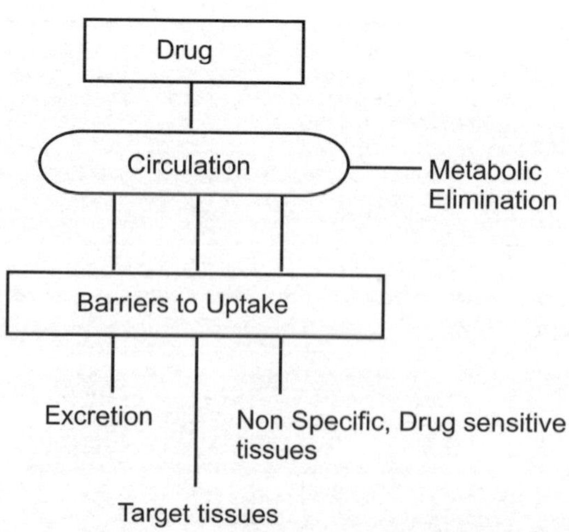

Fig. 1. Barriers encountered in transportation of the drug to active sites in the body.

Table 1. Carrier Systems Used for Targeted Drug Delivery

Colloidal carriers	a. Vesicular systems: liposomes, niosomes, pharmacosomes, virosomes, immunoliposomes, sub-micron emulsions and multiple emulsions b. Particulate systems: micro-particles, nanoparticles, magnetic microspheres and micro- and nanocapsules
Cellular carriers	Resealed erythrocytes, serum albumin, antibodies, leukocytes and platelets
Supramolecular delivery systems	Micelles, reverse micelles, mixed micelles, polymeric micelles, liquid crystals and lipoproteins
Polymer based systems	Signal sensitive, mucoadhesive, biodegradable, bioerodible, soluble synthetic polymeric carriers and hydrogels
Macromolecular carrier	Proteins, glycoproteins, neo-glycoproteins and artificial viral envelopes, toxins and lectins

System	Status of Drug	Figure	Applications
Microspheres	Drug dispersed	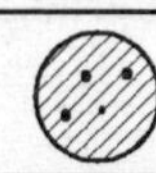	Sustained release Enzyme immobilisation Harmonize at all places. Drug targeting
Nanosphere	Drug adsorbed	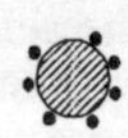	
Microcapsules	Drug entrapped	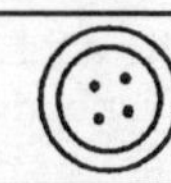	Encapsulation of drugs drug ligands Drug targeting
Nanocapsules	Drug entrapped	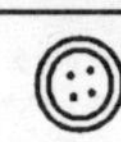	
Core-Shell Particles	Drug dispersed in coated core	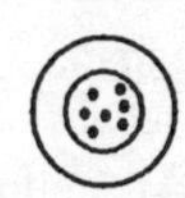	Encapsulation Sustained release

Microspheres: monolithic or matrix-type spherical micro-particles

Nanospheres: matrix system where the drug is absorbed

Microcapsules: micro-spheres having a core surrounded by a material, which is distinctly different from that of the core

Nanocapsules: vesicular system in which drug is surrounded by a polymeric membrane

Core-shell particles: the core is formed of a entirely different material from that of the shell

Applications

Microspheres/nanospheres: Drug delivery and enzyme immobilisation

Microcapsules/nanocapsules: Encapsulation of solid and liquid drugs

Core-shell particles: Encapsulation of anti-tumour drugs

Fig. 2. Differences in structural and biopharmaceutical properties of microparticulate carrier systems.

During the past three decades, however, formulations that control the rate and period of drug delivery (i.e., timed release medications) and target specific areas of the body for treatment have become increasingly common, though complex. Polymeric microspheres, polymeric micelles and hydrogel-type materials have all been shown to be effective in enhancing drug targeting specificity, lowering systemic drug toxicity, improving efficacy absorption rates and providing protection for pharmaceuticals against biochemical degradation. In addition, several other experimental drug delivery systems show exciting signs of promise, including those composed of biodegradable polymers, dendrimers (socalled star polymers), electroactive polymers and modified C-60 fullerenes *(11)*.

1.2. Designing Micro-Particles

Microparticulates are basically designed using polymers or lipids; however, polymeric micro-particles are more popular and are researched extensively. Both biodegradable and non-biodegradable polymers are used to prepare micro-particles and microspheres depending on their application as drug delivery systems and route of administration. Biodegradable polymers have the advantage of controlled degradation in the body, thus avoiding the problem of retrieval (of the ghost carriers) after drug release. Some of the most popular and potential polymers for use in the fabrication of micro-particulate system are summarised as under.

2. POLYMERS USED AND THEIR SELECTION

For the purpose of drug delivery applications, polymers are classified based on the source and biodegradability *in vivo*.

1. Synthetic polymers:
   a. *Non-biodegradable*: Polymethyl methacrylic acid (PMMA), Acrolein, Glycidyl methacrylate, Epoxy polymers, etc.
   b. *Biodegradable*: polylactic acid/polyglycolic acid (PLA/PGA), polyalkyl cyanoacrylate, polyanhydride, etc.
2. Natural polymers:
   a. *Proteins*: Albumin, Gelatin, Collagen, etc.
   b. *Carbohydrates*: Starch, Agarose, Carrageenan, Chitosans, etc.
   c. *Chemically modified carbohydrates*: DEAC cellulose, Polyacryl dextran, Polyacryl starch, etc.

Micro-particles used *in vivo* for drug delivery is not retrievable and so demand biodegradation. In addition, rate of drug release from some of the delivery devices are controlled based on degradation rate of the polymer used. Hence, in this chapter, the discussion is restricted to the biodegradable polymers only.

2.1. Biodegradable Polymers

Early research into biodegradable systems was focused on naturally occurring polymers (collagen, cellulose, etc.) but has recently moved into the area of chemically synthesized polymers also. Examples of such polymers include polyanhydrides, polyesters, polyacrylic acids, poly(methyl methacrylates) and polyurethanes. As a result of extensive experimentation with these materials, several key factors have emerged to help scientists to design biodegradable polymers with varying degradation rate to control rate of release of the loaded drug. Specifically, a fast-degrading matrix consisting of a hydrophilic, amorphous, low-molecular-weight polymer that contains hetero-atoms (i.e., atoms other than carbon) in its backbone has received greater interest. In addition to research on carrier systems composed of single polymeric networks, researchers are also investigating the properties of block co-polymers (networks formed through the joint polymerisation of two or more different monomers) and their potential application as drug carriers.

2.2. Natural Biodegradable Polymers

2.2.1. Chitosan

Chitosan is a natural polymer obtained by the hydrolysis of chitin, a native polymer present in shellfish. Together with chitin, chitosan is considered as second most abundant polysaccharide after cellulose. However, unlike cellulose, the use of chitosan as an excipient in pharmaceutical formulations is a relatively new development. Chitosan is structurally poly(-[1,4]-2-amino-2-deoxy-D-glucopyranose) (Fig. 3) and differs from chitin in that a majority of the *N*-acetyl groups in chitosan are hydrolysed. The degree of hydrolysis (deacetylation) has a significant effect on the solubility and rheological properties of the polymer. The amine group on the polymer has a pK_a in the range of 5.5 to 6.5, depending on the source of the polymer and pH *(12)*. At low pH, the polymer is soluble, with the sol–gel transition occurring at approximately pH 7.0. The pH sensitivity, coupled with the reactivity of the primary amine groups, make chitosan a unique polymer for oral drug delivery applications.

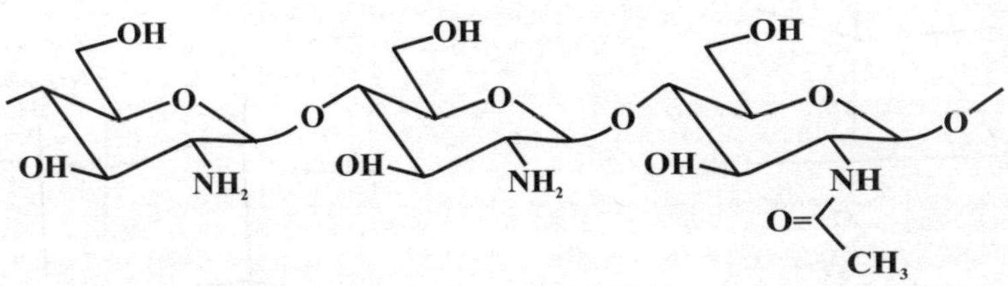

Fig. 3. Chemical structure of chitosan obtained by partial deacetylation of chitin. [Reprinted from Polymer, 37, Payne, GF., Chaubal, MV., Barbari, T. Enzyme-catalyzed polymer modification: reaction of phenolic compounds with chitosan films, 4643–4648, 1996, with permission from Elsevier. *(12)*.]

Chitosan's film forming abilities are well exploited as a coating agent for conventional solid dosage forms such as tablets *(12,13)*. Furthermore, its gel- and matrix-forming abilities make it useful for solid dosage forms such as granules, micro-particles, etc. *(14)*. Crystallinity, molecular weight and degree of deacetylation are the factors that affect release rates from the chitosan-based granules and micro-particles. Combination of positively charged chitosan with negatively charged biomolecules, such as gelatin, alginic acid and hyalouronic acid, has been tested to yield novel matrices with unique characteristics for controlled release of drugs. The pH sensitive nature of chitosan is exploited for colon-specific delivery of the drug like 5-aminosalicylic acid encapsulated in microcapsules *(15)*. It was observed that chitosan capsules disintegrated specifically in the large intestines as compared with the control formulation (in absence of chitosan), which demonstrated absorption of the drug in small intestines. While the mechanism of chitosan disintegration is speculative at this point of time, the excipient has promise for site-specific delivery *(16)*.

Chitosan, due to its cationic nature is also capable of opening tight junctions in between cell membranes. This property has led to a number of studies to investigate the use of chitosan as a permeation enhancer for hydrophilic drugs that may otherwise have poor oral bioavailability, such as peptides *(17)*. Because the absorption enhancement is caused by interactions between the cell membrane and positive charges on the polymer, the phenomenon is pH and concentration dependant. Furthermore, increasing the charge density on the polymer by quaternising the amine functionality on chitosan, would lead to higher permeability. Chitosans are also evaluated as mucoadhesive excipients. Bioadhesivity is often used as an approach to enhance the residence time of a drug in the gastrointestinal (GI) tract, thereby increasing the oral bioavailability. A comparison between chitosan and other commonly used polymeric excipients indicates that the cationic polymer like chitosan has higher bioadhesivity compared with other natural polymers, such as cellulose, xantham gum and starch *(18)*.

2.2.1.1. Derivitatives of Chitosan

While chitosan provides a number of excellent properties, further derivatisation of the amine functionalities can be carried out to obtain polymers with a wide range of properties. A number of approaches, both chemical and enzymatic, have been tried to exploit the reactivity of the amine functional groups *(12)*.

2.2.1.1.1. N-*Trimethylene Chloride Chitosan (TMC)*

A number of studies demonstrated that the charge on chitosan has a role in providing intestinal permeability. A quaternary amine derivative of chitosan, TMC was shown to demonstrate higher intestinal permeability than chitosan alone. The TMC derivative was used as a permeation enhancer for large molecules, such as octreotide, a cyclic peptide. Hamman and co-workers *(19)* showed that the degree of quaternisation of TMC influences its drug absorption-enhancing properties. Polymers with higher degree of quaternisation (>22%) were able to reduce the *trans*-epithelial electrical resistance and thereby epithelial transport (*in vitro*) in a neutral environment (pH 7.4). The maximum reduction in *trans*-epithelial resistance was reached with TMC with a degree of quaternisation of 48%. This degree of quaternisation was also seen to be optimum for *in vitro* transport of model drugs across a human colon adenocarcinoma (CaCO-2) cell monolayer.

2.2.1.1.2. Chitosan Esters

Chitosan esters, such as chitosan succinate and chitosan phthalate have been used to change the solubility profile of chitosan significantly. The modified polymers were insoluble under acidic conditions and provided sustained release of the encapsulated agent under basic

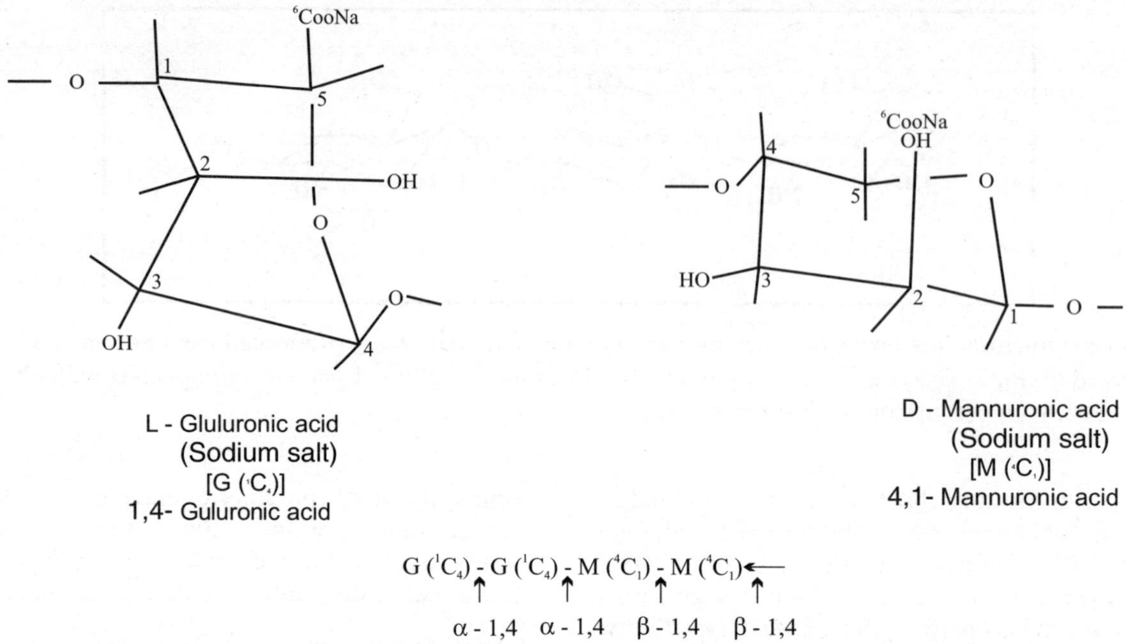

Fig. 4. Structure of sodium alginate.

conditions. The same researchers also synthesised an iron cross-linked derivative of hydroxamated chitosan succinate, as a matrix for oral theophylline beads *(20)*. Chitosan esters were evaluated successfully as potential matrices for the colon-specific oral delivery of sodium diclofenac *(21)*.

2.2.1.1.3. Chitosan Conjugates

Reactivity of the amine functionality can be exploited to covalently conjugate functional excipients to the polymer backbone. For example, Guggi and Bernkop *(22)* prepared a complex of an enzyme inhibitor with chitosan. The resulting polymer retained the mucoadhesivity of chitosan and further prevented drug degradation by inhibiting enzymes, such as trypsin and chymotrypsin. This conjugated chitosan demonstrated a promise for delivery of sensitive peptide drugs, such as calcitonin.

2.2.1.2. Safety and Regulatory Status of Chitosan

Chitosan has been used in multiple nutritional supplement products due to its ability to bind fat. However, no controlled studies have been found that test the safety and tolerability of the polymer. Chitosan has an ability to bind metal ions—a property that has led to the use of chitosan for wastewater treatment. This property may also cause mineral depletion in the GI tract. In addition, vitamin depletion may be a side effect of chitosan *(23)*. According to the documents obtained from the National Toxicology Program, two Type IV Drug Master Files (DMFs) has been submitted for chitosan. The excipient is not listed on the Food and Drug Administration (FDA) Inactive Ingredient Database. In addition, safety and toxicology studies in accordance with the FDA's guidelines for new excipient development would however be desired to further promote the use of this polymer as a pharmaceutical excipient.

2.2.2. Sodium Alginate

Alginate is a naturally occurring polysaccharide commonly derived from brown seaweed. Depending on the source, this linear polymer is composed of different proportions of L-guluronic acid (G) and D-mannuronic acid (M) in variable sequential arrangement *(24)*. It is the sodium salt of alginic acid. The formula is $(C_6H_7NaO_6)_n$ and the structure is shown in fig. 4.

Soluble sodium alginate can be converted to an insoluble form by cross-linking the polymer with polyvalent cations such as dicalcium phosphate. The non-toxic alginates have the potential for many pharmaceutical applications, including the preparation of drug delivery systems *(24,25)*. Drug release from calcium alginate microspheres is generally fast. More than 90% of sulphaguanidine, with aqueous solubility of 1:1000 at 25°C, was released from calcium alginate microspheres within 1 h in dissolution test *(26)*. Co-polymers were used with alginate for controlling the release of water-soluble drugs *(27)*, stomach-irritant drugs *(28)*, site-specific colon targeting *(29)* and for oral delivery of peptides and proteins *(30)*.

Alginate gel micro-particles can be prepared by using different grades of alginates depending on the flow properties. First, a bubble free suspension of drug in sodium alginate solution is to be prepared. The suspension is then required to be added drop wise into $CaCl_2$ solution at room temperature using a peristaltic pump with a polyethylene tubing nozzle and a pumping rate of 1 mL/min. The micro-particles formed in this manner are to be allowed to stand in the 0.1 *M* $CaCl_2$ solution to cure for 12 h. Separate the micro-particles, wash it with distilled water, dry in air for 48 h and then screen through a standard sieve *(31)*.

Sodium alginate is widely applied to food, medicine, textile, printing, dyeing, paper making and dairy chemicals as thickener, emulsifier, stabiliser and binder. It is explored more in food industry especially since 1980s. It is not only a safe food additive, but also a basic material for modeling food or dietary food. As it is a natural cellulose, it can slow the absorption of fatty sugar and bile salts, reduce serum cholesterol and triglycerides in the blood and blood sugar to prevent high blood pressure, diabetes and adiposity, the modern diseases, as well as control the accumulation of noxious metals, such as Sr, Cd and lead. Its importance has been increasingly recognised at home and abroad, and therefore the Japanese call the food rich in sodium alginate as "longevity food", while Americans call it "magic food" additive.

More recently, Murata *et al. (32)* investigated alginate gel bead containing chitosan salt. When the bead was placed in bile acid solution, it rapidly took bile acid into itself. The uptake amount of taurocholate was about 25 μmol/0.2 g dried gel beads. The phenomena was observed in case of the beads incorporating cholestyramine instead of chitosan. From the studies reported, it appears that ion-exchange reaction accompanying the insoluble complex formation between chitosan salt and bile acid occurs in alginate gel matrix.

2.2.3. Chitosan+Calcium Alginate Systems

Cationic amino group of chitosan can react with anionic carboxy terminals in alginate to form micro-particles. However, chitosan has amino groups that are very close to the polysaccharide backbone and so interaction between the charged amino groups of chitosan and carboxylate groups of alginate may be lessened due to steric repulsion between the two molecules. Encapsulation of calcium alginate beads with poly-L-lysine is the most promising encapsulation system.

Chitosan and calcium alginate was used by Huguet *et al. (33)* to encapsulate haemoglobin. One of the methods in making the beads is by adding the mixture of haemoglobin and sodium alginate dropwise to the solution of chitosan and the interior of capsules thus formed hardens in the presence of $CaCl_2$. The other method is where the droplets are directly pulled off in a chitosan–$CaCl_2$ mixture. Both procedures lead to beads containing a high concentration of haemoglobin [>90% of the initial concentration (150 g/L) were retained inside the beads] provided chitosan concentration is sufficient. Likewise, the encapsulation of various molecules (Hb, bovine serum albumin [BSA] and dextrans with various molecular weights) in calcium alginate beads coated with chitosan has been reported *(33,34)*. The ionic interaction between alginate and chitosan is pH dependent and is depicted in Fig. 5.

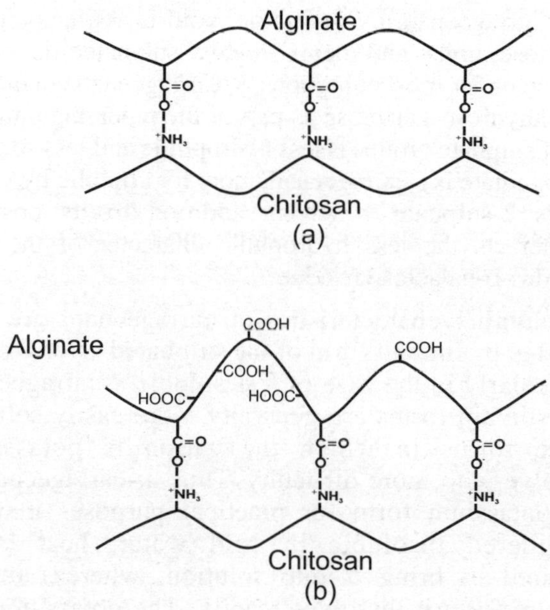

Fig. 5. Schematic representation of the ionic interactions between alginate and chitosan (a) pH 5.4 and (b) pH 2.0.

2.2.4. Carrageenan

Carrageenan is an anionic polymer of hemi-sulphate galactose and 3,4- anhydro galactose residues alternatively linked by α-1,3 and β-1,4 glycosidic linkage. Negative charge is imparted due to the presence of hemi-sulphate group. There are three main types of carrageenan: λ-, κ- and ι-carrageenan.

These types of carrageenan, possible through variation in structural detail provide much variability regarding solubility properties. For practical purposes, however, it is convenient to classify it in terms of several general structural types and to equate solubility with the overall balance of hydrophilicity as provided by the hydrophilic sulphate and hydroxyl groups on one hand and the more hydrophobic 3,6-anhydro-D-galactose residues on the other.

λ-Carrageenan, by definition, void of 3.6-anhydro-D-galactose units and being highly sulphated is easily soluble under most conditions. κ-Carrageenan containing 3.6-anhydro-D-galactose as part of the repeating unit and fewer sulphate groups is less hydrophilic and less soluble. Intermediate is ι-carrageenan, more hydrophilic by virtue of its 2-sulphate which in addition to its position counteracts the less hydrophilic character of the 3.6-anhydro-D-galactose residue.

Solubility characteristics of carrageenans are also affected by the salt form of the sulphated ester groups, particularly in the case of less soluble κ-carrageenan. The sodium forms are generally more easily soluble, while forms in which the cation is potassium, dissolve with more difficulty. Thus, κ-carrageenan in the potassium form for practical purposes may be considered insoluble in cold water, heat being required to bring it into solution, whereas in the sodium form it dissolves readily. The potassium salt of ι-carrageenan is also insoluble in cold water although it swells markedly. λ-Carrageenan is soluble in all its salt forms.

Both the dissolution rate and solubility of carrageenan are affected by the presence of other solutes, the effect mainly being to compete for available water and thus to alter the state of hydration of polysaccharide. Sensitivity to other solutes parallels solubility with κ-carrageenan being the most sensitive to the presence of solutes. Inorganic salts are most effective in altering the hydration of carrageenan, particularly, when the cation is potassium. 1.5–2% potassium chloride is sufficient to prevent the dissolution of κ-carrageenan at normal temperatures while sodium chloride solutions of 4–4.6% and above are also non-dissolving. Considerably higher concentrations of non-ionics are required before similar effects are noted. Sucrose shows little effect on hydration of κ-carrageenan until present in concentrations of 50% and above, while glycerol must be present in very high amounts before appreciable effects are seen. In cases, where more than one solute is present, their combined effect on hydration is generally additive and may be predicted from a knowledge of individual effects. For example, in the presence of high amounts of glycerol, solubility is markedly influenced by traces of potassium ions.

Of practical importance is the fact that κ-carrageenan due to its solubility variation mediated through temperature, ionic concentration is suitable for the preparation of micro-particles. ι-Carrageenan will dissolve with heating in solutions containing relatively high concentrations of salts and thus is able to provide gelation in certain applications.

Being a water soluble polysaccharide, carrageenan is difficult to disperse in water due to the formation of a film layer around each carrageenan particle. This leads to the formation of large agglomerates (lumps), which (due to the protective film layer) are very difficult for the water molecules to penetrate. Hence, less soluble the carrageenan, easier the dispersion, for example, a potassium κ-carrageenan being insoluble in cold water is much easier to disperse in cold water than a sodium κ-carrageenan. Both, however, are soluble in hot water and therefore equally difficult to disperse in hot water. Other factors which decrease the solubility of carrageenan will improve the dispersibility.

In most applications, carrageenan may be pre-blended with other ingredients such as sugar, and in order to achieve complete dispersion, one part of carrageenan should be blended with 10 parts of sugar. In applications where carrageenan cannot be pre-blended with other ingredients, a high speed mixer is necessary in order to break up the lumps formed by adding the carrageenan to the water. Although potassium or calcium carrageenans are insoluble or only slightly soluble, they swell in cold water producing viscous dispersion. Thus, dispersing carrageenan in cold water using a high speed mixer limits the strength of dispersion to approximately 3% depending on the type of mixer.

In hot (60–75°C) water, carrageenan can be dissolved to make 7–8% solution. This on cooling forms lumps, but high speed mixers are available which easily break these lumps. In hot water the carrageenan goes into true solution, and in this state the viscosity is much lower than in the state of hydration. Solubility properties of all the three types of carrageenans in different medium is summarised in Table 2.

Ozsoy and Bergişadi *(35)* used natural polymers such as sodium alginate, pectin, chitosan and carregeenan, as barriers to affect the drug release to formulate sustained release mefanamic acid-beads based on κ-carrageenan in order to reduce daily oral dose and to minimise GI disturbances caused by the drug.

Sankaliya *et al. (36)* prepared papain entrapped cross-linked κ-carrageenan beads for improvement of its stability. A Doehlert shell design (DSD) was employed to investigate the effect of three process variables, namely κ-carrageenan concentration, KCl concentration, and hardening time on the time required for 50% enzyme release (*T[50]*), time required for 90% enzyme release (*T[90]*), and particle size. The beads were prepared by dropping the κ-carrageenan containing papain into a magnetically stirred KCl solution. Beads of spherical

Table 2. Solubility Properties of Three Types of Carrageenans

Medium	κ	ι	λ
Hot water	Soluble above 60°C (140°F)	Soluble above 60°C (140°F)	Soluble
Cold water	Sodium salt soluble, Potassium and calcium salt, insoluble	Sodium salt soluble, Calcium salts gives thixotropic dispersions	Soluble
Concentrated sugar solutions	Soluble hot	Not easily soluble	Soluble hot
Concentrated salt solutions	Insoluble	Soluble hot	Soluble hot

disc shape with a collapsed centre devoid of aggregates were formed with an entrapment of 82.75%. The shelf-life of the enzyme-loaded beads was found to increase upto 3.63 yr compared with 1.01 yr for the conventional formulation. A similar study by the same authors on cross-linked κ-carrageenan beads *(37)* containing α-amylase also showed sustained release of the enzyme from the beads (T[90] of 74.4 min). Shelf-life of the enzyme loaded in the beads was found to increase up to 3.53 yr compared with 0.99 yr of the conventional α-amylase formulation.

The inter-polymeric complexation of carrageenan and chitosan was investigated by Bani-Jaber and Al-Ghazawi *(38)* for its effect on drug release from matrices in comparison to single polymers. Matrices with carrageenan:chitosan (CG:CS) ratios of 100, 75, 50, 25 and 0%, respectively, were prepared at 1:1 drug to polymer ratio with two model drugs: diltiazem HCl (DZ) and diclofenac Na (DS). When tested for dissolution profiles, three dissolution media were used: water, simulated gastric fluid (SGF), and simulated intestinal fluid (SIF). Some combinations of the two polymers showed remarkable sustained release effect on DZ in comparison to the single polymers in water and SGF. With DS, the polymer combinations had similar dissolution profiles to those of the single polymers in water and SIF, which was explained by the lack of chitosan ionisation by the medium or the drug basic salt. The importance of chitosan ionisation for its interaction with CG to have an effect on the release of DS was demonstrated by performing dissolution of SGF presoaked tablets of DS in SIF, which showed an effect of combining the two polymers on sustaining the drug release.

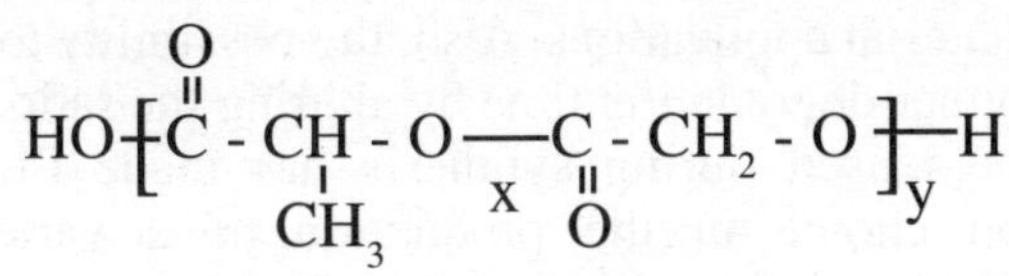

x : Number of Lactic acid units

y : Number of Glycolic acid units

Fig. 6. Structure of PLGA.

2.3. Synthetic Biodegradable Polymers

2.3.1. Poly(Lactic-co-Glycolic Acid)—PLGA

PLGA is an FDA approved co-polymer which is used in a most of therapeutic devices, owing to its biodegradability and biocompatibility. PLGA is synthesised by means of random ring-opening co-polymerisation of two different monomers, glycolic acid and lactic acid. Common catalysts used in the preparation of this polymer include Tin(II) 2-Ethylhexanoate, Tin(II) alkoxides or aluminium isopropoxide. During polymerisation, successive monomeric units (of glycolic or lactic acid) are linked together in PLGA by ester linkages, thus yielding linear, aliphatic polyester.

Depending on the ratio of lactide to glycolide used for the polymerisation, different forms of PLGA can be obtained: these are usually identified by monomer's ratio used (e.g., PLGA 75:25 identifies a co-polymer whose composition is 75% lactic acid and 25% glycolic acid; Fig. 6). All PLGAs are amorphous and show a glass transition temperature in the range of 40–60°C. Unlike the homopolymers of lactic acid (polylactide) and glycolic acid (polyglycolide) which show poor solubility, PLGA can be dissolved by a wide range of common solvents, including chlorinated solvents, tetrahydrofuran, acetone or ethyl acetate.

PLGA degrades by hydrolysis of its ester linkages in presence of water. It has been shown that the time required for degradation of PLGA is related to the monomer's ratio used in production: higher the content of glycolide units, lower the time required for degradation. An exception to this rule is the co-polymer with 50:50 monomers' ratio which exhibits faster degradation (about 2 mo).

PLGA has been as a biodegradable polymer because it undergoes hydrolysis in the body to produce i.e. original monomers, i.e. lactic acid and glycolic acid. These two monomers under normal physiological conditions are by-products of various metabolic pathways in the body. Since the body effectively deals with the two monomers, there is very minimal systemic toxicity associated with using PLGA for drug delivery or biomaterial applications. Also, the possibility to tailor the polymer degradation time by altering the ratio of the monomers used during synthesis has made PLGA a common choice in the production of a variety of biomedical devices. As an example, a commercially available drug delivery device using PLGA is Lupron Depot® for the treatment of advanced prostate cancer.

As the ester bond cleavage is catalysed by protons, PLGA degradation decreases micro-environmental pH and can lead to accelerated polymer degradation (auto-catalysis) *(39,40)*. This phenomenon affects drug stability (especially in the case of protein-based drugs) and also significantly increases the mobility of drug molecules (due to the accelerated decrease in the average of polymer molecular weight), resulting in increased drug release rates. It has recently been shown in a quantitative way that these auto-catalytic effects are of major importance in non-porous, PLGA-based micro-particles *(41)*. Different strategies can be used to avoid/reduce auto-catalytic effects in PLGA-based micro-particles, including a decrease in the length of the diffusion pathways for the acids and bases (reduced micro-particle size) *(42)*, the addition of bases to the formulation *(43)*, and an increase in the mobility of the involved diffusing species by increasing the porosity of the system *(44)*. Using adequate preparation techniques (e.g., water-in-oil-in-water [W/O/W] solvent extraction/evaporation methods), highly porous PLGA-based micro-particles can be obtained. Fan *et al.* also studied the method to prepare highly porous, drug-loaded PLGA-based micro-particles of different size and physicochemically characterised the systems before and upon exposure to phosphate buffer pH 7.4. They also studied the effects of the porosity and size of the micro-particles on the drug release kinetics and polymer degradation behaviour to understand the underlying drug release mechanisms, in particular, the importance of auto-catalytic effects.

2.3.2. Ethylcellulose

Ethylcellulose (EC) microspheres were prepared Dhawan *et al. (45)* by adding the solution of EC in acetone to mineral oil containing an emulgent at high stirring speed for a predetermined time at room temperature. Excess mineral oil was added to the dispersion, filtered and washed the microspheres recovered with petroleum ether to remove the traces of mineral oil and dried.

Micro-particulate systems for sustained release of ketoprofen were prepared using ketoprofen in the form of calcium salt (KP-Ca) and EC. Simple EC micro-particles of KP-Ca (EC-MP) exhibited the fairly rapid release in the first phase with slower release in the late period. For polymer-coated micro-particles of ketoprofen, Eudragit® micro-particles of KP-Ca (ER-MP) were first prepared, and then coated with EC (EC-coat) or with a mixture of carboxymethyl ethylcellulose and EC (CMEC/EC-coat). Some polymer-coated micro-particles showed drug release at nearly zero-order rate, especially, CMEC/EC-coat prepared at a CMEC:EC ratio of 1:1 (w/w). This formulation when administered intraduodenally to rats, showed that plasma concentration of ketoprofen was maintained at a nearly constant level *(46)*.

Li *et al. (47)* prepared EC micro-particles with super-critical CO_2 as the dry medium using an experimental spray drying apparatus and studied the influences of spray nozzle diameter, mass ratio of gas to liquid, solution concentration, temperature and pressure on the physical characteristics of EC micro-particles. The results indicated that the average size of the dried particles ranged from 1.07 to 9.84 μm. The average particle size increased with the increase in ratio of gas to liquid. Also, the average size and distribution of the micro-particles increased with the rise of temperature and solution concentration, but decreased with the increase in pressure *(48)*.

Zandi *et al. (49)* prepared microcapsules containing perphenazine by solvent evaporation using EC of three different molecular weights (mol. wt. = 47,000, 71,000 and 99,000). The drug was dissolved in a polymer solution and emulsified into an aqueous phase to form microcapsules. Covalent bonding of drugs to polymers via hydrolytically or enzymatically cleavable covalent bond was achieved for sustained drug delivery.

Metformin hydrochloride floating microspheres, were prepared and evaluated for *in vitro* release, and optimisation of floatation. Floating microspheres were prepared by non-aqueous emulsification solvent evaporation technique using EC as the rate controlling polymer. In most cases, good *in vitro* floating behaviour was observed and a broad variety of drug release pattern could be achieved by variation of the polymer and solvent ratio, which was optimised to match the target release profile *(50)*.

Salib *et al. (51)* prepared EC coated particles by two relatively recent techniques, namely microencapsulation by phase separation co-acervation, induced by temperature change, and drug entrapment by flocculation, induced by non-solvent addition using chloramphenicol as a model drug. Results of this study revealed the fact that EC proved to be a potential sustained-release coating for oral dosage forms and could help in the design of programmed or timed-release drugs.

Microcapsules of phenylpropanolamine hydrochloride with core: wall ratios of 1:1, 2:1 and 1:2 were prepared by the co-acervation-phase separation method, using EC as the coating material. Two batches of PPA.HCl powder with different particle sizes (>58 μm and <28 μm) were used as the core material. The effects of drug particle size, the media pH and the core:wall ratio on the dissolution kinetics were studied, and evaluated kinetically *(52)*. These microcapsules were also tabletted and dissolution study of both suspended microcapsules and tablets was conducted in simulated gastric and intestinal fluid without enzyme. The dissolution of PPA.HCl was found to be governed by the core: wall ratio, drug particle size, media pH and type of disintegrating agent *(53)*.

Mukherjee *et al. (54)* encapsulated verapamil with EC and cellulose acetate in various ratios of drug and polymer by the hot melt technique and prepared microcapsules were evaluated for size range, drug content, drug release profiles and kinetics of drug release. All the microcapsules were discrete, free flowing and reproducible with respect to size distribution and drug content. The microcapsules of both types having a drug:polymer ratio of 1:1 had the slowest release rate in their respective categories. The drug release data of microcapsules, when examined kinetically, showed to follow Higuchian kinetics.

Singh and Robinson *(55)* prepared captopril microcapsules using four different viscosity grades of EC (core: wall ratios 1:1, 1:2 and 1:3) by temperature induced co-acervation from cyclohexane. *In vitro* dissolution studies in 0.1 *M* hydrochloric acid showed that the drug release was dependent on core to wall ratio, viscosity grade of the EC and the total viscosity of the co-acervation system. Viscosity grade of greater than 100 c.p. was unsuitable for microencapsulation by co-acervation method at concentrations used. Scanning electron microscopy (SEM) showed that the surface of the microcapsules prepared with 10 c.p. viscosity grade (1:2 core to wall ratio) was comparatively more porous with larger pores than 50 c.p. viscosity grade of EC. However, 300 c.p. viscosity grade showed incomplete wall formation.

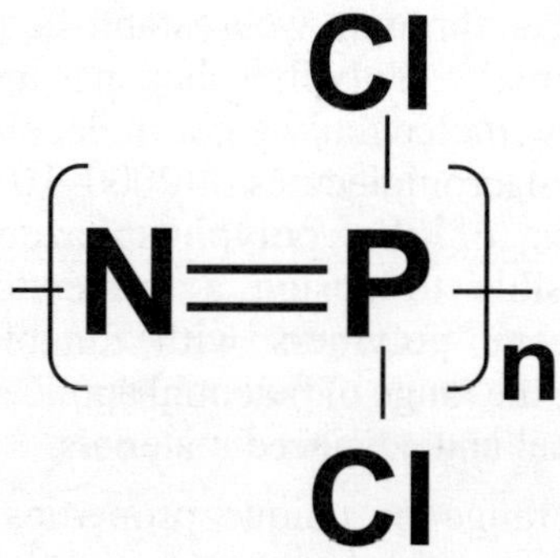

Fig. 7. Polyphosphazene 'backbone' polymer.

EC coating (core:wall ratios 1:1, 1:2 and 1:3) was used to mask the taste and to eliminate odour of phenethicillin potassium micro-particles. Results of the release study *(56)* showed a linear relation between the amount of EC and the time for 60% release of drug, and the release pattern was analogous to that from insoluble porous matrices. Scanning electron micrographs showed the microcapsules to be irregularly shaped with circular surface pores.

Sanjeev *et al. (57)* formulated and evaluated microencapsulated controlled release preparations of diclofenac sodium (DS) using different proportions of EC as the retardant material to extend the release by phase separation-co-acervation. *In vitro* release pattern of the designed microcapsules studied in triple distilled water showed the duration of DFS release from microcapsules to be directly proportional to the proportion of EC and, thus, coat thickness.

2.3.3. Polyphosphazenes

Polyphosphazenes, a unique class of polymers developed in 1960's represent the single largest class of polymers (Fig. 7). They are differentiated from most conventional polymers by their route of synthesis, their synthetic versatility, tunable hydrolytic degradability, high thermal and oxidative stability and broad range of physical, chemical and mechanical characteristics.

Polyphosphazenes consist of an inorganic phosphorous– nitrogen backbone and reactive pendant side groups that may be organic, organometallic or inorganic in nature. Polyphosphazenes are constructed by initially synthesising a polymer backbone called polydichlorophosphazene. The backbone's highly reactive side groups are then substituted with chosen building blocks through well-established methods of organic chemistry. Polyphosphazene molecules can range from low molecular weight molecules of 1–2 KD to very large macromolecules of 2000–10,000 KD. The characteristics of the polyphosphazene backbone make it possible to design a tremendous range of Polyphosphazene polymers with tunable properties. Consequently, the range of potential applications includes both biomedical and advanced materials.

The wide range of unique properties that can be generated from polyphosphazenes has made these polymers the focus of interest for numerous advanced applications, especially where no other polymers exist with the required combinations of characteristics. These applications include several challenging areas of biomedical research, utilisation as ion conductive membranes for re-chargeable polymer lithium batteries and fuel cell membranes, as advanced elastomers for applications in the aerospace engineering, as photonic materials and fire-resistant polymers. Members of our group design the polymer synthesis and characterisation studies, and we then collaborate with specialists in each of the applications areas.

2.3.3.1. Polyphosphazenes in Biomedical Research

A number of polyphosphazenes have been proved to have properties that are particularly important in medical research. These include solid polymers that bioerode to harmless products and which have many advantages as scaffolds for tissue regeneration, macromolecules that form responsive hydrogels and membranes, polymers that serve as microsphere delivery vehicles for drugs and vaccines, and block co-polymers for micelle formation. The following are illustrative examples.

2.3.3.2. Polyphosphazene Scaffolds for Bone Regeneration

Polyphosphazenes can serve as resilient but bioerodible supports for *in vivo* bone regeneration. The strongest emphasis has been placed on polymers that have carboxylic acid function groups that can form ionic cross-links with calcium ions and polyphosphazenes with amino acid ethyl ester side groups that bioerode to phosphate, ammonia, amino acid and ethanol. The phosphate/ammonia combination is a pH-buffered system, which overcomes many of the disadvantages of the polyesters that have been investigated intensively for this application. The fibre matrices seeded with the patient's own osteoblast cells will serve as a support for broken or diseased bones. The polymer erodes hydrolytically as the osteoblast cells multiply and fill the space between the fibres. Eventually the polymer will disappear and be replaced completely by living bone.

Designing polyphosphazenes that hydrolyse at a specific rate and maintain their strength as the erosion process proceeds is a challange. Polymers with different amino acid ester side groups either alone or in combination with hydrophobic co-substituents forms most promising materials which can be used for varieties of drug delivery applications.

2.3.3.3. Membranes and Hydrogels

Polyphosphazenes with alkyl ether side groups, such as– $OCH_2CH_2OCH_2CH_2OCH_3$, are soluble and stable in water. When lightly cross-linked by γ-radiation, they absorb water and swell to hydrogels, but do not dissolve. The hydrogels show a lower critical solution temper-ature (LCST), which means that below a certain temperature they are expanded. Above that temperature they contract and expel the water. The LCST depends on the length, branching and end groups of the side chains. The LCST for several of these hydrogels is near human body temperature which means that, in the form of membranes, they may be used for the stepped delivery of drugs or to control the activity of trapped enzymes or cells. In the expanded state, molecules in solution can reach or leave the enzymes. In the contracted state of the membrane, the activity of the enzyme is curtailed. The behaviour of the membrane can be tuned further by the incorporation of aryloxy co-substituent group that bear carboxylic acid functional units. These hydrogels expand and contract in response to changes in pH, cation charge or the ionic strength of the medium. The possibility of using phosphazene hydrogels in the development as artificial muscles is under investigation.

2.3.3.4. Microspheres

Polyphosphazenes with carboxylic acid functional groups are soluble in water as their sodium salts but insoluble as calcium salts because the divalent cations form ionic cross-links between the chains.

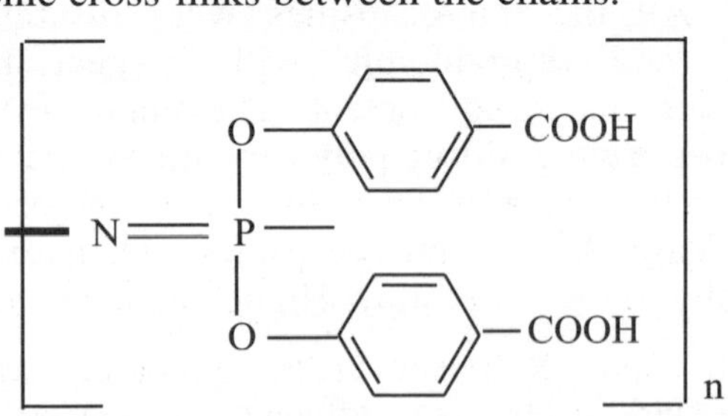

Thus, treatment of solutions of the sodium salt with soluble calcium salts can bring about precipitation of the polymer in the form of microspheres. Biological agents present as co-solutes in the polymer solution will be trapped in the microspheres and will be released in the presence of sodium ions, which decross-link the chains. This phenomenon was first developed for mammalian

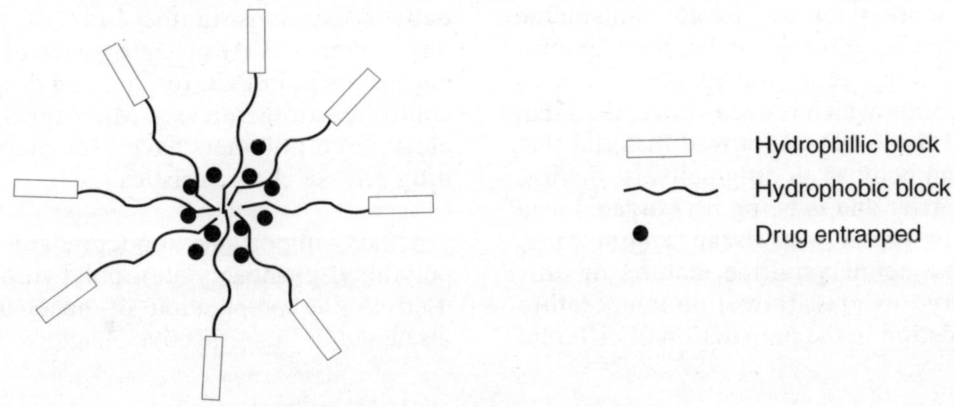

Fig. 8. Polymeric micelle.

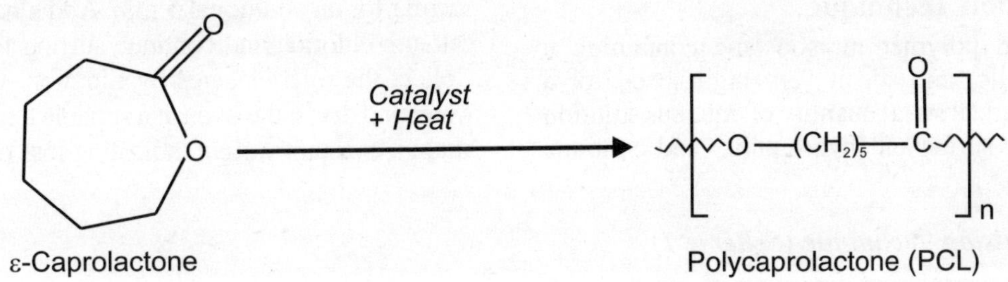

Fig. 9. Ring opening polymerisation of ε-caprolactone to PCL.

cell encapsulation, but it has been utilised specifically for the oral delivery of vaccines.

Polyphosphazene (PP) micro-particles were also prepared by reaction with calcium chloride by adding 2.5% (w/v) polyphosphazene solution as droplet to a 7.5% (w/v) aqueous solution of calcium chloride to form micro-particles in size range of 0.5–1.5 μm. It is also prepared by spraying the PP solution through an ultrasonic spray nozzle at 40 psi pressure to form cloud. The cloud when collides with $CaCl_2$ solution instantaneously gels to form the microspheres. Polyphosphazene microspheres are sensitive to ionic environment and are generally stabilised by coating with positively charged polyelectrolytes like poly-L-lysine.

2.3.3.4.1. Micelles

Phosphazene diblock co-polymers formed via living cationic polymerisation technique can also be designed to show amphiphilic character, with one block hydrophilic and other hydrophobic. Such polymers form nanometer-size micelles in aqueous media, with the hydrophilic block on the outside and the hydrophobic block in the interior (Fig. 8).

This phenomenon is utilised in developing controlled delivery of hydrophobic drugs via the circulatory system. Block co-polymers that have been investigated include species with two different phosphazene blocks, or a phosphazene block and organic polymer or silicone block. The phosphazene block can be hydrophilic or hydrophobic, and may also be bioerodible, for example, with amino acid ester side groups.

2.4. Polycaprolactone

Polycaprolactone (PCL) is a biodegradable polyester with a low melting point of around 60°C and a glass transition temperature of about 40–60°C. PCL can be prepared by ring opening polymerisation of ε-caprolactone using a catalyst such as stannous octanoate (Fig. 9).

This polymer is often used as an additive for resins to improve their processing characteristics and their end use properties (e.g., impact resistance). Being compatible with a range of other materials, PCL can be mixed with starch to lower its cost and increase biodegradability or it can be added as a polymeric plasticiser to Poly Vinyl Chloride (PVC).

PCL is degraded by hydrolysis of its ester linkages in physiological conditions and has therefore received a great deal of attention for use as an implantable biomaterial. In particular, it is especially interesting for the preparation of long term implantable devices, owing to its degradation which is even slower than that of polylactide. PCL is an FDA approved material that is used in the human body as an drug delivery, device, suture, adhesion barrier and is being investigated as a scaffold for tissue repair via tissue engineering. Biocompatible and semicrystalline nature of this polymer with a very low glass transition temperature has led to its application in the preparation of different delivery systems in the form of microspheres and nanospheres. Various categories of drugs have been encapsulated in PCL for targeted drug delivery and for controlled drug release. Microspheres of PCL either alone or co-polymers have been prepared to obtain the drug release characteristics *(58)*.

Other important biodegradable polymers like poly(alkyl cyanoacrylate), polyhydroxy acids, etc. are used in the preparation of nanoparticle and so are discussed in the respective chapters.

3. GENERAL METHODS OF PREPARATION

3.1. Emulsification Technique

Disperse drug and polymer in isooctane containing a surfactant (lipophilic) and stir at very high speed for a period of 10 min. Add a small quantity of aqueous solution containing another surfactant (hydrophilic) and continue stirring for an additional 5 min. Add a hardening agent like calcium chloride and continue stirring for another 10 min. Collect the microspheres by filtration, wash with distilled water and dry in the oven at a sutiable temperature until they attain a constant weight indicating loss of moisture *(59)*.

3.1.1. Single Emulsion Technique (Scheme 1)

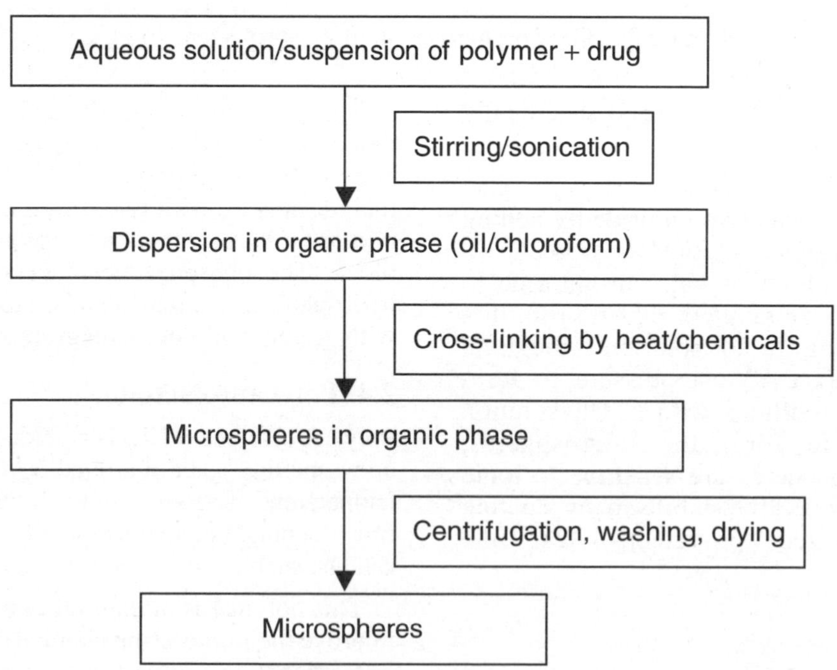

3.1.2. Double Emulsion Technique (Scheme 2)

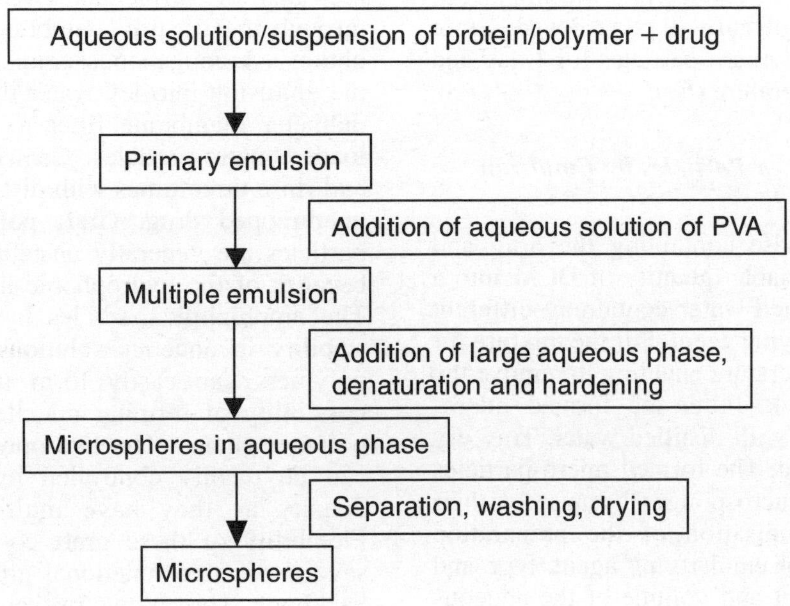

3.1.3. Multiple Emulsion (W/O/W) Process

Micro-particles can be prepared using the W/O/W emulsion technique according to the following procedure *(60)*.

Dissolve PLGA at room temperature in a small quantity of dichloromethane (DCM). Cool it to 4°C. Take Bovine Serum Albumin (BSA) of a suitable strength and sonicate into 1 mL solution of PLGA in DCM for 15 min to obtain the primary W/O emulsion. Vortex this into 10 mL of cooled aqueous polyvinyl alcohol (PVA) solution and prepare W/O/W emulsion. Stir for a sufficient period of time to remove the solvent. Isolate the formed micro-particles by filtration and then wash them with successive quantities of deionised (DI) water. Freeze dry the washed micro-particles. Blank micro-particles are prepared, which are devoid of BSA *(61)*.

Lidocaine-loaded, PLGAbased micro-particles were prepared by a W/O/W solvent extraction/evaporation technique: de-mineralised water was emulsified into a solution of lidocaine and PLGA in methylene chloride using an Ultra-Turrax® (Ika, Germany) at 13,000 rpm. This primary water-in-oil (W/O) emulsion was dispersed within an outer aqueous polyvinyl alcohol solution (0.5% w/w) under stirring with a three-blade propeller for 30 min (2000 rpm), inducing micro-particle formation. The latter were hardened by adding further outer aqueous phase. The particles were separated by filtration and subsequently freezedried to minimise the residual solvents content.

Porous, PLGA based micro-particles were prepared using a W/O/W solvent extraction/evaporation technique with lidocaine as the model drug. A study was conducted by subjecting the particle fractions to various studies. In contrast to non-porous micro-particles of identical composition, the relative drug release rate was found to decrease with increasing system size. All studies showed that the degradation rate of the polymer increased with increasing micro-particle dimension, indicating that autocatalytic effects play an important role even in small and highly porous PLGA based micro-particles. As PLGA based micro-particles are bulk-eroding, acids are generated throughout the devices and diffuse out into the surrounding release medium or human body fluids, where they are neutralised. In addition, bases from the bulk fluid diffuse into the micro-particles, neutralising the generated acids. The diffusional mass transport is relatively slow, especially in polymer based matrices. The rate at which the acids are generated within the micro-particles can be higher than the rate at which they are neutralised. Consequently, the pH within the system can significantly drop *(62,63)*.

3.1.4. Preparation of Micro-Particles by a W/O/O Emulsion-Solvent Evaporation Method

Prepare the polymer solution from PLGA and poly D-lactic acid (PLA) with acetone to achieve a required concentration range. Add the drug previously dissolved in water to provide a final loading in W/W. Mix the drug phase with the organic phase by sonication. Pour the W/O emulsion immediately into light white oil containing lecithin and stir at a high rpm with a low temperature for around 6 h. Harvest the micro-particles by washing with hexane and filter the same with a suitable media. Care must be taken while washing to see that the remnants of the solvent will be removed before filtration. Vacuum dry the micro-particles for 1 day and store at appropriate temperature *(64)*.

3.1.5. Preparation of Micro-Particles by Emulsion Solvent Diffusion Method

Add organic internal phase containing the drug and polymer like EC in a sutiable quantity of DCM into a healthy quantity of distilled water containing different concentrations of emulsifying agent. Stir the mixture for a long time at a low temperature enabling to remove the DCM form reaction flask. Filter the formed micro-particles and wash them with distilled water. Tray dry them at room temperature. The formed micro-particles can also be termed as microsponges because of their characteristics. For optimisation of the preparation method, concentrations of emulsifying agent, type and volume of organic solvent and volume of the aqueous phase can be varied and tested *(65)*.

3.1.6. Melting Emulsion Method

Micro-particles with sizes smaller than 5 μm can be prepared by a melting emulsion method using graft polymers. A suitable quantity of graft co-polymers and a particular amount of drug is to be mixed well. Immerse the mixture in hot water at 80°C with the presence of surfactant Tween-80 and then extrude through a 0.45 μm membrane filter several times to obtain a homogeneous emulsion. Subsequently, inject the emulsion into icy water through the 0.45 μm pore diameter membrane filter to recover the solid drug-loaded micro-particles. Centrifuge the micro-particles and rinse three times with distilled water to remove the unentrapped drug. Graft polymers are used as the particles are generally unstable and tend to aggregate because of the hydrophobic nature of these polymers. The amphiphilic particles have good thermodynamic stability in aqueous solutions. Amphiphilic graft co-polymers can easily form micelles because of the possibility of forming micelles within one or several polymer chains. The hydrophilic/hydrophobic balance can be readily controlled by adjusting the grafting density as they have multigrafted branches *(66)*. Flexibility of these graft co-polymers is that of the several reactive functional groups existing along each backbone. This allows further incorporation of various biorecognisable ligands to achieve the enhanced cell adhesion and recognition. All these properties make amphiphilic graft co-polymers of special interest as biomaterials *(67)*.

3.2. Polymerisation Technique

3.2.1. Suspension Polymerisation (Scheme 3)

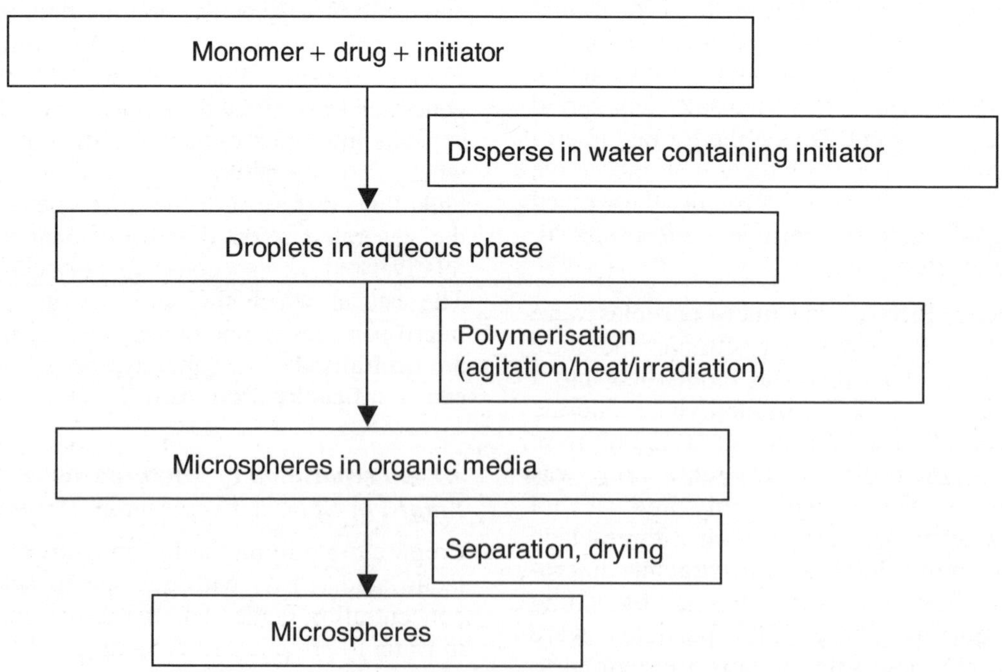

3.2.2. Interfacial Polymerisation (Single Monomer) (Scheme 4)

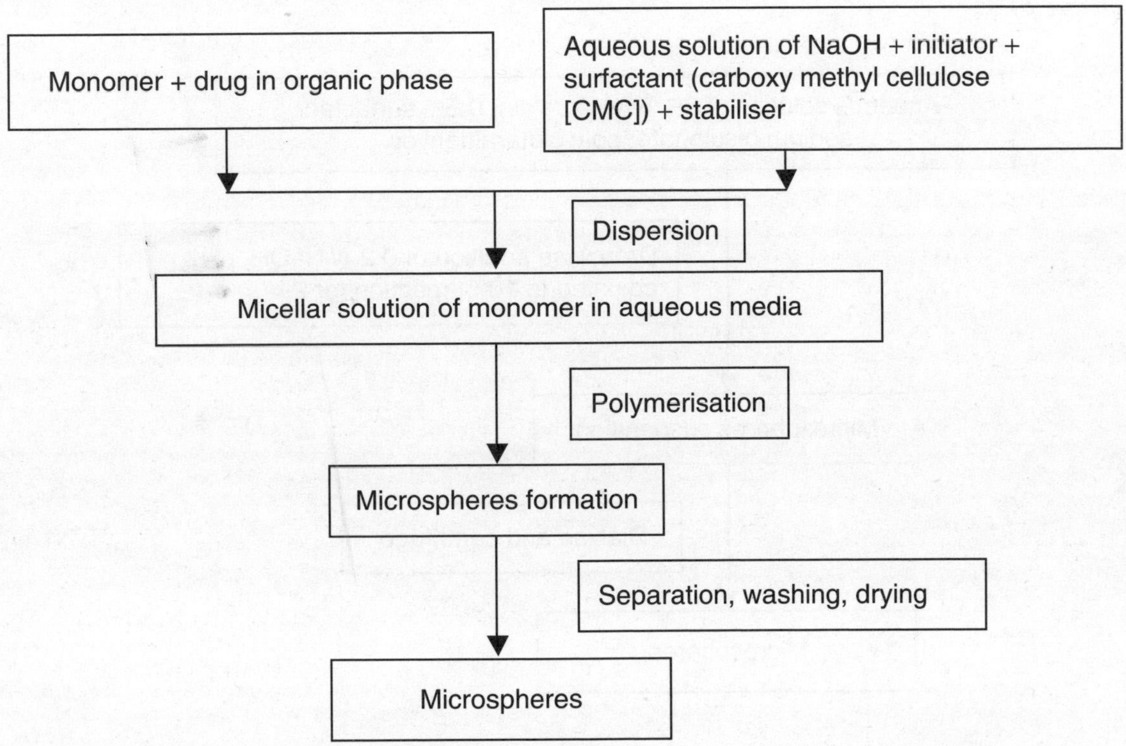

3.2.3. Interfacial Polymerisation (Two Monomers) (Scheme 5)

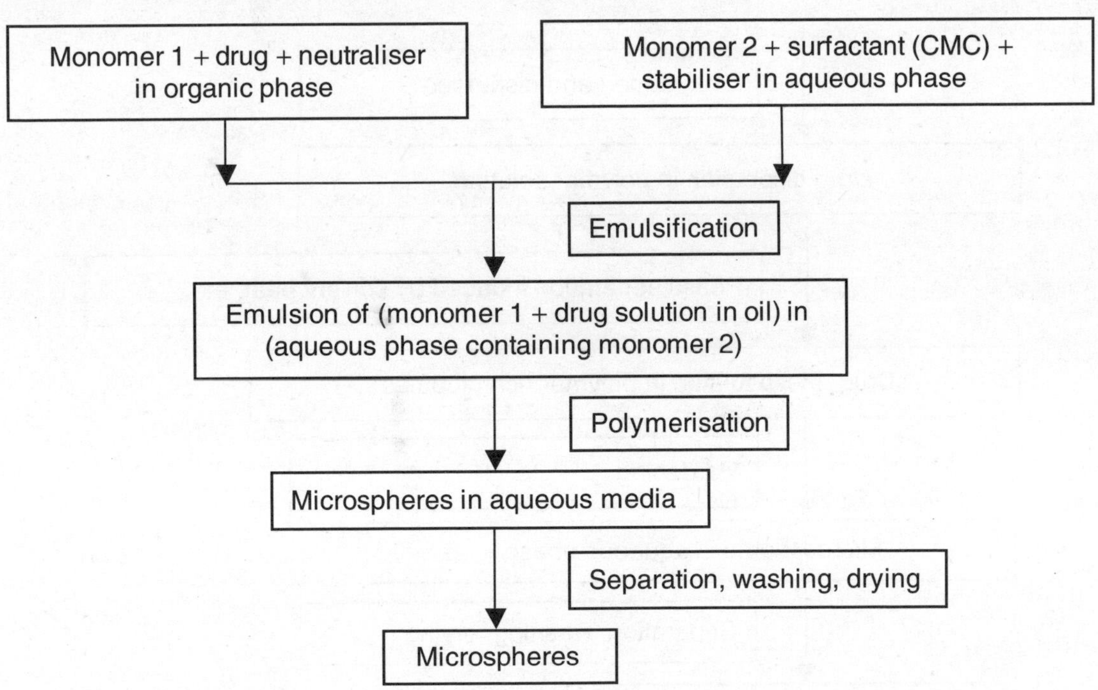

3.2.4. Alkaline Polymerisation (Radical) of One Monomer With Other Monomers: Example Acrolein Microparticles (Scheme 6)

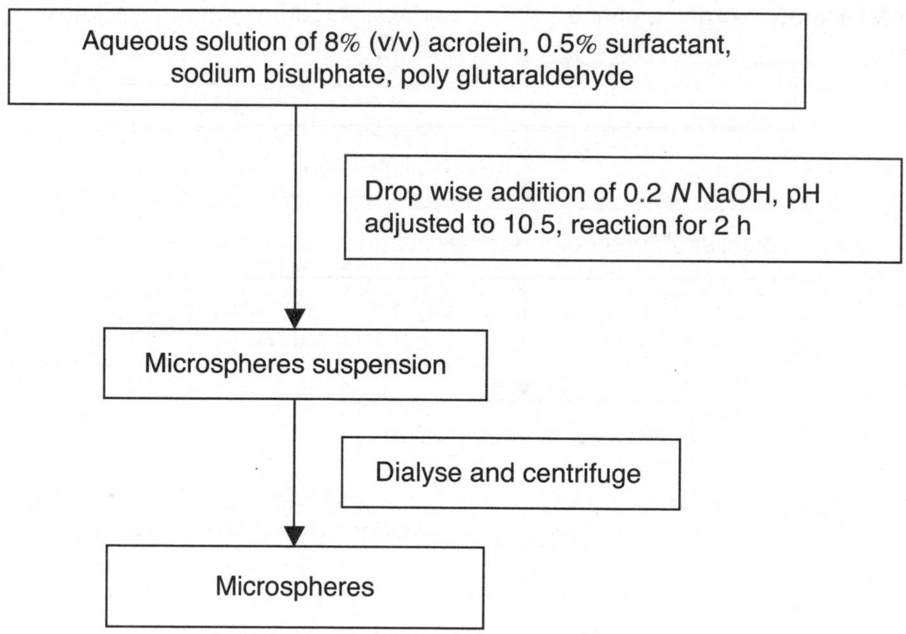

3.2.5. Phase Separation and Co-Acervation Technique (Scheme 7)

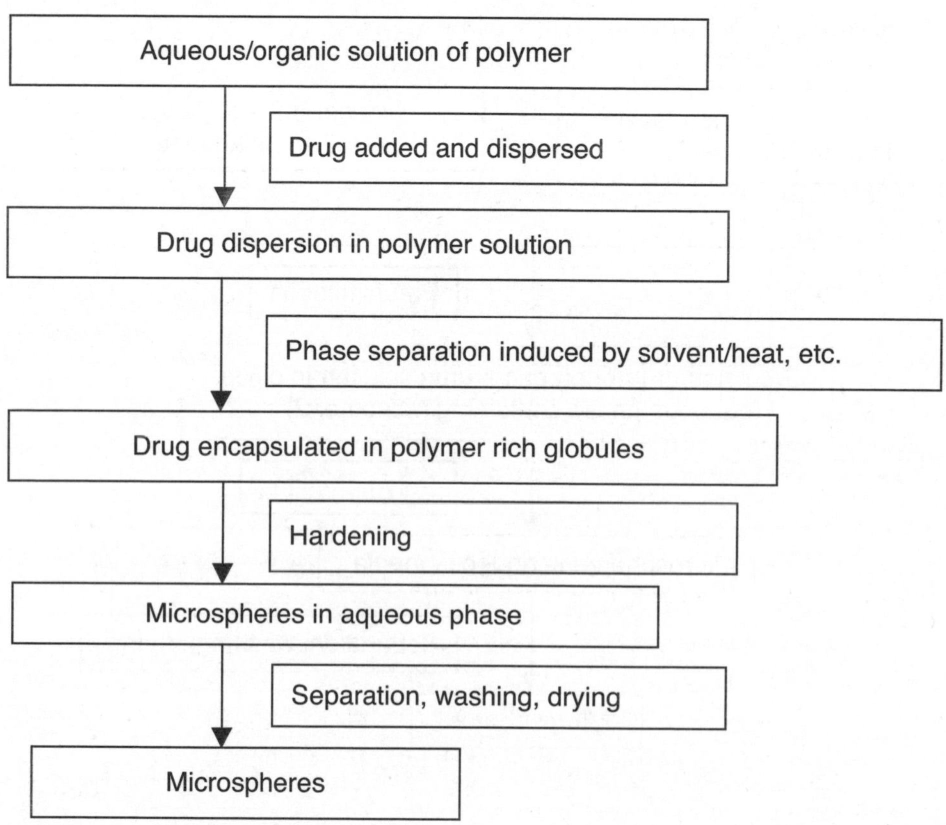

3.2.6. *Organic Phase Separation Process (Co-Acervation)*

Dissolve a polymer in DCM in a glass reactor provided with a glass stirrer. Dissolve an appropriate amount of drug substance in methanol and introduce with stirring to solution of polymer followed by addition of a phase separation inducer (silicon fluid). Soft embryonic microspheres will result from this procedure and can be hardened by transferring into a heptane/water emulsion with ongoing stirring. The formed microspheres are collected on a suitable sintered glass filter and dried. Mannitol can be added prior to the drying step to prevent agglomeration of the formed microcapsules. The formed polymeric particles may be porous in nature and the porosity depends on several factors *(68)*.

3.3. Physical Methods of Preparation

3.3.1. *Spray Drying*

Micro-particles less than 5 μm can be prepared by this method. Dissolve drug in water and add a sufficient quantity of PLGA or poly L-lactic acid in DCM. Sonicate the mixture for a suitable time at a suitable speed using a sonicator. Spray dry the formed emulsion maintaining the inlet temperature, outlet temperature, pump flow rate, aspiration, etc. appropriately. Vacuum dry the resulting micro-particles at the right temperature and store them for further use.

Spray-dried particles can also be prepared by coating with a W/O/W emulsion-solvent extraction method. Spray dried micro-particles with drug are dispersed in sufficient quantity of water and mixed with the solution of PLGA dissolved in ethyl acetate. Sonicate the mixture to form W/O emulsion and pour this into aqueous PVA solution stirred at the set rpm. After 5 min, reduce the stirring rate to a lesser rpm for 30 min allowing the micro-particles to harden. Add a large quantity of aqueous PVA solution dropwise at 3 mL/min to extract the organic solvent. Filter the micro-particles and wash with water. Harvest the particles after vacuum drying for 24 h and store them at appropriate temperature *(64)*.

3.3.2. *Preparation of Micro-Particles by Spray–Coagulation Method*

Spray the polymer solution into calcium chloride solution through a nozzle at a set air pressure. Stir the micro-particles for about an hour, filter and wash them with DI water. Disperse the crosslinked micro-particles in water and freeze them using liquid nitrogen. Lyophilise the frozen micro-particles using a freeze dryer for 48 h. Collect the dried micro-particles and sieve them according to the size. Porosity of the micro-particles can also be checked and studied by varying the concentration of calcium chloride *(69)*.

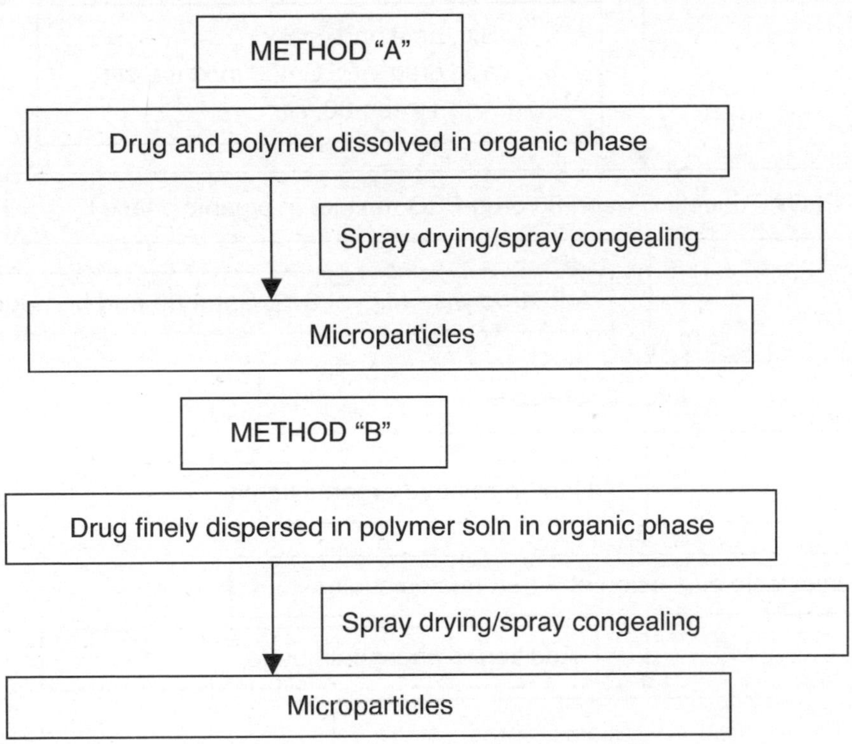

3.3.3. Spray Coagulation Method

A spray–coagulation method was developed for the preparation of large scale of porous alginate micro-particles. The effect of three variables on porosity was evaluated: (1) alginate solution concentration (2) the concentration of $CaCl_2$ in the coagulation medium and (3) the ratio of guluronic acid to mannuronic acid of the alginate. Methylene blue (MB), a highly water-soluble compound and a practically water-insoluble compound, 4-phenylazoaniline (PAA) were used as the model drugs to study drug loading and release characteristics from alginate micro-particles. The release of the model compounds from the micro-particles was found to depend upon the release medium. Incomplete *in vitro* release of both model drugs in DI water was observed. The release of MB in simulated GI fluid (0.1 *N* HCl) was fast and complete, while the release of PAA was slow in 0.1 *N* HCl and fast in phosphate buffer solution (pH 6.8) *(69)*.

3.3.4. Solvent Extraction Method (Scheme 9)

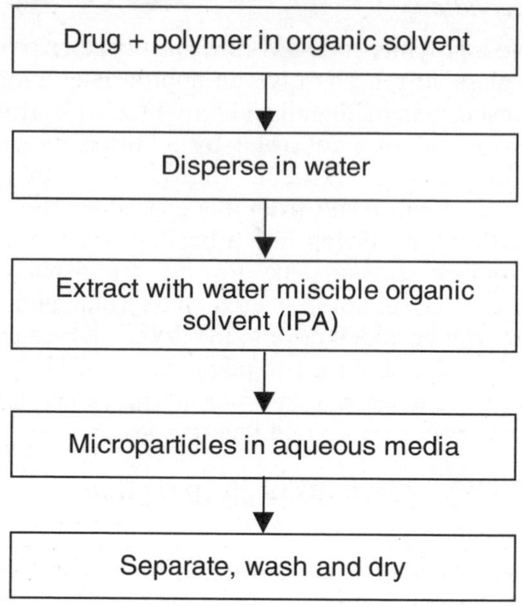

Examples:

3.3.4.1. Method to Prepare PLGA Microspheres (Scheme 10)

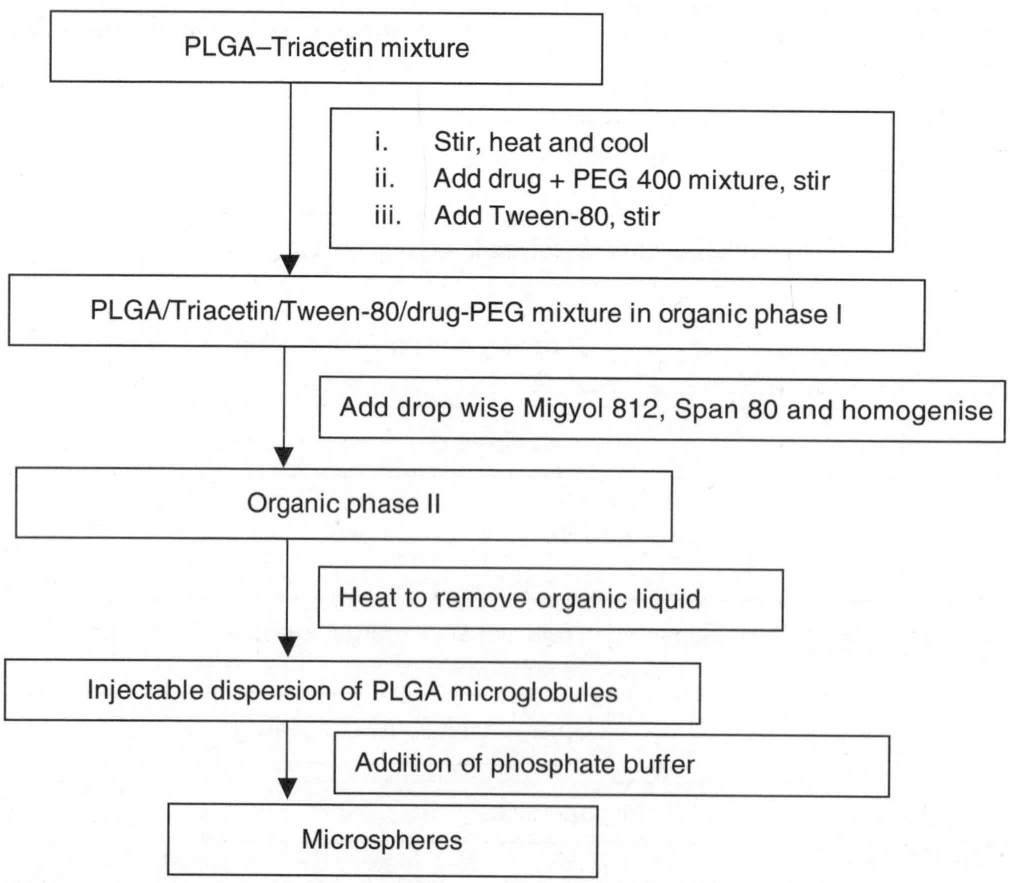

3.3.4.2. Dextran Microspheres (Scheme 11)

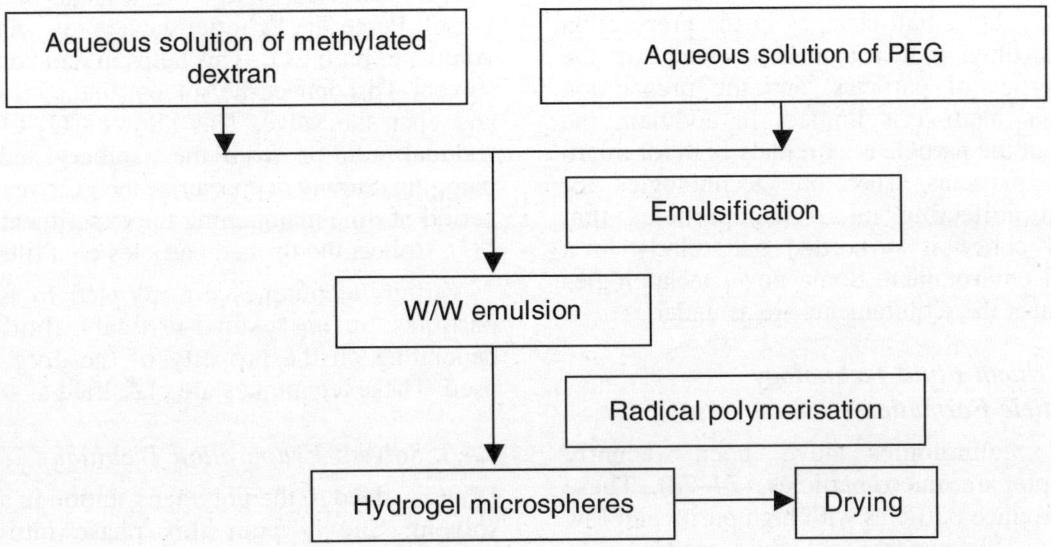

3.3.4.3. PLGA Double-Walled Microspheres (Scheme 12)

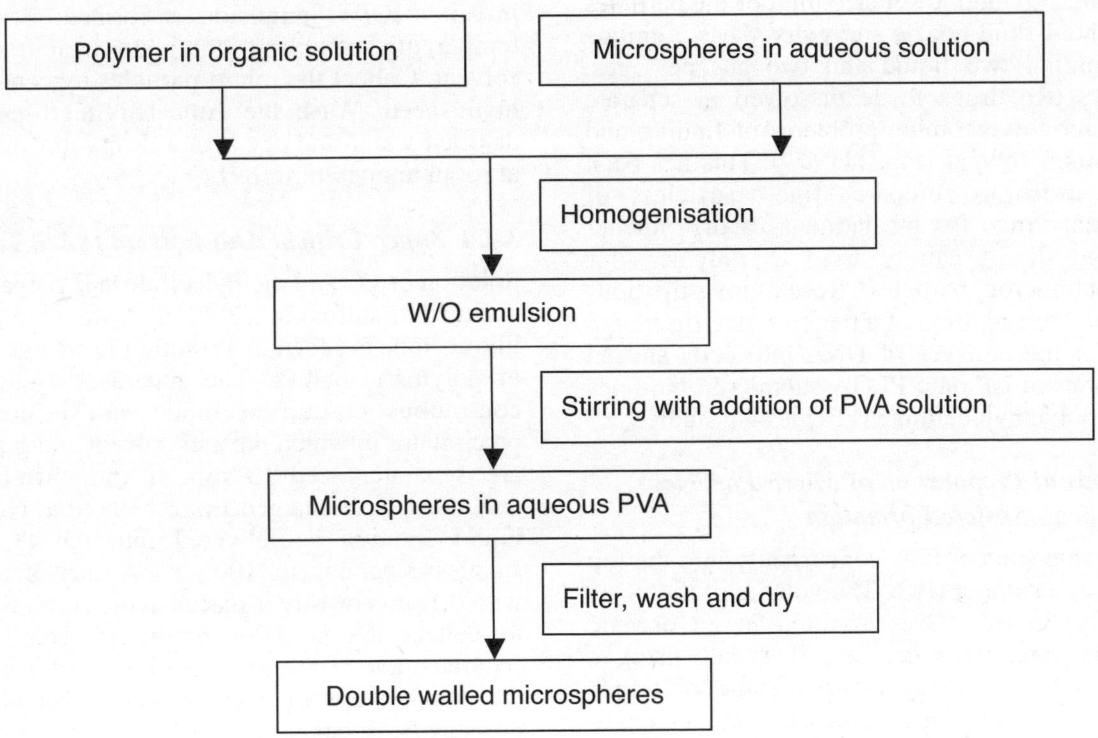

3.4. Some Special Methods of Production of Micro-Particles

Traditional methods for the production of particles include pulverisation of large particles using a ball or jet mill, and solidification of emulsions by in-water drying methods. The first method is often used to improve the solubility of water insoluble drugs. The dry grinding method may be limited to the preparation of particles down to several microns in diameter. Although the preparation of particles down to several hundreds of nanometers in diameter may be possible with wet grinding method *(70,71)*, IT requires a large amount of co-grinding agents or surfactants, and the products are usually supplied as a suspension in which the solvent remains. These products are also susceptible to contamination by particles of ground metal. The second method can prepare particles from one to several hundreds of nanometers in diameter *(72,73)*, but small changes in the preparation conditions may often induce a marked change in the physical properties of particles, and the preparation scale using this method is limited. In addition, the surface energy of the particle is extremely high for micro and nanoscale particles. Therefore, technologies for preparing and collecting micro-/nanoparticles that avoids mutual cohesion is needed particularly in a pharmaceutical environment. Some novel technologies developed to meet the requirements are as under.

3.4.1. Super-Critical Fluid Technology for Micro-Particle Formation

Super-critical technologies have been recently employed to prepare micro-particles *(74–78)*. These technologies produce particles with high purity and low surface energy. This supercritical fluid technique is suitable for preparing particles of several microns, but is limited by the scale of preparation, the solubility of compounds in CO_2, and lower size limit of the particles produced. The 4-fluid nozzle spray dryer has a unique nozzle containing two liquid and two gas passages, which allows two drugs to be dissolved in separate solvents, thereby overcoming problems of finding and using a common solvent (Fig. 11) *(79)*. This has been previously used to prepare fine particles of pharmaceutical drugs for inhalation as a dry powder *(80)*. EC and PLGA can be used as polymers for producing submicron particles. Recent investigations have examined the addition of a positive electric charge to carriers for the delivery of DNA into cells and an attempt to prepare cationic PLGA submicron particles loaded with polyethyleneimine (PEI) is also studied.

3.4.2. Methods of Preparation of Micro-Particles by SuperCritical Particle Formation

CO_2 and organic solvent flow concurrently into the top of precipitation chamber (PC). The volume of the PC is approximately 80 mL. Drug solution in an organic solvent is delivered at a constant flow rate using a metered pump. Using a spray nozzle, organic solution is allowed to enter the PC. Deliver the CO_2 anti-solvent to the PC at the desired operating temperature and pressure using a digitally controlled high pressure syringe pump. The flow rate of CO_2 can be controlled using a back pressure regulator on the outlet line of the PC. To prevent the freezing due to CO_2 expansion, the regulator can be heated by hot water circulation. The temperature of the PC can be controlled using strip heaters attached to the sides of the vessel. The temperature inside the PC and the pressure is monitored *(81)*.

Allow CO_2 to flow through the PC and when the flow rate is stabilised, spray the organic solution into the vessel. Purge the PC after each spray with 1 equivalent volume of pure CO_2. This helps in removing any residual solvent. Disconnect the solvent line after the final purge and open the valve. This allows CO_2 to push out any residual solution from the capillary and thus prevent plugging. Slowly depressurise the PC over a considerable period of time maintaining the experimental temperature *(81)*. Collect the formed particles on a filter.

Various techniques are adopted to prepare micro-particles using super-critical fluid technology depending on the property of the drug and polymers used. These techniques are classified as under.

3.4.3. Solvent-Evaporation Technique

Drug is added to the polymer solution in a super-critical solvent. Slowly pour this phase into the aqueous solution of the polymer that acts as an emulsifying agent. Stir with a two baffled rotator for a sufficient period of time at high speed. Then stir gently till oil-in-water (O/W) emulsion is formed. Bring to room temperature enabling complete evaporation of the solvent. Collect the micro-particles by centrifugation at high speed. Wash the collected micro-particles with distilled water and dry it in a desiccator under vacuum at room temperature *(82)*.

3.4.4. Super-Critical Anti-Solvent (SAS) Technique

Solution of EC and methylcellulose is prepared in DCM + dimethyl sulfoxide (DMSO). A water soluble solvent like acetone is added to a solution to change the porosity of polymeric matrix. The apparatus used works in a continuous co-current mode and it consists of a precipitator in which the anti-solvent and liquid solution are separately fed to top of the chamber and are continuously discharged from the bottom (Fig. 10). The liquid solution is delivered into the PC through a stainless steel nozzle (100 μm). A filter of sintered steel with 0.1 μm porosity is placed at the bottom of the vessel to collect the particles produced. The solvents are separated and recovered from a second vessel. Usually the temperature of the vessel is around 15°C and pressure 5–10 bar.

3.4.5. SuperCritical Impregnation Process

The impregnation is performed in a semi-continuous apparatus described schematically in Fig. 11.

A tubular batch extraction cell is initially loaded with the pharmaceutical compound and packed between a sequence of a filter paper, cotton and net metallic discs that work as filters of small particles. The

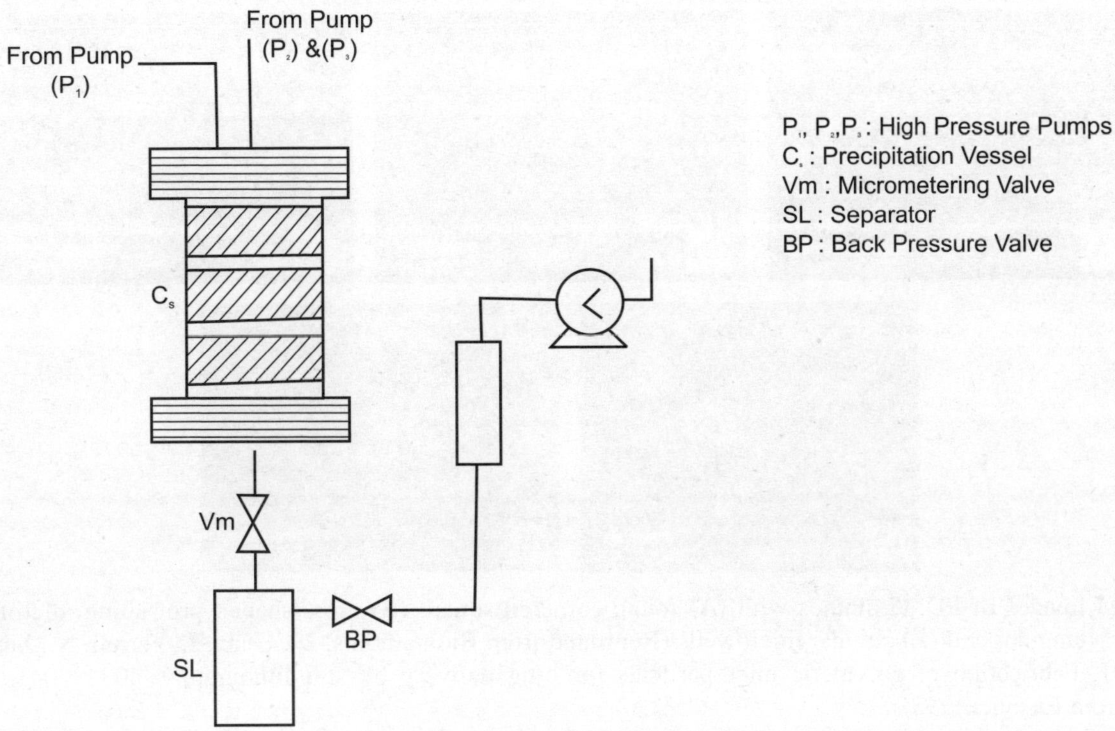

Fig. 10. SAS Apparatus.

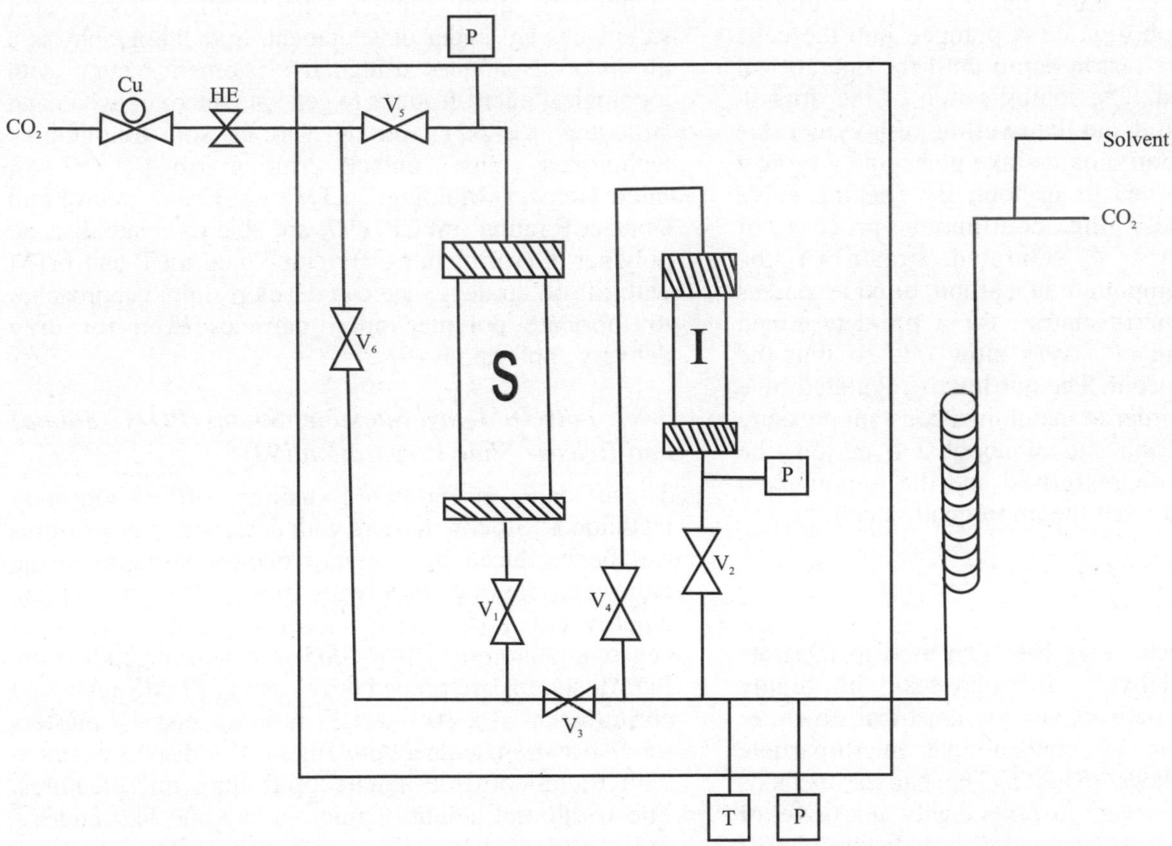

Fig. 11. Schematic representation of the impregnation apparatus.

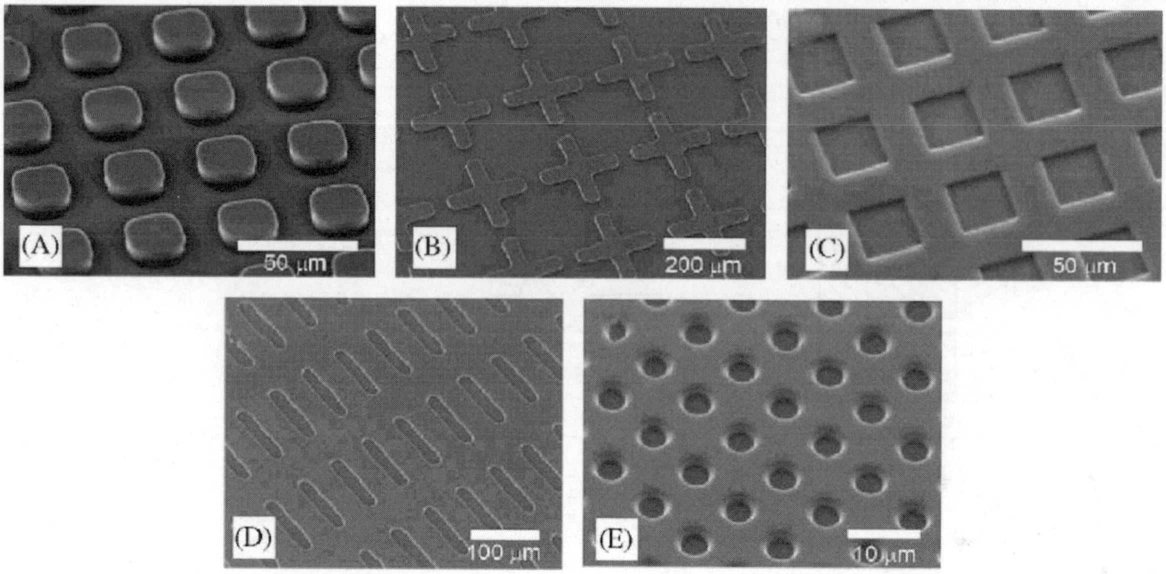

Fig. 12. SEM images of PDMS stamps with **(A)** round-cornered square **(B)** cross-shaped protruding microfeatures **(C)** square, **(D)** rectangular and **(E)** circular microwells (Reprinted from Biomaterials, 27, Guan, J., Ferrell, N., James Lee, L., Hansford, DJ. Fabrication of polymeric microparticles for drug delivery by soft lithography, 4034–4041, 2006, with permission from Elsevier.) *(93)*.

polymer is loaded, in same manner, in the impregnation cell. The cells are then immersed in a thermostated water bath heated to a suitable temperature. Carbon dioxide is pumped into the cells using high pressure piston pump until the operational pressure is attained. The solubilisation of the drug in the supercritical fluid and the swelling of polymer due to presence of carbon dioxide take place and a typical equilibrium is attained in an hour. By opening valve between the cells, the continuous process of impregnation starts. A saturated stream of the pharmaceutical compound in carbon dioxide passes through the polymeric matrix, for a pre-determined period of time and at a very slow rate so that the impregnation can occur. The outflow is regulated by a metering valve in order to maintain a constant pressure in the system. At the end of about 2 h period, the system is quickly depressurised and the impregnated sample is collected from the impregnation cell.

3.4.6. Preparation of Micro-Particles by Soft Lithography Technique

Microfabrication technology has been used to fabricate particulate drug delivery microdevices with highly uniform sizes, well-defined, and asymmetrical structures that are impossible by conventional micro-particle manufacturing methods *(83–85)*. The current methods described here, however, involve highly corrosive or etching solutions, toxic solvents, ionising radiation, plasma etching and/or elevated temperatures. A limiting factor in using these techniques may be the involvement of high cost of materials, facilities and practicability of the technology even though, many other lower cost techniques are under development. Soft lithography is a group of techniques using an elastomeric stamp with topological micro-features to generate micro or even nano structures *(86–92)*. Among various soft lithographic techniques, microContact Printing (mCP) *(87,88)*, microTransfer Molding (mTM) *(89)* and microFluid Contact Printing (mFCP) *(90)* are able to create discrete polymer microstructures. By combining mCP and mTM with lift-off strategy, one can develop simple approaches to fabricate polymer micro-particles even for drug delivery applications *(91)*.

3.4.7. Poly(DiMethyl Siloxane) Stamp (PDMS Stamp) and Release Slide Preparation (93)

These can be prepared using soft lithography techniques. Silicon masters with designed microfeatures can be produced by standard photolithography using either chrome or transparency masks. The process can employ either positive photoresist (Shipley S1813) or negative photoresist (SU8-2005) for pattern production. PDMS stamps are prepared by casting PDMS resin and curing agent at a 10:1 weight ratio against the masters for 48 h at room temperature. Figure 13A displays a stamp with round-cornered square protruding microfeatures. The width and height of micropillars are 24.7 and 6.5 µm, respectively. The centre-to-centre distance between the adjacent microfeatures is 40 µm in the

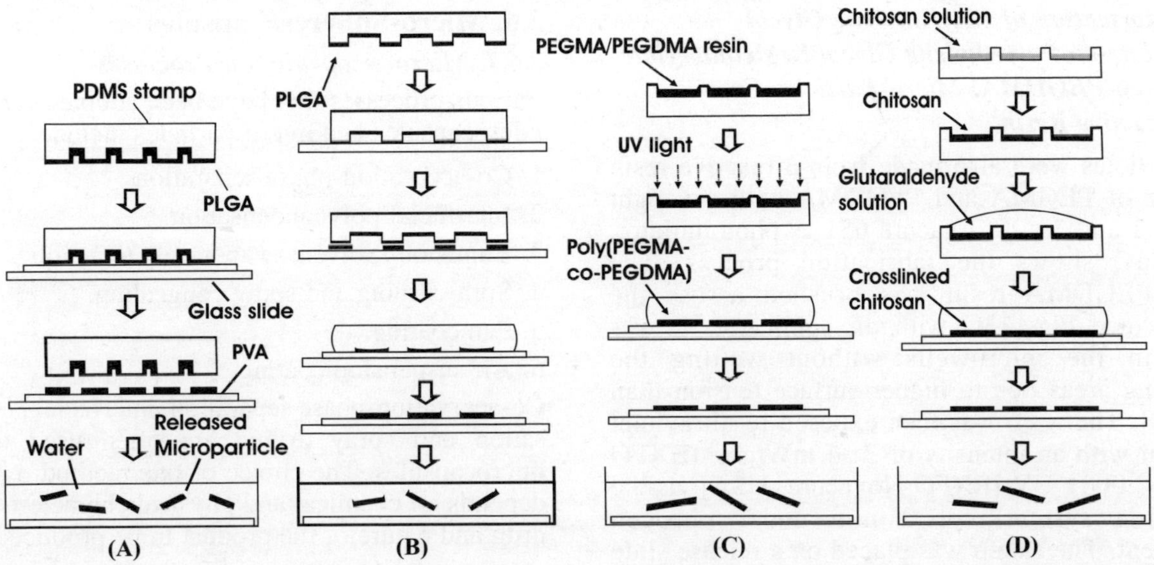

Fig. 13. Schematic illustrations of processes for the fabrication of PLGA micro-particles using stamps with **(A)** protruding and **(B)** recessed microfeatures, respectively, **(C)** poly(PEGMA-*co*-PEGDMA) micro-particles from liquid reactive resin and **(D)** chitosan micro-particles from aqueous polymer solution (Reprinted from Biomaterials, 27, Guan, J., Ferrell, N., James Lee, Hansford, DJ. Fabrication of polymeric microparticles for drug delivery by soft lithography, 4034–4041, 2006, with permission from Elsevier) *(93)*.

prepared slides. A stamp with cross-shaped protruding microfeatures is shown in Fig. 13B. The microfeatures had an end-to-end length of 197 μm, arm width of 40 μm, and height of 6.8 μm. Figure 13C shows a stamp consisting of 30 μm wide, and 1.22 μm deep square recessed microfeatures, or microwells, separated by 20 μm-wide ridges. Figure 13D shows a stamp bearing rectangular microwells 95 μm long, 20 μm wide and 6.9 μm deep. The last stamp was an array of circular microwells with 5.0 μm-diameter opening, 3.5 μm-diameter bottom, 8.0 μm centre-to-centre distance and 1.94 μm depth as shown in Fig. 12E. Release slides fabricated provide a substrate, which released the fabricated particles into water following fabrication. The slides are prepared casting a 2%wt polymer/water solution on a standard glass slide.

3.4.8. Fabrication of PLGA Micro-particles Using Stamps

Figure 13A illustrates the process for the fabrication of PLGA micro-particles using stamps with protruding microfeatures shown in Fig. 13A and B. First, the stamp is immersed in a PLGA/acetone solution for 30 s and pulled out at a speed of approximately 1 cm/s. Low concentration solutions of PLGA formed isolated structures on the microfeatures, while higher concentrations formed a continuous PLGA film. The stamp was dried in air for about 20 s and placed on a release slide. After maintaining the contact for about 20 s, the stamp was peeled away, leaving the PLGA micro-particles on release slide. Water was then added to release the micro-particles. The printing temperatures used were 80°C for a 5 wt% and 120°C for a 7 wt% solution, respectively.

3.4.9. Fabrication of Chitosan Micro-Particles Using Stamp

The chitosan solution was brushed across the stamp surface (Fig. 13D) with an applicator. The solution was trapped in the discrete microwells due to discontinuous dewetting. Water in the solution evaporated immediately, leaving a chitosan film at the bottom of microwells. Glutaraldehyde aqueous solution (50 wt%) was added on the PDMS stamp to cross-link the chitosan in the microwells for 10 min. The sample was then rinsed with DI water and dried in air. To transfer the chitosan microstrips from the microwells, the stamp was placed on a release slide immediately after (<5 s) the slide was briefly (~5 s) exposed to water vapor from a 90°C water bath. A solid weight was set on the PDMS stamp to generate a pressure of approximately 30 kPa for 5 min. The stamp was then peeled away with the microstrips stuck to the release slide. Water was added to release the microstrips from the PVA film.

3.4.10. Fabrication of PolyEthylene Glycol Methacrylate-co-Polyethylene Glycol DiMethacrylate (PEGMA-co-PEGDMA) Micro-Particles From Liquid Reactive Resin

Micro-particles were also made from a reactive resin consisting of PEGMA and PEGDMA with a weight ratio of 1:1 and 3 wt% Irgacure 651 as photoinitiator. Figure 26C shows the fabrication process. The PEGMA/PEGDMA resin was brushed across the stamp surface Fig. 13C with an applicator. It was trapped in the microwells without wetting the surrounding areas due to higher surface tension than the PDMS. The resin was then exposed to ultraviolet (UV) light with an intensity of 31.4 mW/cm^2 (EXFO Novacure 2000® UV [EXFO Novacure, USA]/visible spot curing system) for 2 min under nitrogen environment. The stamp was placed on a release slide immediately (<5 s) after the slide was briefly (~5 s) exposed to water vapor from a 90°C water bath. The stamp and slide were then maintained on the hot plate at 100°C for 1 min. After they cooled down to room temperature, the stamp was peeled off, leaving the micro-particles on the slide. Finally, the micro-particles were released by adding water.

3.5. Specialised Micro-Particulate Systems

3.5.1. Solid-Lipid Micro-Particle Preparation

Solid-Lipid Micro-Particle (SLM) were obtained by O/W emulsification employing the phase inversion technique *(94,95)*. It requires use of a lipophilic component (Compritol®) and an emulsifying agent (Poloxamer®). Heat the lipophilic component and the surfactant to 100°C. Add this and hot purified water at the same temperature slowly to the oily phase. Prepare emulsion using a suitable mixer at a very high rpm for a specified period of time. The time allowed for mixing can be varied and tried for a better emulsion. This depends on the constituents of the mixture. Cool the obtained emulsions at room temperature under magnetic stirring until solidification of the micro-particles occurs *(96)*.

3.5.2. Solid Lipid Micro-Particle Lyophilisation

Select a formulation on the basis of particle size and continue the modification of the particles obtained. Aliquots of solid lipid micro-particles (SLM) are selected. Freeze rapidly in an ethanolic bath at negative temperatures for 10–15 min. Carry out lyophilisation at negative temperatures for more than a day in Heto Holten apparatus (Heto, Denmark) *(96)*.

3.6. Micro-Spheres/Capsules

3.6.1. Microencapsulation Processes

Various processes that have been adopted for preparing microcapsules and micro-particles include:

1. Co-acervation-phase separation.
2. Interfacial polycondensation.
3. Emulsion /Solvent evaporation technique.
4. Spray drying and spray congealing.
5. Pan coating.
6. Air suspension coating.

Co-acervation-phase separation, interfacial polycondensation and spray drying are often used to prepare microcapsules. The choice of one method over another depends on chemical and physical characteristics of the drug and nature of the product to be produced *(97)*.

3.6.1.1. Co-Acervation Phase Separation Technique (98)

This is one of the oldest techniques of preparing micro-particles. The phenomenon is based on the properties of colloids to separate into colloid rich and colloid poor regions just before coagulation, at which point it can be made to coat the core material. The method basically involves three steps:

Step I: formation of three immiscible chemical phases.
Step II: deposition of coating around the core.
Step III: rigidisation of the coat.

Step I: Formation of three immiscible chemical phases

This step involves formation of three distinct chemical phases, namely, the liquid manufacturing phase (which is the solvent for the coating material), the core material phase (which is insoluble in the solvent) and the coating material phase (which is made by inducing separation of the polymer from the solvent). The drug or core material is dispersed in the liquid manufacturing phase which consists the dissolved coating material (polymer or colloid) and then the colloid is made to separate out into the third phase by means of a suitable phase separation-*co*-acervation technique like: (i) temperature change, (ii) salt addition, (iii) incompatible polymer addition, (iv) non-solvent addition and (v) polymer-polymer interaction.

During this process, the solvent becomes poorer while the core material becomes richer with respect to the coating material. Thus, during co-acervation, the colloidal dispersion of the polymer separates into colloid-rich and colloid-poor regions, provided the co-acervation-inducing conditions are carefully controlled.

Step II: Deposition of coating around the core

The phase separated polymeric coating material deposits around the core material, provided the interfacial tension of coat is less than that of the core. The rate of deposition can be controlled by controlling the mixing conditions like viscosity, speed, temperature, etc.

Step III: Rigidisation of the Coat

The coat is rigidised by desolvation, thermal or cross-linking techniques to make it resistant to thermal, physical and mechanical shocks.

Based on the number of coating polymers involved, co-acervation techniques can be classified as simple (single polymer) or complex (two or more polymers). Simple co-acervation is based on thermal change, desolvation, salt addition, incompatible polymer addition techniques whereas complex co-acervation usually involves polymer–polymer interaction, most often by charge neutralisation of oppositely charged colloids, for example, gelatin and acacia. In both processes, two-solution phase formation begins with the colloidal species aggregating to form sub-microscopic clusters which coalesce to form microscopic droplets which are then finally recovered as micro-particles.

3.6.1.1.1 Techniques of Phase Separation and Co-Acervation

Co-acervation is induced by subjecting the biphasic system to conditions which bring about coalescence of the polymer by withdrawing the solvent away from colloidal particles under controlled conditions. If the rate of withdrawal is too fast, the colloid tends to precipitate rather than coalesce. Hence, phase diagrams are used to identify various regions and exact conditions for bringing about phase separation-*co*-acervation. Co-acervation is usually marked when the concentration of polymer is less than 3% and can be detected as haziness or cloudiness in the clear colloidal dispersion. Also, the process has to be carried out above the gelation temperature of colloid. If the co-acervation occurs around a single drug particle, a mononuclear microcapsule will be formed and if it occurs around multiple particles, a multinuclear product will be formed.

The techniques by which separation can be induced include addition of non-solvent, change in temperature, addition of salt or addition of incompatible polymer.

3.6.1.1.2 Non-Solvent Addition

This method is widely used for hydrophilic colloids in which, the water associated with polymer is removed by adding a solvent that is miscible with, and has a greater affinity for water but is a non-solvent for the polymer. For example, acetone, ethanol or methanol are all non-solvents for gelatin and can bring about coalescence. This phase separation will be visible in terms of haziness or cloudiness. But if the non-solvent is added at a fast rate or too much in excess, it will cause precipitation rather than separation of the polymer *(99)*.

Other examples include acetone for agar and methylcellulose, isopropyl alcohol for pectin. The method can also be applied to lyophilic colloids. For example, isopropyl ether acts as the non-solvent for cellulose acetate butyrate dissolved in methyl ethyl ketone. Similarly, for solutions of EC dissolved in various organic solvents, various non-solvents can be used, for example, chloroform for petroleum ether, ether for heptane, benzene for corn oil, ethyl acetate for liquid paraffin, DCM for *N*-hexane, etc. Graves *et al. (100)* prepared EC microcapsules containing bovine insulin with cyclodextrins by co-acervating a solution of EC in DCM with *N*-hexane. Briefly, 900 mg of EC was dissolved in 20 mL DCM. *N*-hexane was added drop-wise to the resulting dispersion to induce phase separation and co-acervation. Stirring was continued for 1 h to harden the particles that were then air dried for 24 h, followed by lyophilisation for an additional 15 h. The microcapsules appeared to be in the form of loose irregular aggregates.

3.6.1.1.3 Salt Addition

As hydrophilic colloids are unstable in presence of relatively high concentrations of inorganic salts or electrolytes, they tend to salt out from their aqueous dispersions. When the addition of the salt is controlled, phase separation can be brought about instead of coagulation. The most widely applied example is that of 5% gelatin gel which coacervates upon addition of 25% sodium sulphate salt solution *(101,102)*. The choice of the salt can be made based on the charge carried by the colloid and hydration affinity. Monovalent ionic salts are preferred to multivalent ones as the higher salts bring about coagulation rather than co-acervation. Hence, among the cations, sodium, potassium and ammonium salts are preferred whereas amongst the anions, sulphate, citrate or tartarate salts are used.

3.6.1.1.4 Temperature Change Method

In this technique, the polymer is dissolved in a suitable solvent at a temperature above its upper (or below its lower) consolute temperature and core material is dispersed in it. Then temperature is lowered (or increased) at a controlled rate till the phase boundary is crossed. As the temperature reduces further, the polymer separates into two distinct regions. The core material region becomes polymer rich and the solvent region becomes polymer poor, leading to deposition of the coat around the core material. The most widely studied example is that of EC in cyclohexane which is dissolved around the boiling point of the solvent and reduction in temperature brings about co-acervation. In case of methylcellulose, the polymer is dissolved in cold water and then the temperature is slowly increased to bring about co-acervation.

3.6.1.1.5 Incompatible Polymer Addition

This technique involves the addition of a second polymer, which is also soluble in the solvent used for dissolving the first polymer but incompatible with the first polymer, Thus, addition of second polymer to solution of a polymer brings about something similar to salting out of the first polymer due to chemical incompatibility between the two polymers, which repel each other and form two distinct phases. Here too, a help of ternary phase diagram is taken to bring about controlled co-acervation and to prevent coagulation.

Example: Addition of polybutadiene to a solution of EC in toluene or addition of low molecular weight polyethylene to a solution of EC in cyclohexane, for encapsulating drugs like aspirin.

3.6.1.1.6 Polymer–Polymer Interaction (Complex Co-Acervation) (103)

This technique basically involves interaction between two oppositely charged polymers which results in charge neutralisation. The most widely used pair is that of gelatin and acacia. Gelatin, below its isoelectric point in acidic media (pH ≅ 4.0–4.5) carries a net positive charge due to protonated amino groups whereas acacia, under all conditions, carries a net negative charge due to free carboxylic groups. Hence, when a solution of acacia is added to an acidic solution of gelatin, the two react with each other, forming a complex co-acervate, accompanied by loss of water molecules bound to the colloids. In this case, the colloid-rich region usually contains a 1:1 ratio of the two colloids in about 20% concentration while the aqueous phase contains hardly 0.5% polymers.

Microspheres designed to control drug delivery using a single polymeric material are sometimes unable to fulfill all the required physical properties, encapsulation efficiency, or rate and mechanism of drug release. Thus, a combination of two or more polymers offers an acceptable means of avoiding such problems in order to achieve optimum control of drug release. Hence, this method has been widely studied *(104–106)*. Microcapsules of methoxybutropate solid particles or of an oily saturated solution of the same drug were prepared by complex co-acervation between gelatin and acacia and dried with three different methods: isopropanol addition, spray-drying and freeze-drying by Palmieri *et al. (107)*. Results highlighted that the most appropriate drying method for industrial purposes was spray-drying, particularly for oil-containing microcapsule formulations.

3.6.1.1.7 Hardening or Rigidisation of the Coat

As the co-acervation is induced, there is gradual gelation of the colloid, resulting in a rise in viscosity of the core material phase. As a result, the formed microcapsules may undergo cohesion or aggregation. These may be stabilised by shock preventing agents or polyelectrolytes that reduce the viscosity of the gel by charge repulsion. Examples include sodium CMC, sodium carboxy methyl starch, acrylic acid-methacrylate co-polymer, anionic or cationic surfactants, etc. Inert fillers like silica dioxide can also be used to prevent cohesion and aggregation by providing mechanical barrier and separation between the two particles.

However, these are unable to reduce the mechanical fragility of the walls as they are associated with moisture, residual solvent and porous, permeable coats. Hence, hardening of walls is done by removing the residual moisture/solvent by desolvation which can be done by complete drying or removal of the solvent or by treating with a solvent withdrawing liquid (dehydration or desolvation). It can also be accomplished by reducing the temperature, which causes complete salting out and separation of solvent molecules from the coat.

These approaches are not able to completely control porosity of the coat as inter-molecular distance between the coat molecules tends to remain. This is often undesirable for sustained release applications as it tends to result in rapid drug escape from the porous walls. In such cases, chemical cross-linking technique is most widely preferred to ensure a compact, non-porous coat. These are small molecular weight, reactive compounds which form an inter-molecular linkage with the polymer molecules and thereby ensure a tight, compact coat. Aldehydes like glutaraldehyde and formaldehyde are most frequently used as wall hardening chemical cross-linkers, of which glutaraldehyde is safer and less toxic as compared with formaldehyde. Hardening can also be enhanced by increasing the temperature to 40–60°C for a short period.

3.6.1.2 Interfacial Polycondensation (108)

This is a specialised type of microencapsulation technique that was initially reported by Chang and Co workers for encapsulation of proteins and enzymes. The technique involves the principle of interfacial polymerisation based on the preparation of an emulsion containing two monomers in each of the immiscible phases. The two monomers meet only at or near the interface and rapidly and spontaneously polymerise to produce the coat around the inner phase globules which contain the core material. Most applications are based on a step growth polymerisation based on the Schotten–Baumann reaction between a diacid chloride and a substance with functional groups like amine, alcohol or thiol. Some degree of cross-linking is obtained with the carboxy groups of the diacid reacting to form anhydride linkages, which help to strengthen the microcapsule walls. As this is a polycondensation type of polymerisation, a byproduct is usually formed that is taken up by the external continuous phase.

The speed of reaction, degree of polymerisation and nature and thickness of coat can be controlled by the reactivity of monomers chosen, their concentration, composition of two immiscible phases and temperature of polymerisation.

The size of the microcapsules can be controlled by controlling globule size, speed of stirring, time of emulsification and concentration of emulsifier. The thickness of coat can be controlled by controlling the reaction through concentration of reactants, by product formation and the rate and extent of reaction. Usually, it is not advisable to have an excessively thick coat and hence the polymerisation is not allowed to proceed till completion but is rather quenched after 3–5 min, which is sufficient to form a uniform coat around the globules. This technique is widely applied to microcapsules based on polyamides, polyesters, polyurethanes, etc.

In general, all these are formed by interaction between two different types of monomer—one water soluble, and another oil or organic phase soluble. The water soluble monomer can be a diamine, amino acid or protein while diacid chloride can be sebacoyl chloride, azeloyl chloride, terephthaloyl chloride, adipoyl chloride, phosgene, etc. The general reaction is as under:

1. *For polyamide*:

$$_2HNR_1NH_2 + Cl\ COCR_2\ COCl = -[HNR_1NHOCR_2CO]_n + HCl$$

Diamine Diacid chloride Polyamide

2. *For polyester*:

$$HOR_1OH + HOOCR_2COOH = -[HOR_1OOCR_2COO]_n + H_2O$$

Diol Diacid Polyester

3. *For polyurethane*:

$$_2HNR_1NH_2 + Cl\ OOCR_2\ COOCl = -[HNR_1NHOOCR_2OOC]_n + HCl$$

Diamine Bischloroformate Polyurethane

The common procedure involves dissolving the water soluble monomer in water or an aqueous buffer and dissolving or dispersing the core material in this phase. Then it is emulsified into an external organic phase containing a suitable W/O emulsifier (Span 85 is the universally used emulsifier). The second monomer is dissolved in the same external organic phase and this solution is added to the emulsion under continuous stirring. The two monomers meet at the interface and spontaneously react to form the polymer. The by product formed is taken up by the phase in which it is more soluble. The reaction is allowed to proceed till the desirable coat thickness is achieved and then is quenched by adding excess of the continuous phase. The resultant microcapsules are separated by centrifugation and decantation or filtration. Nowadays, they are usually lyophilised for better shelf life.

The aqueous phase comprises of sodium hydroxide, sodium carbonate or sodium bi-carbonate solution or buffer. The organic phase is usually benzene, toluene, chloroform, cyclohexane or carbon tetrachloride, alone or in combination.

The advantages of this technique is that it is quite simple in approach, the coating is instantaneous, the product quality is very good and reproducible, process parameters can be controlled and very fine product can be produced. Most importantly, no heat is involved during the process and hence, it can be used safely for thermolabile drugs. Chang *(109)* was the first to report the use of this technique for encapsulation of erythrocyte haemolysate for use as artificial red cells. Shigeri *(110)* prepared biocompatible and biodegradable polyphthalamide microcapsules using various diamino acids instead of the diamine, which offered additional advantage of mechanical strength due to cross-linking between the amino and carboxy groups of the amino acids. Thereafter, it was used for encapsulation of proteins *(111,112)* (BSA, fibrinogen) and enzymes *(113–116)* (carbonic anhydrase, asparaginase, urease, invertase and arginase) for improving their stability and activity. Thereafter, they have been widely applied for encapsulation of drugs for sustained release applications. Microcapsules based on cross-linked proteins like lysozyme, haemoglobin, albumin, casein, etc. have also been investigated as biodegradable and mechanically stable drug carriers *(117–120)*.

3.6.1.3 Emulsion–Solvent Evaporation Technique (121–125)

A commonly reported laboratory technique for preparing microspheres is the emulsion-solvent evaporation method or double emulsion technique, which is commonly used to prepare biodegradable, hydrophobic micro-particles containing hydrophilic proteins or polypeptides for sustained-release applications. Encapsulation or entrapment of drugs in microspheres occurs by evaporation of a solvent from an O/W or an oil-in-oil (O/O) emulsion, respectively, depending on solubility properties of the drug being encapsulated. If the drug is water soluble, an O/O emulsion achieves higher encapsulation efficiency. On the other hand, for lipophilic drugs, O/W emulsion is better. Briefly, this technique requires preparation of a solution of polymer in an organic solvent first, to which then the drug is added. When drug is not soluble in polymer solution, a homogeneous suspension is usually formed by sonication, but with care to avoid raise in temperature of the mixture. Once mixed, the drug–polymer dispersion is added as inner phase to a previously prepared external or continuous phase of emulsion that contains a surfactant. Depending on nature of the external phase (an aqueous, or a non-aqueous solvent that is not a solvent for the polymer), the emulsion formed would be an O/W, W/O or O/O emulsion, respectively. In some cases, such as with polypeptides, a W/O/W emulsion is formed *(126)*.

Evaporation of organic solvent is carried out while the emulsion is being stirred at constant speed in a hood, at room temperature, under atmospheric or reduced pressure *(127)*. The process yields a suspension of solidified microspheres loaded with drug. Once formed, the microspheres are washed with an inert solvent to remove any residual organic cosolvent and, in some cases; they are filtered through sieves to separate the microspheres in fractions of different sizes. Finally, the microspheres are dried by lyophilisation or over anhydrous $CaSO_4$ in a vacuum desiccator for storage until they are needed.

Generally, the amount of encapsulated drug depends on the physicochemical properties of the polymer and drug, as well as of the technique used in the preparation of microspheres. The evaporation rate of polymer solvent also influences the entrapment of drug in microspheres. Albumin microspheres containing recombinant human macrophage colony-stimulating factor were prepared by polymerisation from a W/O emulsion and their use with methotrexate demonstrated a significant increase ($p < 0.05$) in the survival time *(128,129)*.

Many authors have prepared micro-particles using this technique for loading proteins and peptides. However, this approach generally results in low protein entrapment levels (usually <10% w/w) due to partition of hydrophilic proteins into the aqueous continuous phase. Non-uniform protein release is common and the delivery capacity is low, usually less than 1 mg/mg micro-particles/d.

In one report, selected polymer (PLGA) and the drug were dissolved in a small quantity of DMSO/methylene chloride mixture of equal concentration. The above solution was emulsified in sufficient quantity of a polymer like PVA with homogenisation for a very short duration of time. Emulsion formed was incubated for required length of time with further stirring at lower rpm. Micro-particles formed were recovered and freeze-dried *(130)*.

The W/O/W-encapsulated process, which is simple but has a large number of reaction control parameters, involves many parameters that may affect the properties of micro-particles such as particle size, morphology and release characteristics. Some factors including homogenisation intensity, viscosity of inner water and organic phase, volume size and surfactant were used to control the particle size *(131,132)*. Also, change of viscosity resulted from different volume and polymer concentrations of inner and organic phases, and pH in the external continuous water phase have been investigated to improve drug loading efficiency *(133,134)*. Choi *et al.* *(135)* encapsulated the drug into micro-particles by the double emulsion (W/O/W) and solvent evaporation method. The drug was dissolved in a buffer solution and emulsified in methylene chloride phase containing a polymer like PLGA. The primary emulsion was homogenised at a very high rpm and added to 25 mL of another polymer solution (e.g., PVA) with subsequent homogenisation at a lower rpm. The double emulsion was incubated for a specified period of time as per requirements with continuous homogenisation at a much lesser rpm. The hardened micro-particles were collected, washed three times with DI water and then freeze dried *(136)*.

3.6.1.4 Ionotropic Gelation Method

Weigh required quantity of drug and add to a polymer solution. Stir for 4 min to form a uniform dispersion. Select more than 2/3 quantity of the formed dispersion and extrude through a suitable size needle drop wise into around 50 mL of fluid containing a hardening agent (e.g., calcium chloride). Maintain the extrusion flow rate in a proper manner. Allow the formed particles to remain in the hardening solution for a period of 10 min. Filter the formed particles, wash, dry at 40°C for 1 d. These can be used to prepare beads of even size and the syringe selection makes the difference *(137)*.

3.6.1.5 Cross-Linking Process

Polymer microspheres/micro-particles are hardened by thermal or chemical cross-linking process.

3.6.5.1. Preparation of Microspheres by Thermal Cross-Linking

The method involves the addition of a cross-linking agent to an aqueous acid solution of polymer, maintaining a constant molar ratio between the polymer and added acid. The polymer solution is cooled to 0°C and added to the oily phase maintained at a very high temperature. The cross-linking is performed in a glass receptacle under vigourous stirring at high speed for 40 min.

3.6.5.2. Cross-Linking by Chemical Method (45)

Generally, aldehydes like glutaraldehyde or tripolyphosphate (TPP) is used for cross-linking.

3.6.5.2.1. Preparation of Microspheres by Glutaraldehyde Cross-Linking

In this method, the polymer solution in aqueous acid media is added to oil phase consisting of both light and heavy liquid paraffin in equimolar ratios containing surfactants and stirred to form an W/O emulsion. Continue stirring at high speed while adding a measured quantity of aqueous glutaraldehyde solution dropwise at different time intervals. Microspheres obtained are separated and washed, first, with petroleum ether and then with distilled water to remove the adhered liquid paraffin and glutaraldehyde. Vary the volume of glutaraldehyde to achieve effective cross-linking efficiency. Dry microspheres finally in a vacuum desiccator.

3.6.5.2.2. Preparation of Microspheres by TPP Cross-Linking

Here, the polymer solution is prepared and the bubble free solution/dispersion of the polymer is dropped through a disposable syringe into a gently agitated solution of TPP. Separate the formed microspheres after 2 h by filtration and rinse with distilled water. Air dry the separated microspheres.

3.6.5.2.3. Preparation of Microspheres by Emulsification and Ionotropic Gelation by NaOH

Add disperse phase containing polymer in acid solution to the continuous phase consisting of an organic phase and surfactant to form a W/O emulsion. Add sodium hydroxide solution at a predetermined rate after 20 min of mechanical stirring at 15 min intervals. Maintain stirring speed at a very high rpm. Separate the formed microspheres by filtration and subsequently wash with petroleum ether followed by distilled water and air dry.

3.7. Paramagnetic Micro-Particles

3.7.1. Synthesis Through Emulsion-Templated Free Radical Polymerisation

Paramagnetic micro-particles have been widely used for biological affinity separations because they offer a simple and efficient method for purification of cells, viruses and macromolecules *(138–142)*. These micro-particles have to be stable in water, uniform in size and should respond to magnetic field gradients. The paramagnetic particles are typically composed of maghemite or magnetite distributed in a polymer matrix. The particles prepared like this can be coated with a polymer and then stabilised in aqueous solution. This further provides chemical groups to which conjugation of proteins and polynucleotides can be done. Magnetisation of the particles is measured in emu and can range from 2–18 emu/g. These types of particles can be used in the fields of drug delivery *(143,144)*, analytical measurement, diagnosis, hyperthermia therapy, etc. *(145–149)*. The first paramagnetic particles were prepared by the oxidation of Fe^{2+} to Fe^{3+}, which gave nanoparticles of maghemite within the pores of swollen polystyrene particles *(150)*. After this method, several other methods were used to prepare paramaganetic and magnetic micro-particles for drug delivery. One of the methods called as ‘core-shell’ processing had nanometer-scale magnetic particles, which were chemically or physically adsorbed onto a polymer particle of micrometer sizes. This provided with an advantage of producing micro-particles with uniform size or which can be called as ‘monodispersed’ particles. The particles produced with this technique had a low loading of magnetic material as the major portion of the particle was of polymer core *(151)*. Another approach was by heterogenous polymerisation of nanosize magnetic particles with a polymer monomer. Particles can also be prepared by spinning a mixture of polymers and nanoparticles *(152)*, co-polymerisation of cobalt particles with poly(dimethylsiloxane) *(153)*, co-polymerisation of methylmethacrylate with oleic acid modified magnetite particle *(154)*, suspension polymerisation of polystryrene with ferrofluid *(155)* or the encapsulation of magnetite through a microemulsion process *(156)*. Micro-particles prepared by these techniques have been used in DNA purification *(157)* and the substance used was agarose. Highly uniform micrometer size magnetic particles from ferrofluids were prepared using solvent evaporation *(158,159)*. In this technique, hydrophobic magnetic nanoparticles are suspended in a volatile hydrophobic solvent to form an emulsion in a non-ionic surfactant solution. This emulsion is exposed to a defined shear force to produce particles of highly uniform size. Monodispersed micrometer size assemblies can be obtained after the evaporation of solvent because of aggregation of nanoparticles. The size of particles is limited by the shear technique and hydrophobic interactions can reversibly assemble the resultant particles.

3.7.2. Emulsion Templated UV-Initiated Polymerisation Technique for Formation of Paramagnetic Micro-Particles

This method gives an opportunity to control the surface chemistry of micro-particles by controlling the concentration of species in aqueous phase before cross-linking. High-magnetisation paramagnetic micro-particles functionalised with a controlled density of poly ethylene glycol (PEG) and carboxyl groups can be prepared by a unique and novel method as described below:

The synthesis involves four steps

1. Creation of an O/W emulsion in which hydrophobic iron oxide nanoparticles and a UV-activated initiator were distributed in hexane.
2. Formation of uniform micro-particles through emulsion homogenisation and evaporation of hexane.
3. Functionalisation of the micro-particle with a PEG-functionalised surfactant and acrylic acid.
4. Polymerisation of micro-particles.

The size of micro-particles can be controlled by pore size of the membrane used to homogenise the emulsion. The concentration of surfactant and acrylic acid can be used to optimise the surface chemistry, iron content and magnetisation of the micro-particles. The micro-particles prepared like this can be functionalised with antibodies and exhibited a low propensity for non-specific protein adsorption. These micro-particles can also be useful for magnetic tweezers measurements and bioanalytical devices that require micro-particles with a high magnetisation.

3.7.3. Size-Templated Synthesis of Paramagnetic Micro-Particles

The magnetite particles can be prepared by co-precipitation of ferric and ferrous salt solutions using concentrated ammonia *(160,161)*. Ferrous chloride tetrahydrate is dissolved in ferric chloride and deoxygenated water to prepare an aqueous Fe^{2+}/Fe^{3+} solution. Add a small amount of ammonium hydroxide rapidly to this solution under vigorous stirring and heat it for 30 min at 70°C. The resultant mixture is a black slurry which is then washed with water and perchloric acid. Dialyze the particles against water to remove excess acid and filter with a suitable media. Make these particles hydrophobic by coating with oleic acid in water for a suitable time. Remove excess oleic acid by rinsing with ethanol and re-suspend the particles in hexane. Mix the particles in suitable concentrations of RN-10 and acrylic acid and then polymerise by exposing the particles to a 20 mW/cm^2 UV light for 10 min. Collect the particles on a permanent magnet, rinse with water sufficiently and store them at 4°C *(162)*.

4. CHARACTERISATION OF MICRO-PARTICLES

The micro-particles are generally subjected to a variety of evaluation tests. The tests range from measuring the size of micro-particles to identifying the structure and surface characteristics. The characterisation tests with a brief description are given below.

4.1. Scanning Electron Microscope (SEM)

SEM is a microscope that uses electrons rather than light to form an image. There are many advantages of using SEM instead of a light microscope. SEM has a large depth of field, which allows a large amount of the sample to be in focus at one time. SEM also produces images of high resolution, which means that closely spaced features can be examined at a high magnification. Preparation of samples is relatively easy since most SEMs only require the sample to be conductive. The combination of higher magnification, larger depth of focus, greater resolution, and ease of sample observation makes SEM one of the most heavily used instruments in research areas today. In addition, SEM images have a characteristic three-dimensional (3D) appearance and are useful for judging surface structure of the sample.

In a typical SEM, electrons are thermionically emitted from a tungsten or lanthanum hexaboride (LaB6) cathode and are accelerated towards an anode; alternatively electrons can be emitted via field emission. The electron beam, which typically has an energy ranging from a few 100 eV to 50 keV, is focused by one or two condenser lenses into a beam with a very fine focal spot sized 1–5 nm. The beam passes through pairs of scanning coils in the objective lens, which deflect the beam in a raster fashion over a rectangular area of the sample surface. As primary electrons strike the surface, they are inelastically scattered by atoms in the sample. Through these scattering events, the primary electron beam effectively spreads and fills a teardrop-shaped volume, known as the interaction volume, extending from less than 100 nm to around 5 μm into the surface. Interactions in this region lead to the subsequent emission of electrons which are then detected to produce an image.

However, the most common imaging mode monitors low energy (<50 eV) secondary electrons. Due to their low energy, these electrons originate within a few nanometers from the surface. The electrons are detected by a scintillator-photomultiplier device and the resulting signal is rendered into a two-dimensional (2D) intensity distribution that can be viewed and saved as a digital image. This process relies on a raster-scanned primary beam. The brightness of the signal depends on the number of secondary electrons reaching the detector. If the beam enters the sample perpendicular to the surface, then the activated region is uniform about the axis of the beam and a certain number of electrons "escape" from within the sample. As the angle of incidence increases, the "escape" distance of one side of the beam will decrease, and more secondary electrons will be emitted. Thus steep surfaces and edges tend to be brighter than flat surfaces, which results in images with a well-defined, 3D appearance. Using this technique, resolutions less than 1 nm are possible.

4.1.1. Detection of Backscattered Electrons

In addition to the secondary electrons, back scattered electrons can also be detected. Back scattered electrons may be used to detect contrast between areas with different chemical compositions. These can be observed especially when average atomic number of various regions are different. Back scattered electrons can also be used to form an electron backscatter diffraction image. This image can be used to determine the crystallographic structure of specimen.

4.1.2. Resolution of SEM

The spatial resolution of SEM depends on the size of the electron spot, which in turn depends on the magnetic electron-optical system which produces the scanning beam. The resolution is also limited by the size of interaction volume, or the extent of material which interacts with the electron beam. The spot size and interaction volume are both very large compared with the distances between atoms, so the resolution of SEM is not high enough to image down to the atomic scale, as is possible in the transmission electron microscope (TEM). SEM has compensating advantages, though, including the ability to image a comparatively large area of the specimen; the ability to image bulk materials (not just thin films or foils); and the variety of analytical modes available for measuring the composition and nature of the specimen. Depending on instrument, the resolution can fall somewhere between less than 1 nm and 20 nm. In general, SEM images are much easier to interpret than TEM images.

4.2. X-Ray Diffractometry

X-ray crystallography is one of the most useful methods for exploring the nature of matter. X-ray diffractometry (XRD) is used to determine the phase content in many minerals and materials. As a result, it is used by researchers in a wide range of disciplines. It is used as an adjunct to chemical analysis in the identification of the constituents of mixtures of crystalline phases, for example, in minerals, cements and alloys; for measurements of the lattice parameters of artificially produced structures such as the epitaxially grown materials in modern electronic materials. It is used by the pharmaceutical industry to identify changes in raw materials or methods that might alter a drug's efficacy.

4.3. Fourier Transform-Infrared Spectroscopy (FT-IR)

FT-IR is an analytical technique used to identify organic (and in some cases inorganic) materials. This technique measures absorption of various infrared light wavelengths by the material of interest. These infrared absorption bands identify specific molecular components and structures.

Absorption bands in the range of 4000–1500 wavenumbers are typically due to functional groups (e.g., –OH, C = O, N–H, CH_3, etc.). The region between 1500 and 400 wavenumbers is referred to as the fingerprint region. Absorption bands in this region are generally due to intra-molecular phenomena, and are highly specific for each material. The specificity of these bands allows computerised data searches to be performed against reference libraries to identify a material. In particulate technology, FT-IR is used to assess interaction between the constituents of polymeric micro-/nanoparticles; particularly when one suspects interaction between drug and polymer. Other typical applications include impurity profile analysis, identification and quantification of degradation products, residual monomers/solvents and interaction between constituents.

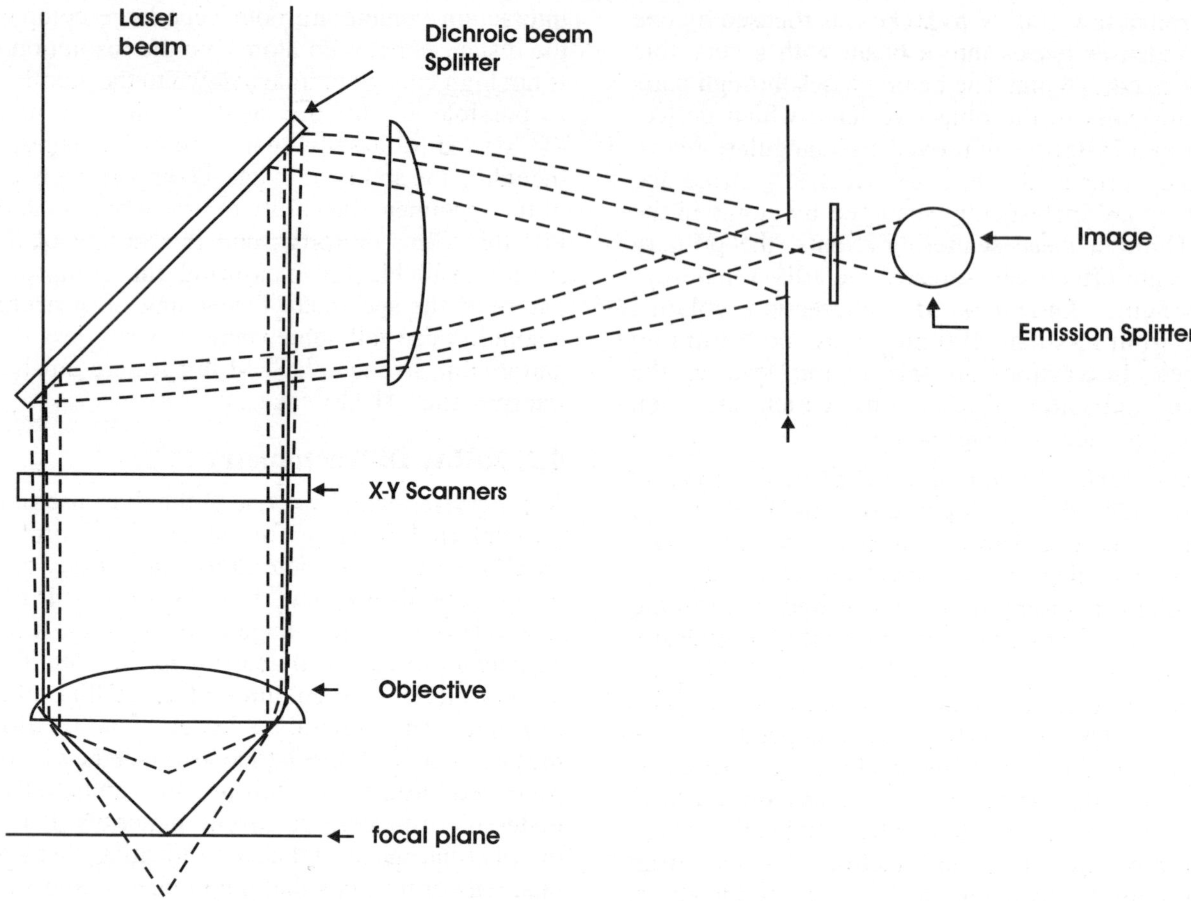

Fig. 14. Principle of confocal microscopy.

4.4. Confocal Microscopy *(163)*

"Confocal" is defined as "having the same focus." What this means in the microscope is that the final image has the same focus as or the focus corresponds to the point of focus in the object. The object and its image are "confocal." The microscope is able to filter the out-of-focus light from above and below the point of focus in object. Normally, when an object is imaged in fluorescence microscope, the signal produced is from the full thickness of specimen which does not allow most of it to be in focus to observer. The confocal microscope eliminates this out-of-focus information by means of a confocal "pinhole" situated in front of the image plane which acts as a spatial filter and allows only the in-focus portion of the light to be imaged. A diagram of the confocal principle is shown in Fig. 14.

While the image that is seen with confocal filtering is all in-focus information, compared with a normal fluorescence microscope, the amount of light that is seen in the final image is greatly reduced by the pinhole, sometimes even up to 90–95%. To compensate for this loss of light, modern confocal microscopes use lasers as light sources instead of the conventional mercury arc lamps. In addition, highly sensitive photomultiplier-detectors (PMTs) are employed as imaging devices to pick up the reduced signal. The signal for detection in the original design of modern confocal microscopes is created by scanning a focussed laser beam across a square or rectangular field. A system of motorised scanner mirrors sequentially scan a horizontal beam across the specimen. The computer is used to control the microscope's scanner mirrors and motorised focussing mechanism as well as to collect, store and analyse the data. The computer allows the system to scan sequential planes in Z-direction, store them, and create overlays of all the in-focus Z-sections. This information can also be used to create 3D images, or movie rotations of well stained specimens.

Another useful feature of the confocal microscope is the ability to show co-localisations of signals from different fluorochromes. In specimens double-labeled

Table 3. Summary of the Physical and Chemical Properties[a] of Micro-particle

Sample	Fe_2O_4 (wt%)	Fe_3O_4 (vol%)	Mass loss in TGA (%)	Magnetisation (emu/g)	COOH/CCO	C/Fe	Charge density charges/nm^2	Critical coagulation concentration (CCC) (mM)
S1	91	43	8	24.8	2.34	2.52	319	157
S2	81	28	16	18.4	2.22	7.46	304	118
S3	76	24	20	17.1	1.96	4.85	284	76
S4	62	15	28	7.9	1.10	2.64	164	26

[a]*All particles were prepared using 5 μm membrane.*

for different molecules or structures, the different fluorochromes can be collected in different channels and combined to make colour images which along with the 3D information obtained by confocal sectioning can more precisely show co-localisations of the signals than with the normal fluorescence microscope.

Specimens which can be imaged better by the confocal microscope are ones which are brightly stained or too thick to be seen well in the standard fluorescence microscope.

Two types of confocal microscopes are commercially available: confocal laser scanning microscopes (CLSM) and spinning-disk confocal microscopes. Generally speaking, CLSM yields better image quality but the imaging frame rate is very slow (<3 frames/s); spinning-disk confocal microscopes can achieve video rate imaging desired for dynamic observations.

4.4.1. Thermogravimetric Analysis (TGA)

Thermogravimetry (TG) provides a quantitative measurement of any weight change associated with a transition. For example, TG can directly record the loss in weight with time or temperature due to dehydration or decomposition. Thermogravimetric curves are characteristic for a given compound or systems because of the unique sequence of physicochemical reactions which occur over definite temperature ranges and at rates that are a function of the molecular structure. Changes in weight as a result of the rupture and/or formation of various physical and chemical bonds at elevated temperatures that lead to the evolution of volatile products or the formation of heavier reaction products. From such curves, data are obtained concerning the thermodynamics and kinetics of the various chemical reactions, reaction mechanisms and the intermediate and final reaction products. The usual temperature range is from ambient to 1200°C with inert or reactive atmospheres.

Pharmaceutical micro-particles are generally prepared using variety of polymers, drugs and other adjuvants under varied conditions of temperature under specific solvent media. These conditions could cause loss of water molecule, degradation, conjugation, polymerisation and complexation or any interaction which could be characterised by TG.

Table 3 summarises the maximum weight loss of the micro-particles measured with TGA.

The afore-mentioned procedure is one of the methods in estimating characters of the micro-particles and characterising them with appropriate attributes.

4.4.2. Super-Conducting Quantum Interference Device (SQUID) Magnetometry

This is used to measure the magnetic properties of the micro-particles. This can be performed on micro-particles as well as nanoparticles. The requirement is to construct a magnetisation curve for the micro-particles at room temperature.

4.5. X-Ray Photoelectron Spectroscopy (XPS)

This technique can be used to measure the surface chemistry of the micro-particles.

4.6. Estimation of the Stability of the Micro-Particles

This can be characterisd by measuring the CCC of the micro-particles. CCC is defined as the salt concentration at which the log of stability ratio (W) is zero. The stability ratio is defined as K_r/K_s, where, K_r is the rapid aggregation rate constant, and K_s is the slow aggregation rate constant. Aggregation rates can be measured by monitoring the optical density of a particle suspension. K_r can be determined by the rate of decrease in absorbance of a particle suspension in 1 *M* NaCl and K_s can be measured with particles suspended in different milimolar NaCl solutions.

4.7. Optical Microscopy

The method can be used to analyse the morphology and size of the micro-particles. It requires each micro-particle batch to be observed by a suitable optical microscope. SEM can be used to understand the surface and the internal morphology of the micro-particles. The internal morphology of the micro-particles can also be characterised by embedding them in resin with proper sections. Average particle size and their distribution is determined using a Coulter Multisizer (Coultronics, Margency, France). The micro-particles need to be suspended in isotonic saline solution without surfactant and sonicated for a few minutes prior to analysis.

5. KINETICS OF DRUG RELEASE FROM MICRO-PARTICLES

Kinetics of drug release is an important evaluation parameter and the knowledge of mechanism and kinetics of drug release from these microparticlulate systems indicate its performance and gives proof of adequateness of its design. Drug release from microcapsules and micro-particles involve mass transfer phenomenon involving diffusion of drug from higher concentration to lower concentration region in the surrounding liquid.

Application of drug release data is applied basically for:

1. Quality control.
2. Understanding of physicochemical aspects of drug delivery system.
3. Understand release mechanisms.
4. Predict behaviour of system *in vivo*.

However, there are difficulties in modeling drug release data as there is great diversity in the physical form of microcapsules/particles with respect to size, shape, arrangement of core and coat, properties of core like solubility, diffusivity, partition co-efficient, properties of coat like porosity, tortuosity, thickness, crystallinity, inertness, etc. In addition, there are problems in translating kinetics of drug release from "Micro" products of perfect geometry to various irregular micro systems *(165)*.

5.1. Factors Influencing Drug Release

1. *Permeation*: It is the process whereby drug is transported through one or more polymeric membranes corresponding to the coating material, which acts as the barrier to drug release. Permeation depends on crystallinity, nature of polymer, its degree of polymerisation, presence of fillers and plasticisers, matrix properties like thickness, porosity, tortuosity, diffusion layer, etc. *(166)*. Permeation may be reduced by incorporation of dispersed solids, fillers, waxy sealants, etc.
2. *Diffusion*: It is the movement of drug across concentration gradient till equalisation takes place. Governed by Fick's first Law:

   Flux,

$$J = \frac{dM}{dt} = -DA\frac{dC}{dx} \quad (1)$$

where, *dM* is the mass of drug diffused in time (*dt*), *D* is diffusion co-efficient, *A* is diffusion area, *dx* is diffusion layer thickness and $\frac{dC}{dx}$ is concentration gradient.

Negative slope indicates movement from higher to lower concentration. Here *D* and *C* are assumed to be constant. But when *C* varies with distance and time, the equation is given as Fick's second law:

$$J = \left(\frac{\partial c}{\partial t}\right)_x = D\left(\frac{d^2c}{dx^2}\right)_t \quad (2)$$

From integration,

$$\left(\frac{dc}{dt}\right) = D\left[\frac{d^2c}{dx^2} + \frac{d^2c}{dy^2} + \frac{d^2c}{dz^2}\right] = DV^{-2}C \quad (3)$$

This implies that rate of change in concentration in volume element is proportional to rate of change of concentration gradient at that region of the field.

3. *Diffusion co-efficient (167)*: Diffusion co-efficient (*D*) is a measure of rate of drug movement. Diffusion co-efficient, *D* depends on various factors like;

   a. Temperature (given by Arrhenius equation)

$$D = D_0 e^{-Ea/RT} \text{ or } \ln D = \ln D_0 - \frac{Ea}{RT} \quad (4)$$

where D_0 is the temperature independent factor, *Ea* is activation energy, R is gas constant and *T* is absolute temperature. Hence, plot of ln *D* vs $\frac{1}{T}$

gives a straight line, the intercept of which gives the value of D_0.

b. Molecular weight of the molecule,

where

$$D \propto \left(\frac{1}{M_w}\right)^{\frac{1}{3}} \quad (5)$$

c. Radius (for small, electrically neutral and spherical molecules). As per Stokes–Einstein equation:

$$D = \frac{RT}{Na}(6\pi r\eta)^{-1} \quad (6)$$

where, *Na* is the Avogadro's number, η is viscosity and *r* is radius.

d. *Plasticiser concentration*: *D* increases with increase in plasticiser concentration but reduces due to solid additives like fillers, pigments, sealants, etc.

e. *Size of the penetrant*: *D* decreases with increase in size, polymer crystallinity, cross-linking, solid content and viscosity.

f. *Position of the drug in the microsphere*: Surface associated drug diffuses out fast and is associated with burst release whereas if the drug is in the interior of the microsphere, the diffusion decreases due to increased path length.

g. Interaction between polymer and the drug also adversely affect diffusion as the bound or complexed drug will not be free to diffuse out of the matrix or coat.

h. Diffusion may also be affected by simultaneous diffusion of water and other molecules through the coating from the aqueous external environment, as it may dissolve the drug or the carrier and affect the continuum.

When drug diffusion through microcapsules/micro-particles is concerned, drug transport involves dissolution of permeating drug in polymer and diffusion across the membrane,

then, $$J = \frac{DKA\Delta C}{lm} \quad (6a)$$

where ΔC is the concentration difference on either side of membrane, *l*m is membrane thickness, *K* is partition co-efficient of drug toward the polymer. Often, *DK* is permeability co-efficient and DK/*l*m is permeability when *l*m is not known, *D*/*lm* is permeability constant *(168)*.

4. *Partition coefficient*: Partition coefficient between polymer and solvent is referred to as $K_{o/w}$. It will vary if solvent solubility varics. As *K* value becomes very large, flux tends to become diffusion controlled. *K* value may vary if drug concentration continuously changes, for example, weak acid or base in changing pH conditions or when drug binds with some component and in that case, Fick's law would not be followed.

5. *Drug solubility*: As diffusion depends on concentration gradient, drug solubility in penetrant becomes important and then drug release becomes dissolution dependent for sparingly soluble drugs. This can be expressed in various ways:

a. Noyes-Whitney equation *(169)*

$$\frac{dc}{dt} = k(C_s - C) \quad (7)$$

where *dc*/*dt* is the amount of drug released per unit time, k is dissolution rate constant, C_s is saturation solubility in solvent, *C* is concentration in solvent at time (*t*).

$$k = \frac{D_s A}{V l_b} \quad (8)$$

where D_s is the diffusion co-efficient in solvent, *V* is volume of solution, l_b is boundary layer thickness. By substituting the value of k in Eq. (7), we obtain

$$\left[\frac{dc}{dt}\right] = \frac{D_s A}{V l_b}(C_s - C) \quad (9)$$

Thus, water soluble drugs will be released faster than hydrophobic ones.

b. Si-Nang and Carlier *(170)* modified this equation for drug release from microcapsules

$$\left(\frac{dc}{dt}\right) = \frac{D_s A' K'}{V l_m} \quad (10)$$

where *A'* is the internal surface area of coating, *K'* is a constant which includes porosity and tortuosity.

c. Khanna *et al.* *(171)* modified the Noyes-Whitney equation and applied it for characterising dissolution of chloramphenicol from epoxy resins

$$W_0^{\frac{1}{3}} - W_t^{\frac{1}{3}} = kat \quad (11)$$

where W_0 is the initial weight of particles, W_t is weight at time (*t*) and *a* is surface weight fraction at time (*t*).

In this case plot of $\sqrt[3]{W_t}$ vs t gives a straight line and value of *k* can be obtained from the slope.

d. For weakly acidic and basic drugs, the influence of pH on solubility is given by Henderson-Hasselbach equation:

For weak acids,

$$\text{pH} = \text{p}K_a + \log\frac{S - S_0}{S_0} \quad (12)$$

For weak base,

$$\text{pH} = \text{p}K_a + \log\frac{S - S_0}{S_0} \tag{13}$$

where S is the saturation solubility of solute and S_0 is intrinsic solubility of solute.

5. *Coating area and thickness*: Flux is proportional to area. Hence, as size decreases, drug release increases. Also flux $\propto \frac{1}{l}$; so as thickness decreases, flux increases due to reduced diffusional path length. Other factors include type and amount of matrix material, size and density of the micro-particle, presence of additives or adjuvants, extent of polymerisation, denaturation, cross-linking or hardening, diffusion temperature, diffusion medium, its polarity, presence of enzymes, etc.

5.2. Empiric Models of Drug Release

Kinetics of drug release from microparticulates can be understood from various models based on their nature. However, simple empiric models are often used in place of complex models, which are discussed below:

1. Diffusional exponent approach has been given by Peppas et al. *(172,173)*. It is applicable for hydrating or eroding systems where D is not constant, thereby giving anomalous diffusion.

$$\frac{M_t}{M_o} = kt^n \tag{14}$$

where M_t/M_0 is the fractional mass of drug released at time (t), n is diffusional exponent. Values greater than 0.5 indicate non-fickian or anomalous diffusion, which is usually found in swellable systems

For Fickian release, $n = 0.5$ for planar surface and $n = 0.432$ for spheres. For Non-fickian or anomalous diffusion, $n > 0.5$.

2. *Biexponential equation:*

$$\frac{M_t}{M_o} = 1 - [A\exp(-K_1 t) + B\exp(-K_2 t)] \tag{15}$$

where M_t/M_o is the fractional mass of drug released at time (t), A and B are constants, k_1 and k_2 are rate constants for two lifetime exponents into which decay function is being decomposed.

The two exponents consist of rapid or burst phase and slow or sustained release phase respectively.

3. *Diffusion through interfacial barrier:*

For example in emulsified systems, where Guy equation *(174)* is followed:

$$\frac{M_t}{M_o} = 3KT \tag{16}$$

where

$$T = \frac{Dt}{r^2}$$

D is the diffusion co-efficient, t is time and r is radius of particles.

Where K is the reduced interfacial rate constant, and $K = \frac{k_1}{D}$, where k_1 is true interfacial rate constant.

This implies that at short times, zero order release is obtained.

At long times where $T >> 1$, release is given by single exponential decay.

$$\frac{M_t}{M_o} = 1 - \exp\left(\frac{-3k_1 t}{r^2}\right) \tag{17}$$

Converting, $\ln\left(1 - \frac{M_t}{M_o}\right) = \frac{-3k_1 t}{r^2}$ which is equation for straight line

Hence, plot of (1 – Mt/Mo) vs t will give value of k_1 from the slope.

Nowadays, drug release kinetics are determined and better understood from their nature depending on whether they are reservoir, matrix or sandwich type systems.

5.3. Reservoir Type Devices (Microcapsules) *(175–179)*

Various equations have been given depending on different situations.

Case 1. Assuming thermodynamic activity of core material to be constant within the microcapsule which is spherical and has inert homogeneous coating, steady-state release rate is derived from Fick's first law of diffusion:

$$\frac{dM_t}{dt} = 4\pi\, DK\, \Delta C \frac{r_o r_i}{r_o - r_i} \tag{18}$$

where $\frac{dM_t}{dt}$ is the fractional mass of drug released at time (t), r_0 and r_i are outer and inner radii of the coat.

- If right hand side parameters are constant, drug release rate will be zero order.
- However, drug release rate decreases as coating thickness ($r_0 - r_i$) increases.
- If $r_0 >>> r_i$, then equation becomes

$$\frac{dM_t}{dt} = 4\pi\, DK\, \Delta C\, r_i, \tag{19}$$

i.e., drug release rate is independent of coating thickness.

Thus at $\frac{r_o}{r_i} >> 4$, further increase in size will not significantly affect drug release *(175)*.

Case 2. If thermodynamic activity of core is not constant, then release rate is exponential or first order

$$\frac{dM_t}{dt} = \frac{-2\pi(r_i^2 + r_o^2)\, DK}{r_o - r_i}\left(C_{it} - C_{ot}\right) \tag{20}$$

or

$$\frac{dM_t}{dt} = \frac{-2\pi(r_i^2 + r_o^2)\, DK}{r_o - r_i}\left(\frac{M_{ti}V_o - M_{ot}V_i}{V_iV_o}\right) \tag{21}$$

where C_{ot}, C_{it} are the drug concentrations in outer and inner compartment after time (*t*), respectively, M_{it}, M_{ot} is mass of drug remaining in reservoir and sink at any time (*t*), respectively and V_i, V_o is volume of internal reservoir and outer sink, respectively.

From integration,

$$\frac{dM_{it}}{dt} = \frac{-M_{tot}\, 2\pi(r_i^2 + r_o^2)\, DK}{V_i(r_o - r_i)} \exp\left[\frac{2\pi(r_i^2 + r_o^2)\, DK\, (V_o + V_i)\, t}{(r_o - r_i)V_iV_o}\right] \tag{22}$$

This indicates exponential release rate which decreases as coating thickness increases and time increases.

From this, we can calculate time required for 50% drug release $t^{½}$, where

$$t^{\frac{1}{2}} = \frac{-(r_o - r_i)V_i\, V_o}{2\pi(r_i^2 + r_o^2)\, DK\, (V_o + V_i)}\, ln\frac{V_o - V_i}{2V_o} \tag{23}$$

5.3.1. Lag Time and Burst Effect

1. If product is tested immediately after preparation, as fluid takes time to penetrate and attain concentration gradient, there will be a delay or lag time (t_l)

$$t_l = \frac{(r_o - r_i)^2}{6D} \text{ (Crank's equation)} \tag{24}$$

This can be used to find *D* at a particular time and vice versa, if film thickness is known.

2. If product is stored for long period of time before testing or has surface associated drug, it shows burst effect, leading to initial over dosage.

Thus, time necessary to reach steady state depends on coating thickness and *D*.

$$t_b = \frac{(r_o - r_i)^2}{3D} \tag{25}$$

where t_b is the burst time.

5.4. Monolithic Devices (Micro-Particles) (180–183)

Monolithic or matrix systems are those in which the core is uniformly dispersed throughout the matrix polymer. The drug release kinetics will depend on whether the drug is dissolved or dispersed in the polymer.

Case 1. When the drug is dissolved in polymer, matrix the release equations are a series equations which are simplified into early stage and later stage approximations.

Early stage approximation is given by Baker and Lonsdale equation *(175)*

$$\frac{M_t}{M_\infty} = 6\left(\frac{Dt}{r^2\pi}\right)^{½} - \frac{3Dt}{r^2} \tag{26}$$

where M_∞ is the drug dissolved in polymer, M_t is drug released at time (*t*), *r* is radius of particle and *D* is diffusion co-efficient.

This equation is valid for $\frac{M_t}{M_o} < 0.4.$, i.e., for first 40% drug release.

Now, $\frac{Dt}{r^2} = \Gamma$.

Then the equation will convert to

$$\frac{M_t}{M_o} = 6\sqrt{\frac{\Gamma}{\Pi}} - 3\Gamma \tag{27}$$

Total drug release can be obtained by integration of the equation,

$$\frac{d(M_t/M_\infty)}{dt} = 3\left(\frac{D}{r^2\pi^t}\right)^{\frac{1}{2}} - \frac{3D}{r^2} \tag{28}$$

This is equation for straight line and shows that release is inversely proportional to radius, r of the micro-particles.

Later time approximation is given as:

$$\frac{M_t}{M_\infty} = 1 - \frac{6}{\pi^2}\exp\left[\frac{\pi^2\, Dt}{r^2}\right], \tag{29}$$

which is valid for $\frac{M_t}{M_\infty} = > 0.6.$, i.e., for remaining 60% of drug release.

Integration of the equation gives

$$\frac{d(M_t/M_\infty)}{dt} = \frac{6Dt}{r^2}\exp\left[\frac{-\pi^2\, Dt}{r^2}\right] \tag{30}$$

thus, it shows that later drug release is exponential.

Case 2. When the drug is dispersed in coat: here, the drug is insoluble in and is uniformly dispersed throughout the matrix

A. Baker–Lonsdale equation derived from Higuchi equation for homogeneous, spherical matrix

$$\frac{d(M_t/M_\infty)}{dt} = \frac{3C_m D}{r_o^2 C_o}\left[\frac{(1-M_t/M)^{\frac{1}{3}}}{1-(1-M_t/M_\infty)^{\frac{1}{3}}}\right] \quad (31)$$

where C_m is the drug dissolved in membrane and C_o is initial drug concentration.

This is valid when $C_m <<< C_{total}$, i.e., not more than 1% drug is present in the membrane.

This equation assumes that solid drug is dissolved from surface layer first and next layer dissolves only after first layer is exhausted.

B. Simple, uniform equations hold only for spherical, homodisperse systems. However, majority of micro-particulate systems are heterogeneous and drug release is complex.

For irregular particles,

$$\frac{dm}{dt} = \frac{A}{2}\left[\frac{DC_m}{t}(2C_{tot} - C_s)\right]^{\frac{1}{2}} \quad (32)$$

where A is the cross sectional area of matrix, C_{tot} is total drug loading in the polymer matrix, C_s is saturation solubility of drug and C_m is concentration of drug.

Intregrating the equation, we obtain,

$$Q = \frac{M}{A}[DC_m(2C_{tot} - C_s)t]^{\frac{1}{2}} \quad (33)$$

where Q is the mass of drug released per unit area A at time (t). (C_{tot} should be at least equal to $10C_s$.)

The equation implies that drug release is proportional to square root of time and can be simplified to,

$$Q = k_1 t^{1/2}.$$

This is a modified Higuchi equation.

C. For planar surface of granular type matrix having irregular, clustered or aggregated type of product,

$$Q = \left[\frac{D\in}{\Gamma}(2C_{tot} - C_s)C_s t\right]^{\frac{1}{2}} \quad (34)$$

where $\in$ is the porosity, Γ is tortuosity, C_{tot} is total concentration of drug in matrix and C_s is saturation concentration.

This equation assumes that

1. C_{tot} is much greater than C_s, i.e., $C_{tot} >> C_s$.
2. Drug is non-reacting with matrix former.
3. It is uniformly dispersed throughout the matrix.
4. Drug particles are much smaller than matrix particles.
5. Perfect sink conditions are maintained.

This is equation for straight line; so plot of

$$\frac{Q}{t^{\frac{1}{2}}} \text{ vs } (2C_{tot} - C_s)C_s \text{ gives } D \quad (35)$$

or D_m from the slope.

The drawback of this equation is that it is no longer applicable when majority of drug load is released.

D. If C_{tot} is not much larger than C_s, then Fessi equation *(181)* is applied:

$$Q = C_{tot}(Dt)^{\frac{1}{2}},$$

where (36)

$$C_{tot} < \in C_s$$

E. For phase separated system where small quantity of drug is separated from the matrix into pure domains and is released by diffusion through the polymer,

Baker and Lonsdale equation is applied:

$$\frac{3}{2}\left[1-\left(1-\frac{M_t}{M_o}\right)^{\frac{2}{3}}\right] - \frac{M_t}{M_o} = \frac{3C_s Dt}{r^2 A} \quad (37)$$

where C_s is the drug solubility in medium and A is drug loading per unit volume.

5.4.1. Pore Effects

1. Flux of drug passing through pores of certain microcapsules can be a major source of drug release independent of coating and controlled by rate of dissolution of the core in case of large pores.

But in case of very fine pores, resistance is offered by coating to mass transport. Drug release in this case is given by Flynn equation *(182)*;

$$\frac{D_p}{D_s} = \left(1-\frac{r_s}{r_p}\right)^2\left[1 - 2.104\frac{r_s}{r_p} + 2.09\left(\frac{r_s}{r_p}\right)^3 - 0.95\left(\frac{r_s}{r_p}\right)^5\right] \quad (38)$$

where D_p and D_s are the diffusivity in the fine pores and free solution; r_p, r_s are radius of pores and spheres.

This equation shows that release of large molecules is slowed to a much greater extent than smaller ones by fine pores.

In microcapsules produced by interfacial polycondensation, porous membranes act as semi-permeable coatings, allowing transport of low molecular weight solutes but retaining high molecular weight compounds. This concept forms the principle of artificial cells *(183)*.

2. Release of water soluble drug from porous hydrophobic matrix impermeable to drug: here, transport occurs exclusively within water filled pores.

The equation is given by,

$$Q_{ss} = \frac{A \in D_{eff} C_{is}}{l} \quad (39)$$

where C_{is} is the concentration of saturated drug solution inside reservoir and Q_{ss} is steady-state drug release flux out of membrane with area (*A*), porosity (∈) and thickness (*l*). D_{eff} is the effective D in membrane.

If $D_{eff} = FD_{iw}$,

Then,

$$Q_{ss} = \frac{A \in FD_{iw} C_{is}}{l} \quad (40)$$

where *F* is the formation factor which includes pore geometry and topology, D_{iw} is aqueous diffusion coefficient of drug.

The equation assumes that

1. $F < 1$.
2. There is absence of boundary layer.
3. *D* is independent of initial concentration.

For highly water soluble drugs, $D \propto C$, hence

$$D_{eff} = F\left[\frac{1}{C_{is}} \int_{O}^{C_{is}} D_{iw}(C_{iw})\, dC_{iw}\right] \quad (41)$$

where D_{iw} (C_{iw}) is the concentration dependent diffusion co-efficient of drug in water.

5.4.2. Boundary Layer Effects

Stagnant boundary layer of drug concentrated in contact with surface can hinder drug release by diffusion. The effect is more marked for drugs with low aqueous solubility, where their concentration in unstirred layer can tend towards the drug solubility with resultant loss in driving force for diffusion. This is more important in microcapsules with thin coating.

5.5. Erodible and Biodegradable Systems

In many biodegradable polymeric micro-particulate systems, the drug release is controlled by erosion of matrix rather than diffusion of drug within the matrix e.g. polylactic acid, polyglycolic acid, PLGA, polyanhydrides, proteins, polysaccharides, etc. Erosion of the polymer can be caused by a variety of mechanisms. Typically these are cross-link cleavage, ionisation of pendant groups and backbone cleavage *(184)*. Erosion rates are controlled by crystallinity of the polymers, glass transition temperature (T_g), polymer chain length and co-polymer composition, etc. *(185,186)*. Controlled release from protein or polysaccharide particles can be achieved by varying size or degree of cross-linking *(187,188)*.

Theoretically, it is essential that the rate determining step occurs at boundary between the unaffected region of microspheres and degraded material. *(189)*:

Drug release from surface eroding homogeneous particle is given by

$$\frac{M_t}{M_o} = 1 - \left(1 - \frac{k_e t}{C_o r}\right)^3 \quad (42)$$

where k_e is the erosion rate constant, *r* is initial radius of sphere and C_o is drug concentration in sphere.

where $\frac{M_t}{M_o}$ = fractional drug release at time (*t*).

Generally, bulk eroding particles lose no mass till critical chain length (Mol.Wt. 15,000) after which breakdown is rapid *(190)*.

However, complications arise in case of: (1) non-sphericity of particles, (2) non-homogeneity of matrix, (3) porosity, (4) tortuosity of pores and (5) phase separation of drug within polymer.

For non spherical particles, the equation is given by

$$\frac{M_t}{M_o} = 1 - \left(1 - \frac{k_e t}{C_o a}\right)^n \quad (43)$$

where *a* is the $\frac{1}{2}$ thickness of slabs or radius of sphere and *n* is shape term, for slab, $n = 1$ and $n = 3$ for cylinder and sphere.

5.6. Swelling Controlled System

For hydrophobic matrix, drug is released as the matrix swells and polymer chains relax. Drug release generally precedes polymer biodegradation in such systems.

Factors affecting drug release kinetics include tortuosity, porosity, diffusion co-efficient, solubility, etc. Diffusion is Fickian under equilibrium conditions but non-Fickian during the swelling process.

For thin, glassy slab, drug release profile obtained under countercurrent diffusion of a swelling agent is given by empirical equation

$$\frac{M_t}{M_\infty} = Kt^n \qquad (44)$$

where K is the matrix constant depending on D and n is constant depending on polymer swelling characteristics and relaxation rate of swelling front.

For hydrophilic matrices, $n = 1$ indicating zero ordered release, which is highly desirable for most ideal controlled release forms.

5.6.1. Hydrogels

Hydrogels are water insoluble hydrophilic matrices having capacity to swell from 10 to 98% of their volume in water. If rate of swelling is constant, they give zero order drug release.

In pre-swelled or rapidly swelled hydrogels, release rate is controlled by rate of drug diffusion through matrix. Drug diffusion depends on diffusion co-efficient in water, molecular weight, percentage of polymer in gel, cross-link density, etc.

5.7. *In Vivo* Performance of a Micro-Particulate System

The pharmacological action of a drug co-rrelates better with the concentration-time course of the drug (or its active metabolites) in the blood or some other biophase than with the absolute dose administered. This proposition is based on empirical evidence demonstrating variability in drug disposition both between and within individuals, particularly in the rates of drug absorption, distribution, metabolism and elimination. Various factors affecting *in vivo* performance of a typical sustained release dosage formulation are listed in Table 4.

The ultimate pharmacological targets of a drug molecule micro-particulate preparation are receptor, enzyme, or other macromolecules in a cell, which in turn lies within a tissue. For micro-particulate carriers, the route of administration may be intravenous (i.v.), nasal, oral, intra-arterial, etc depending on the biological requirement, limitation and site of action. Pharmacokinetic considerations determine the dose, latency of onset, peak time and duration of action and the route(s) of administration. Choice of the route for drug delivery depends on a number of factors including the patient compliance, physicochemical properties of the drug, access to the target tissue(s) or effectiveness in dealing with the disease *(9,10,191)*. Micro-particles continue to remain an important mode of drug delivery especially for local administration. Pulmonary route of delivery is another area typically reserved for micro-particles; however, micro-particles can be easily administrated by injection and those made of biodegradable polymers do not need surgical removal. Drug release rates of micro-particulate formulations can be controlled by manipulation of the particle size, polymer degradation and/or erosion rates, the type of polymer and polymer erosion mechanism. Some salient parameters of *in vivo* assessment of micro-particles are given below;

Table 4. Factors Affecting *In Vivo* Performance of a Dosage Form

Type	*Factors*
Physiological	Prolonged drug absorption Variability in GI emptying and motility GI blood flow Influence of feeding on drug absorption
Pharmacokinetic/ biochemical	Dose dumping First-pass metabolism Variability in urinary pH; effect on drug elimination Enzyme induction/inhibition upon multiple dosing
Pharmacological	Changes in drug effect upon multiple dosing Sensitisation/tolerance

5.8. Biodistribution of Micro-Particulate Systems Administered by Parenteral Route

After parenteral administration, the micro-particulate drug carriers enter systemic circulation and have to find the target site from blood stream. All pharmacokinetic processes involve transport of drug across biological membranes. There are a number of barriers that constrain the *in vivo* distribution and kinetic behaviour of injected micro-particles. These barriers include endothelial barrier of vasculature, the phagocytic cells of reticuloendothelial system (RES), and barrier represented by the complex compartmentalised organisation of cells themselves. Therapeutic approaches which are consistent with the restrictions imposed by these *in vivo* barriers will only be having a high probability of success *(192)*.

5.8.1. Endothelial Barrier

The lumen of vasculature is circumscribed by a layer of endothelial cells, which demarcate the vascular and extravascular (tissue) compartments. These endothelial cells regulate the flow of solutes (including macromolecules and micro-particles) between these compartments. The surface area of systemic capillary bed is enormous; for example, in men it has been estimated to be about 60 M^2. Although the cellular lining of a continuous type capillary will clearly prevent the egress of particles with a diameter in excess of 1000 Å, it is also clear that macromolecules of more modest dimensions can cross these barriers. For a number of years, a debate has proceeded between proponents of the 'pore' theory of trans-capillary transport and those of the 'plasmalemmal vesicle' theory. Most recent evidence supports the view that macromolecules cross the capillary endothelial cell layer by riding in a system of vesicles that engulf fluid and solutes on the luminal side of the capillary and release their content on the tissue side *(192)*. Macromolecules up to a diameter of several 100 Å can cross the capillary endothelial barrier by 'transcytosis vesicles'. On the other hand, micro-particulate carriers will either remain impacted upon the luminal side of capillary endothelium, or may exceed from the circulation in specialised (fenestrated) sites such as sinusoidal vessels of liver and spleen. The relationship between molecular or particle size and the permeation characteristics of circulatory vessels has been nicely summarised by Poste and Kirsh *(193)*.

5.8.2. RES Barrier

The RES is comprised of a set of mononuclear cells, which ingest (phagocytose) foreign particles. These cells are particularly concentrated in the lymph glands, spleen, liver and bone marrow. Monocytes originating from precursors in bone marrow enter the blood stream to pass into various tissues where they form macrophages, which monitor the blood stream and engulf circulating pathogens, tissue debris, damaged macromolecules, and micro-particulate drug carriers and clear them from circulation. The cells involved in particle clearance are macrophages like Kupffer cells of liver and macrophages, which border the splenic sinusoidal vessels. The Kupffer cells actually sit astride channels of liver sinusoidal vessels ideally positioned to intercept circulating particles. The non-specific phagocyte capabilities of macrophages are highly developed and these cells readily take up a variety of micro-particles including liposomes, microspheres, as well as other colloidal particulate systems. In depth understanding of cells of the RES is needed for designing of micro-particulate carriers as the phagocytic activities of RES cells decides the ultimate fate of such carriers *(192)*.

5.8.3. Cellular Barrier

Drugs act at specific sites or 'receptors' within cells. The task of a drug delivery system then is not so much to get a drug to a given tissue or cell type but rather to get drug to the appropriate receptor. Recent advances in cell biology show that cells are highly organised entities, with receptors located in specific sub-cellular compartments, so that the cell itself represents a further barrier to controlled drug delivery. A drug carrier entity binds to a particular cell does not ensure that the drug will have an effect on the cell. For example, Leserman's group has recently used monoclonal antibodies to bind liposomes containing a cytotoxic drug specifically to lymphoid tumour cells *(194)*. When the antibodies were directed against certain cell surface antigens, the liposomes were internalised and the drug was able to exert its effect on the cell. On the other hand, with antibody directed against other determinants, the liposomes were bound to the cells but not internalised and thus the drug was without effect.

5.9. *In Vivo* Fate of Micro-Particulate Drug Delivery Systems

Following i.v. administration, the colloidal carriers first come into contact with plasma/serum proteins before they reach target cells *(195)*. Most notably, the interaction of colloidal carriers with the phagocytes often requires some serum components and then subsequently interaction with complement receptors, F_C receptors and sugar/lectin receptors on the macrophage, lymphocytes or other cells. Soluble carriers can be pinocytosed *via* Fc or lectin receptors. A number of other receptors are expressed on different cell types, which negotiates the transportation of various endogenous ligands or colloidal carriers appended with their synthetic mimics. Normally, i.v. injections of colloidal carriers follow their interactions with at least two distinct groups of plasma proteins. It is now recognised that phagocytosis of particulates by elements of RES (liver, spleen, bone marrow) and especially with reference to liver (Kupffer cells) is regulated by the presence and balance between the two groups of serum components: opsonins that promote phagocytosis and dysopsonins that suppress the process. The so-called opsonins adsorb on the surface of the colloidal carriers and render them recognisable and more palatable to RES. Thus, opsonisation is the process of conditioning/coating by plasma proteins and glycoproteins *(196,197)*. Accordingly, the endocytosis of opsonised particles is mediated by the fixed macrophages of RES and circulating monocytes. Immunoglobulins and components of complement systems (particularly C3 and C5) are known as classical opsonin molecules, while fibronectin, C-reactive proteins and tuftsin are also known to enhance recognisation of various particulates by different macrophages.

Rapid escape of micro-particles from the degradative endo-lysosomal compartment and their sustained intracellular retention suggests that these delivery systems containing encapsulated therapeutic agent could serve as an efficient sustained release drug delivery system. Fate of particles is largely dependent on particle size, shape, surface charge, surface characteristics (hydrophobic or hydrophilic), chemical composition and molecular weight. The structure of capillary endothelium and the phagocytic capabilities of RE cells will tend to eventually cause the accumulation of most micro-particles in organs such as liver and spleen where the endothelium is fenestrated and macrophages are abundant.

5.9.1. Factors Affecting Clearance and Distribution of Micro-Particulate Carriers

The chemical and physical characteristics of the carrier that affect its behaviour *in vivo* have been studied in detail for liposomes. It has been known for many years that both particle size and charge can affect liposome clearance kinetics. Thus, large liposomes are cleared more rapidly than small ones and negatively charged vesicles are cleared more far rapidly than neutral or positive ones. The chemical composition of liposomes, particularly with respect to stabilisation of membrane against the disrupting effects of serum lipoproteins is also an important aspect of liposome behaviour. Another important consideration is the dose or load of liposomes administrated. It has been known for many years that the particle clearance rate of the RES is inversely related to the load of particles. Thus, the fractional rate of clearance of a large dose of liposome (or other micro-particulates) is slower than for a smaller dose. One must also keep in mind changes in clearance due to possible toxicities of liposomes and other micro-particles to RES, although, except for the case of sphingomyelin liposomes, the toxicity reported so far have been rather minimal. There have been a number of studies of kinetic behaviour of liposomes in humans *(198)*. The literature on factors controlling the *in vivo* behaviour of drug containing microspheres is currently somewhat limited, although some analyses are beginning to appear. An interesting recent development is the observation that coating microsphere with certain detergents can result in a markedly prolonged circulation lifetime. Nonetheless, one must keep in mind possible detergent toxicities to RES. Thus, a variety of physical factors including particle size, surface charge, surface chemistry and load of particle will all affect the particle clearance rate.

5.9.2. Particle Engineering for Altering the Biopharmaceutics of Micro-Particles

The release profile of encapsulated species can be altered by modifying different formulation parameters like polymer and protein molecular weight, composition, method of preparation, particle size, type of emulsifier used, addition/subtraction of additives, surface modification, etc. In other words the micro-particulate systems for a particular application can be tailor – made. The fabrication protocol of each particle differs considerably and the scale-up could be a challenge for some of these devices. An important issue to be considered when fabricating these systems is the drug load that the reservoir can carry. Furthermore, it is essential that drug will not be altered during the fabrication process and storage. Finally, interactions between drug and the reservoir must be optimised to facilitate drug release only in the target where it is needed and at the desired dose.

'Tailored' micro- and nanoparticles can be exploited to control or avoid, in a predictable manner, their tropism for RES, particularly the tissues of mononuclear phagocyte system (MPS), mainly macrophages of liver and spleen. Surface coating, HLB are the mainly used physical methods and alteration of charge and derivatisation are among the most commonly used chemical methods available for changing their biopharmaceutics. Steric stabilised (stealth) micro-particles, antibody coated micro-particles, surfactant coated micro-particles, bioadhesive (mucoadhesive) micro-particles, magnetically guided micro-particles and biomimetic micro-particles are examples of surface tailoring of micro-particulate drug delivery systems. The uptake of microspheres and nanoparticles by macrophages can be altered by varying parameters like surface properties, composition, concentration and hydrophilicity of the carriers. The particles first come into contact of pseudopodes of macrophages and are engulfed into cytoplasm via lamellipods.

Hydrophobic and relatively large microspheres as well as nanoparticles with lipophilic protein are better phagocytosed than their hydrophilic counterparts. A coating of opsonic materials can exhibit enhanced phagocytosis. Macrophages play an important role in host defense against many infectious agents including bacteria, virus and pathogens. But at the same time, they are the potential reservoirs of some microorganisms that use them as a safe haven. Here rises the need of macrophage targeting for an efficacious prevention and treatment of infectious diseases like leishmaniasis, schistosomiasis, brucellosis, cancer, tuberculosis, etc. *(4,199)*.

The process of particle recognition and capture can be modulated by particle size and surface properties of micro-/nanoparticles. Particles with sizes less than 100 nm in diameter and having a hydrophilic surface are able to have higher residency time in blood and hence possess a greater ability to get targeted to the desired site. Negatively charged and hydrophobic carriers undergo extensive opsonisation and distribute into the RES organs while, positively charged particles act as long-circulating carriers in blood and can also be useful for cancer therapy. They also distribute to brain at relatively higher concentrations and could be useful to deliver drugs to brain for therapeutic purposes. Particles less than 100 nm and having a hydrophobic surface are efficiently removed from the circulation but hydrophilic nanoparticles less than 100 nm can resist this coating process and consequently cleared more slowly. Micro-/nanoparticles can be used to extend the time window of bioavailability along with various sustained and controlled release applications and to protect the drug from chemical and enzymatic decomposition. This can result in reduction of peripheral side effects of drugs by decreasing the overall dose of drugs in body.

The influence of surface charge and size of microspheres on their phagocytosis by mouse peritoneal macrophages were studied by using polystyrene and phenylated polyacrolein microspheres of different diameters as well as modified cellulose microspheres with different surface charge *(200,201)*. The maximum phagocytosis took place when their size was in the range of 1–2 mm and the uptake was a maximum within the range of 1 h period of incubation. The workers assumed that macrophages have the ability to recognise the size of foreign materials by an unknown mechanism. For both negatively and positively charged particles, the extent of phagocytosis were increased with increasing ζ-potentials, and were the lowest when the ζ-potential was zero. However, there was no significant difference in the phagocytosis between the cationic and anionic surfaces when compared at a ζ-potential of same absolute value. Modified cellulose microspheres with different water wettabilities were added to macrophages in order to study the influence of hydrophobicity on macrophage phagocytosis. Hydrophobic microspheres prepared from benzoyl cellulose were most susceptible to phagocytosis and the non-ionic hydrophilic one was least *(200,201)*. It was observed that an optimal surface hydrophobicity is necessary for microspheres to be phagocytosed.

The repeated use of a drug coupled to a protein microcarrier may elicit an immune response. The antibodies formed would then bind to the micro-particle and promote rapid uptake via the Fc receptor of macrophages. Highly charged anionic particles can trigger the alternate pathway of complement activation thereby causing complement components to bind to the particle and hastening its uptake via macrophage C3 receptor. Alternatively, microparticulates may simply adsorb certain serum proteins, such as fibronectin, which can interact with macrophage receptors and thus promote particle clearance.

Magnetically modulated particulate systems have recently attracted much attention for *in vivo* imaging and targeted drug delivery. In this approach, the imaging agents or drugs can be localised to specific sites through the application of an external magnetic field. Particulate systems are rendered magnetic by incorporating Fe_3O_4 particles (10–20 nm) simultaneously with the drug during the preparation stage.

The coating of micro-/nanoparticles with endogenous serum components may circumvent their uptake through MPS. These biomimetic particles mimic the biological environment and disguise the recognition from RES components. The rationale for using albumin and complement components as biomimetic ligands has been proposed by some workers. Albumin is the main protein present in the blood (40 g/L), whereas complement moieties are among the most important opsonins involved in clearance mechanisms. Sialic acids may also serve as a biomimetic ligand to prevent the drug carrier from being recognised by RES, by imitating the sialylated surface. Human orosomucoid, sialic acid rich serum glycoprotein, has been recently used to coat polyalkyl cyanoacrylate nanoparticles. However, the biomimetic coatings were found to provide inadequate protection against opsonin adsorption and RES uptake, presumably due to rapid desorption of these ligands, which turns out to be insufficient in negotiating the stealthing effect *(202)*.

6. EVALUATION OF EFFICACY OF MICRO-PARTICULATE DRUG DELIVERY SYSTEMS

6.1. Conventional/Traditional Methods

Pharmacokinetics (PK) is the quantitative study of drug movement in, through and out of the body. The necessity of *in vivo* evaluation of any drug delivery system lies in the fact to differentiate the action of free drug and encapsulated drug. For *in vivo* evaluation, the drug-loaded carrier is administrated to the animal model of disease by the desired route. With the availability of sensitive assay methods, blood levels of drugs can be measured at pre-determined intervals following administration. Measurement of plasma drug concentration can give an estimate of pharmacokinetic variables. Computer programs are available to analyse pharmacokinetic data on single as well as multi-compartment models. The *in vivo* distribution of drug in different organs/tissues can be studied by scarifying the test animals followed by analysing the desired tissues for drug concentration and other pharmacokinetic parameters.

6.2. Pharmacoscintigraphy

Non-invasive techniques such as nuclear medicine techniques and magnetic resonance imaging and spectroscopy have been utilised for monitoring drug pharmacology. γ-Scintigraphy and positron emission tomography (PET) are basic nuclear medicine tools to investigate life, its function and structure in health and disease. Pharmacoscintigraphy is the application of nuclear medicine techniques for tracing the radiolabeled ingredient of active component of drug/device or the formulation excipient. It can provide vital information regarding the extent, rate, site and mode of drug release in animals. In context of evaluation of micro-particulate drug delivery systems, pharmacoscintigraphy technique appears to be very promising as it is non-invasive, permits repeated measurements and allows use of same organism as its own pre-treatment control. It is possible to extend pharmacoscintigraphy studies in human patients also, thereby making it a pre-clinical screening modality of choice.

Radiotracers have been traditionally used in drug research for the determination of presence of desired effects and untoward side effects, drug–target interaction and drug-delivery studies. Radiopharmaceuticals are radioactive drugs that, when used for the purpose of diagnosis or therapy, typically elicit no physiological response from the patient. The design of these compounds is based solely upon physiological function of the target organ. Unlike radiographic procedures, which depend almost entirely on tissue density differences, external imaging of radiopharmaceutical is essentially independent of density of the target organ. The mechanism of localisation of a radiopharmaceutical in a particular target organ can be as simple as the physical trapping of particles or as sophisticated as an antigen–antibody reaction or chemisorption of an inorganic phosphate on the hydroxyapatite crystals deposited in an acute myocardial infection.

Basic steps in the assessment of biopharmaceutics by nuclear medicine methods are design and synthesis of labeled drug, followed by imaging, determination of parameters of interest and finally data interpretation. Medical diagnostic modalities currently in use include the application of γ-emitting radioactive materials, such as Technetium-99m (^{99m}Tc), Indium-111 (^{111}I), Iodine-125 (^{125}I), Iodine-131 (^{131}I) and Gallium-67 (^{67}Ga). Nearly 80% of all radiopharmaceuticals used in nuclear medicine are ^{99m}Tc-labeled compounds. In terms of physical properties, ^{99m}Tc is the radionuclide of choice for diagnosis in nuclear medicine.

It is possible to get an insight of PK and pharmacodynamics (PD) using nuclear medicine techniques. It permits non-invasive monitoring of PK and functional processes in intact organisms at tracer concentration. Rational use of PK/PD (absorption, transport kinetics, plasma binding, partitioning and biodistribution studies, metabolism, efflux pump activity, etc.) allows for better decision making and streamlines dose optimisation.

Transit and release characteristics of a variety of pharmaceutical dosage forms and quantification of drug release could be followed using the pharmacoscintigraphic studies. It also provides insight into the fate of delivery system and its morphology and integrity, and enables examination of relationship between resultant PK and *in vivo* performance.

For purpose of evaluation of novel drug delivery systems, active ingredient or excipient of formulation/drug delivery system are tagged with a radioisotope and the movement of these carriers traced by *in vivo/ex vivo* studies. The ultimate pharmacological and/or therapeutic response at the region of interest could be obtained from the information at site of release, integrity of formulation and percentage of drug released/absorbed. Pharmacoscintigraphic evaluation of micro-particulate drug delivery system carried out at the Institute of Nuclear Medicine and Allied Sciences, Delhi revealed many interesting findings *(203–211)*. Reddy and co-workers studied influence of administration route on tumour uptake and biodistribution of etoposide loaded tripalmitin nanoparticles (ETPL) in Dalton's lymphoma tumour bearing mice *(212)*. The negatively charged and ^{99m}Tc radiolabeled ETPL nanoparticles were administered by i.v. or intraperitoneal (i.p.), and sub-cutaneous (s.c.) routes and their biodistribution and tumour uptake was evaluated. They found that sub - cutaneous route exhibited reduced distribution in all the tissues studied whereas after i.p. injection, the distribution of ETPL nanoparticles to tissues was higher than the free etoposide. The i.v. injection resulted in lower concentrations of ETPL nanoparticles in the organs of RES compared with free etoposide. It was found that after i.p. injection ETPL nanoparticles were showing a high brain distribution, this finding can be utilised for targeting etoposide to brain tumours. After s.c. injection, the tissue distribution of ETPL nanoparticles increased with time indicating accumulation at the injection site for a longer time. The tumour uptake of both etoposide and ETPL nanoparticles was significantly high after subcutaneous injection compared with other routes of injection. The tumour concentrations of ETPL nanoparticles after s.c. injection was 59-folds higher than that obtained after i.v. injection and eightfolds higher than after i.p. route at 24 h post-injection. The tumour concentration of ETPL nanoparticles increased with time after s.c. injection indicating slower and progressive penetration from the injection site into tumour. The study signifies the advantage of incorporating etoposide into tripalmitin nanoparticles in controlling its biodistribution and enhancing the tumour uptake by several folds. The study also reveals that, of the three routes investigated, s.c. injection is the route of preference for facilitating high tumour uptake and retention.

7. APPLICATIONS

Micro-particles are one of the most exploited carrier system for delivery and modulation of release of therapeutic agents from small molecule drugs to therapeutic proteins and peptides *(213)*. Micro-particle systems can be designed for administration by various routes like oral, injectable (intramuscular [IM]), topical, nasal, pulmonary, etc. They are also potential carriers for target delivery in the form of ligand mediated micro-particles, magnetic micro-particles or microspheres. There is enormous research conducted in this area with an objective of improving the therapeutic efficacy of drug candidates by various strategies including improving release profiles, site specific delivery and extra-corporal modulation for targeting. Some of these micro-particle systems have attracted much attention and are extensively researched and even commercialised. Table 6 enlists few micro-particulate drug delivery systems available in the market.

In addition, micro-particulate systems technology is expected to impact almost all aspects of life. There are numerous biological applications of micro-particles like enzyme immobilisation, cell immobilisation for multi-enzyme reactions, transportation of tracers in biological studies (radioactive marker, fluorescent markers, electron-dense markers), etc.

7.1. Micro-Particles in Oral Drug Delivery

Oral route is the most preferred route for administration of bioadhesive micro-particles, but is associated with poor bioavailability for a number of drugs. To circumvent this problem, it has been proposed to associate drugs to polymeric bioadhesive micro-particulate systems because they adhere to mucosal surface (bioadhesion) and provide better opportunity for drug absorption in a controlled manner. The fate of micro-particles in GI tract follows one or more of these different pathways; bioadhesion, mucosal translocation and transit and direct fecal elimination. The bioadhesion offered by micro-/nanoparticles could be attributed to several factors like an increase of adhesive force due to decrease in size (nanoscopic), or a prolongation of GI transit time leading to higher bioavailability of drugs. The bioadhesive properties can be optimised by reducing the size of the micro-particulate systems. Kriwet et al., prepared bioadhesive micro- and nanoparticles of polyacrylic acid by inverse emulsion polymerisation method and found their adhesive forces comparable with those of polycarbophil *(214)*.

The application of tomato lectin as a bioadhesive ligand has been demonstrated to enhance subsequent intestinal transcytosis of colloidal particulates to which it is bound to gliadin nanoparticles (GNP) compared with control GNP *(215,216)*. Gliadin is rich in neutral amino acids that can promote hydrogen-bonding interactions with mucosa, and lipophilic residual components, which can interact with biological tissue through hydrophobic interactions.

Chitosan is a unique polymer that has demonstrated utility in a number of applications for oral drug delivery. This excipient can serve a number of purposes, including

Table 5. Micro-Particulate Drug Delivery Systems in the Market

Name/Manufacturer	*Application*
Doxil/Alza (liposome encapsulated doxorubicin)	Cancer
Ocusert/Alza	Depot for ocular delivery of pilocarpine
Zoladex/Astra Zenecea	Cancer
Oncospar/Enzon (PEG-L-asparaginase)	To treat acute lymphocytic leukemia
Lupron Depot/Tap Pharma	Luteinising hormone releasing hormone treatment of prostate cancer
Capronor	1-yr release of levonorgestrel (contraceptive)

as a coating agent, gel former, controlled-release matrix, in addition to inducing desirable properties, such as mucoadhesion and permeation enhancement to improve oral bioavailability of a drug. Additional safety and toxicology studies in accordance with the FDA's guidelines for new excipient development however, are going on to further promote the use of this polymer as a pharmaceutical excipient.

Sharma *et al. (208)* prepared microbeads for oral sustained delivery of nifedipine, ampicillin and various steroids by co-acervation process. The beads can be hardened by cross-linking with glutaraldehyde or epoxychlorpropane to produce rotundine microcapsules. The release profiles of all these drugs when investigated showed higher release rates at pH 1.0–2.0 than at pH 7.2–7.4.

Chitosan derivatives like *N*-trimethyl chitosan chloride (TMC) holds a lot of promise to deliver drugs. The formed micro-particles are non-toxic, bioadhesive and biodegradable. Chitosan can also be used as an absorption enhancer for poorly absorbable hydrophilic and/or macromolecular drugs. Chitosan, when linked with oppositely charged ions, lead to polymer matrix formation with decreased hydrophilicity and subsequent modified drug release properties. Ibuprofen was incorporated into the micro-particles and were evaluated using Caco-2 cell monolayers in order to determine and screen the compound for intestinal transport. Astonishing results were observed when the drug– chitosan, drug–TMC and drug–cetosteryl alcohol were compared.

Magnetically modified particulate systems have shown prolonged drug retention in the intestine and also, is used for oral delivery of therapeutic proteins. Cheng and co-workers performed an interesting experiment to achieve the oral route for therapeutic proteins *(217)*. Using BALB/c mouse model, they checked the therapeutic potential of oral intake of insulin assuming that the application of magnetic forces (using a magnetic belt in the intestinal region) in the intestinal area will localise insulin drug carrier containing magnetites to prolong the residence time of orally ingested micro-particles by slowing down their transit and finally increase the absorption of protein drugs. They co-encapsulated magnetite nanocrystals and insulin into poly(lactic-*co*-glycolic acid) (PLGA) micro-particles and studied their effects on hypoglycemia in mice in presence of circumferentially applied external magnetic field. Upon orally ingesting 100 U/kg of insulin– magnetite–PLGA micro-particles to fasted mice, they observed reduction of blood glucose levels of 43.8% in the presence of an external magnetic field for 20 h and subsequently obtained higher bioavailability.

7.2. Micro-Particles in Ocular Drug Delivery

Microspheres can also be used for ocular drug delivery In ocular drug delivery, high rate of tear turnover, and the blinking action of eyelids lead to short pre-corneal residence times for applied eye drops. Typically, the washout rate reduces concentration of the drug in a tear film to one-tenth of its starting value in 4–20 min. As a result, the eye absorbs only a few percent of administered drug and the duration of therapeutic action may be quite short. Early reports showed that the formulation of eye drops is decisive for availability of an ocular drug *(218)*. The absorbed amount of model substance, fluoro metholone, and duration in aqueous humor increased when a suspension was used instead of a solution, and the best result was obtained when the drug was formulated in an ointment. Similar results as with an ointment were obtained when a suspension formulated in a hydrogel was used *(219)*. The combination of particles with a hydrogel thus increases the bioavailability of an ocular drug. A hydrogel may increase pre-corneal residence time of a suspension, and the residence time of the hydrogel, therefore, sets the maximal achievable residence time for a given drug. Water-soluble drugs are generally not retained by hydrogels because of their high diffusion co-efficients. One way of solving this problem is to incorporate these drugs into polymeric micro-particles.

A novel microsphere-gel formulation was investigated aiming to extend pre-corneal residence times for ocular drugs *(220)*. Poly(adipic anhydride) was used for microencapsulation of timolol maleate. A non-aqueous method for the microsphere preparation was employed due to hydrolytical sensitivity of the polymer. Microspheres were prepared with an average diameter of 40 μm. The polymer and the microspheres were characterised before and during degradation using size exclusion chromatography, differential scanning calorimeter, X-ray diffraction, infrared spectroscopy and SEM *(220)*. The microspheres had a smooth external surface and a hollow centre surrounded by a dense outer shell. Degradation of the microspheres resulted in a constant release of adipic acid, the degradation product, indicating a surface-eroding degradation mechanism. The surface erosion of polymer controlled the release of incorporated substance, timolol maleate. The drug release rate profile appeared to be suitable for ocular drug delivery. However, the initial drug release rate was decreased to some extent when the PAA–microspheres were incorporated into an *in situ* gelling polysaccharide Gelrite® *(220, 221)*. The authors claimed that improved ocular bioavailability of these novel microsphere-gel delivery formulations remains to be compared with that of ordinary eye drops.

7.3. Micro-Particles in Parenteral Drug Delivery

Faisant *et al.* prepared and studied 5-fluorouracil (5-FU)-loaded, PLGA based micro-particles for brain tumours and evaluated them for drug release kinetics and to understand the release mechanisms *(222)*. The micro-particles were prepared by a solvent extraction method. PLGA based micro-particles offer various important advantages compared with conventional pharmaceutical dosage forms as to control accurate release of drug over prolonged periods of time, easy administration and good biocompatibility. It also included complete biodegradation avoiding the removal of empty remnants of the polymer. Drug release was studied in various types of release media, differing in osmolarity, buffer concentration, pH, temperature, etc. Stability studies showed that 5-FU was stable in all release media during the entire observation periods. The obtained micro-particles were spherical in shape, with a mean diameter of 47 μm and an intial drug loading of 26%. The 5-FU was located in the form of small crystals in different sized cavities, which were distributed throughout the micro-particles. The experimentally determined release kinetics of 5-FU in phosphate buffer pH 7.4 at 37°C showed three phasic patterns—at early time points, the release rate was high with an initial high burst; a second phase with an approximately constant 5-FU release rate with zero order kinetics, and the last with a final rapid release phase leading to complete exhaust of the drug.

7.4. Micro-Particles as Immunologicals

The cellular immune response against tumours, viruses or intracellular bacteria requires adequate antigen delivery to professional phagocytes, their processing and presentation of antigenic peptides to T-cells. Biodegradable micro-particles to enhance antigen phagocytosis and the response of cytotoxic lymphocytes have been proposed. The study was conducted by Wischke *et al.* to formulate poly(lactide-*co*-glycolide) (PLGA) micro-particles using a W/O/W solvent evaporation procedure in order to obtain suitable vehicles for vaccination. BSA bearing fluorescein isothiocyanate (FITC–BSA) was used as a model antigen. For micro-particle preparation, a static micromixer was employed. Micro-particles of 2–3 μm can be produced with good reproducibility by applying high flow rates of the micromixer. Micro-particles with a smooth surface and only one pore were observed using SEM. CLSM revealed the localisation of FITC–BSA near the surface of micro-particle. Microencapsulation of FITC–BSA did not alter the polymer characteristics, as determined by measuring the glass transition temperature. The studies also showed that the micro-particles were able to deliver the model antigen to human dendritic cells (DC) *(223)* micro-particles for the antigen delivery to DCs using a static micromixer *(224)*.

7.5. Micro-Particles in Vaccine Delivery

The pre-requisite of a vaccine is protection against the microorganism or its toxic product(s). An ideal vaccine must fulfill the requirement of efficacy, safety, convenience in application and cost. The aspect of safety and minimisation of adverse reaction is a complex issue. The aspect of safety and degree of production of antibody responses are closely related to mode of application. Biodegradable delivery systems for vaccines that are given by parenteral route may overcome the shortcoming of the conventional vaccines. The interest in parenteral (s.c, IM and intradermal) carrier is due to specific advantages like (1) improved antigenicity by adjuvant action, (2) modulation of antigen release and (3) stabilisation of antigen (225).

Immunisations are an essential tool for the prevention of many infectious diseases. DNA vaccines offer great promise for safer and more effective vaccines when compared with traditional protein immunisations. Current technologies for the delivery of DNA vaccines involve the simple injection of DNA in solution, use of cationic polymers or lipids, or use of gene guns. Efficient, targeted delivery of nucleic acids to antigen processing cells could significantly enhance the efficacy of nucleic acid based immunotherapy for cancer and infectious diseases. Nucleic acids, surface adsorbed on cationic particles, have been shown to produce superior immune responses compared with existing methods. Currently, such cationic particles are synthesised by non-covalent incorporation of cationic polymers or surfactants on the surface of polymer micro-particles, which suffer from easy and premature dissociation of the cationic polymer and nucleic acids. In addition, cationic surfactants are often toxic and do not possess any intrinsic mechanism to enhance DNA delivery inside the cells. Improved non-toxic formulations, with built-in properties for enhancing gene transfer efficacy, are therefore needed for successful clinical translation of nucleic acid based immunotherapy.

7.6. Micro-Particles Containing Bacterial Antigens

Micro-particles encapsulating bacterial antigens are prepared using a standard bacterial antigenic pool. The live cells are dispersed in physiological saline with heating in flowing steam for 15 min. After centrifugation, dialyse the supernatant for 5 d at 4°C between several changes of DI water. Centrifuge the dialysed material and suspend the same in ultra pure water and freeze dry. Determine the required components by standard methods and use the antigen to prepare micro-particulate vaccine formulation.

Loaded micro-particles are prepared using a three step procedure as follows:

1. Homogenisation of antigenic extract.
2. Preparation of micro-particles by multiple emulsion followed by a solvent evaporation method.
3. Purification and lyophilisation.

Homogenisation is achieved by mixing in a mortar for 5–30 min. Disperse the mixture in an aqueous solution containing Pluronic F-68 for 2 min. Determine the size after filtering and the final product is studied physicochemically.

7.7. Chemoembolisation

Chemoembolisation is an extension of percutaneous embolisation techniques. With chemoembolisation, investigators embolise tumours with micro-particles soaked with chemotherapeutic agents. In chemoembolisation, the biodegradable particle is administered to the liver tumours using a catheter that passes directly into an artery of the tumour *(202)*. The theoretical advantage is that such embolisations not only provide vascular occlusion but will bring about sustained therapeutic levels of chemotherapeutics in the areas of tumour. Generalised ischemia so created would reduce the ability of the cell to relieve itself from the toxicity of chemotherapy. Degradable starch microspheres injected intra-arterially are trapped in an extra capillary network formed in liver metastases. Drug dissolved in the microsphere suspension gets retained in the blood vessel of the target organ as long as the blood flow remains blocked and then gradually releases the drugs, resulting in a longer duration of drug exposure to the tumour. The technique of chemoembolisation is a combination of beneficial effects of embolisation and local chemotherapy. Intra-arterial injections of microspheres increase the therapeutic efficacy of anti-mitotic drugs by causing temporary embolisation. Spherical particles are most useful in achieving distal homogenous and effective embolism. The kinetics of drug release from the emboli and biodegradation rate of drug carriers are important in determining the bioavailability of the drug in restricted area. The biodegradable microspheres of starch, PLA or PLGA may be used for the purpose of achieving the occlusion. The microspheres of size less than 40 μm are injected intra-arterially, which causes blockade of the arterioles at the tumour sites. This blockade of the arterioles and the capillary bed may be beneficial in two ways; first, it increases the time of absorption of the drugs at the tumour site and second, due to blockade of feeder vessels it causes ischemia and hence leads to the tumour regression.

7.8. Imaging

Medical diagnostic imaging requires that an appropriate intensity of a certain signal from an area of interest be achieved to differentiate this area from surrounding tissues. Currently used medical imaging techniques are γ-imaging, magnetic resonance, computed tomography and ultrasonography. The microspheres have been extensively studied and used for the targeting purposes. Various cells, cell lines, tissues and organs can be imaged using radiolabeled microspheres. The particle size range of microsphere is an important factor in determining the imaging of particular sites. The particles injected intravenously apart from the portal vein will become entrapped in the capillary bed of the lungs. This phenomenon is exploited for scintiographic imaging of the tumour masses in lungs using labeled human serum albumin microspheres *(202)*. Oldenburg *et al.* recently prepared serum albumin microspheres and modified its surface by layer-by-layer electrostatc adhesion of peptides containing an integrin-receptor specific sequence *(226)*. They showed that these modified microspheres can be used as an effective target for integrin expressing cells and colon tumour cells *in vivo*. They proposed that a generalised method can be developed for labeling the microspheres with peptide ligands to other important cell membrane receptors and thus a new approach towards both targeted imaging and targeted drug delivery can be developed *(227)*.

Vyas and Khar *(202)*, Vyas and Malaiya *(228)*, studied the *in vivo* magnet responsiveness and kinetics of distribution of indomethacin entrapped in magnetic poly (methylmethacrylate) nanoparticles on a rat tail model and periodically monitored drug concentration in various visceral organs after intra-arterial and i.v. administration. Upto 60 min post-injection time, 60-fold higher concentration could be achieved in tail target segment which resulted in considerably reduced drug concentration in other organs like liver and spleen. Guimaraes and co-workers, have been used super-paramagnetic iron oxide nanoparticles as pathologic basis for contrast enhancement by MR lymphography. After i.v. injection of super-paramagnetic nanoparticles, a decrease in signal intensity indicates active uptake of particles by macrophages, whereas an increase signal intensity indicates altered capillary permeability to the tumour. These findings in rats may prove to be clinically useful for differentiating benign from malignant enlarged lymph nodes. Moore and co-workers, investigated the accumulation and cellular uptake of long-circulating dextran-coated iron oxide (LCDIO) particles in malignant neoplasms *in vivo*. LCDIO was preferentially localised in tumour cells (49.0% ± 4.6) but was also taken up by macrophages in tumours (21.0% ± 3.1) and by endothelial cells in the area of active angiogenesis *(230)*.

7.9. Immobilisation

The chitosan micro-particles are prepared by simple co-acervation method by dissolving the polymer in aqueous acetic acid or formic acid and the solution is blown into NaOH, NaOH–methanol or ethanediamine solution using a suitable device like compressed air nozzle. This helps in the formation of co-acervates which are porous beads with porosity depending on the concentration of chitosan-acid solution and the degree of N-acetylation of chitosan. Apart from these, type and concentration of co-acervation agents used also decide the nature of porosity of formed beads. These beads have applications in various fields like enzymatic immobilisation, chromatograph support, adsorbent of metal ions, lipoprotein and cell cultures. The porous surface of the beads make good cell culture carriers. Protease was immobilised into the porous chitosan beads and the immobilised enzyme was found to have higher thermal storage stability and a higher activity toward the smaller ester substrate, *N*-benzyl-L-arginine ethyl ester (231).

8. SUMMARY AND FUTURE PERSPECTIVES

Each person responds to a drug therapy in a unique manner *(229)*. Drug absorption, distribution, metabolism can vary widely from person to person, even within the same family. These facts have raised the need of individualised drug therapy and use of chemical biosensors for monitoring level of important marker molecules for guiding the therapeutic process and hence improving drug safety and efficacy. The solution for this lies in 'Responsive drug delivery' whereby the system located inside the patient's body could sense continuously, detect the early onset of a crisis and immediately respond with the remedial measure causing minimal discomfort to the patient's daily routine *(232)*.

Till date responsive drug delivery have included *ex vivo* detection of a marker molecule and *in vivo* delivery of drug or *in vivo* detection of a marker molecule coupled to an external delivery system. Both the systems have merits and are advantageous but the complete *in vivo* system where both, the detection and delivery occurs *in vivo* is a distant reality till date *(232)*.

Few other approaches to drug delivery systems are osmotic pumps, gene delivery. With availability of various biodegradable and bioinspired polymers it shall be now possible to design micro-particulate systems for protracted drug release, organ imaging, effective immunisation and in development of bioimplantable devices, bioreactors, biochips, biosensors and tissue surrogates prosthesis. Furthermore, in future by combining various other strategies, micro-particles will find their central place in novel drug delivery systems, particularly in disease cell sorting, diagnostics, gene and genetic materials, safe, targeted and effective *in vivo* delivery, which may have its implications in gene therapy, genetic customisation and supplements as miniature versions of the diseased organs and tissues in the body. Particulate dosage forms are an area where new technologies and better fundamental understanding is required to design newer drug delivery systems. For tailored micro-particulate systems to gain momentum, surface chemistry research is expected to contribute in designing dosage forms and routes of administration. By using micro-particulate system, we can avoid the inconvenient surgical insertion of large implants. Till date, the biomedical potential of micro-particulate formulations is far from being fully exploited and future steps may lead to further and better products and offer novel therapeutic and economic technologies *(233)*.

9. REFERENCES

1. **Birnbaum, DT. and Peppas, LB.** Microparticle drug delivery systems, in Drug delivery System in Cancer Therapy, (Brown, DM., ed.), Humana Press Inc., Totowa, NJ, 2004, pp. 117–137.
2. **Delie, F. and Blanco-Prieto, MJ.,** Polymeric particulates to improve oral bioavailability of peptide drugs. *Molecules* 2005;10:65–80.
3. **Orive, G., Hernandez, RM., Gascon, AR., and Pedraz, JL.** Micro and nano drug delivery systems in cancer therapy. *Cancer Ther.* 2005;3:131–138.
4. **Ahsan, F., Rivas, IP., Khan, MA., and Suarez, AIT.** Targeting to macrophages: role of physicochemical properties of particulate carriers-liposomes and microspheres- on the phagocytosis by macrophages. *J. Control. Release* 2002;79:29–40.
5. **Soppimath, SS., Aminabhavi, TM., Kulkarni, AR., and Rudzinski, WE.** Biodegradable polymeric nanoparticles as drug delivery devices. *J. Control. Release* 2001;70:1–20.
6. **Alexandridou, S., Kiparissides, C., Kotti, K., and Chaitidou, S.** Recent advances in drug delivery systems, In: proceedings of the 8th polymers for Advanced Technologies International Symposium, Budapest, Hungary, 13–16th September, 2005.
7. **Soni, S., Babbar, AK., Sharma, RK., Banerjee, T., and Maitra, AN.** Pharmacoscintigraphic evaluation of polysorbate80 coated chitosan nanoparticles for brain targeting #653, In: proceedings of the 32nd Annual Meeting Controlled Release Society, Miami Beach, FL, USA, 2005.
8. **Gregoriadis, G. (ed.)** Drug Carriers in Biology and Medicine, Academic Press Inc., (London) Ltd., 1979, pp. viii–xi.
9. **Dunn, RL. and Ottenbrite, RM. (eds.),** Polymeric drugs and drug delivery systems, American Chemical Society, Washington, DC, 1991.
10. **Langer, R.** Drug delivery and targeting. *Nature* 1998;392(Supp):5–10.
11. **Bhalla, HL.** Drug delivery research in India: a challenge and an opportunity. *J. Control. Release* 1999;62:65–68.
12. **Payne, GF., Chaubal, MV., Barbari, T.,** Enzyme-catalyzed polymer modification: reaction of phenolic compounds with chitosan films. *Polymer* 1996;37:4643–4648.
13. **Park, HS., Lee, JY., Cho, SH., Baek, HJ., and Lee, SJ.** Colon delivery of prednisolone based on chitosan-coated polysaccharide tablets. *Arch. Pharm. Res.* 2002;25(6):964–968.
14. **Sakkinen, M., Linna, A., Ojala, S., Jurjenson, H., Veski, P., and Marvola, M.** In vivo evaluation of matrix granules containing microcrystalline chitosan as a gel-forming excipient. *Int. J. Pharm.* 2003;250(1):227–237.
15. **Tozaki, H., Odoriba, T., Okada, N., et al.** Chitosan capsules for colon-specific drug delivery: enhanced localization of 5-aminosalicylic acid in the large intestine accelerates healing of TNBS-induced colitis in rats. *J. Control. Release* 2002;82(1):51–61.
16. **Sinha, VR. and Kumria, R.** Polysaccharides in colon-specific drug delivery. *Int. J. Pharm.* 2001;224(1–2):19–38.
17. **Thanou, M., Verhoef, JC., Marbach, P., and Junginger, HE.** Intestinal absorption of octreotide: N-trimethyl chitosan chloride (TMC) ameliorates the permeability and absorption properties of the somatostatin analogue in vitro and in vivo. *J. Pharm. Sci.* 2000;89(7):951–957.
18. **Kotze, AF., Luessen, HL., Thanou, M., et al.** Chitosan and chitosan derivatives as absorption enhancers for peptide drugs across mucosal epithelia, in Bioadhesive Drug Delivery Systems, (Matiowitz, E., Chickering, DE., and Lehr, CM., eds.), New York, NY., Marcel Dekker, 1999, pp. 341–386.
19. **Hamman, JH., Schultz, CM., and Kotze, AF.** N-trimethyl chitosan chloride: optimum degree of quaternization for drug absorption enhancement across epithelial cells. *Drug Dev. Ind. Pharm.* 2003;29(2):161–172.

20. **Aiedeh, K. and Taha, MO.** Synthesis of iron-cross-linked chitosan succinate and iron-cross-linked hydroxamated chitosan succinate and their in vitro evaluation as potential matrix materials for oral theophylline sustained-release beads. *Eur. J. Pharm. Sci.* 2001;13(2):159–168.
21. **Aiedeh, K. and Taha, MO.** Synthesis of chitosan succinate and chitosan phthalate and their evaluation as suggested matrices in orally administered, colon-specific drug delivery systems. *Arch. Pharm.* (Weinheim). 1999;332(3):103–107.
22. **Guggi, D. and Bernkop-Schnurch, A.** *In vitro* evaluation of polymeric excipients protecting calcitonin against degradation by intestinal serine proteases. *Int. J. Pharm.* 2003;252(1–2):187–196.
23. National Toxicology Program Document. http://ntp.niehs.nih.gov/index.cfm?objectid; accessed on 1st September, 2007.
24. **Tonnesen, HH. and Karlsen, J.** Alginate in drug delivery systems. *Drug Dev. Ind. Pharm.* 2002;28:621–630.
25. **Kim, CK. and Lee, EJ.** The controlled release of blue dextran from alginate beads. *Int. J. Pharm.* 1992;79:11–19.
26. **Wan, LSC., Heng, PWS., and Chan, LW.** Influence of hydrophile-lipophile balance on alginate microspheres. *Int. J. Pharm.* 1993;95(1–3):77–83.
27. **Patel, YL., Sher, P., and Pawar, AP.** The effect of drug concentration and curing time on processing and properties of calcium alginate beads containing metronidazole by response surface methodology. *AAPS PharmSciTech.* 2006;7(4):86.
28. **Gonzalez-Rodriguez, ML., Holgado, MA., Sanchez Lafuente C., Rabasco, AM., and Fini, A.** Alginate/chitosan particulate systems for sodium diclofenac release. *Int. J. Pharm.* 2002;232:225–234.
29. **Lin, SY. and Ayres, JW.** Calcium alginate beads as core carriers of 5-aminosalicyclic acid calcium alginate beads as core carriers of 5-aminosalicyclic acid. *Pharm. Res.* 1992;9(9):1128–1131.
30. **Lee, B., Min, G., and Kim, T.** Preparation and in vitro release of melatonin loaded multivalent cationic alginate beads. *Arch. Pharm. Res.* 1996;19:280–285.
31. **Takka, S. and Acartürk, F.** Calcium alginate microparticles for oral administration. I. Effect of sodium alginate type on drug release and drug entrapment efficiency; *J. Microencapsul.* 1999;16(3):275–290.
32. **Murata, Y., Toniwa, S., Miyamoyo, E., and Kawashima, S.** Preparation of alginate gel beads containing chitosan salt and their functions. *Int. J. Pharm.* 1999;176;265–268.
33. **Huguet, ML. and Dellacherie, E.** Calcium alginate beads coated with chitosan: effect of structure encapsulated materials on their release. *Process Biochemistry* 1996;31:745–751.
34. **Huguet, ML., Neufeld, RJ., and Dellacherie, E.** Calcium alginate beads coated with polycationic polymers: comparison of chitosan and DEAE-dextran. *Process Biochemistry* 1996;31:347–353.
35. **Ozsoy, Y. and Bergişadi, N.** Preparation of mefenamic acid sustained release beads based on kappa-carrageenan. *Boll. Chim. Farm.* 2000;139:120–123.
36. **Sankalia, MG., Mashru, RC., Sankalia, JM., and Sutariya, VB.** Physicochemical characterization of papain entrapped in ionotropically cross-linked kappa-carrageenan gel beads for stability improvement using Doehlert shell design. *J. Pharm. Sci.* 2006;95(9):1994–2013.
37. **Sankalia, MG., Mashru, RC., Sankalia, JM., and Sutariya, VB.** Stability improvement of alpha-amylase entrapped in kappa-carrageenan beads: physicochemical characterization and optimization using composite index. *Int. J. Pharm.* 2006;312(1–2):1–14.
38. **Bani-Jaber, A. and Al-Ghazawi, M.** Sustained release characteristics of tablets prepared with mixed matrix of sodium carrageenan and chitosan: effect of polymer weight ratio, dissolution medium, and drug type. *Drug Dev. Ind. Pharm.* 2005;31(3):241–217.
39. **Grizzi, I., Garreau, H., Li, S., and Vert, M.** Biodegradation of devices based on poly (D,L-lactic acid): size-dependence. *Biomaterials* 1995;16:305–311.
40. **Li, S.** Hydrolytic degradation characteristics of aliphatic polyesters derived from lactic and glycolic acids. *Biomed. Mater. Res.* 1999;48:342–353.
41. **Siepmann, J., Elkharraz, K., Siepmann, F., and Klose, D.** How autocatalysis accelerates drug release from PLGA-based microparticles: a quantitative treatment. *Biomacromolecules* 2005;6:2312–2319.
42. **Dunne, M., Corrigan, OI., and Ramtoola, Z.** Influence of particle size and dissolution conditions on the degradation properties of polylactide-co-glycolide particles. *Biomaterials* 2000;21:1659–1668.
43. **Kang, J. and Schwendeman, SP.** Comparison of the effects of $Mg(OH)_2$ and sucrose on in poly(lactide-co-glycolide) microspheres. *Pharm. Res.* 2000;17(6):677–683.
44. **Fan, LT. and Singh, SK.** Diffusion controlled release, in Controlled release—A Quantitative Treatment, (Fan, LT. and Singh, SK., eds.), Berlin, Germany, Springer-Verlag, 1989, pp. 61–79.
45. **Dhawan, S., Singla, AK., and Sinha, VR.** Properties of chitosan microspheres prepared by different methods. *AAPS Pharm Sci Tech.* 2004;5(4):67.
46. **Tomofumi, Y., Hiraku, O., and Yoshiharu M.** Sustained release ketoprofen microparticles with ethylcellulose and carboxymethylethylcellulose. *J. Control. Release* 2001;75(3): 271–282.
47. **Li, B., Wu, Y., and Pan, Z.** Experimental study on preparation of microparticles using supercritical CO_2 spray drying: Paper number. 066204, 2006 ASAE Annual Meeting., Portland, Oregon, July 9–12.
48. **Vikova, M., Rak, J., and Chalabala, M.** Matrix type tablets formed from microparticles coated with ethylcellulose. *Euro. J. Pharm. Sci.* 1996;4(1):186–186(1).
49. **Zandi, M., Pourjavadi, A., Hashemi, SA., and Arabi, H.** Preparation of ethyl cellulose microcapsules containing perphenazine and polymeric perphenazine based on acryloyl chloride for physical and chemical studies of drug release control. *Polym. Int.* 1998, 47(4):413–418.

50. **Tanwar, YS., Gupta, GD., and Ramawat, KG.** Development and evaluation of microparticles of gugulipid. *Pharm. Rev.* 2006;124–132.

51. **Salib, NN., El-menshaway, ME., and Ismail, AA.** Ethyl cellulose as a potential sustained release coating for oral pharmaceuticals. *Pharmazie.* 1976;31(10):721–723.

52. **Sevgi, F., Ozyazici, M., and Guneri, T.** Sustained-release dosage form of phenylpropanolamine hydrochloride. Part I: Microencapsulation and *In vitro* Release Kinetics. *J. Microencapsul.* 1994;11(3):327–334.

53. **Sevgi, F., Ozyazici, M., and Guneri, T.** Sustained-release dosage form of phenylpropanolamine hydrochloride. Part II: Formulation and *In vitro* Release Kinetics from tableted microcapsules. *J. Microencapsul.* 1994;11(3):335–344.

54. **Mukherjee, B., Mahanti, B., Panda, P., and Mahapatra, S.** Preparation and evaluation of verapamil hydrochloride microcapsules. *Am. J. Ther.* 2005;12(5):417–424.

55. **Singh, J. and Robinson, DH.** Controlled release captopril microcapsules: effect of ethyl cellulose viscosity grade on the *in vitro* dissolution from microcapsules and tableted microcapsules. *J. Microencapsul.* 1990;7(1):67–76.

56. **Alpar, HO. and Walters, V.** The prolongation of the *in vitro* dissolution of a soluble drug (phenethicillin potassium) by microencapsulation with ethyl cellulose. *J. Pharm. Pharmacol.* 1981;33(7):419–422.

57. **Sanjeev, C., Vinay, G., Archna, R., and Saha, RN.** Oral controlled release formulation of diclofenac sodium by microencapsulation with ethyl cellulose. *J. Microencapsul.* 2002;19(6):753–760.

58. **Sinha, VR., Bansal, K., Kaushik, R., Kumria, R. and Trehan, A.** Poly-ε-caprolactone microspheres and nanospheres: an overview. *Int. J. Pharm.* 2004;278(1):1–23.

59. **Chan, LW., Liu, X., and Heng, PW.** Liquid phase coating to produce controlled-release alginate microspheres. *J. Microencapsul.* 2005;22(8):891–900.

60. **Herrero-Vanrell, R. and Refojo, MF.** Biodegradable microspheres for vitreoretinal drug delivery. *Adv. Drug Deliv. Rev.* 2001;52:5–16.

61. **Porjazoska, A., Goracinova, K., Mladenovska, K., et al.** Poly(lactide-co-glycolide) microparticles as systems for controlled release of proteins—preparation and characterization. *Acta Pharm.* 2004;54(3):215–229.

62. **Brunner, A., Mader, K., and Gopferich, A.** pH and osmotic pressure inside bio-degradable microsphere during erosion. *Pharm. Res.* 1999;6:847–853.

63. **Li, L. and Schwendeman, SP.** Mapping neutral microclimate pH in PLGA microspheres. *J. Control. Release* 2005;101(1–3):163–173.

64. **Chaw, CS., Yang, YY., Lim, IJ., and Phan, TT.** Water-soluble betamethasone-loaded poly(lactide-coglycolide) hollow microparticles as a sustained release dosage form. *J. Microencapsul.* 2003;20(3):349–359.

65. **Jelvehgari, M., Siahi-Shadbad, MR., Azarmi, S., Martin, GP., and Nokhodchi, A.** The microsponge delivery system of benzoyl peroxide: preparation, characterization and release studies. *Int. J. Pharm.* 2006;308(1–2):124–132.

66. **Jeong, JH., Byun, Y., and Park, TG.** Synthesis and characterization of poly(L-Lysine)-g-poly(D,L-lactic-co-glycolic acid) biodegradable micelles. *J. Biomater. Sci. Polym.* 2003;14:1–11.

67. **Miao, ZM., Cheng, SX., Zhang, XZ., and Zhuo, RX.** Study on drug release behaviors of poly-alpha, beta-[n-(2-hydroxyethyl)-L-aspartamide]-g-poly(epsilon-caprolactone) nano- and microparticles. *Biomacromolecules* 2006;7(6):2020–2026.

68. **Petrov, O., Furó, I., Schuleit, M., Domanig, R., Plunkett, M., and Daicic, J.**, Pore size distributions of biodegradable polymer microparticles in aqueous environments measured by NMR cryoporometry. *Int. J. Pharm.* 2006;309(1–2):157–162.

69. **Tu, J., Bolla, S., Barr, J., Miedema, J. Li, X., and Jasti, B.** Alginate microparticles prepared by spray–coagulation method: preparation, drug loading and release characterization. *Int. J. Pharm.* 2005;303(1–2):171–181.

70. **Merisko-Liversidge, E., Liversidge, GG., and Cooper, ER.** Nanosizing: a formulation approach for poorly-water-soluble compounds. *Eur. J. Pharm. Sci.* 2003;18:113–120.

71. **Patravale, VB., Date, AA., and Kulkarni, RM.** Nanosuspensions: a promising drug delivery strategy. *J. Pharm. Pharmacol.* 2004;56(7):827–840.

72. **Krause, KP., Kayser, O., Mäder, K., Gust, R., and Müller, RH.** Heavy metal contamination of nanosuspension produced by high-pressure homogenisation. *Int. J. Pharm.* 2000;196: 169–172.

73. **Coppola, D.** Nanocrystal technology targets poorly water-soluble drugs. *Pharm. Technol.* 2003;(11):20.

74. **Rehman, M., Shrkunov, BY., York, P., et al.** Optimisation of powders for pulmonary delivery using supercritical fluid technology. *Eur. J. Pharm. Sci.* 2004;22:1–17.

75. **Schiavone, H., Palakodaty, S., Clark, A., York, P., and Tzannis, ST.** Evaluation of SCF-engineered particle-based lactose blends in passive dry powder inhalers. *Int. J. Pharm.* 2004;281:55–66.

76. **Okamoto, H., Sakakura, Y., Shiraki, K. et al.** Stability of chitosanYpDNA complex powder prepared by supercritical carbon dioxide process. *Int. J. Pharm.* 2005;290:73–81.

77. **Liu, H., Finn, N., and Yates, MZ.** Encapsulation and sustained release of a model drug, indomethacin, using CO_2-based microencapsulation. *Langmuir* 2005;21:379–385.

78. **Whiraker, MJ., Hao, J., Davies, OR., et al.** The production of protein-loaded microparticles by supercritical fluid enhanced mixing and spraying. *J. Control. Release* 2005;101:85–92.

79. **Ozeki, T., Beppu, S., Mizoe, T., Takashima, Y., Yuasa, H., and Okada, H.** Preparation of polymeric submicron particle-containing microparticles using a 4-fluid nozzle spray drier. *Pharm. Res.* 2006;23(1):177–183.

80. **Beppu, S., Ozeki, Y., Sasaki, T., et al.** Preparation of particles for dry powder inhalation using a novel 4-fluid nozzle spray drier. *J. Pharm. Sci. Technol. Jpn.* 2003;63:228–237.

81. **Martin, TM., Bandi, N., Shulz, R., Roberts, CB., and Kompella, UB.** Preparation of budesonide and budesonide-PLA microparticles using supercritical fluid precipitation technology. *AAPS PharmSciTech.* 2002;3(3):E18.

82. **Duarte, AR., Costa, MS., Simplício, AL., Cardoso, MM., and Duarte, CM.** Preparation of controlled release microspheres using supercritical fluid technology for delivery of anti-inflammatory drugs. *Int. J. Pharm.* 2006;308(1–2):168–174.

83. **Tao, SL., Lubeley, MW., and Desai, TA.** Bioadhesive poly(methyl methacrylate) microdevices for controlled drug delivery. *J. Control. Release* 2003;88:215–228.

84. **Ahmed, A., Bonner, C., and Desai, TA.** Bioadhesive microdevices with multiple reservoirs: a new platform for oral drug delivery. *J. Control. Release* 2002;81:291–306.

85. **Ahmed, A., Bonner, C., and Desai, TA.** Bioadhesive microdevices for drug delivery: a feasibility study. *Biomed. Microdevices* 2001;3:89–96.

86. **Xia, Y. and Whitesides, GM.** Soft lithography. *Angew. Chem. Int. Ed.* 1998;37:550–575.

87. **Granlund, T., Nyberg, T., Roman, LS., Svensson, M., Inganas, O.** Patterning of polymer light-emitting diodes with soft lithography. *Adv. Mater.* 2000;12:269–273.

88. **Yan, L., Huck, WTS., Zhao, XM., and Whitesides, GM.** Patterning thin films of poly(ethylene imine) on a reactive SAM using microcontact printing. *Langmuir* 1999;15:1208–1214.

89. **Yang, H., Deschatelets, P., Brittain, ST., and Whitesides, GM.** Fabrication of high performance ceramic microstructures from a polymeric precursor using soft lithography. *Adv. Mater.* 2001;13:54–58.

90. **Wang, MT, Braun, HG., Kratzmuller, T., and Meyer, E.** Patterning polymers by micro-.uid-contact printing. *Adv. Mater.* 2001;13:1312–1317.

91. **Guan, J., Chakrapani, A., and Hansford, DJ.** Polymer microparticles fabricated by soft lithography. *Chem. Mater.* 2005;17:6227–6229.

92. **Jackman, RJ., Duffy, DC., Ostuni, E., Willmore, ND., and Whitesides, GM.** Fabricating large arrays of microwells with arbitrary dimensions and filling them using discontinuous dewetting. *Anal. Chem.* 1998;70:2280–2287.

93. **Guan, J., Ferrell, N., James Lee, L., and Hansford, DJ.** Fabrication of polymeric microparticles for drug delivery by soft lithography. *Biomaterials* 2006;27:4034–4041.

94. **Prinderre, P., Piccerelle, P., Cauture, E., Kallantzis, G., Reynier, JP., and Joachim, J.** Formulation and evaluation of O/W emulsions using experimental designs. *Int. J. Pharm.* 1998;163:73–79.

95. **Roland, I., Piel, G., Delattre, L., and Evrard, B.** Systematic characterization of O/W emulsions for formulation design. *Int. J. Pharm.* 2003;263:85–94.

96. **Sanna, V., Kirschvink, N., Gustin, P., et al.** Preparation and in vivo toxicity study of solid lipid microparticles as carrier for pulmonary administration. *AAPS PharmSciTech.* 2004;5(2):e27.

97. **Genta, I., Perugini, P., Pavanetto, F., et al.** Enzyme loaded biodegradable microspheres *in vitro ex vivo* evaluation. *J. Control. Release* 2001;77(3):287–295.

98. **Bakan, JA. and Anderson, JL.** "Part III, Microencapsulation," in The Theory and Practice of Industrial Pharmacy, (Lachman, L., Lieberman, HA., and Kanig, JL., 2nd ed. 1976, Lea and Febi, eds.), Philadelphia, pp. 420–438.

99. **Nixon, JR., Khalil, SA., and Carless, JE.** Phase relationships in simple coacervation isoelectric gelatin:ethanol:water systems. *J. Pharm. Pharmacol.* 1966;18:409–416.

100. **Graves, RL., Makoid, MC., Jonnalagadda, S.** The effect of coencapsulation of bovine insulin with cyclodextrins in ethylcellulose microcapsules. *J. Microencapsul.* 2005;22(6):661–670.

101. **Phares, RE. and Sperandio, GJ.** Coating pharmaceuticals by coacervation. *J. Pharm. Sci.* 1964;53:515–518.

102. **Nixon, JR., Khalil, SAH., and Karless, JE.** Gelatin coacervate microcapsules containing sulfamerazine: preparation and *in vitro* release of drug. *J. Pharm. Pharmacol.* 1968;20:528–538.

103. **Luzzi, LA. and Geraughty, RJ.** Effects of selected variables on the encapsulation of solids. *J. Pharm. Sci.* 1967;56:634–638.

104. **Harris, MS.** Preparation and release characteristics of potassium chloride microcapsules. *J. Pharm. Sci.* 1981;70:391–394.

105. **Madan, PL., Madan, DK., and Price, JC.** Clofibrate microcapsules: preparation and release rate studies. *J. Pharm. Sci.* 1976;65:1476–1479.

106. **Takeda, Y., Nambu, N., and Nagai, T.** Microencapsulation and bioavailability in beagle dogs of indomethacin. *Chem. Pharm. Bull.* 1981;29:264–267.

107. **Palmieri, GF., Lauri, D., Martelli, S., and Wehrle, P.** Methoxybutropate microencapsulation by gelatin-acacia complex coacervation drug development and industrial pharmacy. *Drug Dev. Ind. Pharm.* 1999;25(4):399–407.

108. **Deasy, PB.** Microencapsulation and related drug processes, Marcel Dekker Inc., NY, 1984, 119 p.

109. **Chang, TMS.** Semipermeable Microcapsules. *Science* 1964;146:524.

110. **Tomizawa, SM., Takahashi, K., Koishi, M., and Kondo, T.** Studies on microcapsules. XII. Preparation and characterization of carboxylated polyphthalamide microcapsules. *Can. J. Chem.* 1971;49(22):3623.

111. **Arakawa, M. and Kondo, T.** Preparation of hemolysate-loaded poly(N alpha, N epsilon-L-lysinediylterephthaloyl) nanocapsules. *J. Pharm. Sci.* 1981;70:354.

112. **Wood, DA. and Whateley, TL.** A study of enzyme and protein microencapsulation—some factors affecting the low apparent enzymic activity yields. *J. Pharm. Pharmacol.* 1982;34:552–557.

113. **Shiba, M., Tomoika, S., Koishi, M., and kondo, T.** Studies on microcapsules. V. Preparation of polyamide microcapsules containing aqueous protein solution. *Chem. Pharm. Bull.* 18(4);803:1970.

114. **Chang, TMS.** The *in vivo* effects of semipermeable microcapsules containing L-asparaginase on 6C3HED lymphosarcoma. *Nature* 1971;229:117.

115. **Sundaram, PV.** The kinetic properties of microencapsulated urease. *Biochim. Biophys. Acta* 1973;321:319.

116. **Rambourg, P., Levy, J., and Levy, MC.** Microencapsulation III: Preparation of invertase microcapsules. *J. Pharm. Sci.* 1982;71:753.

117. **Luzzi, LA., Zoglio, MA and Maulding, HV.** Influences of matrixes on nylon-encapsulated pharmaceuticals. *J. Pharm. Pharmacol.* 1970;59:338.

118. **Mcginity, JW., Martin, A., Cuff, GW., and Combs, AB.** Influences of matriceson nylon w/o/w microcapsules formed by a multiple emulsion technique. *J. Pharm. Pharmacol.* 1981;70:372.

119. **Desoize, B., Jardillier, JC., Kanoun, K., Guerin, D., and Levy, MC.** *In-vitro* cytotoxic activity of cross-linked protein microcapsules. *J. Pharm. Pharmacol.* 1986;38:8.

120. **Levy, MC., Lefebvre, S., Rahmouni, M., Andry, MC., Manfait, M.** Fourier transform infrared spectroscopic studies of human serum albumin microcapsules prepared by interfacial cross-linking with terephthaloylchloride: Influence of polycondensation pH on spectra and relation with microcapsule morphology and size. *J. Pharm. Sci.* 1991;80:578–585.

121. **Maa, Y. and Hsu, C.** Effect of promary emulsions on microsphere size and proteinloading in the double emulsion process. *J. Microencapsul.* 1997;14:225–241.

122. **Nihant, N., Schugens, C., Grand les, C., Jerome, R., and Teyssie, P.** Polylactide microparticles prepared by double emulsion/evaporaion technique. I. Effect of primary emulsion stability. *Pharm. Res.* 1994;11:1479–1484.

123. **Ogawa, Y., Yamamoto, M., Okada, H., Yashiki, T., and Shimamoto, T.** A new technique to efficiently entrap leuprolide acetate into microcapsules of polylactide acid or copoly(lactic/glycolic) acid. *Chem. Pharm. Bull.* 1988;36:1095–1103.

124. **Uchida, T., Yoshida, K., Ninomiya, A., and Goto, S.** Optimization of preparative conditions for polylactide (PLA) microspheres containing ovalbumin. *Chem. Pharm. Bulletin,* 1995;43:1569–1573.

125. **Yeh, M., Coombes, A., Jenkins, P., and David, S.** A novel emulsifiation solvent extraction technique for vaccine and drug delivery. *J. Control. Release* 1995b;33:437–445.

126. **Lee, M., Cho, YW., Park, JH., et al.** Size control of self-assembled nanoparticles by an emulsion/solvent evaporation method. *Colloids Polym. Sci.* 2006;284(5):506–512.

127. **Zydowicz, N. and Nzimba-Ganyanad, E.** PMMA microcapsules containing water-soluble dyes obtained by double emulsion/solvent evaporation technique, Polymer bulletin, 2002;47(5):457–463.

128. **Pourfarzib, R. and D'Souza, MJ.** Preparation of albumin microspheres containing macrophage colony stimulating factor. *Pharm. Res.* 1992;9:S-68.

129. **D'Souza, MJ. and Pourfarzib, R.** Improved efficacy of a microencapsulated macrophage colony stimulating factor and methotrexate in melanoma. *Drug Dev. Ind. Pharm.* 1999;25(5):583–590.

130. **Choi, SH. and Park, TG.** G-CSF loaded biodegradable PLGA nanoparticles prepared by a single oil-in-water emulsion method. *Int. J. Pharm.* 2006;311(1–2):223–228.

131. **Yan, N., Zhang, M., and Ni, P.** Study on polyamide microcapsules containing oily liquids. *J. Microencapsul.* 1994;11:365–372.

132. **Maa, Y. and Hsu, C.** Liquid-liquid emulsification by static mixer for use in microencapsulation. *J. Microencapsul.* 1996;13:419–433.

133. **Alex, R. and Bodmeier, R.** Encapsulation of water-soluble drugs by a modified solvent evaporation method. I. Effect of process and formulation variables on drug entrapment. *J. Microencapsul.* 1990;3:347–355.

134. **Dos Santos, N., Cox, KA., McKenzie, CA., et al.** pH gradient loading of anthracyclines into cholesterol-free liposomes: enhancing drug loading rates through use of ethanol. *Biochim. Biophys. Acta* 2004;1661(1):47–60.

135. **Choi, Y., Kim, SY., Kim, SH., Lee, KS., Kim, C., and Byun, Y.** Long term delivery of all trans Retinoic acid using biodegradable PLLA/PEG-PLLA blended microspheres. *Int. J. Pharm.* 2001;215:67–81.

136. **Barichello, JM., Morishita, M., Takayama, K., and Nagai, T.** Encapsulation of hydrophilic and lipophilic drugs in PLGA nanoparticles by the nanoprecipitation method. *Drug Dev. Ind. Pharm.* 1999;25(4):471–476.

137. **Sharma, S. and Pawar, A.** Low density multiparticulate system for pulsatile release of meloxicam. *Int. J. Pharm.* 2006;150–158;313(1–2).

138. **Kemshead, JT., Ugelstad, J., Rembaum, A., and Gibson, F.** The potential use of monoclonal antibodies and microspheres containing magnetic compounds to remove neuroblastoma cells from bone marrow to be used in autologous transplantation programmes. *Eur. J. Cancer Clin. Oncol.* 1982;18:1043.

139. **Dirami, G., Poulter, LW., and Cooke, BA.** Separation and characterization of Leydig cells and macrophages from rat testes. *J. Endocrinol.* 1991;130:357.

140. **Ahmed, ARH., Olivier, GWJ., Adams, G., et al.** Isolation and partial purification of a melanocyte-stimulating hormone receptor from B16 murine melanoma cells: a novel approach using a cleavable biotinylated photoactivated ligand and streptavidin-coated magnetic beads. *Biochem. J.* 1992;286:377.

141. **Ito, T., Smith, CL., and Cantor, CR.** Sequence-specific DNA purification by triplex affinity capture. *Proc. Natl. Acad. Sci. USA* 1992;89:495.

142. **Wahlberg, J., Holmberg, A., Bergh, S., Hultman, T., and Uhlen, M.** Automated magnetic preparation of DNA templates for solid phase sequencing. *Electrophoresis* 1992;13:547.

143. **Devineni, D., Blanton, CD., and Gallo, JM.** In vivo imaging. *Bioconjug. Chem.* 1995;6:203.

144. **Dodd, CH., Hsu, HC., Chu, WJ., et al.** Normal T-cell response and in vivo magnetic resonance imaging of T cells loaded with HIV transactivator-peptide-derived superparamagnetic nanoparticles. *J. Immunol. Methods* 2001;256:89.

145. **Shang, H., Kirkham, PM., Myers, TM., Cassell, GH., and Lee, GU.** The application of magnetic force differentiation for the

measurement of the affinity of peptide libraries. *J. Magn. Magn. Mater.* 2005;293:382–388.

146. **Strick, TR., Allemand, JF., Bensimon, D., Bensimon, A., and Croquette, V.** The elasticity of a single supercoiled DNA molecule. *Science* 1996;271:1835.

147. **Smith, SB., Finzi, L., and Bustamante, C.** Direct mechanical measurements of the elasticity of single DNA molecules by using magnetic beads. *Science* 1992;258:1122.

148. **Baselt, DR., Lee, GU., Natesan, M., Metzger, SW., Sheehan, PE., and Colton, RJ.** A biosensor based on magnetoresistance technology. *Biosens. Bioelectron.* 1998;13:731.

149. **Lao, LL. and Ramanujan, RV.** Magnetic and hydrogel composite materials for hyperthermia applications. *J. Mater. Sci. Mater. Med.* 2004;15:1061.

150. **Ugelstad, J., Soderberg, L., Berge, A., and Bergstrom, J.** Monodisperse polymer particles-a step forward for chromatography. *Nature* 1983;303:95.

151. **Bizdoaca, EL., Spasova, M., Farle, M., Hilgendorff, M., and Caruso, F.** Magnetically directed self assembly of submicron sphere with a Fe_3O_4 nanoparticle shell. *J. Magn. Magn. Mater.* 2002;240:44.

152. **Moller, W., Scheuch, G., Sommerer, K., and Heyder, J.** Preparation of spherical monodisperse ferrimagnetic iron-oxide microparticles between 1 and 5 mu m diameter [radiolabeled particles]. *J. Magn. Magn. Mater.* 2001;225:8.

153. **Stevenson, JP., Rutnakornpituk, M., Vadala, M., et al.** Magnetic cobalt dispersions in poly(dimethylsiloxane) fluids *J. Magn. Magn. Mater.* 2001;225:47.

154. **Khng, HP., Cunliffe, D., Davies, S., Turner, NA., and Vulfson, EN.** The synthesis of sub-micron magnetic particles and their use for preparative purification of proteins. *Biotechnol. Bioeng.* 1998;60:419.

155. **Rana, S., White, P., and Bradley, M.** Synthesis of magnetic beads for solid phase synthesis and reaction scavenging. *Tetrahedron Lett.* 1999;40:8137.

156. **Ramirez, LP. and Landfester, K.** Magnetic polystyrene nanoparticles with a high magnetite content obtained by miniemulsion processes. *Macromol. Chem. Phys.* 2003;204:22.

157. **Levison, PR., Badger, SE., Dennis, J., et al.** Recent developments of magnetic beads for use in nucleic acid purification. *J. Chromatogr. A* 1998;816:107.

158. **Mason, TG. and Bibette, J.** Emulsification in viscoelastic media. *Phys. Rev. Lett.* 1996;77:3481.

159. **Mason, TG. and Bibette, J.** Shear rupturing of droplets in complex fluids. *Langmuir* 1997;13:4600.

160. **Suter, JJ.** Process for preparing magnetically responsive microparticles. U.S. Patent 5,648,124, 1997.

161. **Elmore, WC.** The magnetization of ferromagnetic colloids. *Phys. Rev.* 1938;54:1092.

162. **Shang, H., Chang, WS., Kan, S., Majetich, SA., and Lee, GU.** Synthesis and characterization of paramagnetic microparticles through emulsion-templated free radical polymerization. *Langmuir* 2006;22:2516–2522.

163. **Lamprecht, A., Schafer, U., and Lehr, CM.** Structural analysis of microparticles by confocal lazer scanning microscopy. *AAPS PharmSciTech.* 2000;1(3):E-17.

164. **Fernández-Barbero, A., Martín-Rodríguez, A., Callejas-Fernández, J., and Hidalgo-Álvarez, R.** On the calculation of electrokinetic potential and Hamaker constant of model colloids. *J. Colloid Int. Sci.* 1994;162:257.

165. **Washington, C.** In drug release from microparticulate systems, in Microencapsulation: Methods and Industrial Applications, (Benita, S., ed.), Marcel Dekker, NY, 1996, pp. 156–175.

166. **Si-Nang, L., Carlier, PF., Delort, P., Gazzola, J., and Lafont, D.** Determination of coating thickness of microcapsules and influence upon diffusion. *J. Pharm. Sci.* 1973;62:452–455.

167. **Lippoid, BC.** Solid dosage forms: mechanism of drug release, in Formulation and Preparation of Dosage Forms, (Polderman, J., ed.), Elsevier, Amsterdam, 1977, pp. 215–236.

168. **Crank, J.** The Mathematics of Diffusion, 2nd ed, Clarendon Press, 1975, 414 p.

169. **Noyes, AA. and Whitney, WR.** The rate of solution of solid substances in their own solutions. *J. Amer. Chem. Soc.* 1897;19:930–934.

170. **Si-Nang, L. and Carlier, PF.** Some physical chemical aspects of diffusion from microcapsules, in Microencapsulation, (Nixon, JR., ed.), Dekker, NY, 1976, pp. 185–192.

171. **Khanna, SC., Soliva, M., and Speiser, P.** Epoxy resin beads as a pharmaceutical dosage form II: dissolution studies and release of drug. *J. Pharm. Sci.* 1969;58:1385–1388.

172. **Sinclair, GW. and Peppas, NA.** Analysis of non-fickian transport in polymers using simplified exponential equation. *J. Membr. Sci.* 1984;17:329–331.

173. **Ritger, PL. and Peppas, NA.** A simple equation for description of solute release II Fickian and anamolous release from swellable devices. *J. Control. Release* 1987;2:37–42.

174. **Guy, RH., Hadgraft, J., Kellaway, IW., and Taylor, MJ.** Calculation of drug release rates from spherical particles. *Int. J. Pharm.* 1982;11:199–207.

175. **Baker, RW. and Lonsdale, HK.** Controlled Release: mechanism and rates, in Controlled Release of Biologically Active Agents, (Tanquary, AC. and Lacey, RE. eds.), Plenum Press, NY, 1974, pp. 15–71.

176. **Yeo, Y. and Park, K.** Characterization of reservoir-type microcapsules made by the solvent, exchange method. *AAPS PharmSciTech.* 2004;5(4):e52.

177. **Rhine, WD., Hseih, DST., and Langer, R.** Polymers for sustained acromolecular release: procedures to fabricate reproducible delivery systems and control release kinetics. *J. Pharm. Sci.* 1980;69:265–270.

178. **Lui, H., Magron, P., Bouzon, J., and Vergnaud, JM.** Spherical dosage form with a core and a shell, experiments and modeling. *Int. J. Pharm.* 1988;45:217–227.

179. **Lu, SM. and Chen, SR.** Mathematical analysis of drug release from a coated particle. *J. Control. Rel.* 1993;23:105–121.

180. **Higuchi, T.** Mechanism of sustained action medication: theoretical analysis of rate of release of solid drugs dispersed in solid matrices. *J. Pharm. Sci.* 1963;52:1145–1149.

181. **Fessi, H., Marty, JP., Puisieux, F., and Carstensen, JT.** Square root of time dependence of matrix formulations with low drug content. *J. Pharm. Sci.* 1982;71:749–752.

182. **Flynn, GL., Yalkowsky, SH., and Roseman, TJ.** Mass transport phenomena and models: theoretical concepts. *J. Pharm. Sci.* 1974;63:479–510.

183. **Chang, TMS.** Artificial Cells, Thomas, Springfield, III, 1972.

184. **Langer, RS.** Polymeric delivery systems for controlled drug release. *Chem. Engg. Commun.* 1980;6:1–48.

187. **Izumikawa, S., Yoshioka, S., Aso, Y., and Takeda, Y.,** Preparation of PLA microspheres of different morphology and its effect on drug release rate. *J. Control. Rel.* 1991;15:133–140.

186. **Le Corre, P., Le Guevello, P., and Gajan, V.** Preparation and characterization of bupivacaine-loaded PLGA microspheres. *Int. J. Pharm.* 1994;107:41–49.

187. **Rubino, OP., Kowalsky, R., and Swarbrick, J.** Albumin microspheres as a drug delivery system: relation among turbidity ratio, degree of crosslinking and drug release. *Pharm. Res.* 1993;10:1059–1065.

188. **Jayakrishnan, A., Knepp, WA., and Goldberg, EP.** Casein microspheres: preparation and evaluation as a carrier for controlled drug delivery. *Int. J. Pharm.* 1994;106:221–228.

189. **Hopfenberg, HB.** Controlled release from erodible slabs, cylinders and spheres, in Controlled Release Polymeric Formulations, (Paul, DR. and Harris, FW., eds.), *Am. Chem. Soc.* Washington, DC, 1976, pp. 182–194.

190. **Pitt, CG., Gratzl, MM., Kimmel, GL., Surles, J., Schindler.** Aliphatic polyesters II: the degradation of PLA, poly caprolactone and their copolymers in vivo. *Biomaterials* 1981;2:215.

191. **Wise, DL. (ed.)** Handbook of Pharmaceutical Controlled Release Technology, Marcel Dekker, Inc., New York, 2000, pp. 99–130.

192. **Juliano, RL. (ed).** Microparticulate drug carriers: liposomes, microspheres, and cells, in Controlled Drug Delivery: Fundamentals and Applications, 2nd ed., Drugs and The Pharmaceutical Sciences Series, vol. 29, Marcel Dekker, Inc., New York, 1987, pp. 556–565.

193. **Poste, G. and Kirsh, R.** Site-specific drug delivery in cancer therapy. *Biotechnology* 1983;1:869–878.

194. **Machy, P., Pierres, M., Barbet, J., and Leserman, LD.** Drug transfer into lymphoblasts mediated by liposomes bound to distinct sites on H-2 encoded I-A, I-E, and K molecules. *J. Immunol.* 1982;129:2098–2101.

195. **Davis, SS., Illum, L., Moghimi, SM., et al.** Microsphere for targeting drugs to specific body sites. *J. Control. Release* 1993;24:157–163.

196. **Owens III, DE. and Peppas, NA.** Opsonization, biodistribution, and pharmacokinetics of polymeric nanoparticles. *Int. J. Pharm. Sci.* 2006;307:93–102.

197. **Moghimi, SM., Hunter, AC., and Murray, JC.** Long-circulating and target-specific nanoparticles: theory to practice. *Pharm. Rev.* 2001;53(2):283–318.

198. **Lopez-Berestein, G., Kasi, L., Rosenblum, MG., et al.** Clinical pharmacology of 99m Tc-labeled liposomes in patients with cancer. *Cancer Res.* 1983;47:19–37.

199. **Leroux, JC., Allemann, E., Jaeghere, FD., Doelker, E., and Gurny, R.** Biodegradable nanoparticles–from sustained release formulations to improved site specific drug delivery. *J. Control. Release* 1996;39:339–350.

200. **Tabata, Y. and Ikada, Y.** Effect of the size and surface charge of polymer microspheres on their phagocytosis by macrophage. *Biomaterials* 1988;9:255–263.

201. **Tabata, Y. and Ikada, Y.** Phagocytosis of polymer microspheres by macrophages. *Adv. Polym. Sci.* 1994;11:261–269.

202. **Vyas, SP. and Khar, RK.** Targeted and Controlled Drug Delivery: Novel Carrier Systems, 1st edition, CBS Publishers and Distributors, New Delhi, 2002, pp. 359–379, 444–454.

203. **Banerjee, T., Singh, AK., Mitra, S., Sharma, RK., and Maitra, AN.** Comparative evaluation of stannous chloride and sodium borohydride as reducing agents for preparation of Technetium-99m labeled chitosan nanoparticles. *Ind. J. Nucl. Med.* 2002;17(4):11.

204. **Reddy, LH., Sharma, RK., and Murthy, RSR.** Tumor retention and biodistribution studies of etoposide loaded tripalmitin nanoparticles in Dalton's Lymphoma bearing mice. *Alasbimn J.* 2004;6: paper no.25: (http://www2.alasbimnjornal.cl/alasbimn/CDA/ sec_b/0,1206,SCID%253D11063,00.html); accessed on 3rd September 2007.

205. **Soni, S., Babbar, AK., Sharma, RK., Banerjee, T., and Maitra, AN.** Pharmacoscintigraphic evaluation of polysorbate80 coated chitosan nanoparticles for brain targeting. *Ind. J. Nucl. Med.* 2004;19(4):144.

206. **Reddy, LH., Sharma, RK., Mishra, AK., Chuttani, K., and Murthy, RSR.** Etoposide incorporated tripalmatin nanoparticles with different surface charge: formulation, characterization and biodistribution studies. *AAPS J.* 2004;6(3):e23; (http://www.aapsj.org); accessed on 3rd September 2007.

207. **Reddy, LH., Sharma, RK., and Murthy, RSR.** Enhanced tumour uptake of doxorubicin loaded poly(butyl cyanoacrylate) nanoparticles (DPBC) in mice bearing Dalton's lymphoma tumor. *J. Drug Target* 2004;12(7):443–451.

208. **Sharma, RK.** In health technology as fulcrum of development for the nation: the road ahead. NISCAIR, New Delhi, 2005, pp. 214–218.

209. **Banerjee, T., Singh, AK., Sharma, RK., and Maitra, AN.** Labeling efficiency and biodistribution of Technetium-99m labeled nanoparticles: interference by colloidal tin oxide particles. *Int. J. Pharm.* 2005;289(1–2):189–195.

210. **Soni, S., Babbar, AK., Sharma, RK., and Maitra, AN.** Delivery of hydrophobised 5-fluorouracil derivative to brain tissue through intravenous route using surface modified nanogel. *J. Drug Target.* 2005;14(2):87–95.

211. **Jain, S., Sharma, RK., and Vyas, SP.** Chitosan nanoparticles encapsulated vesicular systems for oral immunization: preparation, in vitro and in vivo characterization. *J. Pharm. Pharmacol.* 2006;58:303–310.

212. **Reddy, LH., Sharma, RK., Mishra, AK., Chuttani, K., and Murthy, RSR.** Influence of administration route on the uptake and biodistribution of etoposide loaded tripalmitin nanoparticles in Dalton's Lymphoma tumor bearing mice. *J. Control. Release* 2005;105(3):185–198.

213. **Ravi Kumar, MNV.** Nano and microparticles as controlled drug delivery devices. *J. Pharm. Pharm. Sci.* 2000;3(2):234–258.

214. **Kriwet, B., Walter, E., and Kissel, T.** Synthesis of bioadhesive poly(acrylic acid) nano- and microparticles using an inverse emlusion polymerization method for the entrapment of hydrophilic drug candidates. *J. Control. Release* 1998;56:149–158.

215. **Florence, AT., Hillery, AM., Hussain, N., and Jani, PU.** Nanoparticles as carriers for oral peptide absorption: studies on particle uptake and fate. *J. Control. Release* 1995;36:39–46.

216. **Hussain, N., Jani, PU., and Florence, AT.** Enhanced oral uptake of tomato lectin conjugated nanoparticles in the rat. *Pharm. Res.* 1997;14:613–618.

217. **Cheng, J., Teply, BA., Jeong, SY., Tong, R., Luther, G., Sherifi, I., Yim, C.H., Khademhosseini, A., Farokhzad, O.C., Langer, R.** Magnetically responsive polymeric nanoparticles for oral delivery of protein drugs. *Pharm. Res.* 2006;23(3):557–564.

218. **Seig, JW. and Robinson, JR.** Vehicle effect on ocular drug bioavailability. 1. evaluation of fluorometholone. *J. Pharm. Sci.* 1975;64:931–936.

219. **Lee, VHL. and Robinson, JR.** Review: topical ocular drug delivery: recent developments and future challenges. *J. Ocul. Pharmacol.* 1986;2:67–108.

220. **Albertsson, AC., Carlfors, J., and Sturesson, C.** Preparation and characterization of poly (adipic anhydride) microspheres for ocular drug delivery. *J. Appl. Polym. Sci.* 1996;62:695–705.

221. **Liu, L.S., Liu, S.Q., Ng, SY., Froix, M., Ohno, T., and Heller, J.** Controlled release of interleukin-2 for tumour immunotherapy using alginate/chitosan porous microspheres. *J. Control. Release* 1997;43(1):65–74.

222. **Faisant, N., Akiki, J., Siepmann, F., Benoit, JP., and Siepmann, J.** Effects of the type of release medium on drug release on drug release from PLGA—based microparticles: experiment and theory. *Int. J. Pharm.* 2006;314(2):189–197.

223. **Capan, Y., Jiang, G., Giovagnoli, S., Na, K-H., and DeLuca, PP.** Preparation and characterization of poly(D,L-lactide-co-glycolide) microspheres for controlled release of human growth hormone. *AAPS PharmSciTech.* 2003;4(2):E28.

224. **Wischke, C., Lorenzen, D., Zimmermann, J., and Borchert, H-H.** Preparation of protein loaded poly(D,L-lactide-co-glycolide) microparticles for the antigen delivery to dendritic cells using a static micromixer. *Eur. J. Pharm. Biopharm.* 2006;62(3):247–253.

225. **Estevan, M., Gamazo, C., Gonzalez-Gaitano, G., and Irache, JM.** Optimization of the entrapment of bacterial cell envelope extracts into microparticles for vaccine delivery. *J. Microencapsul.* 2006;23(2):169–181.

226. **Oldenburg, AL., Toublan, FJJ., Suslick, KS., Wei, A., and Boppart, SA.** Magnetomotive contrast for *in vivo* optical coherence to-mography. *Opt. Exp.* 2005;13:6597–6614.

227. **Toublan, FJJ., Boppart, S., and Suslick, KS.** Tumor targeting by surface-modified protein microspheres. *J. Am. Chem. Soc.* 2006;128:3472, 3473.

228. **Vyas, SP. and Malaiya, A.** In vivo characterization of indomethacin magnetic polymethyl methacrylate nanoparticles. *J. Microencapsul.* 1989;6:493–499.

229. **Guimaraes, R., Clement, O., Bitton, J., Carnot, F., and Frija, G.** MR lymphography with superparamagnetic iron nanoparticles in rats: pathological basis for control enhancement. *Am. J. Roentgenol. Radium Ther. Nucl. Med.* 1994;162:201–207.

230. **Moore, A., Marecos, E., Bogdanov, A., Jr., and Weissleder, R.** Tumoral distribution of long-circulating dextran-coated iron oxide nanoparticles in a rodent model. *Radiology* 2000;214:568–574.

231. **Hayashi, T. and Ikada, Y.** Protease immobilization on to porous chitosan beads. *J. Appl. Polym. Sci.* 1991;42:85–92.

232. **Deo, SK., Moschou, EA., Peteu, SF., Bachas, LG., and Daunert, S.** Responsive drug delivery systems. *Anal. Chem.* 2003;75(9):207A–213A.

233. **Breimer, DD.** Future challenges for drug delivery. *J. Control. Release* 1999;62:3–6.

7

Nanoparticles

Dr. R.S.R. Murthy, M.PHARM, PhD
Dr. Hariwardhan Reddy, M.PHARM, PhD

CONTENTS

1. INTRODUCTION

Increase in diagnosis of several new diseases has led to the discovery of variety of new potential therapeutic molecules, of which unfortunately many of them possess various disadvantages including poor solubility and physiological absorption, rapid metabolism or severe toxicity resulting in low therapeutic index. It was imagined long ago that successful delivery of such complicated molecules might be possible by incorporation into small-sized carrier systems called micro- and nanocarriers. Basically, nanotechnology is a science of designing smaller and intelligent objects to carry substances of interest for various applications. The aim of pharmaceutical nanotechnology is primarily to deliver the "difficult to deliver drugs" in the form of nanoparticles, to required site of action, thereby enhancing their therapeutic potential. An imaginative proposal of *Magic bullet* by Paul Ehrlich, a very accurate weapon or tool and may refer to a medication that cures a disease without a risk of side effects, a century ago, has turned out into reality and led to the development of several nanotechnological products, which are either at preclinical stage or at clinical level. Though microcarriers have definitely improved therapeutic potential of several drugs, by facilitating controlled drug delivery and resulting in treatment of a variety of diseases, it failed in most circumstances to deliver the therapeutic molecules to site of interest, particularly at the cellular level. This drawback of micro-carriers has led to the development of a variety of novel-nanosized carrier systems including liposomes, niosomes, micelles, nanoparticles, nanogels, dendrimers, etc. All of them are associated with their own advantages and drawbacks. However, in last few decades, the nanoparticles received great attention in the field of drug and gene delivery.

Nanoparticles are solid colloidal particles ranging in size from 10 to 1000 nm. Generally, the definition of nanoparticles include not only the particles described by Birrenbach and Speiser *(1)* by the term nanopellets, but also nanocapsules and polymer lattices such as "molecular scale drug entrapment" products as described by Rhodes and co-workers *(2)* and Boylan and Banker *(3)*. Nanoparticles possess a matrix structure, which incorporates pharmacologically active substance and facilitates controlled release of active agent, while the nanocapsule contains an oily core-incorporating drug surrounded by a membrane structure *(4)* (Fig. 1). Nanoparticles were used to successfully deliver a wide variety of drugs, proteins, peptides and genes to cells, both as non-targeted and targeted forms. Recently, it was shown that drugs can be coupled to nanocarriers that are specific for cells and/or organs *(5)*. These strategies can be used to concentrate drugs in selected target tissues, thus minimising systemic side effects and toxicity. As a result of extensive efforts in the field of nanoparticulate drug delivery, it was possible to develop a nanoparticulate systems to deliver drugs for treatment of various dreadful diseases. In general, the literature in the field of nanoparticles is extensive. This chapter will discuss only important aspects of pharmaceutically employed nanoparticles for disease therapy.

Nanoparticles are prepared from either synthetic or natural macromolecules using two distinct technologies, i.e., bottom up and top down technology. The bottom up technology adopts methods to aggregate molecules into a particle of nanorange, while the top down technology adopts breaking down macro-/micro-particles into particles of nanorange. Pharmaceutical nanoparticles are those where the drug is dissolved, entrapped, encapsulated or adsorbed on surface.

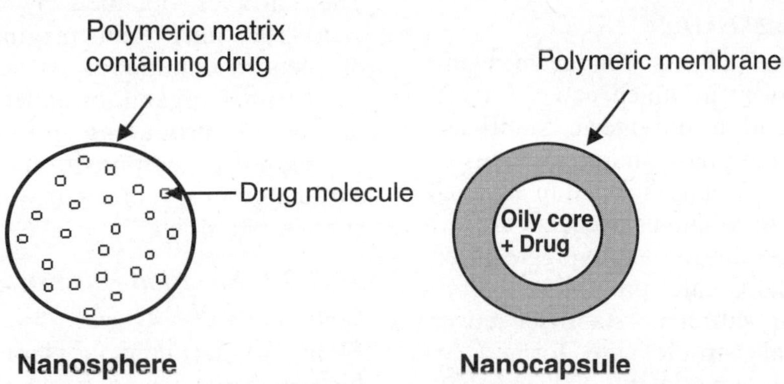

Fig. 1. Schematic representation of nanospheres and nanocapsule.

Pharmaceutical nanoparticles are generally classified based on the type of polymer used, property of end product and its use. The classifications are as follows:

- Polymeric nanoparticles/nanocapsules.
- Solid lipid nanoparticles.
- Hydrogel nanoparticles.
- Peptide nanoparticles.
- Nanocrystals and nanosuspensions.

2. POLYMERIC NANOPARTICLES

In the recent years, biodegradable polymeric nanoparticles have attracted great attention as potential drug carriers in view of their applications in controlled delivery of drugs, ability to target organs/tissues, as carriers for DNA in gene therapy, and their ability to deliver proteins, peptides and genes through peroral route *(4,5)*. Langer opined that construction of fully biomimetic matrices containing all of the required chemical and topographical factors is not yet achieved *(4)*. In this respect, scientists are focusing on design of new polymeric materials in which both topographical features and chemical cues act synergistically to qualify as a drug delivery carrier.

2.1. General Methods of Preparation of Polymeric Nanoparticles

Polymeric nanoparticles can be prepared either by polymerisation of monomers or from the pre-formed polymers.

2.1.1. Nanoparticles Prepared by Polymerisation Process

Polymer chemists first developed methods derived from field of latex engineering to produce nanoparticles. These methods were based on the *in situ* polymerisation of monomer in various media. Birrenbach and Speiser first polymerised nanoparticles for pharmaceutical use adopting two types of polymerisation processes, *(1)* i.e., dispersion polymerisation (DP) and emulsion polymerisation (EP).

2.1.1.1. Dispersion Polymerisation

Dispersion Polymerisation (DP) is conducted using monomer, an initiator solvent in which newly formed polymer is insoluble, and a polymeric stabiliser. Polymer forms in continuous phase and precipitates as a particle. The nucleation is directly induced in aqueous monomer solution. When these chains exceed a critical chain length, small particles are formed by aggregation of growing polymer chains and precipitates from continuous phase. When sufficient stabiliser cover particles, stable colloidal particles are formed by coalescence of these precursor particles with themselves and with their aggregates. In this technique, the monomer is dispersed or dissolved in aqueous medium where formed polymer precipitates out.

Essentially, the initiation of monomer for polymerisation requires an initiator, which may generate ions or radicals to start polymerisation process. If nucleation of monomer is due to ions, then the mechanism is called ionic polymerisation. Here the propagating species is a long chain cation or anion. Depending upon the type of ions produced, ionic polymerisation may be anionic or cationic. Reactions in ionic polymerisation are typically carried out in solvents of low or moderate polarity. If the radical nucleates monomer, then the mechanism is known as radical polymerisation *(6)*.

2.1.1.2. Emulsion Polymerisation

Emulsion Polymerisation (EP) is a method in which the monomer is emulsified in non-solvent containing surfactant, which leads to formation of monomer swollen micelles and stabilised monomer droplets. The polymerisation is performed in presence of initiator, which generates either radicals or ions depending upon type of initiator, and these radicals/ions nucleate the monomeric units and start polymerisation process. It was assumed that once formed, free reactive monomers would more probably initiate reaction within the micelles itself. Being slightly soluble in surrounding phase, the monomer molecules reach the micelles by diffusion from monomer droplets, thus allowing polymerisation to be continued in the micelles *(7,8)*. The particles obtained by EP are usually smaller (100–300 nm) than original stabilised monomer droplets in continuous phase. EP may be performed using either organic or aqueous media, as continuous phase for producing polymer with any desired morphology, composition, sequence distribution, surface groups, molecular weight distribution, particle concentration, etc.

2.1.1.2.1. Emulsion Polymerisation (EP) in an Organic Continuous Phase

EP in organic continuous phase was first process reported for nanoparticle preparation *(2,9)*. In this process, the water-soluble monomers are polymerised. For example,

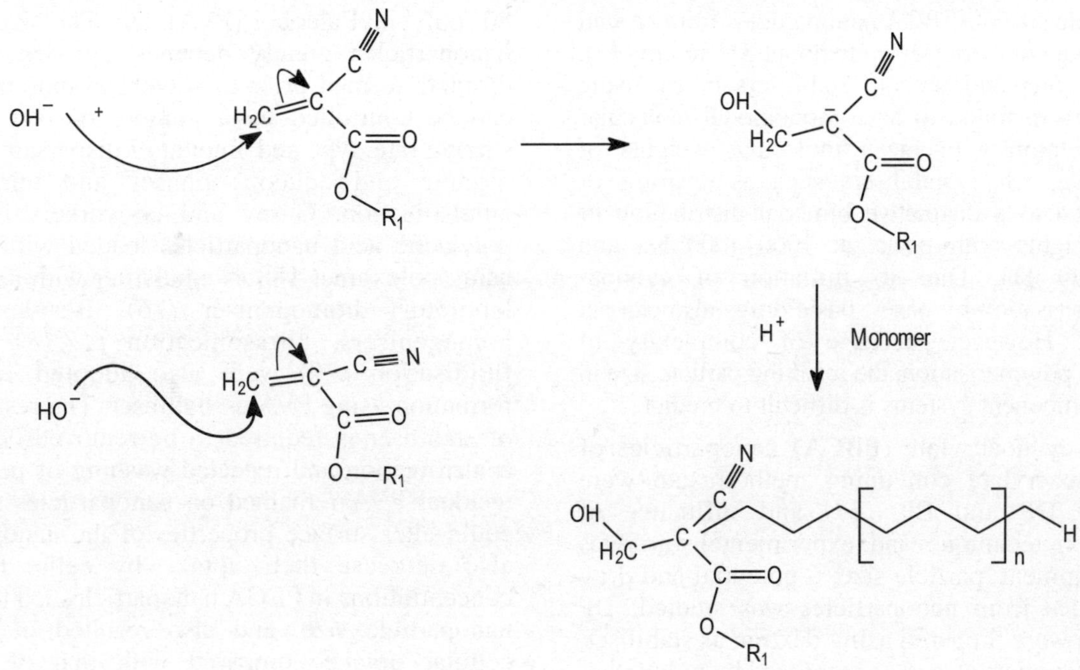

Fig. 2. Mechanism of alkyl cyanoacrylate polymerisation (Reprinted from Biomaterial, 22 Behan, N., Birkinshaw, C. and Clarke, N. poly n-buty1 cyanoacrylate nonoparticles: a mechanistic study of polymerization and particle formation, 1335, 2001 with permission from Elsevier) *(13)*.

acrylamide and cross-linker N,N′-*bis*-acrylamide were prototype monomers to be polymerised using chemical initiators such as N,N,N′N′-tetramethyl ethylene diamine and potassium peroxidisulphate or by light irradiation, γ- and ultraviolet (UV)-radiations. However, high toxicity of monomers and requirement of high amounts of organic solvents and surfactants limits the importance of this technique today.

The cyanoacrylate monomers are relatively less toxic than acrylamide and their polymers are biodegradable. Polyalkyl cyanoacrylate (PACA) nanoparticles were prepared by EP in continuous organic phase.

Depending on condition of preparation, nanocapsule is also formed during polymerisation by this method. The drug dissolved in aqueous phase is solubilised by surfactants within organic phase such as isooctane, cyclohexane-chloroform, isopropyl myristate-butanol and hexane, and resulted in a microemulsion with water-swollen micelles containing drug. The monomer diffuses into swollen micelles and OH^- ions initiate polymerisation. The polymerisation is so rapid that only an impermeable wall may be formed at organic/water interface preventing diffusion of further monomer inside the particles. However, high amounts of organic solvents and surfactants required for this process greatly limit its application.

2.1.1.2.2. Emulsion Polymerisation (EP) in an Aqueous Continuous Phase

This technique is widely adopted for preparation of nanoparticles by polymerisation of wide variety of monomers, including alkylcyanoacrylates. This technique utilises very low quantities of surfactants, and only stabilises newly formed polymer particles. Apart from this, the polymerisation of alkylcyanoacrylates has also been carried out in absence of surfactants *(10)*, in aqueous media containing dextran or hydroxyl propyl β-cyclodextrin. Polyethylcyanoacrylate and polyisobutyl-cyanoacrylate (PIBCA) nanospheres containing metaclopramide have been prepared by this technique. However, the technique resulted in only 9.2% and 14.8% drug loading, respectively due to loss of water soluble drug in aqueous polymerisation media.

The mechanism of polymerisation of cyanoacrylate monomers in aqueous medium by anionic polymerisation *(11,12)* has been depicted in Fig. 2. The cyanoacrylate monomer is initiated by OH^- ions and the polymerisation was performed at low pH to control reaction, which otherwise would lead to rapid polymerisation resulting in precipitation of large polymer aggregates. The stabilisers used were found to have a significant influence on size of formed polymer particles. High concentrations of poloxamer 188 (>2%)

reduced particle size of PIBCA nanoparticles from around 200 nm without emulsifier down to about 31–56 nm *(13)*. Nanoparticles prepared without stabilisers or by using polysorbates were found to have monomodal molecular weight distribution with mean molecular weights of 1000–4000 Da, while stabilisers such as dextrans or poloxamers led to a distinctive bimodal distribution of molecular weights with peaks at 1000–4000 Da and 20,000–40,000 Da. Due to initiation of cyanoacrylate polymerisation by bases, basic drugs also can act as initiators. However, because of complexity of cyanoacrylate polymerisation, the resulting particle size in such multi-component systems is difficult to predict.

Polybutyl cyanoacrylate (PBCA) nanoparticles of *n*-butyl cyanoacrylate containing methotrexate were prepared by DP and EP, *(14)* and influence of polymerisation technique and experimental variables on drug entrapment, particle size, ζ-potential and drug release kinetics from nanoparticles was studied. DP nanoparticles were prepared using dextran as stabiliser, whereas EP nanoparticles were stabilised by poloxamer 188. DP nanoparticles showed high release of methotrexate, suggesting channelising effect of dextran chains incorporated into nanoparticles during polymerisation. Drug release from both nanoparticles followed Fickian diffusion in 0.1 mol/L HCl, while the mechanism was found anomalous in pH 7.4 phosphate buffer. A similar study conducted on PBCA nanoparticles loaded with doxorubicin hydrochloride by incorporation and adsorption techniques *(15)*, showed rapid drug release in 0.001 *N* HCl from both DP and EP nanoparticles and the release kinetics followed Higuchi equation.

2.1.2. Nanoparticles Prepared From Preformed Polymers

Several techniques were employed to prepare biodegradable polymeric nanoparticles from preformed hydrophobic or hydrophilic polymers such as poly(D,L-lactide) (PLA), poly(D,L-glycolide) and poly(D,L-lactide-co-glycolide) (PLGA), chitosan, gelatin, etc.

2.1.2.1. Solvent Evaporation Method

In this method, the polymer solution is prepared in organic solvents such as chloroform, ethyl acetate or dichloromethane. The drug to be encapsulated is dissolved in polymer solution and organic phase is emulsified with an aqueous phase containing surfactant to obtain oil/water (O/W) emulsion. The organic solvent is then evaporated either at elevated temperatures or under reduced pressure. The surfactants used in emulsion formation include poloxamers, polysorbate 80, polyvinyl alcohol [PVA], etc. The size of resulting nanoparticles greatly depends on size of emulsion droplets formed prior to solvent evaporation. The size can be controlled by a number of factors including stirring rate, type and amount of dispersant, viscosity of organic and aqueous phases and temperature of emulsification. Gurny and co-workers reported first polylactic acid nanoparticles loaded with testosterone using poloxamer 188 as emulsifier with a conventional laboratory homogeniser *(16)*. Besides laboratory homogenisers, ultrasonication *(17,18)* and microfluidisation *(19)* were also adopted for emulsion formation using PVA as stabiliser. The residual amount of stabiliser is required to be removed completely by centrifugation and repeated washing of pellet, because residual PVA remained on nanoparticles surface *(20)*, could alter surface properties of the nanoparticles and also decrease their uptake by cells. Higher PVA concentrations in PLGA nanoparticles led to decrease in nanoparticle size, and also resulted in lowering of cellular uptake compared with that of lower PVA concentrations when evaluated in human arterial smooth muscle cells *(21)*.

Incorporation of water-soluble drugs is limited to employing traditional O/W emulsification method. However, Zambaux and co-workers reported W/O/W multiple emulsification method for preparation of nanoparticles loaded with water-soluble drugs, with improved percentage entrapment of water-soluble drugs *(20)*.

2.1.2.2. Emulsification Solvent Diffusion Method

This method is a modified version of solvent evaporation technique *(22,23)*. The technique employs use of water miscible solvents such as acetone or methanol, along with non-polar solvents, which were used as organic phase. Due to solubility of polar organic solvents in water, they spontaneously diffuse into aqueous phase, and an interfacial turbulence is created between two phases leading to precipitation of droplets as small as polymeric nanoparticles.

As above-described techniques utilise organic solvents, which are hazardous to environment as well as physiological system *(24)*; various other techniques such as salting out technique *(25)* and emulsification solvent diffusion technique *(26)* were developed.

2.1.2.2.1. Salting Out Technique

This technique firstly applied to pseudolatexes, was adapted to preparation of drug-loaded biodegradable nanoparticles *(25a)*. This method is based on separation of a water-miscible solvent phase from aqueous solutions promoted by a salting out effect. Water is added to emulsion obtained by addition of an solution of polymer and drug emulsified in an aqueous gel containing salting-out agent and colloidal stabiliser. As a consequence of dilution, acetone diffuses into water resulting in nanoparticle formation. Solvent and salting out agents are then eliminated by cross-flow filtration. This procedure allows incorporation of large amounts of drug with excellent yields, and procedure scale-up is fairly easy. However, this technique can be used only for loading lipophilic drugs.

2.1.2.2.2. Emulsion Diffusion Method

The emulsion diffusion method is a slight modification of salting-out technique. It differs mainly because organic solvent is only partially miscible with water, and it is previously saturated with water, in order to reach an initial thermodynamic equilibrium between water and organic phase. After addition of water, solvent diffusion is observed, and a nanoparticle suspension is formed.

2.1.3. Supercritical Fluid Technology

Several recently discovered hydrophobic drugs presented a problem of low solubility, poor bioavailability and irregular absorption after oral administration. Size reduction of these substances to nanometric range is an interesting approach to overcome associated problems. Particle preparation by size reduction employing wet milling or high-pressure homogenisation (HPH) possess some limitations, such as contamination of product and/or degradation of sensitive products due to high temperatures applied/heat generated during processing. Hence, other techniques such as solution precipitation, emulsion-based particle precipitation and supercritical fluid (SCF) precipitation *(27)* were employed for nanoparticle preparation. These techniques offer small particles; however, the formation of large drug crystals could not be prevented. Of these techniques, SCF technology facilitates rapid precipitation and enables formation of dry nanoparticles. SCFs have presently become the attractive alternatives because they involve use of environment friendly solvents like super critical carbon dioxide or nitrogen and method can be used to process the particles with high purity and very low traces of organic solvents. SCF technique has been widely applied for preparation of microparticles *(28,29)*. However, reports on application of this technique for production of nanoparticles are not extensive.

SCF precipitation techniques can be mainly divided into two major types: rapid expansion of supercritical solution (RESS) for drugs soluble in SCF (generally, CO_2), and supercritical anti-solvent (SAS) process for drugs insoluble in fluid.

In RESS method, the solute is solubilised in a SCF and solution is expanded through a nozzle causing sudden decrease in solubility followed by particle precipitation *(30,31)*. The solvent power of SCF dramatically decreases resulting in eventual precipitation of solute. In this technique, each particle is surrounded by same kind of particles in expansion zone, and hence often results in larger particles due to aggregation. On the other hand, many polymers exhibit little or no solubility in SCFs, thus making the technique less practical.

In SAS method, the solute is dissolved in organic solvent and solution is charged into SCF in precipitation vessel *(32)*. At high pressures, enough anti-solvent enters into liquid phase and as a result solvent power will be lowered and solute precipitates. After precipitation, when final operation pressure is reached, the anti-solvent flows through vessel so as to strip the residual solvent. When solvent content has been reduced to desired level, the vessel is depressurised and solid product is collected. A modified version of afore-mentioned technique known as gas anti-solvent technique has been successfully used in preparation of micron and sub-micron particles *(29)*. Recently, Gupta and Thakur employed modified RESS for preparation of phenytoin nanoparticles (~120 nm). Due to high polarity, the solubility of phenytoin in supercritical CO_2 is low. Using solid menthol as co-solvent, solubility of phenytoin in supercritical CO_2 has been increased by 400-folds. This hindered particle growth resulting in formation of smaller-sized nanoparticles as low as 75 nm depending upon processing conditions. Formation of O/W emulsion of drugs followed by internal phase extraction using SCF has also resulted in aqueous nanosuspensions, with controlled particle size and enhanced dissolution characteristics *(33)*.

SCF technique has also been utilised in preparation of polymeric nanoparticles encapsulating drugs. In this technique, both drug and polymer are co-precipitated using supercritical CO_2 *(34)*. However, during process, solid phase separation or re-crystallisation and non-homogeneous drug distribution may occur. A major challenge associated with this type of technique is plasticisation of polymers in presence of supercritical CO_2. The high viscosity of polymer–CO_2 solutions during atomisation or solvent extraction process leads to strong particle agglomeration, inconsistency of particle size and also poor encapsulation. Hence, a very widely applied class of amorphous polymers, including PLGA, polymethylmethacrylate and polycaprolactone, is not suitable for processing using supercritical CO_2. SCF extraction of emulsions (SCFEE) has been employed to overcome some of the associated problems of afore-mentioned technique *(35)*. In this technique, organic solution containing drug-PLGA/Eudragit RS mixture in ethyl acetate was added into ethyl acetate-saturated PVA solution and homogenised to obtain small droplets. This emulsion was placed in cylindrical extraction cell followed by CO_2 bubbling into cell. This technique enabled greater solvent extraction with residual content as low as 50 ppm and resulted in nanoparticles with 150 nm mean diameter. With SCFEE technique, stable aqueous nanosuspensions could be obtained with very low organic solvent residual content.

2.2. Polymeric Nanocapsules

Nanocapsules are spherical structures, which are formed by an envelope of polymer film surrounding a liquid central cavity. The technique for preparation of PIBCA nanocapsules as reported by Fallaouh and co-workers *(36)*, was by injecting organic phase con-sisting of oil with dissolved drug, isobutylcyanoacrylate and ethanol, into the aqueous phase containing Pluronic F68 (a non-ionic surfactant) under magnetic stirring. The colloidal suspension obtained was concentrated by evaporation under vacuum and filtered to obtain nanocapsules. The nanocapsules possessed shell-like structure with a wall thickness of 3 nm around nanocapsule. Nanocapsules with uniform size and low polydispersity were obtained only between pH 4.0 and 10.0. The mechanism of nanocapsule formation is probably the interfacial polymerisation described by Florence and co-workers for manufacture of PACA microcapsules *(37)*.

A different method was adopted by Chouinard and co-workers for preparation of polyisohexyl cyanoacrylate (PIHCA) nanocapsules, involving treatment of monomer with sulphur dioxide and dissolved in a solution containing Miglyol 810 (caprylic/capric triglyceride) in ethanol *(38)*. This solution was added slowly in 1:2 ratio into aqueous phase containing solution of 0.5% poloxamer 407 and 10 mM phosphate buffer under stirring. The nanocapsules were then purified by centrifugation and washing with distilled water. In this method, sulphur dioxide acts as an inhibitor preventing polymerisation of cyanoacrylates by ethanol. Upon addition of oily phase to aqueous phase, the sulphur dioxide and ethanol migrate to external phase resulting in formation of very fine emulsion. In this case, the nanocapsule size was mainly influenced by Miglyol concentration.

Palumbo and co-workers adopted similar technique for preparation of polyethyl-2-cyanoacrylate nanocapsules containing idebenone (an anti-oxidant) *(39)*. The method was similar to that described earlier. The acetonic solution of Miglyol 812, idebenone and monomer was added to 100 mL aqueous phase (pH 7.0) containing Tween-80. The presence of non-ionic surfactant allowed polymerisation of ethylcyanoacrylate at O/W interface, thus encapsulating Miglyol 812 droplets. The immediate polymerisation triggered formation of drug-loaded nanocapsules. The suspensions were concentrated under vacuum to remove acetone. Tween-80 reduced hydrodynamic size of emulsion droplets as a function of its concentration resulting in smaller-sized nanocapsules. The nanocapsules exhibited negative charge as determined by ζ-potential measurements. The freeze fracture electron microscopy demonstrated presence of internal oil droplet surrounded by polymeric shell of the nanocapsule.

2.2.1. Patents and Patent Filings on Nanoparticle Technology

There are many technologies patented or filed for patents to prepare nanoparticles by various methods. Some of these technologies are in different stages of commercialisation. Table 1 gives list of technologies patented/filed for patent for preparation of nanocrystal and nanosupsension using various homogenisation processes.

In addition there are many nanosuspension products in different stages of clinical trials or commercialisation. They are listed in Table 2.

2.3. Characterisation of Nanoparticles

Nanoparticles are characterised for various physical, biological and pharmaceutical characteristics. The ideal properties demanded by pharmaceutical nanoparticles are listed as follows:

- Particle diameter <100 nm.
- Electrical charge: ζ-potential.
- Pharmaceutical stability.
- Physical stability in blood (no aggregation).
- Non-toxic, biodegradable and biocompatible.

Table 1. Technologies and Patents/Patent Applications on Which Nanocrystal and Nanosupsension are Prepared Using Various Homogenisation Processes

Sr. no.	*Technology*	*Innovator company*	*Patent no.*
1	Hydrosol	Novartis (Sandoz)	GB 22 69 536
2	Nanomorph	Soligs (Abbott)	D 19637517
3	Nanocrystal	Elan Nanosystems	US 5,145,684
4	Dissocubes	SkyePharma	5,858,410
5	Nanopure	PharmaSol	PCT/EP00/0635
6	NANOEDGE	Baxter	US 6,884,436

Table 2. Solid-Particulate-Nanosuspension-Based Formulations in Development and in the Market

Drug	*Indication*	*Drug delivery company*	*Pharma company*	*Route*	*Status*
Paclitaxel	Anticancer	American BioScience	American pharmaceutical partners	Intravenous	Phase III
Undisclosed	Antiinfective	Baxter NANOEDGE	Undisclosed	Oral/multiple intravenous	Preclinical to phase II
Undisclosed	Anticancer	Baxter NANOEDGE	Undisclosed	Intravenous/oral	Preclinical to phase I
Rapamune	Immuno-suppressant	Elan Nanosystems	Wyeth	Oral	Marketed
Emend (drug)	Antiemetic	Elan Nanosystems	Merck	Oral	Marketed
Cytokine inhibitor	Crohn's disease	Elan Nanosystems	Cytokine Pharma Sciences	Oral	Phase II
Diagnostic agent	Imaging agent	Elan Nanosystems	Photogen	Intravenous	Phase I/II
Thymectacin	Anticancer	Elan Nanosystems	NewBiotics./Ilex Oncology	Intravenous	Phase I/II
Fenofibrate	Lipid lowering	SkyePharma	Undisclosed	Oral	Phase I
Busulfan	Anticancer	SkyePharma	Supergen	intrathecal	Phase I
Budesonide	Asthma	Elan Nanosystems	Sheffield Pharmaceuticals	Pulmonary	Phase I
Silver	Eczema, atopic dermatitis	NUCRYST	Self-developed	Topical	Phase I
Calcium phosphate	Mucosal vaccine adjuvant for herpes	BioSante	Self-developed	Oral	Phase I
Insulin	Diabetes	BioSante	Self-developed	Oral	Phase I

From ref. 39a.

- Avoidance of mononuclear phagocytic system (MPS) uptake (no opsonisation), prolonged blood circulation time.
- Scalable and cost-effective manufacturing process.
- Amenable to small molecules, peptides, proteins or nucleic acids.
- Minimal nanoparticle excipient-induced drug alteration (chemical degradation/alteration and protein denaturation).
- Possible modulation of drug release profiles.

2.3.1. Physicochemical Characterisation

2.3.1.1. Particle Size

Particle size is prominent feature of nanoparticles and the fastest and routine methods of size analysis are photon correlation spectroscopy (PCS) and laser diffractometry. The former method is useful for determination of smaller particles *(40)* while latter method is useful for determination of larger particles. PCS determines hydrodynamic diameter of the nanoparticles via Brownian motion. The electron microscopy methods also allow exact particle size determination but require coating of a conductive material such as gold. The gold coating usually results in estimation of particle sizes slightly more than normal and also procedure is limited to dry sample, which are stable under conditions of coating. Transmission electron microscopy (TEM) with or without staining is a relatively easier method of particle size determination. Some nanoparticle materials are not electron dense, and hence could not be stained, or melted and sintered when irradiated by electron beam of microscope, and hence cannot be visualised by this method. Such nanoparticles can be visualised in TEM after freeze fracture or freeze substitution *(41)*. This method is optimal because it also allows fracturing of particles, and consequently, an observation of their interior.

Recently, new types of high-resolution microscopes such as atomic force microscope, laser force microscope and scanning tunnelling microscope are developed *(42–45)*. These techniques are useful especially for investigations of nanoparticle surfaces.

2.3.1.2. Molecular Weight

Molecular weight determination of nanoparticles can be performed after dissolution of particles in an appropriate solvent and analysis by gel permeation chromatography. Accurate results can be obtained only if polymer standards have a similar structure and similar properties as test material. The technique possesses a limitation, i.e., molecular weight of cross-linked polymers and of nanoparticles from natural macromolecules could not be determined.

2.3.1.3. Density

Density measurements can be performed by helium compression pycnometry and by density gradient centrifugation. A comparison of these two methods may offer information about internal structure of nanoparticles.

2.3.1.4. Structure and Crystallinity

Information about the nanoparticle structure and crystallinity may be obtained by X-ray diffraction and thermo-analytical methods such as differential scanning calorimetry, differential thermal analysis, thermogravimetry and thermal optical analysis *(46)*. The charge on nanoparticle surfaces is mainly determined by electrophoretic mobility, laser Doppler anemometry and amplitude-weighted phase structuration.

2.3.1.5. Hydrophobicity

Hydrophobicity of nanoparticles can be determined by two major methods such as contact angle measurements and hydrophobic interaction chromatography. The former can be performed only on flat surfaces, not directly on hydrated nanoparticles in their dispersion media. For this reason, hydrophobic interaction chromatography is better method, wherein a differentiation between nanoparticles with different surface properties can be obtained by loading particles on columns with alkyl-sepharose and eluting them with a Triton X-100 gradient *(47)*.

Kreuter reported that size determination of nanoparticle by PCS spectrometry is very susceptible to errors caused by presence of bigger particles in dispersion, because it gives only mean diameter and so multi-modal size distributions cannot be measured *(40)*. Another disadvantage of this method is that it measures Brownian motion of the particles, and particle diameter is then calculated from measurements via diffusion coefficient *(40)*. Hence, the particle size determined by this method will be affected by surrounding medium such as adsorbed surfactants or hydration layers and may therefore, be different from sizes obtained by electron microscopy where the individual particles can be analysed and measured. According to Kopf and co-workers, the residual surfactants present after separation, coat the nanoparticles leading to change in its surface character and significantly reduce particle surface area *(48)*. Similarly, charge measurements in serum yielded more pronounced decrease caused by adsorption of serum contents. Another parameter that is of great importance for fate of nanoparticles in the blood is hydrophilicity/hydrophobicity of particle surface. The latter has a profound influence on interaction of the particles with blood components *(49–51)*. The hydrophilicity/hydrophobicity of the particles can be determined by measurement of water contact angle *(52)*. This was done by centrifugation, followed by washing with water and drying the nanoparticles. The dried material was dissolved in acetone and casted a film with subsequent solvent evaporation *(40)*. The water contact angles for polymethyl, polyethyl and PBCA nanoparticles were reported to be 55.6°, 64.7° and 68.9°, respectively *(40)*.

2.3.2. Degradation of Polymeric Nanoparticles

Polymeric nanoparticles degrade by two types of degradation, i.e., bulk and surface degradation. The rate of degradation is usually measured by PCS measurements *(47)*. *In vitro* degradation was also determined by turbidimetric measurements *(53)*. In case of surface degradation the particle size should show an immediate decrease whereby the polydisperity index remains constant. If bulk degradation dominates, a lag period should occur, preceding the decrease in mean size due to disintegration of particles. This process of disintegration would lead to more heterogeneous distribution of particle sizes and consequently, to an increase in polydispersity index. Incubation of polyethyl cyanoacrylate nanoparticles within 10^{-4} *N* NaOH led to an immediate and continuous decrease in size of particles and an unchanged polydispersity index indicating predominance in surface degradation. Incubation of PIHCA nanoparticles in 10^{-4} *N* NaOH led to no detectable size decrease and unchanged polydispersity indicating degradation by surface erosion at a much slower rate than polyethyl cyanoacrylate nanoparticles. Coating the particles with poloxamers did not result in acceleration of particle degradation. At low electrolyte concentration, size and dispersity of PIHCA nanoparticles remained unchanged during incubation in 10^{-4} *N* NaOH. At high p*I*, an overall increase in size was observed. This is due to the fact that, increase in size of nanoparticles as a result of flocculation was higher than decrease in size due to degradation. The low toxicity observed with PIBCA and PIHCA was probably due to slow degradation of polymers, thus releasing a low concentration of degradation products over a prolonged period of time.

The stability studies on PBCA nanoparticles reveal that an acidic medium protects nanoparticles against decomposition *(54,55)*. Higher temperatures promoted degradation of nanoparticles. Nanoparticles when incubated in human serum *in vitro* did not show particle agglomeration suggesting their better tolerance *in vivo*.

2.3.2.1. Influence of Enzymes on Degradation

Peroral route is convenient way of drug delivery with better patient compliance especially in long-term treatment. However, many drugs including proteins or peptides are unstable in gastrointestinal tract (GIT) or are insufficiently absorbed. Earlier studies have shown that cyanoacrylate nanoparticles *(56,57)* and nanocapsules *(58,59)*, improve absorption of several drugs like vincamin or insulin from GIT. Maincent and co-workers demonstrated efficiency of PBCA nanoparticles as a drug delivery system for GIT by improving the absorption of vincamin by more than 60% compared with an equimolar solution *(56)*. Investigation of parameters that influence the stability of nanoparticles in GIT is much more difficult due to changing pH from 2.0 in stomach to 7.0–8.0 in small intestine, and due to presence of different enzymes at varied concentrations in different parts of GIT. Degradation studies of cyanoacrylate nanoparticles were performed by Lenaerts and co-workers by incubating PIBCA nanoparticles in rat liver microsomes *(60)*. Scherer and co-workers studied influence of different enzymes like pepsin, amylase and esterase on stability of PBCA nanoparticles *in vitro* *(54)*. The study showed significant degradation of PBCA nanoparticles at 37°C and was dependent on pH of buffer solution, while addition of pepsin and amylase was found to have no influence on stability of nanoparticles. In contrast, the esterase significantly influenced the stability of nanoparticles. Esterase demonstrated highest activity of nanoparticle degradation at neutral pH values, and also degradation of PBCA nanoparticles was proportional to the amount of esterase added. The observations suggest that degradation of PBCA nanoparticles does not occur before they reach small intestine (as esterase is released by pancreas into lumen of small intestine), which is major site for absorption of several drugs.

2.3.3. Drug Release From Polymeric Nanoparticles

Various methods were used to study *in vitro* drug release of nanoparticles. They include side-by-side diffusion cells with artificial or biological membranes, dialysis bag diffusion technique, reverse dialysis sac technique, ultra-filtration, ultra-centrifugation and centrifugal ultra-filtration techniques. Despite the development of afore-mentioned techniques, there are still some technical difficulties, such as nanoparticle separation from the release media during experimentation *(61)*. Leavy and Benita used a reverse dialysis method in which nanoparticles were added directly into dissolution medium *(62)*. The same technique was adopted by Calvo and co-workers for evaluation of nanoparticles, nanocapsules and nanoemulsions *(63)*. However, this method is not very sensitive for studying rapid release formulations. The dialysis bag technique is relatively better method of assessing *in vitro* drug release and is generally used in product development and quality control *(64,65)*.

2.4. Applications of Polymeric Nanoparticles in Drug Delivery

2.4.1. Ophthalmic Delivery of Nanoparticles

Eyes are sensitive and are prone to several bacterial and viral infections, as well as age-related macular degeneration (ARMD). Due to tight junctions both on inner (in retinal pigment epithelium [RPE]) and outer side (in retinal pigment) of blood retinal barrier (BRB) of eye *(66)*, delivery of drugs to the eye is often limited. The success of oral and intravenous (i.v.) administration of drugs for treatment of ocular diseases is very little, due to poor concentrations attained in retina and other essential parts of the eye. Generally, lipophilic drugs have better access to BRB, while hydrophilic drugs are poorly penetrated. The treatment of diseases such as ARMD is difficult due to poor access of drugs to posterior part of macula. Delivery of drugs to macula was partly successful by injection through various routes such as subconjunctival *(67)*, juxtascleral *(68)* or direct intravitreal injection *(69)*. Intravitreal injection was widely employed to deliver several drugs and to localise relatively higher concentrations at their site of action. For instance, the drugs such as ganciclovir and foscarnet for treatment of cytomegalo virus retinitis *(70,71)*, triamcinolone acetonide for treatment of cystoid macular edema *(72,73)* and as adjunct in therapy of ARMD *(74)* were used. However, this mode of therapy, apart from rapid onset of action, also results in rapid clearance of drugs and demands multiple doses at frequent intervals, which is not always advisable. Intraocular implants (Vitrasert®, Retisert®) were developed for drug delivery *(75–77)*, but surgical implantation of these systems for routine management of common macular diseases is not ideally acceptable. Polymeric systems such as microparticles or nanoparticles could solve this problems due to their ease of administration and injectability. Microparticles were tried for delivering budesonide to subconjunctival space, but high polymer load in the vitreous cavity and its possible interference with visual function remained a question. Budesonide was successfully delivered through nanoparticles into subconjunctival space *(78)*, to suppress vascular endothelial growth factor expression, partly responsible for development of retinal vascular disorders.

Intravitreal administration of dye (Rh-6G [Rh] or Nile red [Nr])-loaded PLA nanoparticles resulted in their immediate appearance in vitreal space and in RPE, with significant quantity of nanoparticles localised in RPE cytoplasm at 6 h, and at 24 h post injection. High intracytoplasmic concentrations of nanoparticles were observed at least up to 4 months after a single intravitreal injection in rat eye (79), indicating prolonged retention and suggesting possible improvement in therapy of incorporated drugs.

Cyclosporine A, a cyclic undecapeptide is widely used as immunosuppressive agent *(80)* in surgical cases of organ transplantion, intraocular inflammation, peripheral ulcerative keratitis, severe grave's opthalmopathy, etc. *(81,82)* as oil-based formulations administered orally or by i.v. injection *(83,84)*. The treatment is often compromised by poor tolerability, low ocular bioavailability *(85)* and severe toxicity associated with cyclosporine A *(86)*. Improved delivery of cyclosporine A to eye was observed when polycaprolcatone nanocapsules loaded with cyclosporine A in oily core was administered topically with fivefold higher corneal levels of drug, compared with oily solution *(87,88)* in rat model. However, the objective of maintaining prolonged drug concentration was not possible with this formulation *(89)*. On the other hand, *ex vivo* corneal absorption of Cyclosporine A-loaded PIBCA nanoparticles dispersed in poly(acrylic) acid (carbopol) gel, was significantly higher than nanoparticles alone and oily solution when evaluated in bovine corneas *(90)*. Chitosan nanoparticles loaded with cyclosporine A showed relatively high concentrations in periocular tissues of rabbit after topical administration, which was attributed to positive charge of nanoparticles *(91)*. Though an improvement in ocular delivery has been attained with the nanoparticles formulations, still there is a long way to go to obtain a better nanoparticulate system for the eye, with beneficial properties in terms of tolerance, sustained drug release and targetability.

2.4.2. Brain Delivery of Polymeric Nanoparticles

Blood brain barrier (BBB) is a tight endothelial junction, highly selective and prevents transport of several therapeutic molecules into brain. A significant volume of research has been focused on delivery of drugs to brain. Especially, the large molecular therapeutics such as proteins, peptides, antisense nucleotides, etc. are poorly transported into brain, and require delivery carriers for their transport into brain. Drug transport through BBB is essentially complex, and depends on various factors such as lipophilicity, molecular weight, substrates for efflux pumps, etc. Various approaches have been tried to improve transport of drugs to the brain, of which nanoparticles are promising carriers for such application. The success of delivery of nanoparticles across BBB may depend on various factors such as smaller size (<100 nm), prolonged circulation, transport by transcytosis, etc. Polysorbate 80-coated PBCA nanoparticles were shown to successfully deliver associated hexapeptide dalargin (antinociceptive agent) to the brain, as determined by its therapeutic effect *(92,93)*. Biodistribution studies demonstrated longer plasma half-life and increased brain concentration of coated nanoparticles compared with uncoated ones *(94)*. Later, other peptides such as kytorphin *(95)* and loperamide *(96)* were also successfully delivered to brain, and brain transport of some drugs like amitryptylline (anti-depressant) was enhanced after i.v. injection using polysorbate-coated nanoparticles. Experiments involving doxorubicin-loaded PBCA nanoparticles coated with polysorbate 80 demonstrated that coating modified tissue distribution of nanoparticles, and decreased the distribution of nanoparticles to organs of reticulo-endothelial system (RES). At the same time, coated nanoparticles resulted in significantly higher concentration of associated doxorubicin in brain. Confocal microscopic studies revealed much higher cellular uptake of coated nanoparticles than uncoated ones *(97)*. The mechanisms proposed for the observed enhancement of brain transport of nanoparticles after coating with polysorbate 80 include *(98)*:

1. Temporary destabilisation of endothelial wall by dissolution of membrane lipids due to surfactant effect of polysorbate 80.
2. Increased retention and adsorption of nanoparticles in brain capillaries.
3. Opening up of tight endothelial junctions to allow penetration of drug as free form or as associated with nanoparticles.
4. Inhibition of p-glycoprotein (P-gp) associated with efflux process.

The involvement of apolipoprotein E (Apo E) in transport of coated PBCA nanoparticles has been realised both *in vitro* in plasma, as well as *in vivo* in Apo E-deficient ApoEtm1Unc mice, in which a decreased nociceptive effect was observed with coated PBCA nanoparticles. Also possibility of endocytosis triggering by Apo E has been proposed.

Olivier in his recent review *(99)*, raised few queries about efficacy and clinical potential of polysorbate 80-coated PBCA nanoparticles. They include:

1. Adsorption of Apo E onto surface of PEGylated PLA nanoparticles (not only onto polysorbate 80-coated nanoparticles) indicating nonspecific adsorption *(100,101)*.
2. Polysorbate 80-coated polystyrene nanoparticles did not result in enhancement of efficacy of loaded dalargin *(102)*.
3. Rapid degradation of nanoparticles in plasma/serum followed by the release of associated drugs indicated their pharmacokinetic profiles similar to those of free drugs.

Apart from strategy of nanoparticle coating by surfactants, other approaches such as PEGylation and employment of PEGylated cationic nanoparticles was also attempted for enhancing brain-related therapeutic effect. Conjugation with poly(ethylene glycol) (PEG) has also improved brain transport of nanoparticles. PEG-coated-PACA nanoparticles showed greater brain penetration without any modification of BBB, compared with the nanoparticles coated with polysorbate 80 after i.v. injection in mice and rats *(103)*. Brigger and co-workers reported a significant accumulation of (^{14}C)-poly(MePEG2000cyanoacrylate-co-hexadecylcyanoacry late) nanoparticles compared with non-pegylated nanoparticles in gliosarcoma after i.v. injection in rats *(104)*. Alzheimer's disease is a type of brain-related disorder accompanied by learning and memory impairment with a concomitant loss of choline acetyl transferase in cerebral cortex *(105)*. Arginine vasopressin fragment 4-9, a peptide, is used for treatment of spatial memory deficits and promotes memory by modulating cholinergic system in central nervous system *(106)*. However, i.v. administration to diseased patients is poorly acceptable. The cationic bovine serum albumin (BSA)-conjugated PEGylated nanoparticles (<100 nm diameter) entrapping arginine vasopressin fragment 4-9, exhibited great improvement in memory impairments and then to normal level in mice after i.v. injection, compared with unconjugated nanoparticles *(107)*.

2.4.3. Delivery of Nanoparticles to Cancer Cells

The main limitations associated with therapy using anticancer agents are their non-specific distribution leading to severe toxicity and development of resistance upon chronic dosage. Also some anticancer agents are substrates to P-gp and multidrug resistant associated protein (MRP) efflux pumps and are poorly diffused into cancer cells. For instance, doxorubicin and paclitaxel a potential anticancer drugs, are substrates of P-gp. These limitations were partly overcome by incorporation of such drugs into nanoparticulate carriers. PLGA nanoparticles improved cytotoxicity of incorporated paclitaxel *(108)*. Doxorubicin conjugated to PLGA nanoparticles showed greater anti-tumour activity after single dose injection in subcutaneously implanted EL4 thymoma tumour in mice *(109)*. Poly(ε-caprolactone) nanoparticles enhanced cellular penetration and cytotoxicity of the loaded tamoxifen in cancer cells *(110)*. Similar observations were made in case of gelatin nanoparticles. PEGylated gelatin nanoparticles showed enhanced blood circulation time and uptake into Lewis lung carcinoma grown as solid tumour in mice *(111)*. Chitosan nanoparticles incorporated with doxorubicin-dextran conjugate, greatly enhanced the survival of tumour-bearing mice *(112)*. Also, smaller-sized chitosan nanoparticles (of 64 nm mean diameter) by themselves were found to possess anti-tumour activity when tested in MGC803 human gastric carcinoma cells *(113)*.

Several types of cancers show resistance to conventional chemotherapy. Resistance to cancer chemotherapy involves both altered drug activity at designated target and modified intratumour pharmacokinetics. The membrane transporter P-gp plays a major role in pharmacokinetic resistance by preventing sufficient intracellular accumulation of several anti-cancer agents. PACA nanoparticles were found to overcome MDR phenomena both at cellular and non-cellular level *(114,115)*. Complete reversion of drug resistance *in vitro* was observed with doxorubicin-loaded PACA nanoparticles in terms of cell growth inhibition *(114)*. These nanoparticles significantly prolonged survival of doxorubicin-resistant P388 tumour-bearing mice after intraperitoneal injection. PACA nanoparticles enhanced the efficiency of treatment of doxorubicin in M5076 murine hepatic tumour metastasis in mice *(116)*. The PIHCA nanoparticles improved antitumour efficacy of doxorubicin *in vivo*, in hepatocellular carcinoma-bearing transgenic mice over-expressing *mdr1* and *mdr3* genes. It was hypothesised that the nanoparticles adhere to cell surface, followed by release of doxorubicin and nanoparticle degradation products that combine as an ion-pair able to cross the cell membrane without being recognised by P-gp *(117,118)*. PIHCA nanoparticles also increased cellular penetration and nuclear and cytoplasmic accumulation in resistant human breast adenocarcinoma cells, i.e., MCF7/VP and MCF7/doxorubicin over-expressing multidrug resistance associated protein 1 (MRP1) and P-gp, respectively *(119)*. Similarly, the PACA nanoparticles were also used for delivering drugs to lymphatic carcinoma *(120)* and gastric carcinoma *(121)*. Solid lipid nanoparticles (SLN) also improved the anticancer effect of etoposide in dalton's lymphoma ascites-bearing mice *(122,123)*.

Thiolation of polymeric nanoparticles is another strategy employed to improve the delivery of incorporated agents. For instance, in case of gelatin nanoparticles, free thiol groups form disulfide bonds with gelatin and also stabilise the particles. These disulfide bonds cleave in presence of excess glutathione or other redox enzymes present in hypoxic regions such as that of tumour cells. Generally, the cytoplasmic concentrations of glutathione are about 1000-folds greater than that present extracellularly *(124)*. The thiolated-gelatin nanoparticles entrapped with plasmid DNA-encoding enhanced green fluorescent protein (EGFP-N1) showed efficient gene expression and transfection in NIH3T3 cells (murine fibroblasts) *(125)*.

2.4.4. Delivery of Nanoparticles to Macrophages

The applications of unmodified nanoparticles are limited due to their recognition by RES followed by rapid clearance from blood after i.v. injection. Macrophages also act as reservoirs for microorganisms responsible for a variety of infectious diseases. Hence, the macrophages represent potential target for delivery of drugs to such diseases. The nanoparticles are extensively taken up by the macrophages by endocytosis, through macrophage phagocytic receptors such as mannose receptors *(126)*, D-galactose receptors *(127)* and scanvenger receptors *(128)*. Mannose receptors mediate phagocytosis of saccharide-coated particles and pinocytosis of soluble glycoconjugates *(129)*. This characteristic is exploited in delivering nanoparticles for macrophage-mediated therapies by conjugating with selective ligands. Of the various types of receptors, mannose receptor-bound particles are ingested by the macrophages at a faster rate *(130)*. The surface charge and chemistry of nanoparticles are also important for macrophage uptake. Macrophages possess negatively charged sialic acid moieties on surface, and hence positively charged nanoparticles are believed to bind to these moieties and undergo phagocytosis *(131,132)*. Particles having ζ-potential close to zero are found to be less phagocytosed by macrophages compared with charged ones *(133)*. Polymeric nanoparticles have been applied to target drugs to the macrophages. For instance, amphotericin B has been well applied for treatment of leishmania infections. The parasite leishmania localises in lysosomal vacuoles of macrophages, and thus effective therapy is limited due to poor accessibility of drugs when administered in naked form. Poly(ε-caprolactone) nanoparticles incorporating amphotericin B showed improvement in efficacy of the loaded drug *(134)*. The nanoencapsulated quercitin was also found to be effective, and at the same time hepatotoxicity and renal toxicity of the drug were found decreased in nanoencapsulated form *(135)*. PLA nanoparticles encapsulating primaquine exhibited 3.3-folds greater efficacy compared with free drug against leishmania infections *(136)*. The nanoparticles were also effective in delivering antibacterial drugs for treatment of infections caused by bacteria such as staphylococcus, mycobacterium and salmonella species *(137–139)*.

Macrophages also play an important role in immunopathogenesis of acquired immune deficiency syndrome (AIDS), and hence form a mode of target for delivering related drugs. Nucleoside analogues have been employed for treatment of AIDS. These drugs have been delivered through various types of polymeric nanoparticles *(140)*. For instance, poly(hexyl cyanoacrylate) nanoparticles encapsulated with azidothymidine and dideoxycytidine were effective in preventing human immunodeficiency virus (HIV) infection in macrophage cultures *(141)*. The tributionbiodisstudies of ^{14}C-labelled azidothy-midine (AZT) nanoparticles revealed greater distribution of the nanoparticles to RES organs *(142)*. The capsulated nanoensaquinavir (a protease inhibitor) and zalcitabine (a nucleoside analogue) showed increased antiviral activity *in vitro* in infected primary human macrophages in terms of decrease in production of HIV type-1 antigen *(143)*.

Nanoparticles were also employed for treatment of inflammatory diseases like atherosclerosis, rheumatoid arthritis and neuro-inflammatory conditions. The nanoencapsulated coenzyme Q10 (compound with anti-atherogenic effect) underwent higher uptake when tested in J-774 macrophages compared with free coenzyme Q10 *(144)*. In case of rheumatoid arthritis, the tissue necrosis factor-α (TNF-α) plays a major role in inflammatory process. Apart from different strategies, the inhibition of TNF-α has also been suggested for treating rheumatoid arthritis *(145)*. This has been possible by antisense-mediated TNF synthesis inhibition using oligodeoxynucleotides (ODN) *(146)*. For this purpose, the nanoparticles have been employed for encapsulation and delivery of ODN *(147,148)*.

3. SOLID LIPID NANOPARTICLES

Lipid nanoparticles are usually aqueous dispersions of solid lipids or dry powders of nanosize preferably ranging between 50 and 200 nm. Lipid nanoparticles are alternative drug delivery system to emulsions, liposomes and polymeric nanoparticles, as they overcome the problems associated with other delivery systems such as membrane stability and drug leaching in case of liposomes and emulsions, biodegradation and toxicity problems of polymeric nanoparticles, and facilitate prolonged drug release. The inherent property of solid nature of lipids and ability to form smaller particles and their stability has popularised their use in drug delivery. Lipid nanoparticles are prepared from biocompatible lipids like mono-, di- and triglycerides having one or mixed fatty acid moiety, cholesterol and may be phospholipids also. They possess excellent biodegradability and low toxicity.

3.1. General Methods of Preparation of SLN

Several techniques were reported for production of SLN including high-shear homogenisation *(149)*, HPH, emulsification and solvent evaporation *(150,151)*, emulsification and solvent diffusion *(152,153)*, dilution of microemulsions *(154,155)*, etc. Of all the afore-mentioned techniques, HPH is most practical, reliable and industrially feasible technique *(156)*. In HPH technique, liquid to be homogenised is pumped with high pressure (1000–25,000 psi) through a narrow gap (in range of few microns) in high-pressure homogeniser. In the process, fluid accelerates on a very short distance to very high velocity (>1000 km/h). High-shear stress and cavitation forces created during homogenisation disrupt the particles down to sub-micron range. The lipid concentrations up to 40% have been homogenised to lipid nanodispersions *(157)*. HPH method can be subdivided into two types, i.e., hot homogenisation and cold homogenisation technique for production of SLN *(158,159)*. In hot homogenisation technique, a pre-emulsion of drug-loaded lipid melt and aqueous emulsifier phase is homogenised by processing at higher temperatures, which results in lower particle sizes due to decreased viscosity of inner phase *(160)*. The resultant nanoemulsion form solid particles upon cooling the sample to room temperature or still lower temperature. Sometimes due to small particle size and presence of

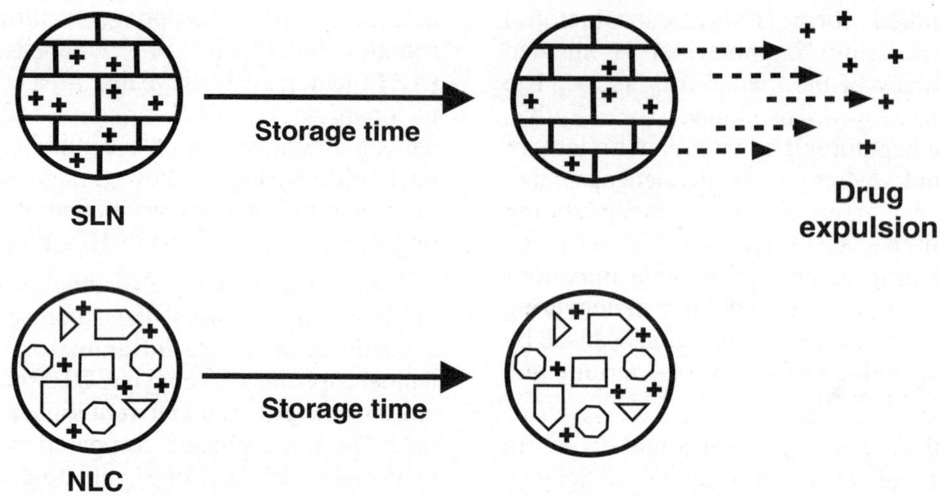

Fig. 3. Formation of a perfect lipid crystal in SLN and a crystal lattice with many imperfections in NLC (Reprinted from Int. J. Pharm., 88, Sjostrom, B. and Bergenstahl, B. Preparation of submicron drug particles in lecithin-stabilized o/w emulsions. I. Model studies of the precipitation of cholesteryl acetate, 53–62, 1992, with permission from Elsevier.) *(150)*.

surfactants, lipid crystallisation may be highly retarded and sample may remain as super-cooled melt (smectic phase) for several months *(161)*. Processing at high temperatures may also cause degradation of thermolabile drugs. In such cases, cold homogenisation is employed in which temperature control is ensured to maintain unmolten state of lipid as a result of increase in temperature during homogenisation. In this technique, the drug is dispersed or solubilised in molten lipid and lipid melt is cooled using dry ice or liquid nitrogen. The solid matrix is then milled into microparticles by means of ball or mortar milling to obtain particles of 50–100 μm size. These microparticles are further dispersed in chilled aqueous emulsifier solution and subjected to HPH. This technique also facilitates entrapment of hydrophilic drugs *(162)* and at the same time suffers from disadvantage of formation of a fraction of microparticles. Recently, a novel core-shell type of SLN was prepared by using cocoa butter as lipid core and curdlan as shell material and stabilised by Tween-80 *(163)*. The SLN remained stable up to 0.5% lipid content, but increased in size at high lipid concentrations and at high pH values. The critical aggregation concentration at pH 7.4 was found to be 6.95×10^{-4} mg/mL. This SLN exhibited sustained release of incorporated verapamil (an antihypertensive agent).

The SLN often suffers from potential problems such as limited drug-loading capacity, adjustment of drug release profile and potential drug expulsion during storage. To overcome the problems associated with SLN, a new type of lipid delivery system called nanostructured lipid matrices (NLM) was developed by mixing solid lipids with spatially incompatible lipids, leading to specialised structures of lipid matrix *(164)*. These structures include imperfect structure, structureless type and multiple types. A prerequisite for good drug accommodation is larger distances between fatty acid chains of glycerides and general imperfections in crystal (e.g., to accommodate amorphous drug crystals). Distances between fatty acid chains can be increased by using glycerides being composed of very different fatty acids. To achieve highest incompatibility, the NLM was produced by mixing solid lipids with chemically different liquid lipids (oils). This leads to more imperfections in the crystal and higher drug load (Fig. 3). By using special mixtures of solid and liquid lipids (e.g., hydroxyoctacosanyl hydroxystearate and isopropyl myristate), the particles become solid after cooling but do not crystallise. NLM usually consists of a high content of liquid lipid, and hence shows higher entrapment efficiency compared with SLN *(165)*. NLM were adopted to improve topical absorption of lipophilic drugs such as clotrimazole and ketoconazole *(166)*.

To obtain the lipid nanoparticles with higher-loading capabilities and controlled drug release characteristics, the systems with liquid crystalline smectic phase may be an interesting alternative. The smectic phase is a layered structure, with an almost parallel arrangement of molecules along their long axes. Due to highly viscous but fluid liquid crystalline state of their matrix lipid, colloidal smectic nanoparticles are expected to offer promising possibilities as delivery systems for lipophilic drugs *(167)*.

3.2. Storage Stability of SLN

Storage stability of SLN involves prevention of physical and chemical degradation and preservation of initial particle size. To improve the stability of SLN, they are either lyophilised, or spray dried. It has been suggested that lipid content of SLN dispersion should not exceed 5% to prevent an increase in particle size. For lyophilisation, the addition of cryoprotectants is necessary to obtain a better redispersion of lyophilised product. Typical cryoprotectants that can be used are sorbitol, mannose, trehalose, lactose, glucose and polyvinyl pyrrolidone (PVP). The cryoprotectants decrease the osmotic activity of water and crystallisation and favour the glassy state of frozen sample *(168,169)*. They also act as placeholders and prevent contact between discrete lipid nanoparticles. Furthermore, they interact with polar head groups of the surfactants and serve as a kind of pseudohydration shell *(170)*. The best cryoprotection was obtained with glucose, mannose, maltose and trehalose in concentrations between 10% and 15% *(171)*.

However, the lyophilisation was not efficient enough to obtain stable, dry nanoparticles with easy redispersibility *(172)*. The average particle sizes of all lyophilised samples with added cryoprotectants (glucose, sucrose, maltose and trehalose were used as cryoprotectants at 5%, 10% and 20% concentrations) were 1.5–2.4 times higher than original dispersions. Cavalli and co-workers observed similar increase in particle sizes (2.1–4.9 times) after lyophilisation *(173)*.

Spray drying may be an alternative procedure to lyophilisation to recover SLN dispersion into dry product. This technique produced redispersible dry powder nanoparticles. Nanoparticle composition containing lipids with high-melting point (>70°C) are generally suitable for spray drying *(174)*. The technique experiences increase in temperature during process, and hence SLN made of low-melting lipids may undergo aggregation. For low-melting lipids, a mixture of water and ethanol can be used as spraying medium, to enable the spray drying process at lower temperature. The best results were obtained with SLN concentrations of 1% in solutions of 30% trehalose in water or 20% trehalose in ethanol–water mixtures (10/90 v/v) *(159)*. In such cases, it is necessary to ensure complete evaporation of employed organic solvents. Carrying out the spray drying using aqueous medium possibly avoids the problems associated with organic solvent mixtures. Spray drying of aqueous SLN dispersion (containing no organic solvent) in presence of lactose resulted in dry nanopowders with excellent redispersibility characteristics, requiring simple hand shaking for obtaining nanoparticles dispersion free from aggregation *(175)*.

3.3. Physicochemical Aspects of SLN

3.3.1. Crystallisation-Polymorphism of Glyceride Lipids

SLN dispersions prepared from glyceride solid lipids often present complex additional stability problems compared with other lipid systems, due to their crystallisation kinetics and polymorphism of dispersed lipids. Crystalline solids have an orderly arrangement of units and show definite melting points, passing from solid to liquid state. The size characteristics of structures can alter the solidification phenomenon of crystalline lipids *(176,177)*. As a result of their smaller particle size, lipid nanoparticles melt at about 3–5°C lower than corresponding bulk material. It is noted that the fusion temperature of bulk lipids is 73, 64, 56 and 47°C for tristearin, tripalmitin, trimyristin and trilaurin, respectively. The re-crystallisation of melted bulk lipid occurs at a lower temperature leading to α-form (51, 42, 28 and 11°C, respectively). In same way, re-crystallisation of molten lipids was delayed by about 20°C in colloidal dispersions compared with bulk lipids (30, 21, 9 and –8°C, respectively for afore-mentioned triglycerides) *(177)*. Consequently, the nanoparticles prepared from triglycerides, which are solid at room temperature can remain liquid for several months without crystallisation *(178)*. Westesen and Bunjes observed that, colloidally dispersed trimyristin and trilaurin particles remained in liquid state for at least several months of storage at room temperature *(177)*. In addition, cooling the dispersion to less than a critical crystallisation temperature did not result in particle crystallisation. In such systems, gradual crystallisation of lipids upon long-term storage is possible and this process might lead to stability problems such as gelling or expulsion of incorporated drug *(179)*. The crystalline re-orientation can result in modification of charge on particle surface and subsequently, on measured ζ-potential and particle size *(180)*.

Polymorphism is defined as the ability to reveal different unit cell structures in crystals, originating from a variety of molecular confirmations and molecular packing *(181)*. Triglycerides often exhibit polymorphism followed by their exposure to changes in temperature. The main polymorphic forms in glycerides are the α, β′ and β *(181)*. α—Hexagonal (H) subcell with a lattice spacing of 0.42 nm.

β′—Orthorhombic (O) perpendicular subcell with wide lattice spacings of 0.42, 0.43 and 0.37, 0.47 nm. β—Triclinic parallel (T) subcell with a wide lattice spacing of 0.46 nm.

The α-form has tendency to be transformed quickly to β′-form with better chain packing. The most stable form is β-form. Therefore, the transition of melt from α to β via β′-form was the pathway for triglycerides to optimum packing form of molecules *(181)*. This unstable form gradually transformed towards most stable form during storage at elevated temperatures while losing initial spherical surface structures *(182)*. This led to crystalline aggregate growth. The change in crystal structure may have influence in release pattern of incorporated drugs *(183)*. Sustained drug release was often related to metastable β′-polymorph. Drug expulsion during polymorph transition was explained by a reduction of amorphous regions in carrier lattice due to a β′ to β-polymorph transition *(184)*.

3.3.2. Gelling Phenomena

Gelling phenomena describes the transformation of a low-viscosity system into a viscous gel causing particle growth. Various studies indicated that gelling phenomena presented some inductors similar to crystallisation phenomena and the degree of gelling was correlated to degree of crystallisation of lipid phase. Westesen and Siekmann related both processes and suggested that crystallisation of tripalmitate in SLN suspension was associated with an increase in specific interfacial area, because platelet-like colloidal crystals with structured surfaces were formed *(185)*. Crystal interfaces with low concentrations of adsorbed emulsifier molecules represented preferred sites of particle aggregation over which gel formation can proceed *(185)*. In most cases, gel formation is an irreversible process, which involves loss of colloidal particle structure. The organisation of lipid dispersions frequently changes over time and exhibits thermodynamic instability. Various other dispersion modifications include phase inversion, Ostwald ripening, flocculation, creaming and sedimentation, and coalescence.

3.4. Characterisation and Determination of Physicochemical Stability of SLN

The destabilisation phenomena results in a non-homogeneous system and may change in viscosity properties. Chemical instability can be observed by classical methods. High performance thin layer chromatography or thin layer chromatography are main techniques used to measure the formation of new entities due to peroxidation or hydrolysis of phospholipids *(186)*. The beginning of destabilisation process can be detected by using appropriate tools.

Differential scanning calorimetric analysis of SLN provides information about crystal behaviour, timing of polymorphic transitions, fusion temperature, enthalpy and degree of crystallinity of melt-homogenised glyceride nanoparticle dispersions *(187,182)*. X-ray scattering (small angle X-ray scattering and wide angle X-ray scattering) studies were used to investigate the crystallisation tendency and polymorphic transitions of triglyceride nanoparticles *(187,188)*. The measurement of ζ-potential allowed predicting the storage stability of a colloidal dispersion. Greater the ζ-potential, more likely the suspension will be stable because charged particles repel each other *(186)*. However, this is not the case when steric stabilisers were employed in nanoparticle preparation, as they may cause shift in surface charge. Shahgaldian and co-workers used atomic force microscopy for characterisation of calixarene-based SLNs in a gel made from four different polymers such as carbopol 980, carbopol 2020, hyaluronic acid and xanthan *(189)*. Imaging showed that SLN were in dispersed state within the gel as discrete particles of 150 nm diameter and showed little or no aggregation. The simultaneous use of topographic and force modulation mode imaging allowed a clear interpretation of observed images, showing presence of nanoparticles in sub-surface region and that SLN affect local mechanical properties of the gels.

Whatever may be the mechanistics of stability of SLN, various factors are also responsible for inducing particle destabilisation. The selection of right composition for formulation is an important aspect and would solve some of the problems involved with stability of final formulation. Process parameters such as temperature and light also appear to be of primary importance for long-term stability. Sometimes, spray drying may result in appearance of unstable polymorphs due to rapid solvent evaporation *(182)*. In same way, sonication has been described as an inductor of oxidation of phospholipids *(190)*. Sterilisation of SLN by autoclaving was reported to preserve ζ-potential of particles *(191,192)*. The pH and electrolytes also appear to be responsible for modification in particle ζ-potential, and influence of a low pH was in general, stronger than influence of electrolyte concentration *(193)*. Drug incorporation into SLN may also induce a major decrease in crystallisation temperature. Incorporation of high amounts of drugs (30–50%) may result in variation of crystallisation of SLN *(179)*. Furthermore; the polymorphic transition can also be accelerated by presence of drug in carrier. These results were attributed to high interaction between drug and lipids *(158)*.

Light causes modification of crystalline state of SLN. Storage of SLN under artificial light in transparent white glass containers led to rapid gelling due to destabilising effect of light radiation *(180)*. Moreover, high energetic radiation (UV, short wavelengths) also increased the particle destabilisation *(180)*. Temperature is another factor responsible for variations in crystalline structure of lipids. Higher temperatures often induce destabilisation. Freitas and co-workers observed rapid growth of SLN when stored at 50°C associated with a decrease in their ζ-potential *(180)*. Temperature of 4°C was found to be most favourable storage temperature. Similar observations were made by Reddy and co-workers in case of glyceride SLN *(194)*. However, in some cases, long-term storage at 20°C did not result in drug-loaded SLN aggregation or loss of drug compared with 4°C storage conditions *(192)*. Storage of spray-dried glyceride SLN in amber coloured (light-resistant) polypropylene containers both at 4–8°C and 25°C at room light conditions, maintained the stability of nanoparticles at least for 5 months and exhibited excellent redispersibility upon gentle shaking *(175)*.

3.5. *In Vitro* Drug Release From SLN

The release experiments with SLN were conducted by different methods by different researchers particularly with sample separation (filtration, centrifugation or by dialysis), and therefore it is not appropriate to compare the results. Every technique has its own advantages and disadvantages *(162)*. Similarly, the release kinetics depends on release conditions (sink or non-sink) and release medium used. However, standard experimental methods of release kinetic study includes use of release medium selected, based on sink condition and sample taken in dialysis bag.

In most cases, SLN showed burst release of the incorporated drugs. The burst release was expected when hot homogenisation was used, and also at high surfactant concentrations, which was attributed to the partitioning effect of drugs between oil and water. SLN produced by hot and cold homogenisation methods exhibited rapid release of tetracaine and etomidate *(158)*. In contrast, the SLN produced by cold homogenisation method resulted in retardation of release of prednisolone *(158,159)*. An appropriate selection of homogenisation parameters permitted the modification of release profile. Similar sustained release behaviour was observed in case of camptothecin-loaded SLN, which showed sustained release of camptothecin over more than 6 days after a slight initial burst release *(195)*. The initial burst followed by sustained drug release was also observed in case of clobetasol propionate-loaded monostearin nanoparticles prepared by solvent diffusion technique *(196)*. The SLN exhibited sustained release at rate of 6% per day.

3.6. Cellular Uptake and Cytotoxicity of SLN

SLN enhanced cellular uptake and internalisation of the incorporated drugs. Especially, in case of anti-cancer agents, the cytotoxicty was enhanced after incorporation into SLNs, either unmodified *(197)* or surface-modified *(198)*. SLN were also reported to enhance cytotoxicity of anti-cancer agents towards P-gp expressing cancer cells. Muller and Olbrich studied the cytotoxicity of compritol and cetyl palmitate nanoparticles in human granulocytes and HL60 cells *(199)*. The uncoated particles were extensively taken up by the cells due to hydrophobicity of particles leading to strong interaction with the cells and subsequent phagocytosis. Surface modification of particles with poloxamers reduced their uptake by the cells. The decrease in cell uptake was more with high molecular weight poloxamers (i.e., poloxamer 188> poloxamer 217> poloxamer 338), which was attributed to increasing thickness of adsorption layer with increasing molecular weight, providing increased steric stabilisation against phagocytosis. Surface modification of compritol and cetyl palmitate SLN with poloxamine 908 and poloxamer 407 reduced the phagocytic uptake in cultures of human granulocytes. In these cells, the SLN were found to be 10-fold less cytotoxic than polylactide nanoparticles and 100-fold less toxic than PBCA nanoparticles *(200)*. The size of SLN was found to have a dramatic influence on cytotoxicity *(201)*. Scholer and co-workers *(201)* investigated influence of lipid matrix, concentration and size of SLN on peritoneal murine macrophages. Marked cytotoxic effects were observed when murine macrophages were incubated with stearic acid SLN, whereas SLN consisting of triglycerides, cetyl palmitate or paraffin did not exert major cytotoxic effects at same concentrations. Hence, the experimental results may also depend on type of lipid matrix and composition chosen for preparation of SLN *(202)*. The surfactants used for stabilisation of SLN often get incorporated in small amounts into nanoparticle matrix or adsorb onto surface. These surfactants if not removed from the formulation may lead to toxicity.

3.7. Applications of SLN in Drug Delivery

Lipid nanoparticles have received great attention as drug carriers in recent years. Striking advantages of lipid nanoparticles as drug delivery system are targetability,

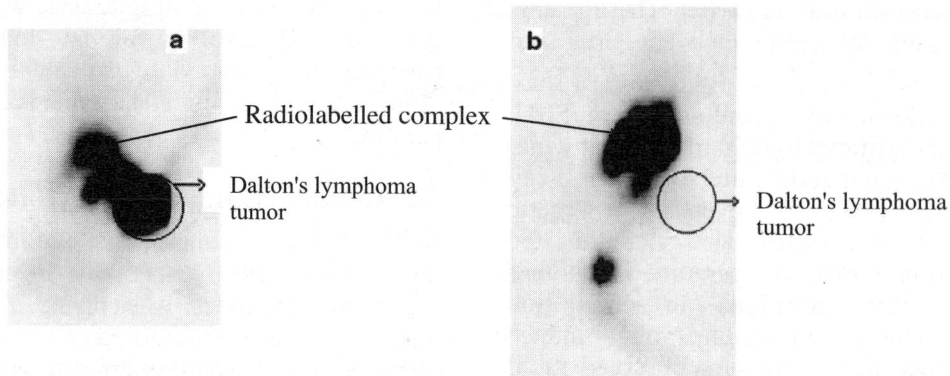

Fig. 4. γ-Scintigraphic images of mice-bearing Dalton's lymphoma tumour at 24-h post-injection of 99mTc-etoposide-loaded tripalmitin SLN by subcutaneous or i.v. route. The circle portions in both the figures indicate Dalton's lymphoma tumour implanted in hind leg of Balb/c mice. **Panel (a)** represents γ-image of tumour-bearing mice after subcutaneous injection of 99mTc-etoposide-loaded tripalmitin SLN taken at 24-h post-injection demonstrating significant tumour uptake and retention (black portion in figure indicates radiolabelled complex). **Panel (b)** represents γ-image of tumour-bearing mice after i.v. injection of 99mTc-etoposide-loaded tripalmitin SLN through tail vein, taken at 24-h post-injection demonstrating poor tumour uptake. The tumour uptake and retention after subcutaneous injection is significantly higher (~59-folds) than after i.v. injection. (Reprinted from J. Control. Release, 105, Reddy, LH., Sharma, RK., Chuttani, K., Mishra, AK., and Murthy, RSR. Influence of administration route on tumor uptake and biodistribution of etoposide loaded solid lipid nanoparticles in Dalton's lymphoma tumor bearing mice, 185–198, 2005, with permission from Elsevier) *(122)*.

sustained drug release, improved stability of entrapped drugs and their feasibility for large-scale production by HPH technique.

Pharmacokinetic studies of doxorubicin incorporated into SLN showed higher blood levels in comparison to commercial drug solution after i.v. injection in rats. Higher distribution of drug was found to organs such as lung, spleen and brain, while the solution led to higher distribution to liver and kidneys *(203)*. Camptothecin-loaded SLN prepared using poloxamer 188 as stabiliser showed 18 times greater mean residence time (MRT) than camptothecin solution in mice upon i.v. injection. Such high difference in MRT was attributed to surface coating of poloxamer 188 on surface of SLN *(195)*. The SLN formulation concentrated mainly in organs of RES and also in heart and brain, the higher brain levels being maintained for a longer time. The C_{max} of camptothecin in brain increased by 180% compared with drug solution, and AUC/dose was 10.4-fold greater than solution. The surface charge of SLN also modified the biodistibution profile after i.v. administration. Positvely charged etoposide SLN (ETP) prepared using stearyl amine as charge modifier showed higher and prolonged blood circulation time and brain distribution than negatively charged etoposide SLN (ETN) *(204)*. Route of administration of SLN was also found to influence the biodistribution and deposition into tumour. When three administration routes were investigated, i.e., i.v., i.p. and subcutaneous, the i.v. injection resulted in lowest tumour concentrations followed by i.p. injection. Subcutaneous injection at lower side away from the tumour region showed maximum tumour concentration (Fig. 4), which increased with time suggesting lymphatic absorption and tumour transport of SLN. The tumour concentration of ETN after subcutaneous injection was 59-folds greater than that obtained after i.v., and eightfolds higher than after i.p. route at 24 h post-injection, indicating the importance of administration route *(122)*. Similarly, Sznitowska and co-workers reported inefficiency of SLN to improve the bioavailability of diazepam after rectal administration *(205)*. They compared three different formulations, i.e., organic solution, sub-micron emulsion made from Miglyol 812 and cetyl palmitate SLN, all containing diazepam. The sub-micron emulsion showed greater bioavailability indicated by high C_{max} and area under curve (AUC) compared with SLN and organic solution. In comparison to previous reports on SLN, this study clearly indicated that route of administration greatly influences the bioavailability of SLN. Hence, a careful choice of route of injection may provide fruitful results.

SLN was also reported to enhance bioavailability of poorly soluble drugs. Followed by intragastric administration, the bioavailability of cyclosporine A was enhanced by SLN (stearic acid nanoparticles) *(206)*. The relative bioavailability of cyclosporine A-loaded SLN over the Sandimmune Neoral® (marketed by Novartis as microemulsion formulation of cyclosporine A) was nearly 80%, and the T_{max} of cyclosporine A after oral administration of cyclosporine A loaded SLN was delayed significantly than the reference. In another study, when cyclosporine A was administered as SLN formulation, it exhibited a mean plasma profile with almost similarly low variations (as variability is an issue in cyclosporine A absorption) compared with commercial microemulsion, and no initial blood peak as observed with commercial formulation *(207)*. However, cyclosporine A administered as drug nanocrystals showed relatively lower blood concentrations. In case of idarubicin-loaded SLN (made from stearic acid), the pharmacokinetic parameters of idarubicin found after duodenal administration of solution and SLN forms were different: AUC and elimination half-life were about 21 times and 30 times, respectively, higher after idarubicin-SLN administration than after solution administration. The idarubicin and idarubicinol concentrations were lower in heart, lung, spleen and kidneys of idarubicin-SLN than idarubicin solution *(208)*. In case of SLN formulation, the idarubicin and its metabolite idarubicinol were detected in brain indicating the possibiblity of transport of SLN through BBB. Surface conjugation of SLN made from emulsifying wax with thiamine ligand (thiamine linked to distearoyl phosphatidylethanolamine via a PEG spacer) significantly increased the brain transport of nanoparticles *(209)*. Most recently, the glycerylmonostearate SLN (<100 nm) were shown to enhance bioavailability of vinpocetine *(210)*, a poorly bioavailable compound *(211)* used in the treatment of cerebral circulatory disorders. The surfactants such as polyoxyethylene hydrogenated castor oil and Tween-80 used for stabilisation of nanoparticles also promoted bioavailability, which was concentration-dependant. Various mechanisms such as bioadhesion to GIT due to smaller size, transient increase in membrane permeability due to surfactants and inhibition of cytochrome P^{450} action on drug by nanoparticles were held responsible for observed bioavailability enhancement of vinpocetine by SLN.

SLN were also employed as carriers for anticancer drugs. Incorporation of paclitaxel into lipid-polysorbate nanoparticles significantly enhanced cytotoxicity of paclitaxel towards P-gp expressing cancer cells *(212)*. Various other reports also demonstrated the potential of SLN in delivering drugs to cancer *(213,214)*. SLN also improved anticancer effect of etoposide in dalton's lymphoma ascites-bearing mice *(123)*. After i.p. injection into ascites-bearing mice, the SLN showed delayed but prolonged apoptotic induction compared with free etoposide. Both etoposide-loaded SLN and free etoposide showed differences in cell cycle, such as expression of hypodiploid peak, shortened S-phase and greater number of dead cells due to significant apoptosis, compared with cells of untreated ascites-bearing mice. However, the effect of etoposide-loaded SLN was more prolonged than free etoposide, resulting in greater survival of ascites-bearing mice, probably due to cell-adhesion effects of SLN followed by sustained drug release, as the etoposide-loaded SLN were shown to exhibit sustained drug release *(175)*.

Apart from their application for i.v. and oral delivery of drugs, the SLN were investigated for their suitability in topical applications, both pharmaceutical and cosmetic. Highly sensitive chemical substances such as coenzyme Q10 and retinol were stabilised in SLN with success *(215,216)*. Various other drugs such as α-lipoic acid *(217)*, N,N-diethyl-m-toluamide and vitamin K *(218)*, flurbiprofen *(219)*, podophyllotoxin *(220)*, etc. were incorporated into SLN for topical delivery purposes. The small size of nanoparticles associated with larger surface area was found suitable for stabilising the sensitive materials.

Cosmetic preparations containing sunscreen agents with UV radiation blocking effect are widely marketed. Use of SLN as carrier for sunscreen agents is an interesting idea, and due to highly crystalline nature and small particle size SLN was found to possess UV blocking activity (physical sunscreen). Also the incorporation of sunscreen agents resulted in formation of stable preparations *(221,222)* possessing synergistic effects, and sometimes making it possible to decrease original concentration of sunscreen agents for required effect *(223)*.

SLN and NLC incorporated into hydrogel enhanced the occlusive properties onto skin, and effectively delivered and sustained the penetration of entrapped ascorbyl palmitate (an anti-oxidant) through excised human skin *(224)*. Tristearin SLN incorporated into hydrogel also enhanced the transdermal penetration of triptolide, an agent possessing anti-inflammatory, anti-fertility and anti-neoplastic activities *(225)*. In comparison to triptolide-loaded normal hydrogel, hydrogel-loaded SLN formulation showed twofold higher anti-inflammatory activity.

4. HYDROGEL NANOPARTICLES

Hydrogels are three-dimensional, macromolecular networks containing a large fraction of water within their structure, insoluble, soft and pliable. Some hydrogels can reversibly swell or shrink up to 1000 times in volume in response to a variety of external stimuli *(226–228)*. Hydrogels can be prepared by co-polymerisation of two different monomers *(229)*, by forming interpenetrating polymer networks *(230)* or by creating networks with microporous structures *(231)*. They can be made in bulk or in nano- or microparticle form. Hydrogel in nanoparticle form react quickly to an external stimulus such as temperature or pH, and are known as stimuli–responsive hydrogel nanoparticles. These types of nanoparticles can be classified into two types: thermo-responsive and pH-responsive.

4.1. Thermo-Responsive Hydrogel Nanoparticles

Thermo-responsive polymers are macromolecular structures, which are soluble in water at low temperatures, while they precipitate out upon heating at more than its lower critical solution temperature (LCST). Hydrogels can be obtained by cross-linking these polymers, which are stable at lower temperature but shrink reversibly at high temperature. Poly(N-isopropyl acrylamide) (PNIPAM) is most widely studied thermo-responsive polymer *(232,233)*, followed by poly(N-vinylcaprolactam) *(234–236)*. Both these polymers possess LCST closer to physiological temperature.

Huang and co-workers synthesised nanoparticles of PNIPAM-co-allylamine and PNIPAM-co-acrylic acid, which are chemically interconnected in presence of dextran, to form three-dimensional macroscopic gels at room temperature and neutral pH *(237)*. The gels have two levels of structural hierarchy, the primary network consisting of cross-linked polymer chains inside each nanoparticle, while the secondary network is a cross-linked system of nanoparticles. The pore sizes of primary and secondary networks were in range of 1–10 nm and 10–500 nm, respectively. This structure allowed unique property of entrapping and releasing the drug between particles. The model compound dextran entrapped between particle cavities in nanoparticle network was released with a rate regulated by their molecular weights and cavity size, while no release was observed from a conventional bulk PNIPAM gel with high cross-linking density. High molecular weight dextran-loaded nanoparticles showed temperature-dependant release, which was faster at 21°C than at 37°C (physiological temperature), indicating their potential in encapsulation and delivery of hydrophilic molecules, and controlled drug release at physiological temperature.

Hydrogel nanoparticles were also employed as oxygen carriers in physiological malfunctions. Several hydrogel-based oxygen carriers were developed having oxygen affinity and comparable osmotic pressure to cellular and acellular oxygen carriers *(238,239)*. The nanoscale hydrogel particles were also developed, which possessed higher haemoglobin encapsulation potential in comparison to that of haemoglobin-loaded liposomal formulations *(240)*. Patton and Palmer synthesised PNIPAM hydrogel nanoparticles loaded with haemoglobin by UV-induced photopolymerisation within liposomal reactors *(241)*. The hydrogel nanoparticles were swollen at LCST of polymer, i.e., 32°C, after which they shrunk and aggregated when temperature was increased to 40°C.

Recently, composite hydrogel nanoparticles made up of a mixture of PNIPAM, other thermo-responsive hydrogels and PEG diacrylate (a photo cross-linking agent) incorporated high amounts of hydrophilic substances and exhibited sustained release property, which was temperature-dependant *(242)*. In composite structure, the PNIPAM nanoparticles were found embedded inside PEG polymeric matrix. Such nanoparticles can be beneficial in targeting and controlled release applications.

4.2. pH-Responsive Hydrogel Nanoparticles

Apart from thermo-sensitive systems, the pH-sensitive hydrogels also gained importance in delivering drugs, especially by oral route. Blanchette and Peppas developed hydrogen bonding-induced complex copolymer networks of poly(methacrylic acid) grafted with PEG by synthesis through free radical polymerisation *(243)* . The copolymer exhibited pH-dependent swelling behaviour due to formation/dissociation of interpolymer complexes. At acidic pH, the interpolymer complexes were formed due to hydrogen bonding between graft PEG chains and carboxylic acid protons. These complexes serve as temporary, physical cross-links and cause gels to exist in a collapsed conformation. The pK_a of poly(methacrylic acid) is about 4.8. Thus, at neutral pH the methacrylate groups in network are deprotonated. The hydrogen bonds existing at low pH, dissociate at neutral and high pH resulting in swelling of network structure. When loaded with bleomycin (an anticancer peptide), these hydrogel nanoparticles preserved the potency of bleomycin, and also caused a transient increase in permeability Caco-2. Generally, bleomycin undergoes degradation due to bleomycin hydrolase present in cells or is toxic when exposed to nucleus. When incubated with DLD-1 (a human colorectal adenocarcinoma cell line), it resulted in paracellular transport of nanoparticles, and entrapped bleomycin still showed DNA damage suggesting efficacy of nanoparticles in overcoming the toxicity and degradation of bleomycin after oral administration.

The extracellular pH of tumours in patients measured using invasive micro-electrodes was found to be 5.7–7.8 with an average value of 7.0 *(244)*. The acidity off tumour interstitial fluid is mainly attributed to higher rate of aerobic and anaerobic glycolysis in cancer cells compared with normal cells *(245)*. Taking advantage of low tumour pH, the drug delivery systems sensitive to lower pH values were developed for delivering drugs to tumours. Smaller liposomes containing pH-sensitive functional groups as well as hydrophilic surface were successfully delivered to tumour due to greater passive accumulation and selective drug release at tumour pH *(246,247)*. Self-assembled polymeric nanoparticles prepared by conjugating sulphadimethoxine to succinylated pullulan acetate showed excellent pH-responsive property *(248,249)*. These nanoparticles were stable at pH 7.4, but underwent shrinking and aggregation at below pH 7.0. The nanoparticles incorporated with doxorubicin showed pH-dependant release, and release was greater at low pH values (<6.8). Hydrogel nanoparticles of pullulan incorporating pBUDLacZ plasmid were found to be internalised by cells and resulted in efficient gene expression, indicating their potential in gene delivery applications *(250)*.

4.3. Thermo- and pH-Responsive Hydrogel Nanoparticles

Hydrogel nanoparticles with both pH-responsive and thermo-responsive properties are synthesised by co-polymerisation of PVP and acrylic acid *(251)*. The hydrogel nanoparticles were stable to lyophilisation and lyophilised powder was easily redispersed into aqueous medium. The rate of release of entrapped fluorescein isothiocyanate (FITC)-dextran from nanoparticles at 22°C increased with pH. At pH 10.0 and 7.0, 60% burst release was observed, followed by sustained release, whereas at acidic pH values, the release was extremely slow. The nanoparticles also exhibited temperature-dependant increase in release of FITC-dextran, suggesting use of such stimuli–responsive bifunctional systems in controlled drug delivery applications. Another type of temperature/pH dual-responsive colloidal nanogels reported were those which are synthesised by combining PNIPAM with a pH-sensitive polymer in core and shell structure, respectively *(252)*.

Apart from stimuli–responsive hydrogel nanoparticles, various other types of hydrogel nanoparticles were also employed for drug delivery applications and are discussed here.

4.4. Dextran Hydrogel Nanoparticles

Dextran is a polysaccharide consisting of glucose molecules coupled into long branched chains, primarily through a 1,6- and some through a 1,3-glucosidic linkages. Dextrans are inert, non-toxic, colloidal hydrophilic substances. Due to these properties, dextrans have been used for many years as plasma expanders and evaluated as a carrier systems for a variety of therapeutic agents including antidiabetics, antibiotics, anticancer drugs, peptides and enzymes *(253,254)*. Dextrans are degraded by dextranase present in colon *(255)*. Taking advantage of enzymatic degradation, the polymeric prodrugs for colonic drug delivery based on dextran were designed *(256)*. In colon, dextran molecule is degraded by microbial dextranases making the ester bond accessible to hydrolysis, and thereby releasing incorporated drugs. The hydrogel nanoparticles can complex various hydrophobic substances, including soluble proteins or enzymes *(257,258)*. Recently, the synthesis of self-assembled hydrogel nanoparticles from a mixture of glycidyl methacrylate dextran and dimethacrylate PEG was reported for drug delivery *(259)*. These hydrogel nanoparticles loaded with clonazepam showed rapid drug release in 0.1 *M* pH 7.4 phosphate-buffered saline in presence of dextranase, which was attributed to degradation of dextran portion in DP hydrogel nanoparticles by dextranase. When drug release was evaluated in absence of dextranase at different pH values, the release of clonazepam was higher at low pH values possibly due to formation of hydrogen bonds by hydrogel with water. While the phenomenon was reverse in presence of dextranase, and release was higher at pH 6.0 due to greater activity of the enzyme at this pH, indicating possible application of these hydrogel nanoparticles in drug delivery to colon.

4.5. PolyHydroxy Ethyl Methacrylate Hydrogel Nanoparticles

Opthalmic drug delivery is one of the considerable areas of research focused on delivering drugs locally to the eye, thereby improving drug availability and preventing side effects associated with systemic administration. Many of the available ophthalmic drug formulations are eye drops, and possess limitation of elimination of great amount of formulation through tears, and hence long-term drug availability is not possible. Recently, Gulsen and Chauhan prepared hydrogel in which drug-loaded nanoparticles were mixed with hydroxy ethyl methacrylate (HEMA) and polymerised by free radical polymerisation *(260)*. PolyHEMA hydrogels are biocompatible and are used since several decades for biomedical applications. PolyHEMA is also widely used in preparation of intraocular lens, vascular prostheses and drug delivery *(261)*. The prepared hydrogels were able to sustain the drug release up to 8 day. On the other hand, incorporation of silica nanoparticles (about 230 nm) into polyHEMA resulted in nanocomposite with improved swelling properties. Here, silica is expected to improve mechanical properties of composite, and hence could be used for biomedical applications such as preparation of tissue scaffolds *(262)*.

4.6. Hydrogel Nanoparticles for Protein Delivery

Protein encapsulation and its active presentation to dendritic cells is in fact a challenging task. Several efforts were made to develop an ideal carrier, in order to maximise antigen loading in carriers, avoid protein denaturation during incorporation into carrier and also during storage, and minimise toxicity associated with the adjuvants and carrier itself. Carriers such as PLGA particles *(263,264)*, latex particles *(265)* and hydrogel particles *(266,267)* resulted in low protein encapsulation (<15%). PEG-based hydrogel nanoparticles have improved the encapsulation and delivery of proteins. These nanoparticles were prepared by cross-linking PEG within polymer-rich phase of an emulsion formed by a poly(ethylene oxide-*b*-propylene oxide-*b*-ethylene oxide) triblock copolymer in saturated aqueous salt solution *(268)*. These nanoparticles (500 nm mean diameter) allowed encapsulation of high amounts of protein (75%), which was selectively released by action of proteolytic enzymes, normally present in endosomal compartments of dendritic cells. Surface modification of these nanoparticles by sequential adsorption of poly(L-arginine) and CpG oligonucleotides, allowed co-delivery of antigen and immunostimulatory ligands responsible for induction of primary immune responses *in vivo*. The dendritic cells pulsed with protein-loaded particles activated T cells *in vitro* about 10-folds more efficiently than dendritic cells incubated with soluble protein, indicating the potential of these hydrogel nanoparticles in improving delivery of non-viral vaccines for therapeutic applications.

Stabilisation and delivery of bioactive proteins is an important issue to date. This is especially true for molecules like insulin, which undergo enzymatic degradation and self-association to form oligomers depending upon various factors *(269)*. Incorporation of such proteins into pullulan nanoparticles improved their stability. Pullulan is a water-soluble, viscous, non-ionic polysaccharide consisting of three α-1,4-linked glucose molecules that are repeatedly polymerised by α-1,6-linkages on terminal glucose. Pullulan possess various advantages such as high water solubility, lack of immunogenicity and usefulness as a plasma expander, and hence was widely studied as a macromolecular carrier for drug delivery applications. Stabilisation of insulin by dodecyl maltoside overcame the self-association and degradation of insulin and the stabilised insulin was effective after oral administration *(270)*. Complexing insulin with hydrophobised cholesterol-bearing pullulan nanoparticles (20–30 nm) resulted in suppression of its thermal denaturation and aggregation *(258)*. The complexed insulin showed improved stability against degradation *in vitro* by α-chymotrypsin, and was completely bioactive after i.v. injection in rats, determined by depression in blood glucose levels.

4.7. PVP Hydrogel Nanoparticles

The presence of hydrophilic surface on delivery carriers avoids their recognition by macrophages, and moreover increases their residence time in blood. Such systems have several applications in field of drug delivery. Various hydrophilic polymers were used for this purpose, and PVP is one such hydrophilic polymer. Cross-linking PVP with N,N′-methylene *bis*-acrylamide in reverse core of micelles resulted in formation of nanoparticles having mean diameter less than 100 nm *(271)*. These hydrogel nanoparticles were able to incorporate hydrophilic substances with high efficiency. The hydrogel nanoparticles underwent swelling in aqueous buffer medium, and released incorporated FITC-dextran at a controlled rate. The extent of release depended upon pH of medium. Low and high pH values caused slow release, while the neutral pH medium resulted in maximum release of FITC-dextran from hydrogel nanoparticles. The release from hydrogel nanoparticles also depended upon degree of cross-linking and loading extent. Such hydrogel nanoparticulate systems could be of great interest for long circulation accompanied by controlled drug delivery.

When entrapped into F-virosomes (a cell membrane fusion protein-F), followed by incubation with the HepG2 cells, cross-linked PVP hydrogel nanoparticles loaded with FITC-dextran were successfully delivered into cells *(272)*. This is result of fusion of F-virosomes with HepG2 cells, followed by microinjection of nanoparticles into the cells. Inside cells, the nanoparticles released entrapped FITC-dextran in a controlled fashion. Such nanoparticles could have possible application in delivering drugs to drug-resistant cancers, where cellular entry of the molecules is highly restricted due to P-gp and MDR.

4.8. PVA Hydrogel Nanoparticles

PVA is another hydrophilic polymer, which is non-toxic, biocompatible and non-carcinogenic, and has been used in preparation of soft contact lenses, implants and artificial organs *(273,274)*, and also in oral-controlled drug delivery applications. Earlier, macroscopic PVA hydrogels were prepared by emulsion technique followed by freeze-thawing at –4°C *(275)*. Employing W/O emulsion using silicone oil, and decreasing the freezing temperature upto –20°C resulted in formation of hydrogel nanoparticles with about 670 nm mean diameter *(276)*. The hydrogel nanoparticles controlled the release rate of incorporated protein, i.e., BSA, and release rate was also influenced by temperature. Incorporation into nanoparticles maintained stability of BSA, suggesting the suitability of PVA hydrogel nanoparticles as protein carriers.

4.9. Curdlan Hydrogel Nanoparticles

Curdlan is a naturally occurring linear (triple helix) polysaccharide composed of 1,3-β-linked D-glucose units produced by a strain of *Alcaligenes faecalis*. Carboxymethylated curdlan (a curdlan derivative) when modified hydrophobically with a carboxylated sulphonylurea derivative having a strong tendency to aggregate in water (due to interactions between phenyl groups, hexyl groups and hydrogen bonding), self-assembled into nanoparticles in aqueous medium *(277)*. Galactosylation of these nanoparticles with lactobionic acid increased their adsorption followed by enhanced uptake by asialoglycoprotein (ASGP) receptor-mediated endocytosis in HepG2 (a hepatoma cell line), while ungalactosylated nanoparticles did not, indicating ligand-mediated interaction of conjugated nanoparticles in hepatoma cells. Such nanoparticles could be possibly applied for hepatic-specific delivery of anti-cancer agents.

4.10. Pluronic Hydrogel Nanoparticles

Poly(ethylene oxide)-poly(propylene oxide)-poly(ethylene oxide) (PEO-PPO-PEO) (Pluronic®) is a triblock co-polymer from BASF possessing the ability to self-assemble in aqueous solution into multi-molecular aggregates in a temperature-dependant manner. The critical micelle temperature (CMT) of pluronic polymers range from 25 to 40°C, over which they self-assemble to form a spherical micellar structure by dehydration of polypropylene oxide block within the structure. At concentrations more than 25% (w/v), the pluronic co-polymers exhibit a sol–gel transition behaviour around CMT *(278)*. Cross-linking pluronic hydrogel nanoparticles withpoly(ethyleneimine) (PEI) showed cellular penetration through endocytosis when incubated with HeLa (human epithelial carcinoma) cells, followed by endosomal breaking due to membrane rupture caused by temperature-dependant swelling of nanoparticles and successive release into cytoplasm *(279)*. The endosomal lysis and escape of nanoparticles was attributed to their swelling in acidic endosomal pH due to protonation of amine functions in PEI. The swelling kinetics of these nanoparticles was influenced by both pH and temperature. Such nanoparticulate systems could be more useful in intracellular delivery of drugs or proteins prone to endosomal degradation.

5. PEPTIDE NANOPARTICLES

Oral route is most preferred route of drug administration. Several peptides exhibit poor bioavailability following oral administration, due to their instability in GIT and low intestinal permeability *(280)*. Due to acidic environment in stomach and presence of proteases in intestine, the peptides undergo degradation in GIT *(281)*. To overcome associated problems and facilitate improved oral delivery of peptides, several approaches were tried. They include use of absorption enhancers *(282)*, protease inhibitors *(283)*, chemical modification of peptides *(284)*, etc. Apart from this, various drug delivery carriers such as microcapsules *(285)*, liposomes *(286)*, emulsions *(287)*, nanoparticles *(288)* and specialised site-directed systems such as colon delivery systems *(289)*, mucoadhesive systems, etc. were employed to enhance bioavailability of peptides *(290)*. Nanoparticles have been widely employed for encapsulation of various peptides such as calcitonin, insulin, cyclosporine A and leutinising hormone releasing hormone (LHRH), etc. *(291)*. The stability of proteins and peptides encapsulated into nanoparticles depend upon several factors such as nature of solvents employed, polymers used, additives such as surfactants/stabilisers and processing parameters *(292)*. Very recently, a new kind of approach of enhancing oral delivery of erythropoietin was attempted *(292,293)*, by absorbing protein on porous adsorbents such as carbon nanotubes, nanohorns, bamboo charcoal and fullurene, in presence of oral absorption enhancers. The resultant nanostructures significantly enhanced the bioavailability of incorporated protein after intrajejunal administration.

The storage stability of calcitonin was improved upon encapsulation into PIBCA nanocapsules *(294)*, and also decreased its degradation compared with free peptide in presence of proteases *(295)*. Co-addition of deoxycholic acid and sodium lauryl sulphate as absorption enhancers into these nanocapsules increased therapeutic effect of calcitonin in terms of decrease in blood calcium level, which was comparable with i.v. injection of similar dose (20 IU/kg) *(296)*.

Cyclosporine A is a hydrophobic cyclic peptide possessing incomplete and variable oral absorption. Cyclosporine A was marketed earlier (Sandimmune®) in form of oily solution, but was then withdrawn and re-introduced in new form Neoral® by Novartis as microemulsion pre-concentrate with improved oral bioavailability and decreased interpatient variability. PIHCA nanocapsules developed for cyclosporine A exhibited a notable increase in bioavailability (32-fold greater AUC) compared with Sandimmune® formulation in NMRI mice *(297)*. Damge and co-workers *(298,299)* observed an increased duration of action of insulin (100 IU/kg) when incorporated into PIBCA nanocapsules, and the effect was more pronounced only when nanocapsules were administered in ileum or jejunum part of intestine.

Hillery and co-workers synthesised a polymer-peptide conjugate of LHRH, by initially preparing a vinylacetate derivative of LHRH, followed by its conjugation with butyl cyanoacrylate *(300)*. The conjugate formed nanoparticles (100 nm) and were stable *in vitro* in luminal contents and serum. Oral administration of these nanoparticles in rats increased their absorption and also resulted in appearance of detectable levels up to 12 h *(301)*. Multiple dosing increased LHRH concentrations and at the same time resulted in prolonged detection, indicating possibility of improved oral delivery of LHRH by these conjugate nanoparticles.

Encapsulation of peptides into nanoparticles often modifies therapeutic properties of the peptides. In case of chronic hepatitis B viral infection, the cell-mediated immune response is considered to be important and curative. When Hepatitis B core antigen (HBcAg) was incorporated along with monophosphoryl lipid A into PLGA nanoparticles, it exhibited strong immune responses compared with free HBcAg *(302)*. Also, the nanoparticles were found capable to alter immune response elicited by the peptide.

5.1. Gene Delivery Using Nanoparticles

Gene therapy using non-viral vectors is associated with safety, low immunogenecity, ease of preparation and ability to accommodate larger DNA than viral vectors *(303)*. However, this strategy is much less efficient in delivering genes compared with viral vectors *(304)*. PEI is a polymer widely employed for gene delivery applications into cells and also neurons *(305,306)*. Owing to its cationic nature, PEI facilitates penetration of gene vectors by binding to negatively charged heparin sulphate proteoglycans present on the cell membrane, followed by their transport into perinuclear space *(307)*. This is especially true in case of transfection permissive cells. But in case of transfection restrictive cells, the gene expression is lower, and to enhance gene expression and to overcome cellular barriers, the polymer/DNA complexes may have to be bound with bioactive ligands. PEI/DNA nanocomplexes carrying plasmid DNA-encoding yellow fluorescent protein transfect showed lower expression in transfection restrictive (differentiated) SH-SY5Y human neuronal cells compared with transfection permissive (undifferentiated) cells *(308)*. Surface PEGylation of PEI/DNA nanocomplexes, followed by linking with either Arginine-Glycine-Aspartate (RGD) sequence or HIV-1 TAT peptides significantly improved transfection, probably as a result of enhanced cellular uptake. Of the two ligands, nanocomplexes conjugated with RGD showed greater enhancement in transfection in differentiated neuronal cells. Similarly, the enhanced gene transfection and expression by TAT–PEG–PEI/DNA complexes was observed, both *in vitro* in human lung epithelial cells (A549) and *in vivo* in mice after intratracheal administration *(309)* In some cases, the nanoparticles were also successfully employed as non-viral vectors for gene delivery by oral route. Poly-L-lysine (PLL)-modified silica nanoparticles, when administered orally were shown to successfully deliver incorporated gene, and efficient reporter gene expression was detected in stomach and intestine mainly in mucous membrane cells *(310)*. On the other hand, the nanoparticles were found to be non-toxic to intestine after oral administration, indicating their potential in oral gene delivery.

Basic fibroblast growth factor (bFGF) is a peptide attempted for angiogenesis therapy. When incorporated into heparin-conjugated PLGA nanoparticles, release of bFGF was greatly controlled and followed zero-order kinetics *(311)*. The release of bFGF was still slowed down when dispersed in fibrin gel.

The acid-degradable cationic acrylamide nanoparticles prepared using acid labile benzyl acetal cross-linker were reported to enhance the delivery of incorporated antigen (ovalbumin) into dendritic cells *(312)*. Due to their cationic nature, the nanoparticles were found to penetrate the cells through endocytosis pathway and direct more ovalbumin antigens to be processed into appropriately trimmed peptide fragments, and presented via major histocompatibility complex class I pathway following hydrolysis within acidic lysosomes.

Delivery of peptides through mucoadhesive nanoparticles was another interesting approach attempted. Generally, proteins and peptides cannot cross mucosal barriers, for instance, after oral administration they are degraded before they reach blood stream *(313)*. The colloidal carriers possessing mucoadhesion properties would improve transmucosal delivery of these therapeutic substances. Mucoadhesive nanoparticles were generally prepared by employing mucoadhesive polmers, or coating nanoparticles with mucoadhesive polymers such as chitosan, PVA and poly(acrylic acid) *(314)*. Mucoadhesive coating can be achieved by either addition of polymer during nanoparticles preparation or by mixing with preformed nanoparticles. Mucoadhesion of nanoparticles to gastric mucosa can be due to electrostatic or hydrophobic interactions or hydrogen bonding *(315,316)*. Following mucoadhesion, the particles remain at site for a longer time, and release drug or are taken up by the cells. Polymerisation of monomers in presence of mucoadhesive polymers result in nanoparticles with modified surface charge. For instance, graft co-polymerisation of methyl methacrylate on chitosan formed positively charged nanoparticles with ζ-potential of 20.2 mV *(317)*. These nanoparticles were able to incorporate hydrophilic compounds such as insulin, by electrostatic interaction, hydrogen bonding, etc. with mucoadhesive polymers. Such nanoparticles protect incorporated drugs or peptides from degradation in GIT and also interact with mucin, thereby assisting in improving the bioavailability.

Nanoparticles made of graft co-polymers possessing hydrophobic backbone and hydrophilic branches were demonstrated to improve oral absorption of calcitonin in rats *(318)*. In these cases, the entrapment occurs by the ionic interactions or by hydrogen bonding between hydrophilic peptide and surface macromonomer chains in water. For instance, high entrapment of calcitonin observed in case of polymethyl acrylamide (PMAA) nanoparticles was attributed to interaction between anionic function of polymer and cationic functional group of calcitonin *(319)*. When administered orally in rats, PMAA nanoparticles, PNIPAM nanoparticles and poly(N-vinyl acetamide) nanoparticles enhanced the absorption of calcitonin, as observed by corresponding decrease in ionised calcium concentration in blood, which was significantly higher in case of PNIPAM nanoparticles *(320)*. The activity of calcitonin-loaded PNIPAM nanoparticles was further enhanced when administered in divided doses *(321)*. The observed efficacy of nanoparticle formulations *in vivo* was attributed to stabilisation of calcitonin against degradation by digestive enzymes, as well as mucoadhesion of nanoparticles. In another study, coating calcitonin-loaded solid lipid nanoparticles with chitosan, resulted in significant and prolonged reduction in serum calcium levels as compared with those obtained for calcitonin solution, after oral administration to rats *(322)*.

Self-assembling block polymers have been widely studied for drug delivery applications. Protein polymers based on peptide sequences (pentameric repeating units) derived from elastin exhibit temperature-dependant self-assembly in aqueous solutions *(323)*. In this process, the polypeptide is converted from a soluble expanded state to a collapsed state over LCST, which in turn depends on polarity of amino acid side chains in pentapeptide sequence *(324)*. Using elastin-mimetic peptide sequences, core-shell type of diblock and triblock, co-polymer nanostructures were designed at more than their transition temperature, especially under physiological temperature *(325,326)* and through genetic engineering *(327,328)*. Such systems are potentials for thermo-sensitive-controlled release reservoirs of protein materials for *in vivo* applications.

6. NANOCRYSTALS AND NANOSUSPENSIONS

Large number of therapeutic molecules that emerged out of research since last two to three decades are lipophilic, and posed problems with respect to solubility, oral absorption and bioavailability. To bring out successful formulation of such drugs to obtain high bioavailability and additional pharmacokinetic benefits is a true challenge *(328)*. Several approaches were adopted to meet this challenge; out of these, micronisation was widely employed especially for oral absorption enhancement. However, this technique generally results in formation of micron-sized particles, and hence the enhancement of bioavailability was not complete, and also posed problems for the i.v. administration of drugs. In early 1990s, Nanocrystal technology (Elan Nanosystems) involving size reduction was employed by Liversidge and co-workers *(329)* leading to development of Nanocrystals.

6.1. Methods of Preparation of Nanocrystals and Nanosuspensions

While the preparation of polymeric and lipid nanoparticle utilises bottom up process, the methods for nanocrystals and nanosuspension preparation adopts both bottom up and top down techniques, preferably, top down approach due to its simplicity and economic viability. Major techniques in top down approach include media grinding and HPH.

6.1.1. Media Grinding Method

Dispersing nanoparticles into liquids can be challenging; tremendous surface area and surface energy, which provides the beneficial effects of nanomaterials also prevents easy dispersion into liquids. Conventional technology for dispersing powders into liquids is not sufficient for dispersing these tiny particles into discrete entities in a liquid.

Production of stable suspensions or dispersions of nanometer size particles is done by utilising a comminution process, like a small media mill. Grinding coarser particles into nanometer range or dispersion of agglomerated nanosized primary particles, which is called dispersion method or top down process, is done on an industrial level with a bead mill, but bead mill process can contaminate the material or worse destroy structure of particle *(330)*. Bead mills are available in various sizes and configurations from Mickle shaker which has a maximum volume of about 40 mL to continuous process equipment capable of handling up to 200 Kg wet yeast or 20 Kg wet bacteria each hour. It has been discovered that by using very fine particle size grinding media beads, in range of 70–125 µm, one can grind materials into nanometer range economically. Or for dispersing nanometer-sized particles using beads even as fine as 30–50 µm shows a significant improvement in process efficiency. List of generally used grinding media along with their specifications are given in Table 3.

The limitation to the process has been that scalable industrial equipment that can use these micron beads on a continuous basis was not well known or well accepted due to the difficulty in handling the small beads, i.e., removing them for suspension after dispersing the particles, or loading and discharging small beads into machine. Bead mills with an improved grinding media separation system have also been developed recently.

Initially, the pearl milling operation encountered erosion problem *(331)*, and was resolved by using pearls made of polymer. Though pearl milling is used in industry for preparation of drug nanosuspension, the process possesses some limitations such as low batch size and longer operation time.

6.1.2. High-Pressure Homogenisation

Another size reduction technique employed for preparation of drug nanosuspensions was high-pressure homogeniser (HPH). Two types of homogenisers were utilised, micro-fluidiser (Microfluidex®) and piston gap homogeniser (Avestine®). The micro-fluidiser employs jet stream principle, in which drug suspension is passed at high speed through homogenisation chamber. Illustrative diagrams of both types of high-pressure homogeniser are given in Fig. 5.

Muller *et al.* reported a relatively feasible technique for preparation of nanosuspensions employing HPH *(332)*. Briefly, the procedure involved dispersion of drug particles into aqueous surfactant solution under high-speed stirring, followed by passing suspension through high-pressure homogeniser. Due to action of cavitation forces created during homogenisation process, the particles are sheared and size reduces into nanosized particles, and resultant particles are stabilised by associated surfactant by adsorption. The size of nanosuspensions mainly depends on homogenisation pressure and number of homogenisation cycles employed. Typically, homogenisation pressure of around 1000–1500 bar, for 3–20 homogenisation

Table 3. Grinding Media Generally Used for Nanoparticle Production

Material	*Size range available*	*Specific gravity*	*Hardness*
Zirconium silicate	0.1–2.0 mm	3.85	MOHS 7
High-purity zirconium oxide (Y203 stabilised)	0.7–1.7 mm 2–25 mm	6	Hv 1280 kg/mm^2
Alumina	2–15 mm	3.4–3.9	Hv 1350 kg/mm^2
Silicon nitride kg/mm^2	2–12 m	3.2	Hv 1400–1500
Mullite	1/16, 1/8 in.	2.8	ROCKWELL 45N 70
Zirconium oxide (rare earth-stabilised)	0.4–2.4 mm	6.1	Hv 1100 kg/mm^2
Tungsten carbide	3/16, 1/4 in.	14.4–14.8	88–89 HRA
Ceramic (steatite)	1/8, 1/4 in.	2.6–2.7	ROCKWELL 45N 60–65
Chrome steel (SAE 52100)	1/8–1/2 in.	7.8	ROCKWELL C 62–66
Glass beads	0.4–11.5 mm	2.5	KNOOP 515 kg/mm^2
Silicon carbide	1/8, 3/16, 1/4 in.	3.1	KNOOP 2800 kg/mm^2
Zirconium oxide (MgO stabilised)	1/4, 3/8, 1/2 in.	5.4	Hv 900–1000 kg/mm^2
Stainless steel (AISI 440-C)	1/8–3/4 in.	7.7	ROCKWELL C 55–64
Carbon steel (SAE 1013—case-hardened, SAE 1065—through-hardened)	1/8–1/2 in.	7.8	ROCKWELL C 60–62

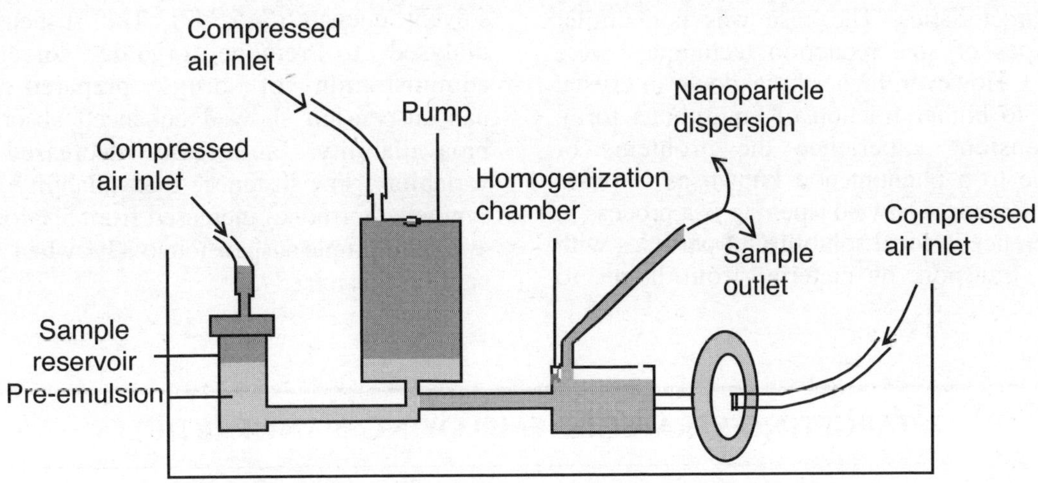

Fig. 5. Representative diagram of high-pressure homogeniser.

cycles, are sufficient to obtain nanosuspensions. This technique was successfully employed to obtain nanosuspensions of various drugs such as budesonide, paclitaxel, clofazimine *(333)*, amphotericin B *(334)*, omeprazole *(335)*, nifedipine *(336)*, spironolactone *(337)*, etc. The solid composition used for processing was up to 10% for i.v. use, and up to 20–40% for other applications.

An interesting feature of nanosuspensions is increase in saturation solubility, and hence the dissolution rate due to increased surface area. Employment of high homogenisation pressures may possibly cause degradation of labile drugs. Initially, the homogenisation technique employed water as a medium for homogenisation process. Later, non-aqueous media (containing PEG or glycerol) along with water was also tried for preparations (isotonic) for i.v. use *(338)*. This technique also resulted in low product contamination *(339)*. In nanopure technology (Pharmasol®), drug suspensions were homogenised in propylene glycol either at room temperature, at 0 or –20°C. For instance, the drug azodicarbonamide underwent degradation when homogenised at room temperature. The degradation was controlled when drug suspension was homogenised at 0°C *(338)*. Another interesting approach was the co-homogenisation of drugs with solid PEG where the drugs were dispersed in solid PEG and homogenised into fine powder and filled in gelatin capsules *(339)*. Drugs such as ibuprofen possessing low melting point was also successfully converted into nanosuspension using homogenisation technique *(340)*. The obtained nanosuspension was further sprayed onto diluents like lactose and microcrystalline cellulose to obtain granules, which exhibited greater dissolution, compared with micronised ibuprofen or its suspension in poloxamer 188 solution.

HPH technique results in break down of crystal structure of crystalline drug substances, and convert them into amorphous form with improvement in dissolution characteristics. The case was not similar when other types of size reduction techniques were employed *(341)*. However, higher breakdown in crystal structure leads to higher fraction of amorphous form; the nanosuspensions experience the problems of aggregation due to a phenomenon known as Ostwald ripening. By definition, Ostwald ripening is a process in which the difference in local solubility of particles with size, facilitate transport of material from larger to smaller particles, and as a consequence results in increase in mean particle size with time *(342)*. Ostwald ripening is a considerable problem resulting in instability of nanosuspensions upon storage. Primarily, the inhibition of Ostwald ripening was demonstrated in O/W emulsions by incorporation of small amount of another component with low aqueous solubility (inhibitor). This leads to a difference in composition between smaller and larger particles during Ostwald ripening, which counterbalance responsible driving force, and consequent termination of process *(343)*. Most recently, Lindfors and co-workers showed that inhibition of Ostwald ripening is possible only when drug and inhibitor (low soluble component) form a homogeneous composite mixture in amorphous particles, and is not inhibited otherwise *(344)*. Also due to large surface area of particles in nanosuspension, they possess adhesion property, which was taken advantage of by enhancing oral absorption of drugs *(345)*. Sterilisation of nanosuspensions is in fact an issue in large-scale operations. Thermal sterilisation of poloxamer 188-stabilised nanosuspension led to aggregation *(345)*. The most appropriate way likely to carry out entire nanosuspension production is under asceptic operation.

6.1.2.1. Desolvation by Particle Precipitation in Aqueous Surfactant Medium

This technique involves dissolution of drug in a water miscible organic solvent, followed by particle precipitation in aqueous surfactant medium after a solvent quench *(346,347)*. The suspension was then dialysed to remove organic solvent. The oral administration of drugs prepared in form of nanosuspension showed enhanced absorption rate and bioavailability, and also decreased inter-patient variability. For instance, bioavailability of Danazol (a synthetic hormone) increased from 5% for commercially available simple suspension to 82% when administered as nanosuspension *(348)*.

7. TARGETING STRATEGIES EMPLOYING NANOPARTICLES

Drug targeting strategies can be classified into two categories, passive and active targeting. Passive targeting involves drug targeting due to physicochemical or pharmacological factors *(349)*. The physiochemical factors including particle size and charge may facilitate the nanoparticle targeting. The nanoparticles due to their colloidal size were able to penetrate arterial capillaries through disrupted epithelium and deliver the drug dexamethasone for prolonged periods in case of angioplasty *(350)*. In case of passive targeting involving pharmacological factors, the pathophysiological conditions such as inflammation of tissues and thereby increased permeability facilitated the nanoparticle targeting *(351)*. Another important case of passive targeting is enhanced accumulation of nanoparticulate systems in tumours by enhanced permeability and retention effect, due to high angiogenesis and increase in tumour vascular permeability *(352)*. Small-sized nanoparticles (<100 nm) can effectively penetrate into liver and can be potential in delivering drugs to macrophages and also to liver for disease therapy. For instance, such nanoparticles were able to efficiently deliver and improve therapeutic index of anti-leishmanial drugs *(353)*. On the other hand, PACA nanoparticles were shown to be effective in delivering sanquinavir (an anti-HIV drug) to HIV-infected human macrophage culture *(143)*. Also, PACA nanoparticles enhanced the efficiency of incorporated doxorubicin in treatment of M5076 murine hepatic tumour metastasis in mice after i.v. injection *(116)*. Though the passive targeting resulted in improvement in drug delivery, the strategy has limited applications.

Active targeting strategy involves surface modification of nanoparticles or conjugating with targeting ligands to facilitate targeting to specific organs of interest. For various applications in disease therapy, the surface of nanoparticles needs to be hydrophilic and able to prevent protein adsorption. Surface modification of nanoparticles helps to create hydrophilic surface, impede opsonisation and aids in prolonged circulation in blood *(354)*. Surface modified nanoparticles with long circulation time have several advantages such as increase in half-life of incorporated active agent, enhancement of delivery of incorporated anti-cancer agents to tumour sites and facilitates greater destruction of tumour cells. Surface modification of nanoparticles was achieved by variety of means, such as physical adsorption and chemical conjugation of surface modifying materials. Recently, a simple method of preparation of surface-modified tamoxifen-loaded poly(ε-caprolactone) nanoparticles by physical adsorption using a triblock co-polymer, Pluronic (PEO-PPO-PEO), has been reported by Shenoy and Amiji *(355)*. These surface-modified nanoparticles showed enhanced blood circulation time and tumour reach. Surface modification has been successfully performed by conjugation with PEG and the process is termed as PEGylation *(356)*. Taking advantage of properties of PEGylation, the nanoparticles have been successfully delivered to tumour regions with increased vascular permeability. As an alternative to PEGylation, surface modification of nanoparticles by polysaccharide coating has been attempted. Biomaterials such as dextran *(357)*, heparin *(358)*, hyaluronic acid *(359)*, chitosan *(360,361)*, etc. were used as polysaccharides for surface coating of nanoparticles. On the other hand, the polysaccharides possess various advantages including tissue targeting. For instance, several mucosal surfaces such as nasal, pulmonary and peroral mucosae are good targets for polysaccharide recognition *(362–364)*. The polysaccharide-coated nanoparticles also showed low macrophage uptake *(365)* and increased half-life of incorporated drugs *(366)*. The polysaccharide-bearing multi-layered nanoparticles were used as carriers for DNA *(367)* and ODN *(368)*. Dextran-coated nanoparticles allowed tissue-specific targeting, such as for lymph nodes and brain tumours *(369)*.

Conjugation of nanoparticles with tissue-directing ligands facilitated targeting to different sites. Various specific cell surface receptors including folate (FOL) receptors, transferrin receptors, low-density lipoprotein receptors, peptide receptors and also surface antigens were targeted by conjugating the nanoparticles with targeting ligands. Targeting to FOL and transferrin receptors was applied especially in cancer therapy. Most successful strategy was conjugation and delivery of nanoparticles with FOL moiety through FOL receptor over-expressed by cancer cells. FOL-binding protein, a glycosylphosphatidylinositol-anchored cell surface receptor for FOL is over-expressed in several human tumours including ovarian and breast cancers, while it has a limited expression in normal tissues *(370)*. The interaction of FOL moiety with FOL receptor on cancer cells leads to endocytic transport of delivery system through various cell organelles involved in endocytic trafficking, and results in cytosolic accumulation *(371)*. FOL receptor-mediated targeting was acheived by surface modification of PLGA nanoparticles with a diblock co-polymer conjugate PLL-PEG-FOL *(372)*. The surface-modified nanoparticles showed low internalisation in A549 (human lung carcinoma) cells, which are FOL receptor-deficient, and higher cell internalisation in KB (human epidermal carcinoma) cells, which are FOL receptor positive. On similar lines, the nanoaggregates of doxorubicin–PEG–FOL nanoparticles showed greater internalisation in KB cells compared with A549 cells *(373)*. The FOL-conjugated shell cross-linked nanoparticles prepared from amphiphilic diblock co-polymers were able to passively accumulate in tumours when injected intravenously into athymic mice-bearing KB tumour cell xenografts, suggesting their interaction with FOL receptors *(374)*.

Transferrin receptors are generally found on cell surface, but are over-expressed by proliferating malignant cells. These receptors are potential sites for delivering several anti-cancer agents, proteins and genes *(375)* Taking advantage of over-expression of transferrin receptors on actively proliferating tumour cells, anticancer agents can be selectively delivered at higher concentrations to cancer cells. Transferrin conjugation can also overcome drug resistance caused by MDR proteins and P-gp *(376)*. Especially, the PLGA and PACA nanoparticles showed improved efficacy of incorporated drugs after transferrin conjugation. Transferrin-conjugated PLGA nanoparticles loaded with paclitaxel showed greater cytotoxicity in human prostate cancer cells, as well as tumour inhibition and regression in human prostate cancer mice model, compared with free drug *(377)*. These nanoparticles also resulted in greater toxicity in MCF-7 breast cancer cells *(378)*. Enhanced anti-tumour effect was also found with PEG-polyhexadecyl cyanoacrylate nanoparticles loaded with paclitaxel after i.v. injection in S-180 solid tumour-bearing mice. The transferrin-conjugated nanoparticles significantly increased life span of tumour-bearing mice compared with unconjugated nanoparticles and free drug *(379)*.

Liver possesses two types of receptors: ASGP receptors in hepatocytes and mannose receptors in Kupffer and liver endothelial cells *(380)*. ASGP receptors are potential targets to deliver anticancer drug delivery systems to liver cancer, and conjugates containing sugar moiety were used to target these receptors for treatment of hepatocellular carcinomas *(381)*. Poly(γ-benzyl L-glutamate) and polylactic acid nanoparticles coated with poly(vinylbenzyl lactonamide), a carbohydrate polymer bearing high density β-galactose residues, showed higher penetration into hepatocytes due to ASGP receptor interaction *(382)*. Conjugation of block co-polymer of poly(γ-glutamic acid) and poly(lactide) with galactosamine also showed enhanced cell penetration in HepG2 cells *(383)*. Upon injection into hepatoma-bearing mice, these nanoparticles underwent greater tumour accumulation and enhanced the efficacy of incorporated paclitaxel in tumour treatment *(384)*. Thus, special drug delivery strategies apart from conventional techniques contribute to the enhancement of therapeutic efficacy of incorporated drugs and decrease associated side effects causing an overall improvement of disease therapy.

8. CONCLUSION

Nanoparticles are solid colloidal particles ranging in the size from 10 to 1000 nm possesing matrix structure, which incorporates the pharmacologically active substance and facilitates the controlled release of active agent. They could be used to successfully deliver a wide variety of drugs, proteins, peptides and genes to cells both as non-targeted and targeted forms.

Nanoparticles are prepared from either synthetic or natural macromolecules using two distinct technologies viz; bottom up and top down technology. The bottom up technology adopt methods to aggregate molecules into a particle of nanorange, while top down technology adopts breaking down macro/micro-particles into particles of nanorange.

Pharmaceutical nanoparticles are those where drug is dissolved, entrapped, encapsulated or adsorbed on surface. In recent years, biodegradable polymeric nanoparticles have attracted great attention as potential drug carriers in view of their applications in controlled delivery of drugs, due to their ability of biodegradation and freedom from hastles of retreival from body after drug release.

Polymeric nanoparticles are prepared either by polymerisation of monomers, or from preformed polymers. Polymerisation is brought about by several methods, which are classified in two catagories, dispersion and emulsion polymerisation. Techniques employed to prepare biodegradable polymeric nanoparticles from preformed hydrophobic or hydrophilic polymers such as poly(D,L-lactide) (PLA), poly(D,L-glycolide) (PLG) and poly(D,L-lactide-co-glycolide) (PLGA), chitosan, gelatin, etc. include solvent evaporation, salting out technique, emulsification-solvent diffusion technique, super critical fluid technique and media grinding. Many of these methods are patented and are established as platform technologies by many companies.

Nanoparticles are characterised for various physical, biological and pharmaceutical characteristics. Physical properties demanded for a pharmaceutical nanoparticle are particle diameter, electrical charge (ζ-potential) and physical and pharmaceutical stability. Biological properties like physical stability in blood, non-toxicity, biodegradability, biocompatibility, avoidance of MPS uptake and prolonged blood circulation time. In addition commercial evaluation includes scalable and cost-effective manufacturing process.

Polymeric biodegradable nanoparticles degrade by either bulk degradation or surface erossion. *In vivo* life of biodegradable nanoparticles ranges from few hours to several months and rate of degradation depends on polymer molecular weight, hydrophobicity, pH of media and presence of enzyme and their concentration. Release rate of drugs from these nanoparticles are generally controlled by adjustment of rate of biodegradation of polymer.

In vivo behaviour of nanoparticulates has made it an important system for drug delivery by various routes for different diseases. Applications of nanoparticles therefore range from oral to injectables covering opthalmic, brain delivery, macrophages, tumours, etc. Site specific targeting capacity of nanoparticles is due to its size, charge and sensitivity/stability with controllable degradation rate at varied *in vivo* biological environment like pH, temperature and ionic strength. In addition, low glass transition temperature, near to body temperature of some carriers like lipids have made these lipid nanoparticles more potential for drug delivery into various domains including intracellular space, which are otherwise difficult to access. Careful designing, meticulous control over their characteristics and quality of solid lipid nanoparticles have proved their potential for industrial scale-up and commercialisation as a succ essful drug delivery system. Exhaustive investigations carried out on nanoparticles for intracellular targeting has opened up hope for gene delivery and to design effective formulations for intracellular infections.

Hydrogel nanoparticulate dispersions have shown their potential in using nanoparticles in mucosal and dermal delivery also. With development of pH and thermal sensitivity of specially designed hydogel nanoparticulate dispersions, dosage forms with unique characteristics are being investigated. Work on different hydrogel nanoparticles using polymers like dextran, poly HEMA, PVP, PVA, curdlan, pluronic, etc. has shown the way for effectve delivery of sensitive proteins as therapeutics.

The most important advantage of nanoparticles as a delivery system is its simple method of production with acceptable impurity profile. Some methods worked out like media grinding have shown that pharmaceutical nanoparticlate delivery systems could be manufactured on mass scale under GMP conditions with economic viability also.

REFERENCES

1. **Birrenbach, G. and Speiser, PP.** Polymerized micelles and their use as adjuvants in immunology. *J. Pharm. Sci.* 1976;65:1763–1766.
2. **Rhodes, CT., Wai, K., and Banker, GS.** Molecular scale drug entrapment as a precise method of controlled drug release II. Facilitated drug entrapment to polymeric colloidal dispersions. *J. Pharm. Sci.* 1970;59:1578–1581.
3. **Boylan, JC. and Banker, GS.** Molecular scale drug entrapment as a precise method of controlled drug release IV. Entrapment of anionic drugs by polymer gelation. *J. Pharm. Sci.* 1973;62:1177–1184.
4. **Langer, R.** Biomaterials in drug delivery and tissue engineering: One laboratory's experience. *Acc. Chem. Res.* 2000;33:94.
5. **Lanza, RP., Langer, R., and Chick, WL.** *Principles of tissue engineering*, Academic press, Austin, TX, 1997, 405 pp.
6. **Gilbert, RG.** *Emulsion Polymerization: A mechanistic approach*, Academic Press, London, 1995, 1 pp.
7. **Zambaux, MF., Bonneaux, F., Gref, R., et al.** Influence of experimental parameters on the characteristics of poly(lactic acid) nanoparticles prepared by double emulsion method. *J. Control. Release* 1998;50:31–40.
8. **Sahoo, SK., Panyam, J., Prabha Bovey, FA., et al.** *Emulsion polymerization*, Interscience publishers, New york. 1955, 1 pp.
9. **Ballard, MJ., Napper, DH., and Gilbert, RG.** Kinetics of emulsion polymerization of methyl methacrylate. *J. Polym. Sci.: Polym. Chem. Ed.* 1984;22:3225–3228.
10. **Ljungstedt, I., Ekman, B., and Sjoholm, I.** Detection and separation of lymphocytes with specific surface receptors by using microparticles. *Biochem. L.* 1978;170:161.
11. **Radwan, MA.** Preparation and *in vivo* evaluation of parenteral metoclopramide-loaded poly(alkylcyanoacrylate) nanospheres in rats. *J. Microencapsul.* 2001;18:467–477.
12. **Couvreur, P., Kante, B., Roland, M., Guiot, P., Bauduin, P., and Speiser, P.** Polycyanoacrylate nanocapsules as potential lysosomotropic carriers: preparation, morphological and sorptive properties. *J. Pharm. Pharmacol.* 1979;31:331.
13. **Behan, N., Birkinshaw, C., and Clarke, N.** Poly n-butyl cyanoacrylate nanoparticles: a mechanistic study of polymerization and particle formation. *Biomaterials* 2001;22:1335.
14. **Seijo, B., Fattal, E., Roblot-Treupel, P., and Couvreur, P.** Design of nanoparticles of less than 50 nm diameter: preparation, characterization and drug loading. *Int. J. Pharm.* 1990;62:1.
15. **Reddy, LH. and Murthy, RSR.** Influence of polymerization technique and experimental variables on the particle properties and release kinetics of methotrexate from poly(butylcyanoacrylate) nanoparticles. *Acta Pharm.* 2004;54:103.
16. **Reddy, LH. and Murthy, RSR.** Study of influence of polymerization factors on formation of poly(butyl cyanoacrylate) nanoparticles and *in vitro* drug release kinetics. *Ars. Pharm.* 2004;45:211.

17. **Gurny, R., Peppas, NA., Harrington, DD., and Banker, GS.** Development of biodegradable and injectable lattices for controlled release of potent drugs. *Drug Dev. Ind. Pharm.* 1981;7:1.

18. **Krause, HJ., Schwarz, A., and Rohdewald, P.** Polylactic acid nanoparticles, a colloidal drug delivery for lipophilic drugs. *Int. J. Pharm.* 1985;27:145.

19. **Tabata, Y. and Ikada, Y.** Protein precoating of polylactide microspheres containing a lipophilic immunopotentiator for enhancement of macrophage phagocytosis and activation. *Pharm. Res.* 1989;6:296.

20. **Coffin, MD. and McGinity, JW.** Biodegradable pseudolatexes: Chemical stability of poly(D,L-lactide) and poly(ε-caprolactone) nanoparticles in aqueous media. *Pharm. Res.* 1992;9:200–205.

21. **Sahoo, SK., Panyam, J., Prabha, S., and Labhasetwar, V.** Residual polyvinyl alcohol associated with poly (D, L-lactide-co-glycolide) nanoparticles affects their physical properties and cellular uptake. *J. Control. Release* 2002;82:105–114.

22. **Wehrle, P., Magenheim, B., and Benita, S.** The influence of process parameters on the PLA nanoparticle size distribution evaluated by means of factorial design. *Eur. J. Pharm. Biopharm.* 1995;41:19–26.

23. **Murakami, H., Yoshino, H., Mizobe, M., Kobayashi, M., Takeuchi, H., and Kawashima, Y.** Preparation of poly(D,L-lactide-co-glycolide) latex of surface modifying material by a double coacervation method. *Proc. Intern. Symp. Control. Release Bioact. Mater.* 1996;23:361–362.

24. **Birnbaum, DT., Kosmala, JD., Henthorn, DB., and Peppas, LB.** Controlled release of β-estradiol from PLGA microparticles: The effect of organic phase solvent on encapsulation and release. *J. Control. Release* 2000;65:375–387.

25. **Allemann, E., Gurny, R., and Doelker, E.** Preparation of aqueous polymeric nanodispersions by a reversible salting-out process: influence of process parameters on particle size. *Int. J. Pharm.* 1992;87:247–253.

25a. **Ibrahim, H., Bindschaedler, C., Doelker, E., and Buri, P.** Aqueous nanodispersions prepared by a salting-out process. *Int. J. Pharm.* 1992;87:239–246.

26. **Leroux, JC., De Jaeghere, F., Anner, B., Doelker, E., and Gurny, R.** An investigation on the role of plasma and serum opsonins on the internalization of biodegradable poly(D,L-lactic acid) nanoparticles by human monocytes. *Life Sci.* 1995;57:695–703.

27. **Pathak, P., Meziani, MJ., and Sun, YP.** Supercritical fluid technology for enhanced drug delivery. *Expert Opin. Drug Deliv.* 2005;2:747–761.

28. **Tom, JW. and Debenedetti, PG.** Particle formation with supercritical fluids-a review. *J. Aerosol. Sci.* 1991;22:555–584.

29. **Randolph, TW., Randolph, AD., Mebes, M., and Yeung, S.** Sub-micron-sized biodegradable particles of poly(L-lactic acid) via the gas antisolvent spray precipitation process. *Biotechnol. Prog.* 1993;9:429–435.

30. **Tom, JW., Debenedetti, PG., and Jerome, R.** Precipitation of poly(l-lactic acid) and composite poly(l-lactic acid)–pyrene particles by rapid expansion of supercritical solutions. *J. Supercrit. Fluids* 1994;7:9–29.

31. **Turk, M., Hils, P., Helfgen, B., Schaber, K., Martin, H-J., and Wahl, MA.** Micronization of pharmaceutical substances by the rapid expansion of supercritical solutions (RESS): a promising method to improve bioavailability of poorly soluble pharmaceutical agents. *J. Supercrit. Fluids* 2002;22:75–84.

32. **Mawson, S., Johnston, KP., Combes, JR., and DeSimone, JM.** Formation of poly(1,1,2,2-tetrahydroperfluorodecyl acrylate) submicron fibres and particles from supercritical carbon dioxide solutions. *Macromolecules* 1994;28:3182–3191.

33. **Shekunov, BY., Chattopadhyay, P., Seitzinger, J., and Huff, R.** Nanoparticles of Poorly Water-Soluble Drugs Prepared by Supercritical Fluid Extraction of Emulsions. *Pharm. Res.* 2006;23:196–204.

34. **Martin, TM., Bandi, N., Schulz, R., Roberts, C., and Kompella, UB.** Preparation of Budesonide and Budesonide-PLA microparticles using supercritical fluid precipitation technology. *AAPS Pharm. Sci. Tech.* 2002;3(3), article 18.

35. **Chattopadhyay, P., Huff, R., and Shekunov, BY.** Drug Encapsulation Using Supercritical Fluid Extraction of Emulsions. *J. Pharm. Sci.* 2006;95:667–679.

36. **Fallaouh, NAK., Roblot-Treupel, L., Fessi, H., Devis-saguet, JP., and Puisieux, F.** Development of a new process for the manufacture of polyisobutylcyanoacrylate nanocapsules. *Int. J. Pharm.* 1986;28:125.

37. **Florence, AT., Whateley, TL., and Wood, DA.** Potentially biodegradable microcapsules with poly-2-cyanoacrylate membranes. *J. Pharm. Pharmacol.* 1979;31:422.

38. **Chouinard, F., Kan, FWK., Leroux, J-C., Foucher, C., and Lenaerts, V.** Preparation and purification of polyisohexylcyanoacrylate nanocapsules. *Int. J. Pharm.* 1991;72:211.

39. **Palumbo, M., Russo, A., Cardile, V., et al.** Improved antioxidant effect of idebenone-loaded polyethyl-2-cyanoacrylate nanocapsules tested on human fibroblasts. *Pharm. Res.* 2002;19:71–78.

39a. **Barrett, ER.** Nanosuspensions in drug delivery. *Nat. Rev. Drug Discov.* 2004;3:785–796.

40. **Kreuter, J.** Physicochemical characterization of polyacrylic nanoparticles. *Int. J. Pharm.* 1983;14:43.

41. **Kreuter, J., Mills, SN., Davis, SS., and Wilson, CG.** Polybutyl cyanoacrylate nanoparticles for the delivery of [^{75}SE]norcholesterol. *Int. J. Pharm.* 1983;16:105.

42. **Magenheim, B. and Benita, S.** Nanoparticle characterization: a comprehensive physicochemical approach, *STP Pharm. Sci.* 1991;1:21.

43. **Edstrom, RD., Yang, XR., Lee, G., and Evans, DF.** Viewing molecules with scanning tunneling and atomic force microscopy. *FASEB J.* 1990;4:3144.

44. **Zasadzinski, JA.** Scanning tunneling microscopy with applications to biological surfaces. *Biotechniques* 1989;7:174.

45. **Fuchs, H. and Laschinski, R.** Surface investigations with a combined scanning-electron scanning tunneling microscope. *Scanning* 1990;12:126.

46. **Gedde, UW.** Thermal analysis of polymers. *Drug Dev. Ind. Pharm.* 1990;16:2465.

47. **Muller, RH., Lherm, C., and Herbort, J.** Alkyl cyanoacrylate drug carriers: I. Physicochemical characterization of nanoparticles with different chain length. *Int. J. Pharm.* 1992;84:1.

48. **Kopf, H., Joshi, RK., Solvia, M., and Speiser, P.** Studium der Mizellpolymerisation in Gegenwart niedermolekularer Arzneistoffe. I. Herstellung und Isolierung der Nanopartikel, Restmonomerenbestimmung, physikalischchemische Daten. *Pharm. Ind.* 1976;38:281.

49. **Andreade, JD., Ma, SM., King, RN., and Gregonis, DE.** Contact angles at the solid-water interface. *J. Colloid Interface Sci.* 1979;72:488.

50. **Baszkin, A. and Lyman, DJ.** The interaction of plasma proteins with polymers. I. Relationship between polymer surface energy and protein adsorption/desorption. *J. Biomed. Mater. Res.* 1980;14:393.

51. **Lindsay, RM., Mason, RG., Kim, SW., Andrade, JD., and Hakim, RM.** Bllod surface interactions. *Trans. Am. Soc. Artif. Intern. Organs* 1980;26:603–610.

52. **Andreade, JD., et al.** Surface characterization of poly (hydroxyethyl methacrylate) and related polymers. I. Contact angle methods in water. *J. Polymer Sci. Polymer Symp.* 1979;66:131.

53. **Muller, RH., Lherm, C., and Herbort, J.** In vitro model for the degradation of alkylcyanoacrylate nanoparticles. *Biomaterials* 1990;11:590.

54. **Scherer, D., Robinson, JR., and Kreuter, J.** Influence of enzymes on the stability of polybutylcyanoacrylate nanoparticles *Int. J. Pharm.* 1994;101:165.

55. **Sommerfeld, P., Schroeder, U., and Sabel, BA.** Long-term stability of PBCA nanoparticle suspensions suggests clinical usefulness. *Int. J. Pharm.* 1997;155:201.

56. **Maincent, P., et al.** Disposition kinetics and oral bioavailability of vincamine-loaded polyalkyl cyanoacrylate nanoparticles. *J. Pharm. Sci.* 1986;75:955.

57. **Kreuter, J.** Peroral administration of nanoparticles. *Adv. Drug Deliv. Rev.* 1991;7:71.

58. **Damge, C., Michel, C., Aprahamian, M., and Couvreur, P.** New approach for oral administration of insulin with polyalkylcayanoacrylate nanocapsules as drug carrier *Diabetes* 1988;37:246.

59 **Damge, C., Michel, C., Aprahamian, M., Couvreur, P., and Devissaguet, JP.** Nanocapsules as carriers for oral peptide delivery. *J. Control. Release* 1990;13:233.

60. **Lenaerts, V., Couvreur, P., Christiaens-leyh, D., et al.** Degradation of poly (isobutylcyanoacrylate) nanoparticles. *Biomaterials* 1984;5:65–68.

61. **Washington, C.** Drug release from monodisperse systems. A critical review. *Int. J. Pharm.* 1990;58:1.

62. **Leavy, MV. and Benita, S.** Drug release from submicron O/W emulsion: A new in vitro kinetic evaluation model. *Int. J. Pharm.* 1990;66:29.

63. **Calvo, P., Vila-jato, JL., and Alonso, MJ.** Comparative *in vitro* evaluation of several colloidal systems, nanoparticles, nanocapsules and nanoemulsions as ocular drug carriers. *J. Pharm. Sci.* 1996;85:530.

64. **El-Samaligly, MS., Rohdewald, P., and Mohmoud, HA.** Polyalkyl cyanoacrylate nanocapsules. *J. Pharm. Pharmacol.* 1986;38:216.

65. **LeRay, AM., Vert, AM., Gautier, M., and Benoit, JC.** End chain radiolabeling and in vitro stability studies of radiolabeled poly(hydroxyl) nanoparticles. *J. Pharm. Sci.* 1994;83:845.

66. **Moshfeghi, AA. and Peyman, GA.** Micro- and nanoparticulates. *Adv. Drug Deliv. Rev.* 2005;57:2047–2052.

67. **Geroski, DH. and Edelhauser, HF.** Drug delivery for posterior segment eye disease. *Invest. Ophthalmol. Vis. Sci.* 2000;41:961–964.

68. **Slakter, JS.** Anecortave acetate as monotherapy for treatment of subfoveal neovascularization in age-related macular degeneration: twelve-month clinical outcomes. *Ophthalmology* 2003;110:2372–2383.

69. **Cochereau-Massin, I., Lehoang, P., Lautier-Frau, M., et al.** Efficacy and tolerance of intravitreal ganciclovir in cytomegalovirus retinitis in acquired immune deficiency syndrome. *Ophthalmol* 1991;98:1348–1353.

70. **Heinemann, MH.** Long-term intravitreal ganciclovir therapy for cytomegalovirus retinopathy. *Arch. Ophthalmol.* 1989;107:1767–1772.

71. **Lieberman, RM., Orellana, J., and Melton, RC.** Efficacy of intravitreal foscarnet in a patient with AIDS. *N. Engl. J. Med.* 1994;330:868–869.

72. **Conway, MD., Canakis, C., Livir-Rallatos, C., and Peyman, GA.** Intravitreal triamcinolone acetonide for refractory chronic pseudophakic cystoid macular edema. *J. Cataract Refract. Surg.* 2003;29:27–33.

73. **Scott, IU., Flynn, HF., Jr., and Rosenfeld, PJ.** Intravitreal triamcinolone acetonide for idiopathic cystoid macular edema. *Am. J. Ophthalmol.* 2003;136:737–739.

74. **Spaide, RF., Sorenson, J., and Maranan, L.** Combined photodynamic therapy with verteporfin and intravitreal triamcinolone acetonide for choroidal neovascularization. *Ophthalmol* 2003;110:1517–1525.

75. **Martin, DF., Parks, DJ., Mellow, SD., et al.** Treatment of cytomegalovirus retinitis with an intraocular sustained-release ganciclovir implant. A randomized controlled clinical trial. *Arch. Ophthalmol.* 1994;112:1531–1539.

76. **Duker, JS., Robinson, M., Anand, R., and Ashton, P.** Initial experience with an eight-month sustained-release intravitreal ganciclovir implant for the treatment of CMV retinitis associated with AIDS. *Ophthalmic Surg. Lasers* 1995;26:442–448.

77. **Lim, JI., Wolitz, RA., and Dowling, AH.** Visual and anatomic outcomes associated with posterior segment complications after ganciclovir implant procedures in patients with AIDS and cytomegalovirus retinitis. *Am. J. Ophthalmol.* 1999;127:288–293.

78. **Kompella, UB., Bandi, N., and Ayalasomayajula, SP.** Subconjunctival nano- and microparticles sustain retinal delivery of budesonide, a corticosteroid capable of inhibiting VEGF expression. *Invest. Ophthalmol. Vis. Sci.* 2003;44:1192–1201.

79. **Bourges, JL., Gautier, SE., Delie, F., et al.** Ocular drug delivery targeting the retina and retinal pigment epithelium using polylactide nanoparticles. *Invest. Ophthalmol. Vis. Sci.* 2003;44:3562–3569.

80. **Noble, S. and Markham, A.** Cyclosporin. A review of the pharmacokinetic properties, clinical efficacy and tolerability of a microemulsion-based formulation (Neoral). *Drugs* 1995;50:924–941.

81. **Georganas, C., Ioakimidis, D., Iatrou, C., et al.** Relapsing Wegener's granulomatosis: successful treatment with cyclosporin-A. *Clin. Rheumatol.* 1996;15:189–192.

82. **Prummel, MF., Mourits, MP., Berghout, A., et al.** Prednisone and cyclosporine in the treatment of severe Graves' ophthalmopathy. *N. Engl. J. Med.* 1989;321:1353–1359.

83. **Nussenblatt, RB., Palestine, AG., Chan, CC., Stevens, G., Mellow, SD., and Green, SB.** Randomized, double-masked study of cyclosporine compared to prednisolone in the treatment of endogenous uveitis. *Am. J. Ophthalmol.* 1991;112:138–146.

84. **Masuda, K., Nakajima, A., Urayama, A., Nakae, K., Kogure, M., and Inaba, G.** Double-masked trial of cyclosporin versus colchicine and longterm open study of cyclosporin in Behcet's disease. *Lancet* 1989;1:1093–1096.

85. **Lallemand, F., Felt-Baeyens, O., Besseghir, K., Behar-Cohen, F., and Gurny, R.** Cyclosporine A delivery to the eye: A pharmaceutical challenge. *Eur. J. Pharm. Biopharm.* 2003;56:307–318.

86. **Li, C., Yang, CW., Ahn, HJ., et al.** Colchicine suppresses osteopontin expression and inflammatory cell infiltration in chronic cyclosporine nephrotoxicity. *Nephron* 2002;92:422–430.

87. **Calvo, P., Thomas, C., Alonso, MJ., Vila-Jato, JL., and Robinson, JR.** Study of the mechanism of interaction of poly(E-caprolactone) nanocapsules with the cornea by confocal laser scanning microscopy. *Int. J. Pharm.* 1994;103:283–291.

88. **Calvo, P., Sanchez, A., Martinez, J., et al.** Polyester nanocapsules as new topical ocular delivery systems for cyclosporin A. *Pharm. Res.* 1996;13:311–315.

89. **Juberias, JR., Calonge, M., Gomez, S., et al.** Efficacy of topical cyclosporine-loaded nanocapsules on keratoplasty rejection in the rat. *Curr. Eye Res.* 2002;17:39–46.

90. **Le Bourlais, CA., Chevanne, F., Turlin, B., et al.** Effect of cyclosporine A formulations on bovine corneal absorption: ex-vivo study. *J. Microencapsul.* 1997;14:457–467.

91. **De Campos, AM., Sanchez, A., and Alonso, MJ.** Chitosan nanoparticles: a new vehicle for the improvement of the delivery of drugs to the ocular surface. Application to cyclosporin A. *Int. J. Pharm.* 2001;224:159–168.

92. **Alyautdin, R., Gothier, D., Petrov, V., Kharkevich, D., and Kreuter, J.** Analgesic activity of the hexapeptide dalargin adsorbed on the surface of polysorbate 80-coated poly(butyl cyanoacrylate) nanoparticles. *Eur. J. Pharm. Biopharm.* 1995;41:44–48.

93. **Ramge, P., Kreuter, J., and Lemmer, B.** Circadian phase-dependent antinociceptive reaction in mice after i.v. injection of dalargin-loaded nanoparticles determined by the hot-plate test and the tail-flick test. *Chronobiol. Int.* 1999;17:767–777.

94. **Schroeder, U., Schroeder, H., and Sabel, BA.** Body distribution of ^{3}H-labelled dalargin bound to poly(butyl cyanoacrylate nanoparticles) after i.v. injections to mice. *Life Sci.* 2000;6:495–502.

95. **Schroeder, U., Sommerfeld, P., Ulrich, S., and Sabel, BA.** Nanoparticle technology for delivery of drugs across the blood-brain barrier. *J. Pharm. Sci.* 1998;87:1305–1307.

96. **Alyautdin, RN., Petrov, VE., Langer, K., Berthold, A., Kharkevich, DA., and Kreuter, J.** Delivery of loperamide across the blood–brain barrier with polysorbate 80-coated poly butylcyanoacrylate nanoparticles. *Pharm. Res.* 1997;14:325–328.

97. **Ramge, P., Unger, RE., Oltrogge, JB., Begley, D., von Briesen, H., and Kreuter, J.** Polysorbate 80-coating enhances uptake of polybutylcyanoacrylate (PBCA)-nanoparticles by human, bovine and murine primary brain capilary endothelial cells. *Eur. J. Neuro.* 2000;12:1935–1940.

98. **Kreuter, J.** Nanoparticulate systems for brain delivery of drugs. *Adv. Drug Deliv. Rev.* 2001;47:65–81.

99. **Olivier, J-C.** Drug transport to brain with targeted nanoparticles. *NeuroRx®* 2005;2:108–119.

100. **Allemann, E., Gravel, P., Leroux, JC., Balant, L., and Gurny, R.** Kinetics of blood component adsorption on poly(D,L-lactic acid) nanoparticles: evidence of complement C3 component involvement. *J. Biomed. Mater. Res.* 1997;37:229–234.

101. **Gref, R., Luck, M., Quellec, P., Marchand, M., Dellacherie, E. and Harnisch, S.** "Stealth" corona-core nanoparticles surface modified by polyethylene glycol (PEG): influences of the corona (PEG chain length and surface density) and of the core composition on phagocytic uptake and plasma protein adsorption. *Colloids Surf. B: Biointerfaces* 2000;18:301–313.

102. **Olivier, JC., Fenart, L., Chauvet, R., Pariat, C., Cecchelli, and Couet, W.** Indirect evidence that drug brain targeting using polysorbate 80-coated polybutylcyanoacrylate nanoparticles is related to toxicity. *Pharm. Res.* 1999;16:1836–1842.

103. **Calvo, P., Gouritin, B., Villarroya, H., Eclancher, F., and Giannavola, C., et al.** Quantification and localization of PEGylated polycyanoacrylate nanoparticles in brain and spinal cord during experimental allergic encephalomyelitis in the rat, *Eur. J. Neurosci.* 2002;15:1317.

104. **Brigger, I., Morizet, J., Aubert, G., Chacun, H., Terrier-Lacombe MJ, Couvreur, P., Vassal, G.** Poly(ethylene glycol)-coated hexadecylcyanoacrylate nanospheres display a combined effect for brain tumor targeting. *J. Pharmacol. Exp. Ther.* 2002;303:928–936.

105. **Wilcock, GK., Esiri, MM., Bowen, DM., and Smith, CC.** Alzheimer's disease. Correlation of cortical choline acetyltransferase activity with the severity of dementia and histological abnormalities. *J. Neurol. Sci.* 1982;57:407–417.

106. **Gaffori, OJW. and De Wield, D.** Time-related memory effects of vasopressin analogues in rats. *Pharmacol. Biochem. Behav.* 1986;25:1125–1129.

107. **Xie, Y-L., Lu, W., and Jiang, X-G.** Improvement of cationic albumin conjugated pegylated nanoparticles holding NC-1900, a vasopressin fragment analog, in memory deficits induced by scopolamine in mice. *Behav. Brain Res.* 2006;173(1):76–84.

108. **Feng, SS., Mu, L., Win KY., and Huang, G.** Nanoparticles of biodegradable polymers for clinical administration of paclitaxel. *Curr. Med. Chem.* 2004;11:413–424.

109. **Yoo, HS., Lee, KH., Oh JE., and Park, TG.** In vitro and in vivo anti-tumor activities of nanoparticles based on doxorubicin-PLGA conjugates. *J. Control. Release* 2000;68:419–431.

110. **Chen, J., Ma, A., Lai, Y., Chen Y., and Cui, M.** The mechanism of degradation for the absorbable biomaterials poly(o-caprolactone) *in vitro* and *in vivo*. *J. Biomed. Eng.* 1997;14:334–337.

111. **Kaul, G. and Amiji, M.** Biodistribution and targeting potential of poly(ethylene glycol)-modified gelatin nanoparticles in subcutaneous murine tumor model. *J. Drug Target.* 2004;12:585.

112. **Mitra, S., Gaur, U., Ghosh PC., and Maitra, AN.** Tumour targeted delivery of encapsulated dextran-doxorubicin conjugate using chitosan nanoparticles as carrier. *J. Control. Release* 2001;74:317–323.

113. **Qi, L.F., Xu, Z-R., Li, Y., Jiang X., and Han, X.Y.** *In vitro* effects of chitosan nanoparticles on proliferation of human gastric carcinoma cell line MGC803 cells. *World J. Gastroenterol.* 2005;11:5136–5141.

114. **Cuvier, C., Roblot-Treupel, L., Millot, JM., et al.** Doxorubicin-loaded nanospheres bypass tumor cell multidrug resistance, *Biochem. Pharmacol.* 1992;44:509–517.

115. **Vauthier, C., Dubernet, C., Fattal, E., Pinto-Alphandary, H., and Couvreur, P.** Poly(alkylcyanoacrylates) as biodegradable materials for biomedical applications, *Adv. Drug Deliv. Rev.* 2003;55:519–548.

116. **Chiannilkulchai, N., Driouich, Z., Benoit, JP., Parodi, AL., and Couvreur, P.** Doxorubicin-loaded nanoparticles: increased efficacy in murine hepatic metastases, *Sel. Cancer Ther.* 1989;5:1–11.

117. **Hu, Y-P., Jarillon, S., Dubernet, C., Couvreur, P., and Robert, J.** On the mechanism of action of doxorubicin encapsulation in nanospheres for the reversal of multidrug resistance, Cancer Chemother. *Pharmacol.* 1996;37:556–560.

118. **Vauthier, C., Dubernet, C., Chauvierre, C., Brigger, I., and Couvreur, P.** Drug delivery to resistant tumors: the potential of polyalkyl cyanoacrylate nanoparticles. *J. Control. Release* 2003;93:151–160.

119. **Aouali, N., Morjani, H., Trussardi, A., Soma, E., Giroux, B., and Manfait, M.** Enhanced cytotoxicity and nuclear accumulation of doxorubicin-loaded nanospheres in human breast cancer MCF7 cells expressing MRP1, *Int. J. Oncol.* 2003;23:1195–1201.

120. **Reddy LH., Sharma, RK., and Murthy RSR.** Enhanced tumour uptake of doxorubicin loaded poly(butyl cyanoacrylate) nanoparticles in mice bearing Dalton's lymphoma tumour. *J. Drug Target.* 2004;12:443–451.

121. **Gao, H., Wang, JY., Shen, XY., Deng, YH., and Zhang, W.** Preparation of magnetic polybutyl cyanoacrylate nanospheres encapsulated with aclacinomycin A and its effect on gastric tumor, *World J. Gastroenterol.* 2004;10:2010–2013.

122. **Reddy, LH., Sharma, RK., Chuttani, K., Mishra, AK., and Murthy RSR.** Influence of administration route on tumor uptake and biodistribution of etoposide loaded solid lipid nanoparticles in Dalton's lymphoma tumor bearing mice. *J. Control. Release* 2005;105:185–198.

123. **Reddy, LH., Adhikari, JS., Dwarakanath, BS., Sharma RK., and Murthy RSR.** Tumoricidal effects of etoposide incorporated into solid lipid nanoparticles after intraperitoneal administration in Dalton's lymphoma bearing mice. *AAPS J.* 2006;8(2):Article 29.

124. **Schafer, FQ. and Buettner, GR.** Redox environment of the cell as viewed through the redox state of the glutathione disulfide/glutathione couple. *Free Radic. Biol. Med.* 2001;30:1191–1212.

125. **Kommareddy, S. and Amiji, M.** Preparation and Evaluation of Thiol-Modified Gelatin Nanoparticles for Intracellular DNA Delivery in Response to Glutathione. *Bioconjug. Chem.* 2005;16:1423–1432.

126. **East, L. and Isacke, CM.** The mannose receptor family. *Biochem. Biophys. Acta* 2002;1572:364–386.

127. **Kolb-Bachofen, V. and Abel, F.** Participation of D-galactose-specific receptors of liver macrophages in recognition of fibronectin opsonized particles. *Carbohydr. Res.* 1991;213:201–213.

128. **Kobzik, L.** Lung macrophage uptake of unopsonized environmental particulates. Role of scavenger type receptors. *J. Immunol.* 1995;155:367–376.

129. **Warr, GA.** A macrophage receptor for (mannose/glucosamine)-glycoproteins of potential importance in phagocytic acticity. *Biochem. Biophys. Res. Commun.* 1980;93:737–745.

130. **Camner, P., Lundborg, M., Lastbom, L., Gerde, P., Gross, N., and Jarstrand, C.** Experimental and calculated parameters on particle phagocytosis by alveolar macrophages. *J. Appl. Physiol.* 2002;92:2608–2616.

131. **Roseman, S.** The synthesis of complex carbohydrates by multiglycosyltrandferase systems and their potential function in intercellular adhesion. *Chem. Phys. Lipids* 1970;5:270–297.

132. **Chellat, F., Merhi, Y., Moreau, A., and Yahia L.** Therapeutic potential of nanoparticulate systems for macrophage targeting. *Biomaterials* 2005;26:7260–7275.

133. **Roser, M., Fischer, D., and Kissel, T.** Surface-modified biodegradable albumin nano- and microspheres. II: effect of surface charges on in vitro phagocytosis and Biodistribution in rats. *Eur. J. Pharm. Biopharm.* 1998;46:255–263.

134. **Espuelas, MS., Legrand, P., Loiseau, PM., Bories, C., Barrat, G., and Irache, JM.** In vitro antileishmanial activity of amphotericin B loaded in poly(epsilon-caprolactone) nanospheres. *J. Drug Target.* 2002;10:593–599.

135. **Sarkar, S., Mandal, S., Sinha, J., Mukhopadhyay, S., Das, N., and Basu, MK.** Quercetin: critical evaluation as an antileishmanial agent *in vivo* in hamsters using different vesicular delivery modes. *J. Drug Target.* 2002;10:573–578.

136. **Rodrigues, JM., Jr., Croft, SL., Fessi, H., Bories, C., and Devissaguet, JP.** The activity and ultrastructural localization of primaquine-loaded poly(D,L-lactide) nanoparticles in *Leishmania Donovani* infected mice. *Trop. Med. Parasitol.* 1994;45:223–228.

137. **Skidan, IN., Gelperina, SE., Severin, SE., and Guliaev, AE.** Enhanced activity of rifampicin loaded with polybutyl cyanoacrylate nanoparticles in relation to intracellularly localized bacteria. *Antibiot. Khimioter.* 2003;48:23–26.

138. **Forestier, F., Gerrier, P., Chaumard, C., Quero, AM., Couvreur, P., and Labarre, D.** Effect of nanoparticle bound ampicillin on the survival of listeria monocytogenes in mouse peritoneal macrophages. *J. Antimicrob. Chemother*. 1992;30:173–179.

139. **Balland, O., Pinto-Alphandry, H., Viron, A., Puvion, E., Andremont, A., and Couvreur, P.** Intracellular distribution of ampicillin in murine macrophages infected with salmonella typhimurium and treated with (^{3}H) ampicillin-loaded nanoparticles. *J. Antimicrob. Chemother.* 1996;37:105–115.

140. **Hillaireau, H., Le Doan, T., and Couvreur, P.** Polymer-based nanoparticles for the delivery of nucleoside analogues. *J. Nanosci. Nanotechnol.* 2006;6:1–10.

141. **Bender, A., Schfer, V., Steffan, AM., et al.** Inhibition of HIV in vitro by antiviral drug-targeting using nanoparticles. *Res. Virol.* 1994;145:215–220.

142. **Lobenberg, R., Araujo, L., von Briesen, H., Rodgers, E., and Kreuter, J.** Bosy distribution of azidothymidine bound to hexyl-cyanoacrylate nanoparticles after i.v. injection to rats. *J. Control. Release* 1998;50:21–30.

143. **Bender, AR., von Briesen, H., Kreuter, J., Duncan, IB., and Rubsamen-Waigmann, H.** Efficiency of nanoparticles as a carrier system for antiviral agents in human immunodeficiency virus-infected human monocytes/macrophages *in vitro. Antimicrob. Agents Chemother.* 1996;40:1467–1471.

144. **Hsu, CH., Cui, Z., Mumper, RJ., and Jay, M.** Preparation and characterization of novel coenzyme Q10 nanoparticles engineered from microemulsion precursors. *AAPA Pharm. Sci. Tech.* 2003;4:E32.

145. **Feldmann M.** Development of anti-TNF therapy for rheumatoid arthritis. *Nat. Rev. Immunol.* 2002;2:364–371.

146. **Taylor, MF., Paulauskis, JD., Weller, DD., and Kobzik, L.** *In vitro* efficacy of morpholino-modified antisense oligomers directed against tumor necrosis factor-αmRNA. *J. Biol. Chem.* 1996;271:17,445–17,452.

147. **Lambert, G., Fattal, E., Brehier, A., Feger, J., and Couvreur, P.** Effects of polyisobutyl cyanoacrylate nanoparticles and lipofectin loaded with oligonucleotides on cell viability and PKC alpha neosynthesis in HepG2 cells. *Biochimie* 1998;80:969–976.

148. **Berton, M., Allemann, E., Stein, CA., and Gurny, R.** Highly loaded nanoparticulate carrier using an hydrophobic antisense oligonucleotide complex. *Eur. J. Pharm. Sci.* 1999;9:163–170.

149. **Ahlin, P., Kristl, J., and Smid-Kobar, J.** Optimization of procedure parameters and physical stability of solid lipid nanoparticles in dispersions. *Acta Pharm.* 1998;48:257–267.

150. **Sjostrom, B. and Bergenstahl, B.** Preparation of submicron drug particles in lecithin-stabilized o/w emulsions. I. Model studies of the precipitation of cholesteryl acetate. *Int. J. Pharm.* 1992;88:53–62.

151. **Siekmann, B. and Westesen, K.** Investigations of solid lipid nanoparticles prepared by precipitation in o/w emulsions. *Eur. J. Pharm. Biopharm.* 1996;43:104–109.

152. **Schubert, MA. and Muller-Goymann, CC.** Solvent injection as a new approach for manufacturing lipid nanoparticles—evaluation of the method and process parameters. *Eur. J. Pharm. Biopharm.* 2003;55:125–131.

153. **Trotta, M., Debernardi, F., and Caputo, O.** Preparation of solid lipid nanoparticles by a solvent emulsification-diffusion technique. *Int. J. Pharm.* 2003;257:153–160.

154. **Gasco, MR.** Solid lipid nanospheres from warm micro-emulsions. *Pharm. Technol. Eur.* 1997;9:52–58.

155. **Boltri, L., Canal, T., Esposito, PA., and Carli, F.** Lipid nanoparticles: evaluation of critical formulation parameters. *Proc. Int. Symp. Control. Release Bioact. Mater.* 1993;20:346–347.

156. **Dingler, A. and Gohla, S.** Production of solid lipid nanoparticles (SLN): scaling up feasibilities. *J. Microencapsul.* 2002;19:11–16.

157. **Lippacher, A., Muller, RH., and Mader, K.** Investigation on the viscoelastic properties of lipid based colloidal drug carriers. *Int. J. Pharm.* 2000;196:227–230.

158. **Zur Muhlen, A. and Mehnert, W.** Drug release and release mechanism of prednisolone loaded solid lipid nanoparticles. *Pharmazie* 1998;53:552–555.

159. **Zur Muhlen, A., Schwarz, C., and Mehnert, W.** Solid lipid nanoparticles (SLN) for controlled drug delivery—drug release and release mechanism. *Eur. J. Pharm. Biopharm.* 1998;45:149–155.

160. **Lander, R., Manger, W., Scouloudis, M., Ku, A., Davis, C., and Lee, A.** Gaulin homogenization: a mechanistic study. *Biotechnol. Prog.* 2000;16:80–85.

161. **Bunjes, H., Siekmann, B., and Westesen, K.** Emulsions of supercooled melts—a novel drug delivery system. *Submicron emulsions in drug targeting and delivery*, (Benita, S., ed.), Harwood Academic Publishers, Amsterdam, 1998, pp. 175–204.

162. **Mehnert, W. and Mader, K.** Solid lipid nanoparticles: Production, characterization and applications. *Adv. Drug. Deliv. Rev.* 2001;47:165–196.

163. **Kim, BD., Na, K., and Choi HK.** Preparation and characterization of solid lipid nanoparticles (SLN) made of cocoa butter and curdlan. *Eur. J. Pharm. Sci.* 2005;24:199–205.

164. **Muller, RH., Radtke, M., and Wissing, SA.** Nanostructured lipid matrices for improved microencapsulation of drugs. *Int. J. Pharm.* 2002;242:121–128.

165. **Souto, EB., Wissing, SA., Barbosa, CM., and Müller, RH.** Development of a controlled release formulation based on SLN and NLC for topical clotrimazole delivery. *Int. J. Pharm.* 2004;278:71–77.

166. **Souto, EB. and Muller, RH.** The use of SLN and NLC as topical particulate carriers for imidazole antifungal agents. *Pharmazie* 2006;61:431–437.

167. **Kuntsche, J., Westesen, K., Drechsler, M., Koch, MHJ., and Bunjes, H.** Supercooled Smectic Nanoparticles: A Potential

Novel Carrier System for Poorly Water Soluble Drugs. *Pharm. Res.* 2004;21:1834–1843.

168. **Crowe, LM., Womersley, C., Crowe, JH., Reid, D., Appel, L., and Rudolph, A.** Prevention of fusion and leakage in freeze-dried liposomes by carbohydrates. *Biochim. Biophys. Acta* 1986;861:131–140.

169. **Madden, T., Bally, M., Hope, M., Cullis, P., Schieren, H., and Janoff, A.** Protection of large unilamellar vesicles by trehalose during dehydration: retention of vesicle contents. *Biochim. Biophys. Acta* 1985;817:67–74.

170. **Mobley, WC. and Schreier, H.** Phase transition temperature reduction and glass transformation in dehydroprotected lyophilized liposomes. *J. Control. Release* 1994;31:73–87.

171. **Schwarz, C. and Mehnert, W.** Freeze-drying of drug-free and drug-loaded nanoparticles. *Int. J. Pharm.* 1997;157:171–179.

172. **Siekmann, B. and Westesen, K.** Melt-homogenized solid lipid nanoparticles stabilized by the nonionic surfactant tyloxapol. II. Physicochemical characterization and lyophilization. *Pharm. Pharmacol. Lett.* 1994;3:225–228.

173. **Cavalli, R., Caputo, O., Carlotti, ME., Trotta, M., Scarnecchia, C., and Gasco, MR.** Sterilization and freeze-drying of drug-free and drug-loaded solid lipid nanoparticles. *Int. J. Pharm.* 1997;148:47–54.

174. **Freitas, C. and Muller, RH.** Spray-drying of solid lipid nanoparticles (SLN™). *Eur. J. Pharm. Biopharm.* 1998;46:145–151.

175. **Reddy, LH. and Murthy RSR.** Etoposide-loaded nanoparticles made from glyceride lipids: formulation, characterization, in vitro drug release, and stability evaluation. *AAPS Pharm. Sci. Tech.* 2005;6(2):Article 24.

176. **Bunjes, H., Koch, MHJ., and Westesen, K.** Effect of particle size on colloidal solid triglycerides. *Langmuir* 2000;16:5234–5241.

177. **Westesen, K. and Bunjes, H.** Do nanoparticles prepared from lipids solid at room temperature always possess a solid lipid matrix. *Int. J. Pharm.* 1995;115:129–131.

178. **Siekmann, B. and Westesen, K.** Submicron-sized parenteral carrier systems based on solid lipids. *Pharm. Pharmacol. Lett.* 1992;1:123–126.

179. **Bunjes, H., Drechsler, M., Koch, MHJ., and Westesen, K.** Phase separation within solid lipid nanoparticles loaded with high amounts of Ubidecarenone (Q10). *Proc. Int. Symp. Control. Release Bioact. Mater.* CRS Press, Paris, 2000, p 27.

180. **Freitas, C. and Muller, RH.** Effect of light and temperature on zeta potential and physical stability in solid lipid nanoparticles (SLN) dispersions. *Int. J. Pharm.* 1998;168:221–229.

181. **Sato, K. and Garti, N.** Crystallization and polymorphism in fats and fatty acids, (Garti, N. and Sato, K., eds.), Marcel Dekker, New York, 1988, pp. 3–87.

182. **Eldem, T., Speiser, P., and Altorfer, H.** Polymorphic behavior of sprayed lipid micropellets and its evaluation by differential scanning calorimetry and scanning electron microscopy. *Pharm. Res.* 1991;8:178–184.

183. **Lukowski, G., Kasbohm, J., Pflegel, P., Illing, A., and Wulff, H.** Crystallographic investigation of cetyl palmitate solid lipid nanoparticles. *Int. J. Pharm.* 2000;196:201–205.

184. **Jenning, V., Schafer-Korting, M., and Gohla, S.** Vitamin A-loaded solid lipid nanoparticles for topical use: drug release properties. *J. Control. Release* 2000;66:115–126.

185. **Westesen, K. and Siekmann, B.** Investigation of the gel formation of phospholipid-stabilized solid lipid nanoparticles. *Int. J. Pharm.* 1997;151:35–45.

186. **Heurtault, B., Saulnier, P., Pech, B., Proust, J-E., and Benoit, J-P.** Physico-chemical stability of colloidal lipid particles. *Biomaterials* 2003;24:4283–4300.

187. **Siekmann, B. and Westesen, K.** Melt-homogenized solid lipid nanoparticles stabilized by the nonionic surfactant tyloxapol. I. Preparation and particle size determination. *Pharm. Pharmacol. Lett.* 1994;3:194–197.

188. **Westesen, B. and Siekmann, K.** Investigations on the physical state of lipid nanoparticles by synchrotron radiation X-ray diffraction. *Int. J. Pharm.* 1993;93:189–199.

189. **Shahgaldian, P., Quattrocchi, L., Gualbert, J., Coleman, AW., and Goreloff, P.** AFM imaging of calixarene based solid lipid nanoparticles in gel matrices. *Eur. J. Pharm. Biopharm.* 2003;55:107–113.

190. **Crommelin, JA. and Schreier, H. Liposomes.** *Colloidal drug delivery systems*, (Kreuter, J., ed.), Marcel Dekker, New York, 1994, pp. 73–190.

191. **Schwarz, C., Mehnert, W., Lucks, JS., and Muller, RH.** Solid lipid nanoparticles (SLN) for controlled drug delivery. I. Production, characterization and sterilization. *J. Control. Release* 1994;30:83–96.

192. **Heitati, H., Tawashi, R., and Phillips, NC.** Drug retention and stability of solid lipid nanoparticles containing azidothymidine palmitate after autoclaving, storage and lyophilization. *J. Microencapsul.* 1998;15:173–184.

193. **Zimmerman, E. and Muller, RH.** Electrolyte- and pH-stabilities of aqueous solid lipid nanoparticle (SLN) dispersions in artificial gastrointestinal media. *Eur. J. Pharm. Biopharm.* 2001;52:203–210.

194. **Reddy, LH., Vivek, K., Bakshi, N., and Murthy RSR.** Tamoxifen citrate loaded solid lipid nanoparticles (SLN): preparation, characterization, in vitro drug release, and pharmacokinetic evaluation. *Pharm. Dev. Technol.* 2006;11:167–177.

195. **Yang, SC., Lu, LF., Cai, Y., Zhu, JB., Liang, BW., and Yang, CZ.** Body distribution in mice of intravenously injected camptothecin solid lipid nanoparticles and targeting effect on brain. *J. Control. Release* 1999;59:299–307.

196. **Hu, FQ., Yuan, H., Zhang, HH., and Fang, M.** Preparation of solid lipid nanoparticles with clobetasol propionate by a solvent diffusion method in aqueous system and physicochemical characterization. *Int. J. Pharm.* 2002;239:121–128.

197. **Fundaro, A., Cavalli, R., Bargonic, A., Vighettob, D., Zara GP., and Gasco, MR.** Non-stealth and stealth solid lipid nanoparticles (SLN) carrying doxorubicin: pharmacokinetics and tissue distribution after i.v. administration to rats. *Pharmacol. Res.* 2000;42:338–343.

198. **Ding JC., Hu, FQ., and Yuan H.** Uptake of monostearin solid lipid nanoparticles by A549 cells. *Yao Xue Xue Bao* 2004;39:876–880.

199. **Muller, RH. and Olbrich, C.** Solid lipid nanoparticles: Phagocytic uptake, *in vitro* cytotoxicity and *in vitro* biodegradation. *Drugs Made Ger.* 1999;42:49–53.

200. **Muller, RH., Maaben, SA., Weyhers, H., Specht, F., and Lucks, JS.** Cytotoxicity of magnetite loaded polylactide, polylactide/glycolide particles and solid lipid nanoparticles (SLN). *Int. J. Pharm.* 1996;138:85–94.

201. **Scholer, N., Hahn, H., Muller, RH., and Lissenfeld, O.** Effect of lipid matrix and size on solid lipid nanoparticles (SLN) on the viability and cytokine production of macrophages. *Int. J. Pharm.* 2002;231:167–176.

202. **Heydenreich, AV., Westmeier, R., Pedersen, N., Poulsen, HS., and Kristensen, HG.** Preparation and purification of cationic solid lipid nanospheres-effects on particle size, physical stability and cell toxicity. *Int. J. Pharm.* 2003;254:83–87.

203. **Zara, GP., Cavalli, R., Fundaro, A., Bargoni, A., Caputo O., and Gasco, MR.** Pharmacokinetics of doxorubicin incorporated in solid lipid nanospheres (SLN). *Pharmacol. Res.* 1999;40:281–286.

204. **Reddy, LH., Sharma, RK., Chuttani, K., Mishra AK., and Murthy RSR.** Etoposide-incorporated tripalmitin nanoparticles with different surface charge: formulation, characterization, radiolabeling, and biodistribution studies. *AAPS* 2004, 6 (3), Article 23.

205. **Sznitowska, M., Gajewska, M., Janicki, S., Radwanska, A., and Lukowski, G.** Bioavailability of diazepam from aqueous-organic solution, submicron emulsion and solid lipid nanoparticles after rectal administration in rabbits. *Eur. J. Pharm. Biopharm.* 2001;52:159–163.

206. **Zhang, Q., Yie, G., Li, Y., Yang, Q., and Nagai, T.** Studies on the cyclosporin A loaded stearic acid nanoparticles. *Int. J. Pharm.* 2000;200:153–159.

207. **Muller, RH., Runge, S., Ravelli, V., Mehnert, W., Thunemann, AF., and Souto, EB.** Oral bioavailability of cyclosporine: Solid lipid nanoparticles (SLN®) versus drug nanocrystals. *Int. J. Pharm.* 2006;317:82–89.

208. **Zara, GP., Bargoni, A., Cavalli, R., Fundaro A., and Vighetto, D.** Pharmacokinetics and tissue distribution of idarubicin-loaded solid lipid nanoparticles after duodenal administration to rats. *J. Pharm. Sci.* 2002;91:1324–1333.

209. **Lockman, PR., Oyewumi, MO., Koziara, JM., Roder, KE., Mumper RJ., and Allen, DD.** Brain uptake of thiamine-coated nanoparticles. *J. Control. Release* 2003;93:271–282.

210. **Luo, Y., Chen, D., Ren, L., Zhao, X., and Qin, J.** Solid lipid nanoparticles for enhancing vinpocetine's oral bioavailability. *J. Control. Release* 2006;114:53–59.

211. **Szakács, T., Veres, Z., and Vereczkey, L.** *In vitro–in vivo* correlation of the pharmacokinetics of vinpocetine. *Pol. J. Pharmacol.* 2001;53:623–628.

212. **Koziara, JM., Lockman, PR., Allen DD., and Mumper, RJ.** Paclitaxel nanoparticles for the potential treatment of brain tumors. *J. Control. Release.* 2004;99:259–269.

213. **Ding, JC., Hu, FQ., and Yuan, H.** Uptake of monostearin solid lipid nanoparticles by A549 cells *Yao Xue Xue Bao* 2004;39:876–880.

214. **Serpe, L., Catalano, MG., Cavalli, R., et al.** Cytotoxicity of anticancer drugs incorporated in solid lipid nanoparticles on HT-29 colorectal cancer cell line. *Eur. J. Pharm. Biopharm.* 2004;58:673–680.

215. **Jenning, V., Schafer-Korting, M., and Gohla, S.** Vitamin A-loaded solid lipid nanoparticles for topical use: drug release properties. *J. Control. Release* 2000;66:115–126.

216. **Muller, RH., Radtke, M., and Wissing, SA.** Solid lipid nanoparticles (SLN) and nanostructured lipid carriers (NLC) in cosmetic and dermatological preparations. *Adv. Drug Deliv. Rev.* 2002;54 Suppl. 1:S131–S155.

217. **Souto, EB., Muller, RH., and Gohla, S.** A novel approach based on lipid nanoparticles (SLN) for topical delivery of alpha-lipoic acid. *J. Microencapsul.* 2005;22:581–92.

218. **Iscan, Y., Wissing, SA., Hekimoglu, S., and Muller, RH.** Solid lipid nanoparticles (SLN) for topical drug delivery: incorporation of the lipophilic drugs N,N-diethyl-m-toluamide and vitamin K. *Pharmazie* 2005;60:905–909.

219. **Jain, SK., Chourasia, MK., Masuriha, R. et al.** Solid lipid nanoparticles bearing flurbiprofen for transdermal delivery. *Drug Deliv.* 2005;12:207–215.

220. **Chen, H., Chang, X., Du, D., et al.** Podophyllotoxin-loaded solid lipid nanoparticles for epidermal targeting. *J. Control. Release.* 2006;110:296–306.

221. **Wissing, SA. and Müller, RH.** A novel sunscreen system based on tocopherol acetate incorporated into solid lipid nanoparticles (SLN). *Int. J. Cosm. Sci.* 2001;23:233–243.

222. **Song, C. and Liu, S.** A new healthy sunscreen system for human: Solid lipid nannoparticles as carrier for 3,4,5-trimethoxybenzoylchitin and the improvement by adding Vitamin E. *Int. J. Biol. Macromol.* 2005;36:116–119.

223. **Wissing, SA. and Müller, RH.** Cosmetic applications for solid lipid nanoparticles (SLN). *Int. J. Pharm.* 2003;254:65–68.

224. **Uner, M., Wissing, SA., Yener, G., and Muller, RH.** Skin moisturing effect and skin penetration of ascorbyl palmitate entrapped in solid lipid nanoparticles (SLN) and nanostructured lipid carriers (NLC) incorporated into hydrogel. *Pharmazie* 2005;60:751–755.

225. **Mei, Z., Wu, Q., Hu, S., Li, X., and Yang, X.** Triptolide loaded solid lipid nanoparticle hydrogel for topical application. *Drug Dev. Ind. Pharm.* 2005;31:161–168.

226. **Tanaka, T.** Collapse of gels and the critical endpoint. *Phys. Rev. Lett.* 1978;40:820–823.

227. **Hirotsu, S., Hirokawa, Y., and Tanaka, T.** Volume-phase transitions of ionized N-isopropylacrylamide gels. *J. Chem. Phys.* 1987;87:1392–1395.

228. **Siegel, RA.** and Firestone, BA. pH-dependent equilibrium swelling properties of hydrophobic polyelectrolyte copolymer gels. *Macromolecules* 1988;21:3254–3259.

229. **Bae, YH., Okano, T., and Kim, SW.** "On–off" thermocontrol of transport. Part 1. Temperature dependence of swelling of Nisopropylacrylamide networks modified with hydrophobic components in water. *Pharm. Res.* 1991;8:531–537.

230. **Qiu, Y., and Park, K.** Environment-sensitive hydrogels for drug delivery. *Adv. Drug Deliv. Rev.* 2001;53:321–339.

231. **Kabra, BG., Gehrke, SH., and Spontak, RJ.** Microporous Responsive HPC Gels 1. Synthesis and Microstructure. *Macromolecules* 1998;31:2166–2173.

232. **Lowe, TL. and Tenhu, H.** Interactions of thermally responsive polyelectrolyte latices with low molar mass organic molecules studied by light scattering. *Macromolecules* 1998;31:1590–1594.

233. **Lowe, TL., Benhaddaou, M., and Tenhu, H.** Partially fluorinated thermally responsive latices of linear and crosslinked copolymers. *J. Polym. Sci. B: Polym. Phys.* 1998;36: 2141–2152.

234. **Gao, Y., Au-Yeung, SCF., and Wu, C.** Interaction between surfactant and poly(*N*-vinylcaprolactam) microgels. *Macromolecules* 1999;32:3674–3677.

235. **Lau, ACW. and Wu, C.** Thermally sensitive and biocompatible poly(*N*-vinylcaprolactam): synthesis and characterization of high molar mass linear chains. *Macromolecules* 1999;32:581–584.

236. **Vihola, H., Laukkanen, A., Hirvonen, J., and Tenhu, H.** Binding and release of drugs into and from thermosensitive poly(*N*-vinyl caprolactam) nanoparticles. *Eur. J. Pharm. Sci.* 2002;16:69–74.

237. **Huang, G., Gao, J., Hua, Z., St. John, JV., Ponderb, BC., and Moro, D.** Controlled drug release from hydrogel nanoparticle networks. *J. Control. Release* 2004;94:303–311.

238. **Patton, JN. and Palmer, AF.** Photopolymerization of bovine hemoglobin entrapped nanoscale hydrogel particles within liposomal reactors for use as an artificial blood substitute. *Biomacromolecules* 2005;6:414–424.

239. **Chang, TMS., Powanda, D., and Yu, WP.** Analysis of polyethylene-glycol-polylactide nano-dimension artificial red blood cells in maintaining systemic hemoglobin levels and prevention of methemoglobin formation. *Artif. Cells Blood Substit. Immobil. Biotechnol.* 2003;31:231–247.

240. **Chang, TMS.** Future generations of red blood cell substitutes. *J. Int. Med.* 2003;253:527–535.

241. **Patton, JN. and Palmer, AF.** Engineering temperature-sensitive hydrogel nanoparticles entrapping hemoglobin as a novel type of oxygen carrier. *Biomacromolecules* 2005;6:2204–2212.

242. **Ramanan, RMK., Chellamuthu, P., Tang, L., and Nguyen, KT.** Development of a temperature-sensitive composite hydrogel for drug delivery applications. *Biotechnol. Prog.* 2006;22:118 125.

243. **Blanchette, J. and Peppas, NA.** Cellular evaluation of oral chemotherapy carriers. *J. Biomed. Mater. Res.* 2005;72A:381–388.

244. **Ojugo, ASE., Mcsheehy, PMJ., M1cintyre, DJO., et al.** Measurement of the extracellular pH of solid tumors in mice by magnetic resonance spectroscopy: a comparison of exogenous ^{19}F and ^{31}P probes. *NMR Biomed.* 1999;12:495–504.

245. **Stubbs, M., Mcsheehy, RMJ., Griffiths, JR., and Bashford, L.** Causes and consequences of tumor acidity and implications for treatment. *Mol. Med.* Today 2000;6:15–19.

246. **Conner, J., Yatvin. MB., and Huang L.** pH-sensitive liposomes: Acid-induced liposomes fusion. *Proc. Natl. Acad. Sci.* USA 2000;81:1715–1718 (1984).

247. **Greidziak, M, Bogdanov, AA., Torchilin, VP., and Lasch, J.** Destabilization of pH-sensitive liposomes in the presence of human erythrocyte ghosts. *J. Control. Release* 1992;20:219–230.

248. **Na, K. and Bae, YH.** Self-Assembled Hydrogel Nanoparticles Responsive to Tumor Extracellular pH from pullulan derivative/sulfonamide conjugate: characterization, aggregation, and adriamycin release *in vitro*. *Pharm. Res.* 2002;19:681–688.

249. **Na, K., Lee, KH., and Bae, YH.** pH-sensitivity and pH-dependent interior structural change of self-assembled hydrogel nanoparticles of pullulan acetate/oligo-sulfonamide conjugate. *J. Control. Release* 2004;97:513–525.

250. **Gupta, M. and Gupta, AK.** Hydrogel pullulan nanoparticles encapsulating pBUDLacZ plasmid as an efficient gene delivery carrier. *J. Control. Release* 2004;99:157–166.

251. **Sahoo, SK., De, TK., Ghosh, PK., and Maitra, A.** pH- and thermo-sensitive hydrogel nanoparticles. *J. Colloid Interface Sci.* 1998;206:361–368.

252. **Kuckling, D., Vo, CD., and Wohlrab, SE.** Preparation of nanogels with temperature-responsive core and pH-responsive arms by photo-cross-linking. *Langmuir* 2002;18:4263–4269.

253. **Molteni, L.** Drug Carriers in Biology and Medicine, Gregoriadis, G. (Ed.), Academic Press, London, 1979, pp. 107–125.

254. **Poznansky, MJ. and Cleland, LG.** Drug Delivery Systems, (Juliano, RL., ed.), Oxford University Press, New York, 1980, pp. 253–315.

255. **Sery, TW. and Hehre, EJ.** Degradation of dextrans by enzymes of intestinal bacteria. *J. Bacteriol.* 1956;71:373–380.

256. **Larsen, C., Harboe, E., Johansen, M., and Olesen, HP.** Macromolecular prodrugs. XVI. Colon-targeted deliverycomparison of the rate of release of naproxen from dextran ester prodrugs in homogenates of various segments of the pig gastrointestinal (GI) tract. *Pharm. Res.* 1989;5:995–999.

257. **Nishikawa, T., Akiyoshi, K., and Sunamoto, J.** Supramolecular assembly between nanoparticles of hydrophobized polysaccharide and soluble protein complexation between the self-aggregate of cholesterol-bearing pullulan and a chymotrypsin. *Macromolecules* 1994;27:7654–7659.

258. **Akiyoshi, K., Kobayashi, S., Shichibe, S., et al.** Self-assembled hydrogel nanoparticles of cholesterol-bearing pullulan as a carrier of protein drugs: complexation and stabilization of insulin. *J. Control. Release* 1998;54:313–320.

259. **Kim, I-S., Jeong, Y-I., and Kim, S-H.** Self-assembled hydrogel nanoparticles composed of dextran and poly(ethylene glycol) macromer. *Int. J. Pharm.* 2000;205:109–116.

260. **Gulsen, D. and Chauhan, A.** Dispersion of microemulsion drops in HEMA hydrogel: a potential ophthalmic drug delivery vehicle. *Int. J. Pharm.* 2005;292:95–117.

261. **Netti, PA., Shelton, JC., Revell, PA., et al.** Hydrogels as an interface between bone and an implant. *Biomaterials* 1993;14(14):1098–1104.

262. **Costantini, A., Luciani, G., Annunziata, G., Silvestri, B., and Branda, F.** Swelling properties and bioactivity of silica gel/pHEMA Nanocomposites. *J. Mater. Sci. Mater. Med.* 2006;17:319–325.

263. **Mestecky, J., Moldoveanu, Z., Novak, M., et al.** Biodegradable microspheres for the delivery of oral vaccines *J. Control. Release* 1994;28:131–141.

264. **Men, Y., Audran, R., Thomasin, C., et al.** MHC class I- and class II-restricted processing and presentation of microencapsulated antigens. *Vaccine* 1999;17:1047–1056.

265. **Shen, ZH., Reznikoff, G., Dranoff, G., and Rock, KL.** Cloned dendritic cells can present exogenous antigens on both MHC class I and class II molecules. *J. Immunol.* 1997;158:2723–2730.

266. **Machluf, M., Apte, RN., Regev, O., and Cohen, S.** Enhancing the immunogenicity of liposomal hepatitis B surface antigen (HBsAg) by controlling its delivery from polymeric microspheres. *J. Pharm. Sci.* 2000;89:1550–1557.

267. **Miyata, T., Asami, N., and Uragami, T.** A reversibly antigen-responsive hydrogel. *Nature* 1999;399:766–769.

268. **Jain, S., Yap, WT., and Irvine, DJ.** Synthesis of Protein-Loaded Hydrogel Particles in an Aqueous Two-Phase System for Coincident Antigen and CpG Oligonucleotide Delivery to Antigen-Presenting Cells. *Biomacromolecules* 2005;6: 2590–2600.

269. **Lougheed, WD., Woulfe-Flanagan, H., Clement, JR., and Albisser, AM.** Insulin aggregation in artificial delivery systems. *Diabetologia* 1980;19:1–9.

270. **Hovgaard, L., Mack, EJ., and Kim, SW.** Insulin stabilization and GI absorption. *J. Control. Release* 1992;19:99–108.

271. **Bharali, DJ., Sahoo, SK., Mozumdar, S., and Maitra, A.** Cross-linked polyvinylpyrrolidone nanoparticles: a potential carrier for hydrophilic drugs. *J. Colloid Interface Sci.* 2003; 258:415–423.

272. **Jana, SS., Bharali, DJ., Mani, P., Maitra, A., Gupta, CM., and Sarkar, DP.** Targeted cytosolic delivery of hydrogel nanoparticles into HepG2 cells through engineered Sendai viral envelopes. *FEBS Lett.* 2002;515:184–188.

273. **Hyon, SH., Cha, WI., Ikada, Y., Kita, M., Ogura, Y., and Honda, Y.** Poly(vinyl alcohol) hydrogels as soft contact lens material. *J. Biomater. Sci. Polym. Ed.* 1994;5:397–406.

274. **Juang, JH., Bonner, WS., Ogawa, YJ., Vacanti, P., and Weir, GC.** Outcome of subcutaneous islet transplantation improved by polymer device. *Transplantation* 1996;61:1557–1561.

275. **Ficek, BJ. and Peppas, NA.** Novel preparation of poly(vinyl alcohol) microparticles without crosslinking agent for controlled drug delivery of proteins. *J. Control. Release* 1993; 27:259–264.

276. **Li, JK., Wang, N., and Wu, XS.** Poly(vinyl alcohol) nanoparticles prepared by freezing–thawing process for protein/peptide drug delivery. *J. Control. Release* 1998; 56:117–126.

277. **Na, K., Park, K-H., Kim, SW., and Bae, YH.** Self-assembled hydrogel nanoparticles from curdlan derivatives: characterization, anti-cancer drug release and interaction with a hepatoma cell line (HepG2). *J. Control. Release* 2000;69:225–236.

278. **Kabanov, AV., Batrakova, EV., and Alakhov, VY.** Pluronic block copolymers as novel polymer therapeutics for drug and gene delivery. *J. Control. Release* 2002;82:189–212.

279. **Choi, SH., Lee, SH., and Park, TG.** Temperature-Sensitive Pluronic/Poly(ethylenimine) nanocapsules for thermally triggered disruption intracellular endosomal compartment. *Biomacromolecules* 2006;7:1864–1870.

280. **Lee, VHL. and Yamamoto, A.** Penetration and enzymatic barriers to peptide and protein absorption. *Adv. Drug Deliv. Rev.* 1990;4:171–207.

281. **Banga, AK.** Therapeutic Peptides and Proteins. Technomic Publishing Company, Lancaster, 1995, pp. 8–12.

282. **Fix, JA.** Absorption enhancing agents for the GI system. *J. Control. Release* 1987;6:151–156.

283. **Lee, VHL.** Protease inhibitors and penetration enhancers as approaches to modify peptide absorption. *J. Control. Release* 1990;13:213–223.

284. **Fujita, T., Fujita, T., Morikawa, K., et al.** Improvement of intestinal absorption of human calcitonin by chemical modification with fatty acids: synergistic effects of acylation and absorption enhancers. *Int. J. Pharm.* 1996;134:47–57.

285. **Morishita, I., Morishita, M., Takayama, K., Machida, Y., and Nagai, T.** Hypoglycemic effect of novel oral microspheres of insulin with protease inhibitor in normal and diabetic rats. *Int. J. Pharm.* 1992;78:9–16.

286. **Fukunaga, M., Miller, MM., and Deftos, LJ.** Liposome-entrapped calcitonin and parathyroid hormone are orally effective in rats. *Horm. Metab. Res.* 1991;23:166–167.

287. **Matsuzaka, A., Morishita, M., Takayama, K., and Nagai, T.** Absorption of insulin using water-in-oil-in-water emulsion from enteral loop in rats. *Biol. Pharm. Bull.* 1995;18: 1718–1723.

288. **Couvreur, P. and Puisieux, F.** Nano- and microparticles for the delivery of polypeptides and proteins. *Adv. Drug Deliv. Rev.* 1993;10:141–162.

289. **Hastewell, J., Lynch, S., Williamson, I., Fox, R., and Mackay, M.** Absorption of human calcitonin across the rat colon *in vivo*. *Clin. Sci.* 1992;82:589–594.

290. **Gruber, P., Longer, M., and Robinson, JR.** Some biological issues in oral, controlled drug delivery. *Adv. Drug Deliv. Rev.* 1987;1:1–18.

291. **Allemann, E., Leroux, J-C., and Gurny, R.** Polymeric nano- and microparticles for the oral delivery of peptides and peptidomimetics. *Adv. Drug Deliv. Rev.* 1998;34:171–189.

292. **Bilati, U., Allemann, E., and Doelker, E.** Strategic approaches for overcoming peptide and protein instability within biodegradable nano- and microparticles. *Eur. J. Pharm. Biopharm.* 2005;59:375–388.

293. **Venkatesan, N., Yoshimitsu, J., Ito, Y., Shibata, N., and Takada, K.** Liquid filled nanoparticles as a drug deliverytool for protein therapeutics. *Biomaterials* 2005;26:7154–7163.

294. **Vranckx, H., Demoustier, HM., and Deleers, M.** Pharmaceutical compositions containing nanocapsules. 1996;US. Patent no. 5,500,224.

295. **Lowe, PJ. and Temple, CS.** Calcitonin and insulin in isobutylcyanoacrylate nanocapsules: protection against pro teases and effect on intestinal absorption in rats. *J. Pharm. Pharmacol.* 1994;46:547–552.

296. **Vranckx, H., Demoustier, M., and Deleers, M.** A new nanocapsule formulation with hydrophilic core: application to the oral administration of salmon calcitonin. *Eur. J. Pharm. Biopharm.* 1996;42:345–347.

297. **Bonduelle, S., Carrier, M., Pimienta, C., Benoıt, JP., and Lenaerts, V.** Tissue concentration of nanoencapsulated radiolabelled cyclosporin following peroral delivery in mice or ophthalmic applications in rabbits. *Eur. J. Pharm. Biopharm.* 1996;42:313–319.

298. **Damge, C., Michel, C., Aprahamian, M., and Couvreur, P.** New approach for oral administration of insulin with poly alkylcyanoacrylate nanocapsules as drug carriers. *Diabetes* 1988;37:246–251.

299. **Damge, C., Hillaire-Buys, D., Puech, R., Hoeltzel, A., Michel, C., and Ribes, G.** Effects of orally administered insulin nanocapsules in normal and diabetic dogs. *Diabetes Nutr. Metab.* 1995;8:3–9.

300. **Hillery, AM., Toth, I., Shaw, AJ., and Florence, AT.** Co-polymerised particles (CPP). I: synthesis, characterization and in vitro studies on a novel oral nanoparticulate delivery system. *J. Control. Release* 1996;41:271–281.

301. **Hillery, AM., Toth, I., and Florence, AT.** Co-polymerised peptide particles. II: Oral uptake of a novel co-polymeric nanopar ticulate delivery system for peptides. *J. Control. Release* 1996;42:65–73.

302. **Lutsiak, ME., Kwon, GS., and Samuel, J.** Biodegradable nanoparticles delivery of a Th2-biased peptide for induction of Th1 immune responses. *J. Pharm. Pharmacol.* 2006;58: 739–747.

303. **Pack, DW., Hoffman, AS., Pun, S., and Stayton, PS.** Design and development of polymers for gene delivery. *Nat. Rev. Drug. Discov.* 2005;4:581–593.

304. **Berry, M., Barrett, L., Seymour, L., Baird, A., and Logan, A.** Gene therapy for central nervous system repair. *Curr. Opin. Mol. Ther.* 2001;3:338–349.

305. **Guerra-Crespo, M., Charli, JL., Rosales-Garcia, VH., Pedraza-Alva, G., and Perez-Martinez, L.** Polyethylenimine improves the transfection efficiency of primary cultures of post-mitotic rat fetal hypothalamic neurons. *J. Neurosci. Methods* 2003;127:179–192.

306. **Wu, K., Meyers, CA., Bennett, JA., King, MA., Meyer, EM., and Hughes, JA.** Polyethylenimine-mediated NGF gene delivery protects transected septal cholinergic neurons. *Brain Res.* 2004;1008:284–287.

307. **Zou, SM., Erbacher, P., Remy, JS., and Behr, JP.** Systemic linear polyethylenimine (L-PEI)-mediated gene delivery in the mouse. *J. Gene. Med.* 2000;2:128–134.

308. **Suka, JS., Suha, J., Choya, K., Laib, SK., Fub, J., and Hanes, J.** Gene delivery to differentiated neurotypic cells with RGD and HIV Tat peptide functionalized polymeric nanoparticles. *Biomaterials* 2006;27:5143–5150.

309. **Kleemann, E., Neu, M., Jekel, N., et al.** Nano-carriers for DNA delivery to the lung based upon a TAT-derived peptide covalently coupled to PEG–PEI. *J. Control. Release* 2005; 109:299–316.

310. **Li, Z., Zhu, S., Gan, K., et al.** Poly-L-lysine-modified silica nanoparticles: A potential oral gene delivery system. *J. Nanosci. Nanotechnol.* 2005;5:1199–1203.

311. **Jeon, O., Kang, SW., Lim, HW., Hyung Chung, J., and Kim, BS.** Long-term and zero-order release of basic fibroblast growth factor from heparin-conjugated poly(L-lactide-co-glycolide) nanospheres and fibrin gel. *Biomaterials* 2006;27:1598–1607.

312. **Kwon, YJ., Standley, SM., Goh, SL., and Frechet, JM.** Enhanced antigen presentation and immunostimulation of dendritic cells using acid-degradable cationinc nanoparticles. *J. Control. Release* 2005;105(3):199–212.

313. **Prego, C., Garcia, M., Torres, D., and Alonso, MJ.** Transmucosal macromolecular drug delivery. *J. Control. Release* 2005; 101:151–162.

314. **Kawashima, Y., Yamamoto, H., Takeuchi, H., and Kuno, Y.** Mucoadhesive DL-lactide/glycolide copolymer nanospheres coated with chitosan to improve oral delivery of elcatonin. *Pharm. Dev. Technol.* 2000;5:77–85.

315. **Gu, JP., Robinson, JR., and Leung, SHS.** Binding of acrylic polymers to mucin/epithelial surfaces: structure–property polymers to mucin/epithelial surfaces: structure–property relationships. *Crit. Rev. Ther. Drug Carrier Syst.* 1988;5:21–67.

316. **Takeuchi, H., Yamamoto, H., Niwa, T., Hino, T., and Kawashima, Y.** Enteral absorption of insulin in rats from mucoadhesive chitosan-coated liposomes, *Pharm. Res.* 1996;13:896–901.

317. **Cui, F., Qian, F., and Yin, C.** Preparation and characterization of mucoadhesive polymer-coated nanoparticles. *Int. J. Pharm.* 2006;316:154–161.

318. **Akashi, M., Kirikihara, I., and Miyauchi, N.** Synthesis and polymerization of a styryl terminated oligovinylpyrrolidone macromonomer. *Angew. Macromol. Chem.* 1985;132:81–89.

319. **Sakuma, S., Hayashi, M., and Akashi, M.** Design of nanoparticles composed of graft copolymers for oral peptide delivery. *Adv. Drug Deliv. Rev.* 2001;47:21–37.

320. **Sakuma, S., Suzuki, N., Kikuchi, H., et al.** Oral peptide delivery using nanoparticles composed of novel graft copolymers having hydrophobic backbone and hydrophilic branches. *Int. J. Pharm.* 1997;149:93–106.

321. **Sakuma, S., Suzuki, N., Kikuchi, H., et al.** Absorption enhancement of orally administered salmon calcitonin by polystyrene nanoparticles having poly(N-isopropylacrylamide) branches on their surfaces. *Int. J. Pharm.* 1997;158:69–78.

322. **Garcia-Fuentes, M., Prego, C., Torres, D., and Alonso, MJ.** A comparative study of the potential of solid triglyceride nanostructures coated with chitosan or poly(ethylene glycol) as carriers for oral calcitonin delivery. *Eur. J. Pharm. Sci.* 2005; 25:133–143.

323. **Wright, ER. and Conticello, VP.** Self-assembly of block copolymers derived from elastin-mimetic polypeptide sequences. *Adv. Drug Deliv. Rev.* 2002;54:1057–1073.

324. **Urry, DW., Luan, CH., Parker, TM., et al.** Temperature of polypeptide inverse temperature transition depends on mean residue hydrophobicity. *J. Am. Chem. Soc.* 1991;113: 4346–4347.

325. **Lee, TAT., Cooper, A., Apkarian, RP., and Conticello, VP.** Thermo-reversible self-assembly of nanoparticles derived from elastin-mimetic polypeptides. *Adv. Mater.* 2000;12: 1105–1110.

326. **Wright, ER., McMillan, RA., Cooper, A., Apkarian, RP., and Conticello, VP.** Thermoplastic elastomer hydrogels via self-assembly of an elastin-mimetic triblock polypeptide. *Adv. Funct. Mater.* 2002;2:149–154.

327. **Panitch, A., Yamaoka, T., Fournier, MJ., Mason, TL., and Tirrell, DA.** Design and biosynthesis of elastin-like artificial extracellular matrix proteins containing periodically spaced fibronectin CS5 domains. *Macromolecules* 1999;32: 1701–1703.

328. **Rabinow, BE.** Nanosuspensions in drug delivery. *Nat. Rev. Drug Discov.* 2004;3:785–796.

329. **Liversidge, GG., Cundy, KC., Bishop, J., and Czekai, D.** Surface modified drug nanoparticles. US Patent no. 5,145,684. 1991.

330. **Enderle, U., Kolb, G., Mende, S., and Way, H.** Technical Proceedings of the 2006 NSTI technology conference and trade show, vol. 1, chapter 4: Nanoparticle processes & applications: Effectively grinding and dispersing nanoparticles using a fine bead mill, in nanotech 2006, pp. 493–496.

331. **Buchmann, S., Fischli, W., Thiel, FP., and Alex, R.** Aqueous microsuspension, an alternative intravenous formulation for animal studies. *42nd Annual Congress of the International Association for Pharmaceutical Technology (APV)*, Mainz 1996, p 124.

332. **Muller, RH., Becker, R., Kruss, B., and Peters, K.** Pharmaceutical nanosuspensions for medicament administration as system of increased saturation solubility and rate of solution. US Patent no. 5,858,410. 1998.

333. **Muller, RH., Jacobs, C., and Kayser, O.** Nanosuspensions as particulate drug formulations in therapy Rationale for development and what we can expect for the future. *Adv. Drug Deliv. Rev.* 2001;47:3–19.

334. **Kayser, O., Olbrich, C., Yardley, V., Kinderlen, AF., and Croft, SL.** Formulation of amphotericin B as nanosuspension for oral administration. *Int. J. Pharm.* 2003;254:73–75.

335. **Moschwitzer, J., Achleitner, G., Pomper, H., and Muller, RH.** Development of an intravenously injectable chemically stable aqueous omeprazole formulation using nanosuspension technology. *Eur. J. Pharm. Biopharm.* 2004;58:615–619.

336. **Hecq, J., Deleers, M., Fanara, D., Vranckx, H., and Amighi, K.** Preparation and characterisation of nanocrystals for solubility and dissolution rate enhancement of nifedipine. *Int. J. Pharm.* 2005;299:167–177.

337. **Langguth, P., Hanafy, A., Frenzel, D., et al.** Nanosuspension formulations for low-soluble drugs: pharmacokinetic evaluation using spironolactone as model compound. *Drug. Dev. Ind. Pharm.* 2005;31:319–329.

338. **Muller, RH., Mader, K., and Krause, K.** Verfahren zur schonenden Herstellung von hochfeinen Micro-/ Nanopartikeln, PCT Application PCT/EP00/06535, Germany, 2000.

339. **Keck, CM. and Muller, RH.** Drug nanocrystals of poorly soluble drugs produced by high pressure homogenization. *Eur. J. Pharm. Biopharm.* 2006;62:3–16.

340. **Kocbek, P., Baumgartner, S., and Kristl, J.** Preparation and evaluation of nanosuspensions for enhancing the dissolution of poorly soluble drugs. *Int. J. Pharm.* 2006;312:179–186.

341. **Liversidge, GC. and Conzentino, P.** Drug particle size reduction for decreasing gastric irritancy and enhancing absorption of naproxen in rats. *Int. J. Pharm.* 1995;125:309–313.

342. **Kabalnov AS. and Shukin, ED.** Ostwald ripening theory: applications to fluorocarbon emulsion stability. *Adv. Colloid Interface Sci.* 1992;38:69–97.

343. **Kabalnov, AS., Pertzov, AV., and Shukin, ED.** Ostwald ripening in two-component disperse phase systems: Application to emulsion stability. *Colloids Surf.* 1987;24:19–32.

344. **Lindfors, L., Skantze, P., Skantze, U., Rasmusson, M., Zackrisson, A., and Olsson, U.** Amorphous drug nanosuspensions. 1. Inhibition of Ostwald ripening. *Langmuir* 2006:22:906–910.

345. **Liversidge, GC.** Drug nanoparticles for improved drug delivery. *23rd Int. Symp. Control. Release Bioact. Mater.* Kyoto, Japan, 1996, 23(2):74–81.

346. **Vitale, SA. and Katz, JL.** Liquid Droplet Dispersions Formed by Homogeneous Liquid-Liquid Nucleation: "The Ouzo Effect." *Langmuir* 2003;19:4105–4110.

347. **Brick, MC., Palmer, HJ., and Whitesides, TH.** Formation of Colloidal Dispersions of Organic Materials in Aqueous Media by Solvent Shifting. *Langmuir* 2003;19:6367–6380.

348. **Liversidge, GC.** Drug nanocrystals for improved drug delivery. Workshop on Particulate Drug Delivery Systems. *Int. Symp. Control. Release Bioact. Mater.* 1996, p 23.

349. **Garnett, MC.** Targeted drug conjugates: Principles and progress. *Adv. Drug Deliv. Rev.* 2001;53:171–216.

350. **Guzman, LA., Labhasetwar,V., Song, C., et al.** Local intraluminal infusion of biodegradable polymeric nanoparticles. A novel approach for prolonged drug delivery after balloon angioplasty. *Circulation* 1996;94:1441–1448.

351. **Schiffelers, RM., Storm, G., and Bakker-Woudenberg, IAJM.** Host factors influencing the preferential localization of sterically stabilized liposomes in Klebsiella pneumoniae-infected rat lung tissue. *Pharm. Res.* 2001;18:780–787.

352. **Matsumura, Y. and Maeda, H.** A new concept for macromolecular therapeutics in cancer chemotherapy: mechanism of tumoritropic accumulation of proteins and the antitumor agent smancs. *Cancer Res.* 1986;46:6387–6392.

353. **Rodrigues, JM., Jr., Fessi, H., Bories, C., Puisieux, F., and Devissaguet, J-P.** Primaquine-loaded poly(lactide) nanoparticles: physicochemical study and acute tolerance in mice. *Int. J. Pharm.* 1995;126:253–260.

354. **Moghimi, SM., Hunter AC., and Murray, JC.** Long-circulating and target-specific nanoparticles: theory to practice. *Pharmacol. Rev.* 2001;53:283–318.

355. **Shenoy DB. and Amiji, MM.** Poly(ethylene oxide)-modified poly(epsilon-caprolactone) nanoparticles for targeted delivery of tamoxifen in breast cancer. *Int. J. Pharm.* 2005;293:261–270.

356. **Gref, R., Minamitake, Y., Peracchia, MT., Trubetskoy, V., Torchilin, V., and Langer, R.** Biodegradable long-circulating polymeric nanospheres. *Science* 1994;263:1600–1603.

357. **Rouzes, C., Gref, R., Leonard, M., and DeSousa Delgado, A.** and Dellacherie, E. Surface modification of poly(lactic acid) nanospheres using hydrophobically modified dextrans as stabilizers in an o/w emulsion/evaporation technique. *J. Biomed. Mater. Res.* 2000;50:557–565.

358. **Chauvierre, C., Labarre, D., Couvreur, P., and Vauthier, C.** Novel polysaccharide-decorated poly(isobutyl cyanoacrylate) nanoparticles. *Pharm. Res.* 2003;20:1786–1793.

359. **Barbault-Foucher, S., Gref, R., Russo, P., Guechot, J., and Bochot, A.** Design of poly-epsilon-caprolactone nanospheres coated with bioadhesive hyaluronic acid for ocular delivery. *J. Control. Release* 2002;83:365–375.

360. **Vila, A., Sanchez, A., Tobio, M., Calvo P., and Alonso, MJ.** Design of biodegradable particles for protein delivery. *J. Control. Release* 2002;78:15–24.

361. **Janes, KA., Calvo, P., and Alonso, MJ.** Polysaccharide colloidal particles as delivery systems for Macromolecules. *Adv. Drug Deliv. Rev.* 2001;47:83–97.

362. **Fernandez-Urrusumo, R., Calvo, P., Remunan-Lopez, C., Vila-Jato JL., and Alonso, MJ.** Enhancement of nasal absorption of insulin using chitosan nanoparticles. *Pharm. Res.* 1999;16:1576–1581.

363. **Illum, L., Farraj, NF., and Davis, SS.** Chitosan as a novel nasal delivery system for peptide drugs. *Pharm. Res.* 1994;11: 1186–1189.

364. **Gurny, R., Ibrahim, H., Aebi, A., et al.** Design and evaluation of controlled release systems for the eye. *J. Control. Release* 1987;6:367–373.

365. **Jaulin, N., Appel, M., Passirani, C., Barratt, G., and Labarre, D.** Reduction of the uptake by a macrophagic cell line of nanoparticles bearing heparin or dextran covalently bound to poly(methyl methacrylate). *J. Drug Target.* 2000; 8:165–172.

366. **Passirani, C., Barratt, G., Devissaguet, JP., and Labarre, D.** Long-circulating nanoparticles bearing heparin or dextran covalently bound to poly(methylmethacrylate). *Pharm. Res.* 1998;15:1046–1050.

367. **Maruyama, A., Ishihara, T., Kim, J-S., Kim, SW., and Akaike, T.** Design of multi-layered nanoparticles as a DNA carrier. *Colloids Surf. A: Physicochem. Eng. Aspects* 1999;153:439–443.

368. **Zimmer, A.** Antisense oligonucleotide delivery with polyhexylcyanoacrylate nanoparticles as carriers. *Methods* 1999;18:286–295.

369. **Lemarchand, C., Gref, R., and Couvreur, P.** Polysaccharide-decorated nanoparticles. *Eur. J. Pharm. Biopharm.* 2004;58:327–341.

370. **Cummings, J. and McArdle, CS.** Studies on the in vivo disposition of adriamycin in human tumours which exhibit different responses to the drug. *Br. J. Cancer* 1986; 53:835–838.

371. **Antony, AC., Kane, MA., Portillo, RM., Elwood PC., and Kolhouse, JF.** Studies of the role of a particulate folate-binding protein in the uptake of 5-methyltetrahydrofolate by cultured human KB cells. *J. Biol. Chem.* 1985;260: 14,911–14,917.

372. **Yoo, HS. and Park, TG.** Bio-degradable nanoparticles containing protein-fatty acid complexes for oral delivery of Salmon calcitonin. *J. Pharm. Sci.* 2004;93:488–495.

373. **Yoo, HS. and Park, TG.** Folate-receptor-targeted delivery of doxorubicin nano-aggregates stabilized by doxorubicin-PEG-folate conjugate. *J. Control. Release* 2004;100:247–256.

374. **Rossin, R., Pan, D., Qi, K., et al.** 64Cu-labeled folate-conjugated shell cross-linked nanoparticles for tumor imaging and radiotherapy: synthesis, radiolabeling, and biologic evaluation. *Nucl. Med.* 2005;46:1210.

375. **Singh, M.** Transferrin As A targeting ligand for liposomes and anticancer drugs. *Curr. Pharm. Des.* 1999;5:443–451.

376. **Lemieux, P. and Page, M.** Sensitivity of multidrug-resistant MCF-7 cells to a transferrin-doxorubicin conjugate. *Anticancer Res.* 1994;14:397–403.

377. **Labhasetwar, V., Song, C., Humphrey, W., Shebuski R., and Levy, RJ.** Arterial uptake of biodegradable nanoparticles: effect of surface modifications. *J. Pharm. Sci.* 1998;87:1229–1234.

378. **Sahoo SK. and Labhasetwar V.** Enhanced antiproliferative activity of transferrin-conjugated paclitaxel-loaded nanoparticles is mediated via sustained intracellular drug retention. *Mol. Pharm.* 2005;2:373–383.

379. **Xu Z., Gu, W., Huang, J., et al.** *In vitro* and *in vivo* evaluation of actively targetable nanoparticles for paclitaxel delivery. *Int. J. Pharm.* 2005;288:361–368.

380. **Ashwell G. and Harford, J.** Carbohydrate-specific receptors of the liver. *Ann. Rev. Biochem.* 1982;51:531–554.

381. **Kopecek, J. and Duncan, R.** Targetable polymeric prodrugs. *J. Control. Release* 1987;6:315–327.

382. **Cho, CS., Jeong, YI., Ishihara, T., et al.** Simple preparation of nanoparticles coated with carbohydrate-carrying polymers. *Biomaterials* 1997;18:323–326.

383. **Liang H.F., Yang, T.F., Huang, C.T., Chen M.C., and Sung, H-W.** Preparation of nanoparticles composed of poly(gamma-glutamic acid)-poly(lactide) block copolymers and evaluation of their uptake by HepG2 cells. *J. Control. Release* 2005;105:213–225.

384. **Liang, H.F., Chen, C.T., Chen, S.C., et al.** Paclitaxel-loaded poly(gamma-glutamic acid)-poly(lactide) nanoparticles as a targeted drug delivery system for the treatment of liver cancer. *Biomaterials* 2006;27:2051–2059.

8

Resealed Erythrocytes

Dr. R.S.R. Murthy, M.PHARM, PhD

CONTENTS

1. INTRODUCTION

Erythrocytes are the most abundant cells in human body amounting to approximately 5.4 million cells/mm^3 bloods in a healthy male and approximately 4.8 million cells/mm^3 blood in a healthy female. Dutch Scientist Lee Van Hock (1674) described these cells in human blood samples. But Hope Seyler in 19th century identified the crucial role of haemoglobin and the oxygen delivery to various parts of body *(1)*. Erythrocytes are biconcave discs with an average diameter of 7.8 μm, a thickness of 2.5 μm in periphery, 1 μm in centre and a volume of 85–91 μm^3 *(2)*. The flexible, biconcave shape enables erythrocytes to pass through narrow capillaries, which may be only 3 μm wide. Mature erythrocytes are quite simple in structure. They lack a nucleus and other organelles. Their plasma membrane encloses haemoglobin, a haem-containing protein that is responsible for O_2–CO_2 binding inside the erythrocytes. The main role of erythrocytes is transport of O_2 from lungs to tissues and of the CO_2 produced in tissues back to lungs. Thus, erythrocytes are a highly specialised O_2 carrier system in body. Because a nucleus is absent, all the intra-cellular space is available for O_2 transport. Also, because mitochondria are absent and because energy is generated anaerobically in erythrocytes, these cells do not consume any of the oxygen they are carrying. Erythrocytes live only about 120 days because of wear and tear on their plasma membranes as they squeeze through narrow blood capillaries. Worn-out erythrocytes are removed from circulation and destroyed in the spleen and liver reticuloendothelial system (RES), and the breakdown products are recycled. The process of erythrocyte formation within body is known as erythropoiesis. In a mature human being, erythrocytes are produced in red bone marrow under the regulation of a haemopoietic hormone called erythropoietin *(3)*.

2. ADVANTAGES OF ERYTHROCYTES AS DRUG CARRIERS

Due to its unique structure (devoid of nucleus), erythrocytes have large intra-cellular space and thus is capable of carrying significant quantity of drugs in it. In addition they have several advantages that are as follows:

- Biocompatibility, particularly when autologous cells are used, hence no possibility of triggered immune response *(4–12)*.
- Biodegradability with out generation of toxic products *(12,13)*.
- Considerably uniform size and shape of carrier *(14)*.
- Relatively inert intra-cellular environment *(15)*.
- Prevention of degradation of loaded drug from inactivation by endogenous chemicals *(16,17)*.
- Wide variety of chemicals that can be entrapped *(16,18–20)*.
- Modification of pharmacokinetic and pharmacodynamic parameters of drug *(5,10,13,16)*.
- Attainment of steady-state plasma concentration decreases fluctuations in concentration *(21,22)*.
- Protection against toxic effects of drugs (e.g., anti-neoplastics *[4,10,16,22]*).
- Availability of techniques and facilities for separation, handling, transfusion and working with erythrocytes *(4,7)*.
- Their ability to target the organs of RES *(4,6,7,23)*.
- Possibility of ideal zero-order drug-release kinetics *(17)*.
- Lack of occurrence of undesired immune response against encapsulated drug *(6,15)*.
- Relatively Large quantity of drug that can be encapsulated within a small volume of cells ensures dose sufficiency *(6,7,12)*.
- A longer life span in circulation as compared with other synthetic carriers *(6,24,25)*, and optimum conditions may result in life span comparable to that of normal erythrocytes *(8,23,26)*.
- Easy control during life span ranging from minutes to months *(11)*.

Erythrocytes, as carrier systems also presents several disadvantages, as under:

- Their removal *in vivo* by RES which limits their useful life as drug carriers and in some cases may pose toxicological problems.

- Rapid leakage of certain encapsulated substances.
- Several molecules loaded may alter the physiology of erythrocyte.
- Encapsulated erythrocytes may present greater variability and lesser standardisation in their preparation, compared to other carrier systems.
- Liable to biological contamination and so demands rigorous controls during collection and handling of the erythrocytes.

3. PREPARATION METHODS

3.1. Source and Isolation of Erythrocytes

Various types of mammalian erythrocytes have been used for drug delivery, including erythrocytes of mice, cattle, pig, dog, sheep, goat, monkey, chicken, rat and rabbit. To isolate erythrocytes, blood is collected in heparinised tubes by venipuncture. Fresh whole blood is typically used for loading purposes because the encapsulation efficiency of erythrocytes isolated from fresh blood is higher than that of the aged blood. Fresh whole blood is the blood that is collected and immediately chilled to 4°C and stored for <2 days. The erythrocytes are then harvested and washed by centrifugation (1000*g* for 5 min). The washed cells are suspended in buffer solution at various haematocrit values as desired and are often stored in acid–citrate–dextrose buffer at 4°C for as long as 48 h before use. Jain and Vyas have described a well-established protocol for isolation of erythrocytes *(6,27)*. In 1953, Gardos called erythrocytes whose intracellular contents are removed as erythrocyte ghost (EG) and loaded them using adenosine triphosphate (ATP) *(28)*. The loading of drugs in erythrocytes was reported separately by Iher *et al. (29)* and Zimmermann *(30)*. In 1979, the term carrier erythrocytes were coined to describe drug-loaded erythrocytes *(5)*.

3.2. Methods of Drug Loading

Several methods can be used to load drugs or other bioactive compounds in erythrocytes, including physical (e.g., electrical pulse method) osmosis-based systems, and chemical methods (e.g., chemical perturbation of the erythrocytes membrane). Irrespective of the method used, optimal characteristics for successful entrapment of compound requires the drug to have a considerable degree of water solubility, resistance against degradation within erythrocytes, lack of physical or chemical interaction with erythrocyte membrane and well-defined pharmacokinetic and pharmacodynamic properties *(31)*.

3.2.1. Hypotonic Haemolysis

This method is based on the ability of erythrocytes to undergo reversible swelling in a hypotonic solution. Erythrocytes have an exceptional capability for reversible shape changes with or without accompanying volume change and for reversible deformation under stress. An increase in volume leads to an initial change in the shape from biconcave to spherical. This change is attributable to absence of superfluous membrane; hence, the surface area of cell is fixed. The cells attain a spherical shape to accommodate additional volume while keeping the surface area constant. The volume gain is approximately 25–50%. The cells can maintain their integrity up to a tonicity of approximately 150 mOsm/kg, above which the membrane ruptures, releasing cellular contents. At this point (just before cell lysis), some transient pores of 200–500 A° are generated on membrane. After cell lysis, cellular contents are depleted. The remnant is called an Erythrocyte Ghost (EG). The principle of using these ruptured erythrocytes as drug carriers is based on the fact that ruptured membranes can be resealed by restoring isotonic conditions. Upon incubation, the cells resume their original biconcave shape and recover original impermeability *(5,32,33)*.

3.2.2. Use of Red Cell Loader

Magnani *et al.* developed a novel method for entrapment of non-diffusible drugs into erythrocytes *(34)*. They developed a piece of equipment called a "red cell loader".

With as little as 50 mL of a blood sample, different biologically active compounds were entrapped into erythrocytes within a period of 2 h at room temperature under blood storage conditions. The process is based on two sequential hypotonic dilutions of washed erythrocytes followed by concentration with a haemofilter and an isotonic resealing of cells. There was approximately 30% drug loading with 35–50% cell recovery. The processed erythrocytes had normal survival *in vivo*. Same cells could be used for targeting by improving their recognition by tissue macrophages.

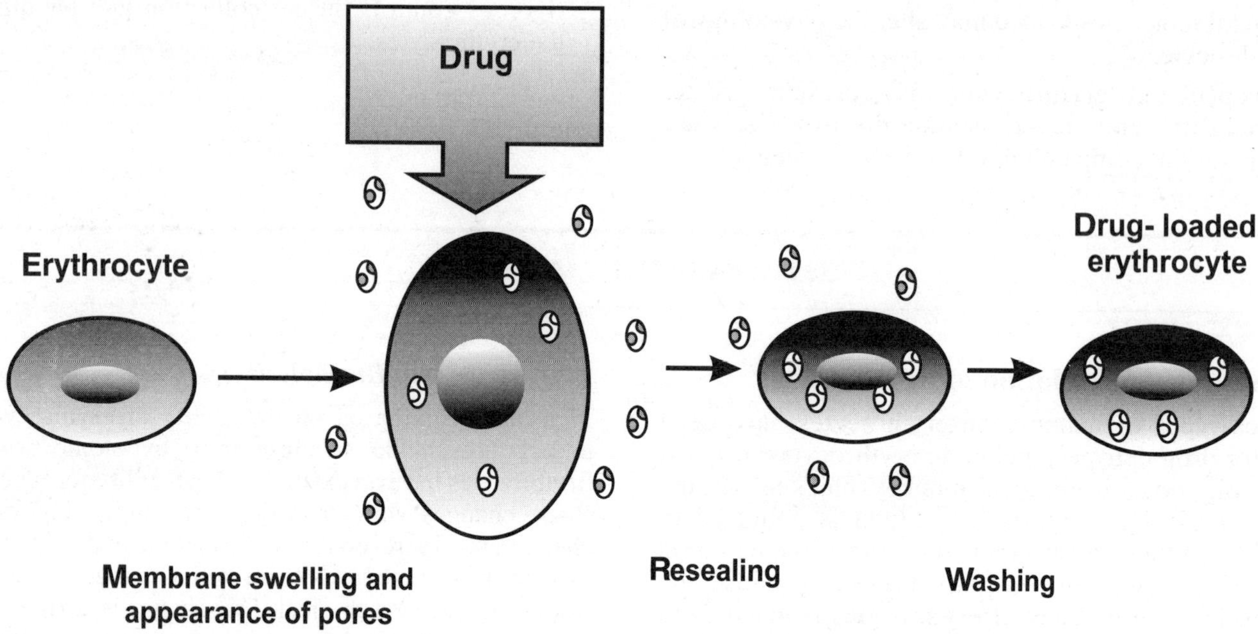

Fig. 1. Encapsulation of drugs within erythrocytes. Human erythrocytes are dialysed against a hypotonic saline solution to permit the opening of pores large enough to be crossed by externally added drugs. The osmolarity is then restored to permit resealing of membrane pores followed by washing out the non-entrapped substances (Reprinted from Antivir. Res., 55, Aquaro, S., Calio, R., Balzarini, J., Bellocchi, MC., Garaci, E., and Perno, CF. Macrophages and HIV infection: therapeutical approaches toword this virus reservior, 209–225, 2002, with permission from Elsevier) *(40a)*.

3.2.3. Hypotonic Dilution

Hypotonic dilution was first method investigated for encapsulation of chemicals into erythrocytes and is simplest and fastest *(5,29)*. In this method, a volume of packed erythrocytes is diluted with 2–20 volumes of aqueous solution of a drug. The solution tonicity is then restored by adding a hypertonic buffer. The resultant mixture is then centrifuged, supernatant is discarded, and the pellet is washed with isotonic buffer solution *(19,29)*. The major drawbacks of this method include a low entrapment efficiency *(7,29,35,36)* and a considerable loss of haemoglobin and other cell components *(13,18,24)*. This reduces circulation half-life of loaded cells. These cells are readily phagocytosed by macrophages of reticulo endothelial system (RES) and hence can be used for targeting RES organs *(19,29)*. Salbutamol encapsulated in resealed erythrocyte by hypotonic dilution showed slow and steady drug release. When the product was lyophilised, release was more rapid between 24–36 h. Release was found to be 56% in both regular formulation and lyophilised product at the end of 72 h. The lyophilised product protected guinea pigs from broncho-constricting effect of histamine for nearly 48 h, indicating prolonged activity of the product as a result of controlled release *(39)*.

Hypotonic dilution is used for loading enzymes such as galactosidase and glucosidase *(11)*, asparginase *(8,38)* and arginase *(15)*.

3.2.4. Hypotonic Pre-Swelling

This method was developed by Rechsteiner *(40)* in 1975 and was modified by Jenner *et al.* *(26)* for drug loading. The technique is based upon initial controlled swelling in a hypotonic-buffered solution *(40a)* as represented in Fig. 1.

This mixture is centrifuged at low rpm. The supernatant is discarded and the cell fraction is brought to lysis point by adding 100–120 L portions of an aqueous solution of drug to be encapsulated. The mixture is centrifuged between the drug-addition steps. The lysis point is detected by disappearance of a distinct boundary between cell fraction and supernatant upon centrifugation. The tonicity of a cell mixture is restored at lysis point by adding a calculated amount of hypertonic buffer. Then, the cell suspension is incubated at 37°C to re-anneal the erythrocytes *(19,35)*. Such cells have a circulation half-life comparable with that of normal cells *(35,41)*. This method is simpler and faster than other methods, causing minimum damage to cells.

The hypotonic pre-swelling method for encapsulating drugs in intact human erythrocytes was evaluated using enalaprilat as a model drug; the effects of various process variables on loading parameters were determined. The probable mechanism of entry of enalaprilat into intact erythrocytes was concentration-based diffusion through pores made on cell membrane at the point of haemolysis. On closure of pores by hypotonic resealing, the drug was trapped in the cells. Validation tests were carried out on loading method, and the results indicated a remarkable degree of accuracy, precision and reproducibility *(42)*.

In vitro characterisation of rat erythrocytes loaded with metronidazole by a method based on hypotonic pre-swelling, haemolysis, isotonic resealing and re-annealing was studied. The effects of glutaraldehyde concentration upon various parameters of loaded cells were also investigated. Encapsulation efficiency of 42–56% was achieved. The loaded cells exhibited elevated osmotic fragility and lower resistance to turbulence shock as compared with normal cells and were found to release encapsulated drug slowly. Glutaraldehyde treatment of cells resulted in the stabilisation of loaded cells, which were found to be highly resistant to osmotic and turbulence shocks. *In vitro* release of metronidazole was also retarded upon treatment, and was dependent upon the concentration of glutaraldehyde *(37)*. Similar studies conducted with primaquin showed increased hepatic concentrations of unmetabolised primaquine and a nearly twofold increase in hepatic half-life when glutaraldehyde treated erythrocytes were administered to rats *(37,12)*. Erythrocytes loaded with thyroxine were found more effective in restoring and maintaining basal metabolic rates than free compound when studied as a slow release system *in vivo* in thyroidectomised rats. Administration of encapsulated thyroxine also allowed a larger increase in body mass over experimental period, compared with control *(41)*. Drugs encapsulated in erythrocytes using this method include propranolol *(9)*, asparginase *(14)*, cycloposphamide, cortisol-21-phosphate *(22,35)*, 1-anti-trypsin *(35)*, methotrexate, insulin *(35,43)*, metronidazole *(37)* and enalaprilat *(42)*.

Using same method with some modifications, magnetically guided rat erythrocytes were loaded with isoniazid, and studied for drug, ferrosoferric oxide (magnetite) and haemoglobin content, percent cell recovery, morphology, osmotic fragility, turbulence shock, drug and haemoglobin efflux and magnetic response in rats. No appreciable detrimental effect on cell morphology, osmotic fragility and turbulence shock in comparison with normal cells was noted. Drug release from system followed approximately zero order kinetics. The drug and ferrosoferric oxide loaded cells effectively responded to an external magnetic field of 8 *K·Oe*. *In vivo* studies demonstrated that the erythrocyte-based system has potential to increase drug concentrations many fold at a target site under influence of an external magnetic field *(44)*.

3.2.5. Hypotonic Dialysis

This method was first reported by Klibansky *(45)* in 1959 and was used in 1977 by Deloach and Ihler *(36)* and Dale *(46)* for loading enzymes and lipids. Several methods are based on the principle that semi-permeable dialysis membrane maximises intra-cellular:extra-cellular volume ratio for macromolecules during lysis and resealing. In the process, an isotonic, buffered suspension of erythrocytes with a haematocrit value of 70–80 is prepared and placed in a conventional dialysis tube immersed in 10–20 volumes of a hypotonic buffer. The medium is agitated slowly for 2 h. The tonicity of dialysis tube is restored by directly adding a calculated amount of a hypertonic buffer to surrounding medium or by replacing surrounding medium by isotonic buffer *(19,36)*. The drug to be loaded can be added by either dissolving the drug in isotonic cell suspending buffer inside a dialysis bag at beginning of experiment *(17,19,47,48)* or by adding the drug to a dialysis bag after stirring is complete *(49–52)*.

The use of standard haemodialysis equipment for loading a drug in erythrocytes was reported by Zanella *et al. (53)*. In this method, the erythrocyte suspension and drug to be loaded were placed in blood compartment and hypotonic buffer was placed in a receptor compartment. This led to the concept of "continuous flow dialysis", which has been used by several other researchers *(53–58)*. The loaded cells exhibit same circulation half-life as that of normal cells *(3,5)*. Also, this method has high entrapment efficiency on order of 30–50% *(24,32,36)*, cell recovery of 70–80%, high-loading capacity *(49,53)* and is amenable to automation with control of process variables *(32,59)*. The drawbacks include a long processing time and need for special equipment *(19)*. This method has been used for loading enzymes such as β-galactosidase, glucocerebrosidase *(35)*, asparginase *(48)*, inositol hexaphosphatase *(55,57,58)*, as well as drugs such as gentamicin *(17)*, adriamycin *(47)*, pentamidine and furamycin *(50)*, interlukin-2 (IL-2) *(51)* and desferroxamine *(49,53,54,56)*.

The effects of encapsulation by hypotonic dialysis method on stability of recombinant human erythropoietin encapsulated resealed erythrocytes were studied. With encapsulation yields of 22% for human erythrocytes and

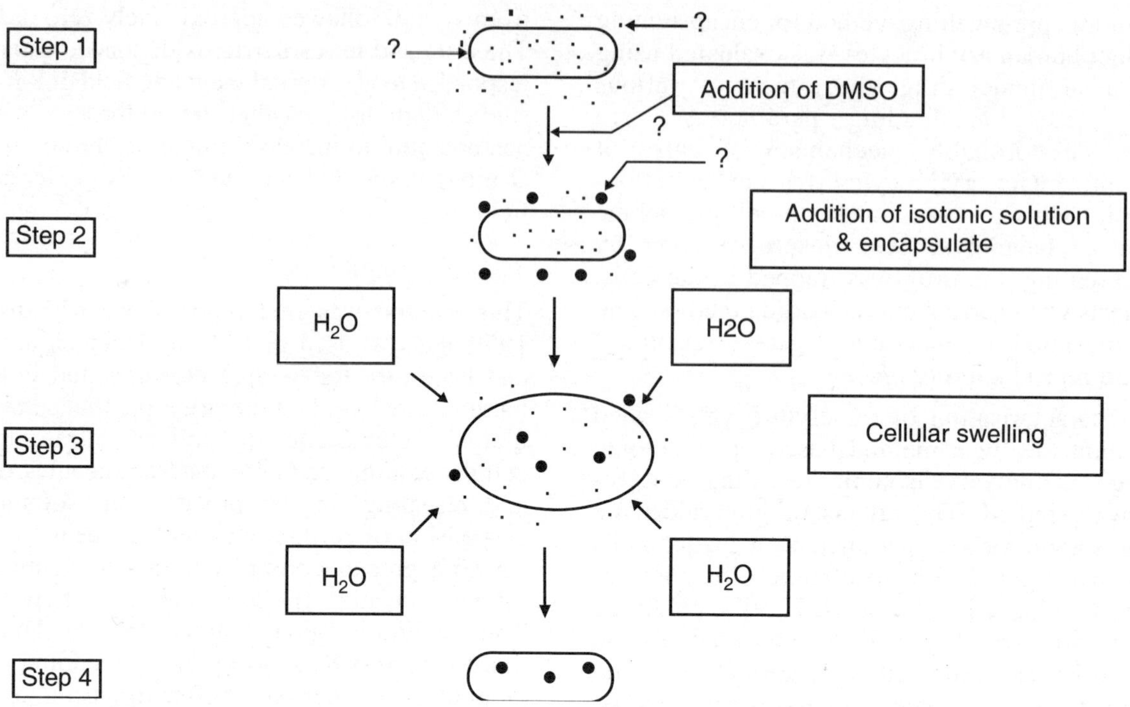

Fig. 2. Schematic representation of drug loading in to ghost erythrocyte by osmotic pulse method.

14% for mouse erythrocytes, the cell recovery was around 70%. Carrier erythrocytes exhibited a tendency to spherocytic morphology and showed higher hypo-osmotic resistance than normal erythrocytes. The presence of erythropoietin inside the carrier erythrocytes was identified. The stability of encapsulated erythropoietin seemed to be related to conditions used during encapsulation *(60)*. Erythrocyte-loaded asparginase was found much more effective in eliminating plasma aspargine, compared with same dose of free asparginase injected in solution during a period of 14 day in mice. It was concluded that use of erythrocytes as carriers for asparginase resulted in increased enzyme efficacy in mice *(48)*.

3.2.6. Isotonic Osmotic Lysis

This method, also known as 'osmotic pulse method', involves isotonic haemolysis that is achieved by physical or chemical means. In physical method, erythrocytes are subjected to transient electric field to cause increase in membrane permeability, in order to allow the solute to diffuse into cells. Kinosita Jr., and Tsong reported haemolysis of human erythrocytes by transient electric field to cause a continuous penetration of solutes toward equilibrium leading to swelling of cells *(60a)*. This effect observed was similar to haemolytic experiments reported earlier with human erythrocytes pulsed in an isotonic NaCl solution *(61,62)*. This effect could be explained by alteration of cell cytoskeleton, due to ATP and GTP leakage during electropulsation.

In chemical method, chemicals such as urea solution *(61)*, polyethylene glycol *(62)* and ammonium chloride have been used for isotonic haemolysis. However, this method also is not immune to changes in membrane structure composition. In 1987, Franco *et al.* developed a method that involved suspending erythrocytes in an isotonic solution of dimethyl sulfoxide *(63)*. The suspension was diluted with an isotonic-buffered drug solution. After the cells were separated, they were resealed at 37°C. A schematic representation of general method (Fig. 2) involving 'osmotic pulse' was described by Magnani *(31a)*.

3.2.7. Chemical Perturbation of Membrane

This method is based on increase in membrane permeability of erythrocytes when the cells are exposed to certain chemicals. In 1973, Deuticke *et al.* showed that the permeability of erythrocytic membrane increases upon exposure to polyene antibiotic such as amphotericin B *(64)*. In 1980, this method was used successfully by Kitao and Hattori *(65)* to entrap anti-neoplastic drug daunomycin in human and mouse erythrocytes. Lin *et al.* used halothane for same purpose *(66)*. However, these methods induce irreversible destructive changes in cell membrane and hence are not very popular.

3.2.8. *Electro-Insertion or Electroencapsulation*

In 1973, Zimmermann tried an electrical pulse method to encapsulate bioactive molecules *(30)*. Also known as electroporation, the method is based on observation that electrical shock brings about irreversible changes in an erythrocyte membrane. In 1977, Tsong and Kinosita *(67)* suggested the use of transient electrolysis to generate desirable membrane permeability for drug loading. The erythrocyte membrane is opened by a dielectric breakdown. Subsequently, the pores can be resealed by incubation at 37°C in an isotonic medium. The procedure involves suspending erythrocytes in isotonic buffer in electrical discharge chamber. A capacitor in an external circuit is charged to a definite voltage and then discharged within a definite time interval through cell suspension to produce a square-wave potential *(24,23)*. The optimum intensity of an electric field is between 1 and 10 kW/cm and optimal discharge time is between 20 and 160 μs *(68–70)*. An inverse relationship exists between electric field intensity and discharge time *(24,27)*. The compound to be entrapped is added to a medium in which cells are suspended from commencement of experiment. The characteristic pore diameter created in membrane depends upon intensity of electric field, discharge time and ionic strength of suspending medium *(68,71)*.

The colloidal macromolecules contents of cell may lead to cell lysis because of increase in osmotic pressure. This process can be prevented by adding large molecules (e.g., tetrasaccharide stachyose and bovine serum albumin) and ribonuclease. One advantage of this method is a more uniform distribution of loaded cells in comparison with osmotic method *(24)*. The main drawbacks are need for special instrumentation and sophistication of the process *(4,17,12,32)*. Entrapment efficiency of this method is approximately 35% *(21)*, and life span of resealed cells in circulation is comparable with that of normal cells *(23,24)*. Various compounds such as sucrose *(23,72)*, urease *(72)*, methotrexate *(70)*, isoniazide *(73)*, human glycophorin *(74)*, DNA fragments and latex particles of diameter 0.2 μm can be entrapped within erythrocytes by this method. Mangal and Kaur achieved sustained release of a drug entrapped in erythrocytes with use of electroporation *(75)*.

3.2.9. *Entrapment by Endocytosis*

This method was reported by Schrier *et al. (76)* in 1975. Endocytosis involves addition of 1 volume of washed packed erythrocytes to 9 volume of buffer containing 2.5 m*M* ATP, 2.5 m*M* $MgCl_2$ and 1m*M* $CaCl_2$, followed by incubation for 2 min at room temperature. The pores created by this method are resealed by using 154 m*M* of NaCl and incubation at 37°C for 2 min. The entrapment of material occurs by endocytosis. The vesicle membrane separates endocytosed material from cytoplasm thus protecting it from the erythrocytes and vice-versa.

Various compounds entrapped by this method include primaquine and related 8-amino-quinolines, vinblastine, chlorpromazine and related phenothiazines, hydrocortisone, propranolol, tetracaine and vitamin A *(77,78)*.

3.2.10. *Loading by Electric Cell Fusion*

This method involves initial loading of drug molecules into erythrocytic ghosts [EGs] followed by adhesion of these cells to target cells. The fusion is accentuated by application of an electric pulse, which causes release of an entrapped molecule. An example of this method is loading a cell-specific monoclonal antibody into EG *(70,79)*. An antibody against a specific surface protein of target cells can be chemically cross-linked to drug-loaded cells that would direct these cells to desired cells.

3.2.11. *Loading by Lipid Fusion*

Lipid vesicles containing a drug can be directly fused to human erythrocytes, which leads to an exchange with a lipid-entrapped drug. This technique was used for entrapping inositol monophosphate to improve oxygen carrying capacity of cells *(80)*. However, the entrapment efficiency of this method is very low (1%).

4. *IN VITRO* CHARACTERISATION

In vivo performance of resealed erythrocytes is affected to a great extent by their biological properties. Hence, *in vitro* characterisation forms an important part of studies involving such cellular carriers. Table 1 summarises various evaluation parameters and techniques applied for their determination. The morphology of erythrocytes decides their life span after administration. Light microscopy reveals no observable change in resealed cells

Table 1. Characterisation Parameters and Methods for Resealed Erythrocytes

Type of characterisation	*Parameter*	*Method/instrument used*
Physical characterisation	Shape and surface morphology	Transmission electron microscopy, scanning electron microscopy, phase contrast microscopy, optical microscopy
	Vesicle size and size distribution	Transmission electron microscopy, optical microscopy
	Drug release	Diffusion cell, dialysis
	Drug content	De-proteinisation of cell membrane followed by assay of resealed drug, radiolabelling
	Surface electrical potential	ζ-potential measurement
	Deformability	Capillary method
Cellular characterisation	Percentage of Hb content	De-proteinisation of cell membrane followed by haemoglobin assay
	Cell volume	Laser light scattering
	Percentage of cell recovery	Neubaur's chamber, haematological analyser
	Osmotic fragility	Stepwise incubation with isotonic to hypotonic saline solutions and determination of drug and haemoglobin assay
	Osmotic shock	Dilution with distilled water and estimation of drug and haemoglobin
	Turbulent shock	Passage of cell suspension through 30-gauge hypodermic needle at 10 mL/min flow rate and estimation of residual drug and haemoglobin, vigorous shaking followed by haemoglobin estimation
	Erythrocyte sedimentation rate (ESR)	ESR methods
Biological characterisation	Sterility	Sterility test
	Pyrogenicity	Rabbit method, limulus amebocyte lysate (LAL) test
	Animal toxicity	Toxicity study

(12,36) but in few cases spherical erythrocytes (spherocytes) are detected *(21,44)*. Scanning electron microscopic studies have shown that a majority of cells maintain their biconcave discoid shapes after loading procedure *(52)*, and few stomatocytes, a form of spherocytes with an invagination in one point are formed *(60)*. In some cases, cells of smaller size (microcyte) are also observed *(58)*.

Shape change (deformability) is another factor that affects life span of cells. This parameter evaluates ease of passage of erythrocytes through narrow capillaries and RES. It determines rheological behavior of the cells and depends on visco-elasticity of cell membrane, viscosity of cell contents, and cellular surface-to-volume ratio *(49)*. The deformability is measured by passage time of definite volume of cells through capillary of 4 μm diameter or polycarbonate filter with average pore size of 45 μm *(49,53)*. Another indirect approach is to evaluate chlorpromazine induced shape changes turbidimetrically *(81)*.

The osmotic fragility of resealed erythrocytes is an indicator of possible changes in cell membrane integrity and resistance of these cells to osmotic pressure of suspension medium. The test is carried out by suspending cells in a media of varying sodium chloride centration and determining the haemoglobin released *(12,81)*. In most cases, osmotic fragility of resealed cells is higher than that of normal cells because of increased intracellular osmotic pressure *(21,30,37,44,60,81)*. The turbulence fragility is yet another characteristic that depends upon changes in integrity of cellular membrane and reflects resistance of loaded cells against haemolysis resulting from turbulent flow within circulation. It is determined by passage of cell suspension through needles with smaller internal diameter (e.g., 30 gauge) *(12,21,37,44)* or vigorously shaking cell suspension *(81)*. In both methods, haemoglobin and drug released after procedure are determined and turbulent fragility of resealed cells is found to be higher. Routine clinical haematological tests also can be carried out for drug-loaded cells, including mean corpuscular volume, mean corpuscular haemoglobin and mean corpuscular haemoglobin content. Studies have shown that average size and haemoglobin content of resealed cells is lower than that of normal cells *(48,52,53,58,60,81)*. Drug content of cells determines entrapment efficiency of method used. The process involves de-proteinisation of packed, loaded cells (0.5 mL) with 2.0 mL acetonitrile and centrifugation at 2500 rpm (~300*g*) for 10 min. The clear supernatant is analysed for drug content *(82)*.

4.1. Drug Release From Loaded Erythrocytes

The most important parameters for evaluation of resealed erythrocytes is drug release pattern. Haemoglobin is also invariably released because drug release involves loss of cell membrane integrity indicating haemolysis. On basis of various *in vitro* release experiments carried out on these cells, three general drug release patterns are observed:

- The rate of drug release is considerably higher than that of haemoglobin. In other words, drug diffuses readily. Such a pattern is shown by lipophilic drugs, including methotrexate, phenytoin, dexamethasone *(10)*, primpquine *(12)* and vitamin B_{12} *(83)*. Cell lysis is not essential for release of such drugs.
- The rate of drug release is comparable with that of haemoglobin. This indicates that cell lysis is essential for drug release and drug can not be released by mere diffusion. Polar drugs such as gentamicin, heparin *(10,17)* and enalaprilat *(33)* and enzymes such as asparginase *(7,14,38,48)*, peptides, including urogasterone and L-lysine-L-phenylalanine *(84)* follow such pattern.
- The rate of drug release lies between aforementioned two extremes; for example, propranolol, isoniazid, metronidazole and recombinant human erythropoietin *(10,21,37,44,60)*.

Two factors that determine drug release pattern are size and polarity of drug molecule *(10)*. The release rate can be modified by cross-linking cell membrane with gluteraldehyde *(26,37)*, which results in a slower drug release. This can also be achieved by entrapping biodegradable prodrug such as *o*-acetyl propranolol, *o*-pivaloyl propranolol, cortisol-21-phosphate, prednisolone-21-sodium succinate and cytosine arabinoside monophosphate *(9,22,35,85)*. The complexation of a drug with macromolecules such as dextran and albumin also retard release rate *(33)*.

5. APPLICATIONS OF RESEALED ERYTHROCYTES

Resealed erythrocytes have several possible applications in various fields of human and veterinary medicine. Such cells could be used as circulating carriers to disseminate a drug within a prolonged period of time in circulation or in target-specific organs, including liver, spleen and lymph nodes. A majority of drug delivery studies using drug-loaded erythrocytes are in the pre-clinical phase. In a few clinical studies, successful results were obtained *(54,86–88)*.

5.1. Modified Release

Erythrocytes have been used as circulating depots for sustained delivery of antineoplastics *(89–92)*, antiparasitics *(11,36,50)*, veterinary antiamoebics *(7)*, vitamins *(83)*, steroids *(26,22,34)*, antibiotics *(21,44,64)* and cardiovascular drugs *(81,93)*. Various mechanisms proposed for drug release include:

- Passive diffusion.
- Specialised membrane associated carrier transport.
- Phagocytosis of resealed cells by macrophages of RES, subsequent accumulation of drug into macrophage, followed by slow release *(5,12)*.
- Accumulation of erythrocytes in lymph nodes upon subcutaneous administration followed by haemolysis to release drug *(51)*.

Routes of administration include intravenous (iv), which is most common, followed by subcutaneous, intra-peritoneal (i.p.), intranasal and oral *(5)*. Studies regarding improved efficacy of various drugs given in this form in animal models have been published. Examples include an enhancement in antiinflammatory effect of corticosteroids in experimentally inflamed rats *(22,26)*, increase in half-life of isoniazid *(21,44)*, levothyroxine *(41)*, cytosine arabinoside *(90)* and IL-2 *(51)* prolongation of plasma half-life of erythropoietin from 30 min to 35 h in mice *(60)*, and can increase in mean survival time of mice with experimental hepatoma after injecting methotrexate loaded erythrocytes *(89)*. Thalassemic patients, because of multiple blood transfusions, are prone to haemosydrosis, a disease state associated with an excess storage of iron *(94)*. This state is treated using subcutaneous (sc) or iv injections of iron-chelating compound desferrioxamine, which causes severe adverse effects in case of multiple injections *(54)*. This agent was loaded on to erythrocytes and performance of these cells upon re-injection was observed and found to be promising *(53,54)*. This therapeutic method is approved in the United States as regular management tool of haemosydrosis since 1984 *(13)*.

Erythrocyte-based bioadhesive system for controlled systemic delivery of propranolol hydrochloride through nasal route was formulated and evaluated *in vitro* for release, diffusion, bioadhesion and morphological characteristics, and for release in rats. Results indicated that propranolol was released slowly, and this rate depended on degree of cross-linking of erythrocytes. The system was found to possess good bioadhesive properties. *In vivo* studies revealed constant plasma levels for up to 10 h. It was concluded that this system may have potential for controlled systemic delivery of propranolol *(82)*.

5.2. Drug Targeting

Ideally, drug delivery should be site-specific and target-oriented to exhibit maximal therapeutic index with minimum adverse effects. Resealed erythrocytes can act as drug carriers and targeting tools as well. Surface-modified erythrocytes are used to target organs of mononuclear phagocytic system/RES because changes in membrane are recognised by macrophages *(95)*. However, resealed erythrocytes also can be used to target organs other than those of RES. Figure 3 presents erythrocyte-mediated delivery of ubiquitin K48R for Inhibition of NF-kB activation in macrophages *(95a)*.

5.2.1. Targeting RES Organs

Damaged erythrocytes are rapidly cleared from circulation by phagocytic Kupffer cells in liver and spleen. Resealed erythrocytes, by modifying their membranes, can therefore be used to target liver and spleen. Various approaches to modify surface characteristics of erythrocytes include:

- Surface modification with antibodies.
- Surface modification with gluteraldehyde.
- Surface modification with carbohydrates such as sialic acid *(95)*.
- Surface modification with sulphydryl.
- Surface chemical cross-linking, for example, delivery of ^{125}I-labelled carbonic anhydrase loaded in erythrocytes cross-linked with *bis*-sulfosuccinimidyl) suberate and 3,3 dithio(sulfosuccinmidyl propionate) *(96)*.

The clearance of gentamicin loaded carrier erythrocytes from circulation that were prepared by hypoosmotic dialysis and sensitised with anti-Rh antibody was studied *(97)*. The results indicated that rapid drug delivery to RES by antibody sensitised carrier erythrocytes is possible, but small volumes of erythrocytes seem more efficient *(17)*.

Two types of surface modified erythrocytes containing methotrexate were prepared for enhanced macrophage uptake, and loaded erythrocytes were studied *in vitro* and in rats. Macrophage uptake was determined *in vitro*, and *in vivo* organ localisation was assessed by recording amount of drug present in different organs. The macrophage uptake of surface modified erythrocytes was enhanced by 3–6 times. These new surface modified carriers were found to be excellent candidates for enhanced macrophage uptake and anticipated to be useful for RES tumours *(98)*.

The usefulness of erythrocyte membrane as a biodegradable carrier for i.v. injection of doxorubicin was studied by examining pharmacokinetics and tissue distribution of doxorubicin hydrochloride in rats following injection of 9.5 mg/kg in suspensions prepared from EG and erythrocyte vesicles (EV). The area under curve of amount in the heart vs time for EG–doxorubicin was approximately same as for the doxorubicin alone. However, the amount of doxorubicin in heart after EV–doxorubicin was below the sensitivity of detection. The fraction of doxorubicin excreted unchanged in urine was quite low for EV–doxorubicin in comparison with EG–doxorubicin and doxorubicin alone. The uptake of drug by spleen was increased after administration of EV–doxorubicin indicating usefulness of these delivery systems for doxorubicin *(91)*.

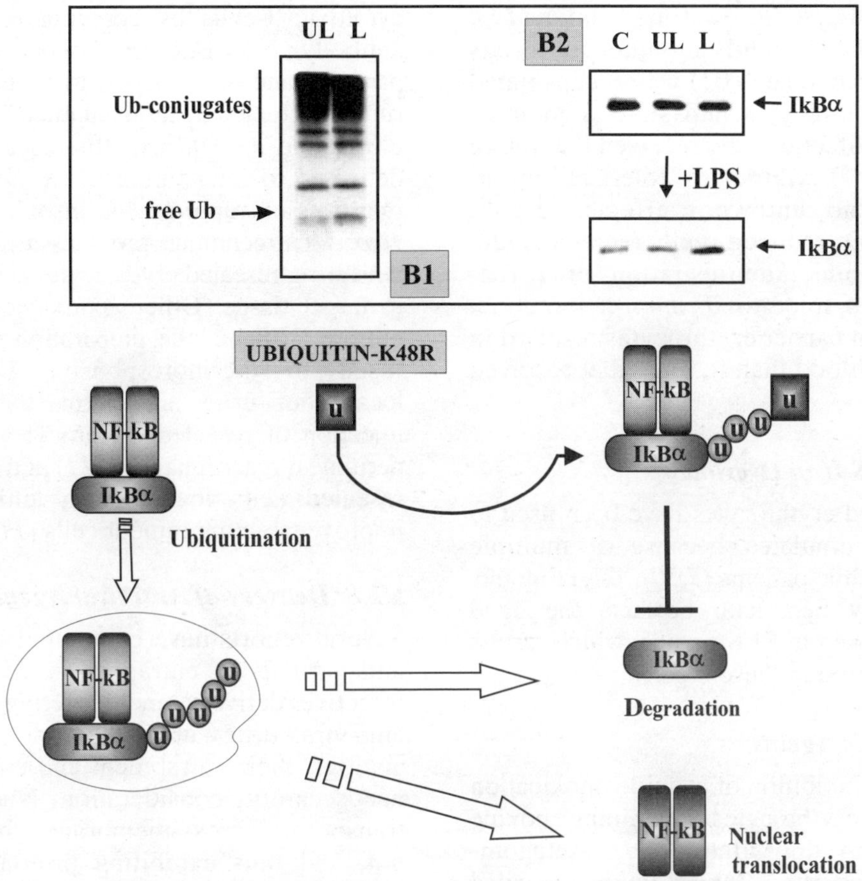

Fig. 3. Inhibition of NF-kB activation in macrophages by erythrocyte-mediated delivery of ubiquitin K48R. Recombinant ubiquitin K48R was encapsulated into human erythrocytes. The loaded erythrocytes were then modified to increase their uptake by macrophages resulting in transfer of ubiquitin K48R into the macrophages (B1). Stimulation of macrophages by lipopolysaccaride (LPS) results in inhibition of IkB degradation (B2) and abrogation of NF-kB activation. In lower panel, the mechanism of action of ubiquitin K48R is shown. The ubiquitin analogue once added to a polyubiquitin chain prevents its further elongation and degradation of target substrate by 26S proteasome *(95a)*.

5.2.2. Targeting Liver: Enzyme Deficiency/ Replacement Therapy

Many metabolic disorders related to deficient or missing enzymes can be treated by injecting these enzymes. However, the problems of exogenous enzyme therapy include a shorter circulation half-life of enzymes, allergic reactions and toxic manifestations. These problems can be successfully overcome by administering enzymes as resealed erythrocytes. The enzymes used include β-glucosidase, β-glucoronidase and β-galactosidase *(7,17,36)*. The disease caused by an accumulation of glucocerebrosides in liver and spleen can be treated by glucocerebrosidase-loaded erythrocytes *(99)*.

5.2.3. Treatment of Hepatic Tumours

Hepatic tumours are one of the most prevalent types of cancer. Anti-neoplastic drugs such as methotrexate, bleomycin, asparginase and adriamycin have been successfully delivered by erythrocytes *(7,8,24,30, 47,91,100)*. Agents such as daunorubicin diffuse rapidly from cells upon loading and hence pose a problem. This problem can be overcome by covalently linking daunorubicin to erythrocytic membrane using gluteraldehyde or cis aconitic acid as a spacer *(101)*. The resealed erythrocytes loaded with carboplatin show localisation in liver *(102)*.

5.2.4. Treatment of Parasitic Diseases

The ability of resealed erythrocytes to selectively accumulate within RES organs make them useful tool during delivery of anti-parasitic agents. Parasitic diseases that involve harbouring parasites in RES organs can be successfully controlled by this method. Results were favourable in studies involving animal models for erythrocytes loaded with antimalarial *(11)*, antileishmanial *(11,17,50)* and antiamoebic drugs *(7,37)*. Imidocarb dipropionate (ID) was encapsulated in murine carrier erythrocytes and studied in mice with *Babesia microti* infection who received 0.2 mg/kg ID by i.p. injection. Erythrocytes tolerated up to 1 mg/mL ID with no untoward effects. Higher concentrations of ID reduced cell recovery and mean cell haemoglobin. Administration of I reduced susceptibility of mice to *B. microti* infection. Encapsulation of ID in carrier erythrocytes resulted in higher drug levels in blood than in mice that received free ID *(103)*.

5.2.5. Removal of RES Iron Overload

Desferrioxamine-loaded erythrocytes have been used to treat excess iron accumulated because of multiple transfusions to thalassemic patients *(7,50)*. Targeting this drug to RES is very beneficial because the aged erythrocytes are destroyed in RES organs, which results in an accumulation of iron in these organs.

5.2.6. Removal of Toxic Agents

Cannon *et al.* reported inhibition of cyanide intoxication with murine carrier erythrocytes containing bovine rhodanase and sodium thiosulfate *(104)*. Antagonisation of organophosphorus intoxication by resealed erythrocytes containing a recombinant phosphodiestrase also has been reported *(105)*.

5.2.7. Targeting Organs Other Than Those of RES

Recently, resealed erythrocytes have been used to target organs outside RES. The various approaches include:

- Entrapment of paramagnetic particles along with drug.
- Entrapment of photosensitive material.
- Use of ultrasound waves.
- Antibody attachment to erythrocyte membrane for site specific drug action.

Zimmermann proposed that entrapment of small paramagnetic particles into erythrocytes might allow their localisation to a particular location under influence of an external magnetic field *(69)*. The loading of ferrofluids (colloidal suspension of magnetite) has been reported by Sprandel *et al.* *(106)*. Jain and Vyas reported entrapment of the anti-inflammatory drugs diclofenac sodium and ibuprofen in magnetoresponsive erythrocytes *(107)* . Photosensitised erythrocytes have been studied as a phototriggered carrier and delivery system for methotrexate in cancer treatment *(108)*. Chiarantini *et al.* have reported *in vitro* targeting of erythrocytes to cytotoxic T-cells by coupling of Thy-1.2 monoclonal antibody *(109)*. Price *et al.* reported delivery of colloidal particles and erythrocytes to tissue through microvessel ruptures created by targeted microbubble destruction with ultrasound *(110)*. i.v. fluorescent erythrocytes were delivered to interstitium of rat skeletal muscle through microvessel ruptures by insonifying microbubbles *in vivo*. This technique provides a non-invasive means for delivering resealed erythrocytes across endothelial carrier to target tissue. Other approaches for targeting organs outside RES include preparation of carrier erythrocytes fused to thermoresponsive liposomes and their localisation using an external thermal source *(24)*, i.p. injection of resealed erythrocytes for drug targeting to peritoneal macrophages *(111)* and lectin pre-treatment of resealed cells loaded with anti-neoplastic drugs to improve targeting tumour cells *(112)*.

5.2.8. Delivery of AntiViral Agents

Several reports have been cited in the literature about anti-viral agents entrapped in resealed erythrocytes for effective delivery and targeting *(33)*. Because most anti-viral drugs are either nucleotides or nucleoside analogs, their entrapment and exit through membrane needs careful consideration. Nucleosides are rapidly transported across membrane whereas nucleotides are not, and thus exhibiting prolonged release profiles. The release of nucleotides requires conversion of these moieties to purine or pyrimidine bases. Resealed erythrocytes have been used to deliver deoxycytidine derivatives, recombinant herpes simplex virus type 1 glycoprotein B *(109)*, azidothymidine derivatives *(113)*, azathioprene, acyclovir *(114)* and fludarabine phosphate *(115)*.

5.3. Protein Delivery

The mode of interaction of human insulin (Humulin R) with erythrocyte membrane in form of ghosts, vesicles (ultrasonicated ghosts), lipid-coated-ghosts or lipid-coated-vesicles, were studied and evaluated for their use as carrier systems for insulin *in vivo*. Humulin R was incubated with either one of four above preparations. Humulin R was found to associate with ghosts by two mechanisms, encapsulation and adsorption on surface. Insulin binding reached equilibrium with a much faster rate with ghosts than other carriers due to these two mechanisms. It was concluded that the use of these carrier-insulin systems may be of value in delivery of insulin for treatment of diabetes *(116)*. Kentaro Kogurea *(116a)* demonstrated the delivery of superoxide dismutase (SOD) or Rhodamine-labelled ovalbumin (R-Ov) by encapsulating it in membrane fusible erythrocyte ghosts (MFEG) in to pretreated monkey kidney normal cells (CV-1) and human cervical tumor cells (HeLa) and studied influence of SOD on adriamycin (ADM) cytotoxicity after pretreatment of cells.

In another study by same author for use of erythrocytes as oral carriers for Humulin R was evaluated in diabetic rats after oral administration of 100 U insulin solution, an erythrocyte-ghosts-insulin suspension, an erythrocyte-vesicles-insulin suspension, a liposomes-ghosts-insulin suspension, a liposomes-vesicles-insulin suspension and control vehicles. All treatment groups, except liposomes-ghosts-insulin, were significantly different statistically from their respective controls. The erythrocyte-ghosts carrier showed highest hypoglycemic response *(117)*.

5.3.1. Enzyme Therapy

Enzymes are widely used in clinical practice as replacement therapies to treat diseases associated with their deficiency (e.g., Gaucher's disease, galactosuria), degradation of toxic compounds secondary to some kind of poisoning (cyanide and organophosphorus) and as drugs *(43)*. The problems involved in direct injection of enzymes into body have been cited. One method to overcome these problems is use of enzyme-loaded erythrocytes *(24,29)*. These cells then release enzymes into circulation upon haemolysis *(8,24)*, act as a "circulating bioreactors" in which substrates enter into the cell, interact with enzymes, and generate products *(118,119)*, or accumulate enzymes in RES upon haemolysis for future catalysis.

The first report of successful clinical trials of resealed erythrocytes loaded with enzymes for replacement therapy is that of β-glucoserebrosidase for treatment of Gaucher's disease *(88)*. The disease is characterised by inborn deficiency of lysosomal β-glucoserebrosidase in cells of RES thereby leading to accumulation of β-glucoserebrosides in macrophages of the RES. The most important application of resealed erythrocytes in enzyme therapy is that of asparginase loading for treatment of pediatric neoplasms. This enzyme degrades aspargine, an amino acid vital for cells. This treatment prevents remission of pediatric acute lymphocytic leukaemia *(120)*. There are reports of improved intensity and duration of action in animal models *(8,14,38,48)* as well as humans *(5)*.

To treat lead poisoning, the concentration of β-aminolevulinate dehydrogenase (ALA-D) in erythrocytes decreases. This leads to an accumulation of β-aminolevulinic acid in tissues, blood and urine. This state leads to acute porphyria and central nervous system related problems *(121)*. An injection of resealed erythrocytes loaded with ALA–D to lead intoxicated animal significantly reduces toxic manifestations *(122)*. Other enzymes used for loading resealed erythrocytes include urease *(72)*, galactose-1-phosphate uridyl transferase *(87)*, uricase *(119)* and acetaldehyde dehydrogenase *(120)*.

5.3.2. Improvement in Oxygen Delivery to Tissues

Haemoglobin is the protein responsible for oxygen-carrying capacity of erythrocytes. Under normal conditions, 95% of haemoglobin is saturated with oxygen in the lungs, whereas under physiologic conditions in peripheral blood stream only 25% of oxygenated haemoglobin becomes de-oxygenated. Thus, the major fraction of oxygen bound to haemoglobin is re-circulated with venous blood to the lungs. The use of this bound fraction has been suggested for treatment of oxygen deficiency. 2,3-diphosphoglycerate (2,3-DPG) is a natural effectors of haemoglobin. The binding affinity of haemoglobin for oxygen changes reversibly with changes in intra-cellular concentration of 2,3-DPG. This compensates for changes in oxygen pressure outside body, as affinity of 2,3-DPG to oxygen is much higher than that of haemoglobin *(122)*.

Other organic polyphosphates can serve as allosteric effectors of haemoglobin with binding affinities higher than those of 2,3-DPG and can compete with 2,3-DPG for binding to haemoglobin *(55)*. Inositol hexophosphate (IHP) is one of the strongest effectors of this type *(123)*. However, because of its ionisation at physiologic pH, it cannot enter erythrocytes *(58,123)*. Hence, it is entrapped by electroporation process. Upon encapsulation, IHP irreversibly binds to haemoglobin, thereby decreasing oxygen affinity to haemoglobin and subsequent shift of oxygen binding isotherm to right *(24)*. As a result, the oxygen pressure corresponding to 50% of total binding capacity of haemoglobin to oxygen (P50 value) increases from 26–27 mmHg to 50 mmHg *(58)*. In presence of IHP encapsulated in erythrocytes, the difference between oxygen bound fraction of haemoglobin in lungs and tissues increases, thereby increasing oxygen concentration in tissues. Also, the extent of carbamate formed in N-terminal amine group of β-chain of haemoglobin decreases, which is compensated by an uptake of H and CO_2 that leads to increased formation of bicarbonate ion. Intravenous injection of IHP-loaded erythrocytes to piglets led to a decrease in cardiac output with a constant oxygen consumption by animals *(58,124)*. This indicates that because of an increased extraction ratio of oxygen by tissues, a given amount of oxygen can be delivered in lower blood flow. In addition, these erythrocytes reduce ejection fraction, left ventricular diastolic volume and heart rate *(57)*. An isolated perfused-heart model showed reduction in coronary blood flow with increased oxygen consumption by myocardium upon administration of IHP-loaded erythrocytes *(125–127)*. The same results are reported when intact animal models were used *(128)*. An application of IHP-loaded erythrocytes for improved oxygen supply is beneficial under following conditions:

- High altitude conditions where partial pressure of oxygen is low.
- Reduction in number of alveoli, where exchange surface of lungs is decreased.
- Increased resistance to oxygen diffusion in lungs.
- Reduction in oxygen transport capacity.
- Mutation or chemical modification, which involves a decrease in oxygen affinity for haemoglobin.
- Increased radiosensitivity of radiation-sensitive tumours.
- Restoration of oxygen-delivery capacity of stored blood.
- Ischemia of myocardium, brain or other tissues *(125)*.

5.3.3. Microinjection of Macromolecules

Biological functions of macromolecules such as DNA, RNA and proteins are exploited for various cell biological applications. Hence, various methods are used to entrap these macromolecules into cultured cells (e.g., microinjection) *(129–131)*. McClung and Kletzien adopted microinjection with chicken erythrocyte ghosts as vehicles for introduction of protein into the cytosol of large populations of cells *(131a)*. The method was used to study the effect of catalytic subunit (C) of cyclic AMP-dependent protein kinase on cell growth kinetics of BHK cells. Schematic diagram of the microinjection procedure is given in Fig. 4. The advantage in using chicken erythrocytes for microinjection is that inactive erythrocyte nuclei serve as a probe for identifying and analyzing microinjection events.

A relatively simple structure and a lack of complex cellular components (e.g., nucleus) in erythrocytes make them good candidates for entrapment of macromolecules *(132)*.

In microinjection, erythrocytes are used as micro-syringes for injection to host cells *(4)*. The micro-injection process involves culturing host eukaryotic cells *in vitro*. The cells are coated with fusogenic agent and

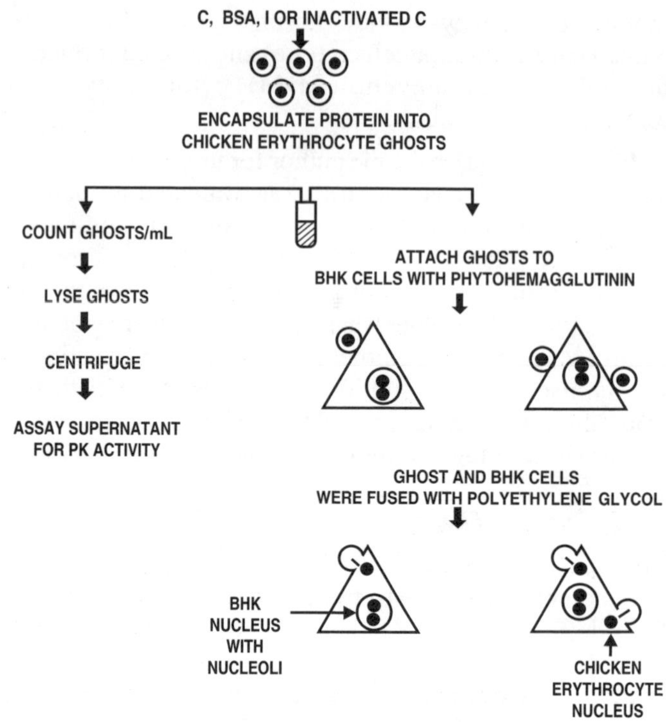

Fig. 4. Schematic diagram of microinjection procedure (PK, protein kinase; C, catalytic subunit of cyclic AMP).

then suspended with erythrocytes loaded with compound of interest in an isotonic medium. Sendai virus (haemagglutinating virus of Japan, HVJ) or its glycoproteins or polyethylene glycol have been used as fusogenic agents *(132,133)*. The fusogen causes fusion of co-suspended erythrocytes and eukaryotic cells. Thus, the contents of resealed erythrocytes and compound of interest are transferred to host cell. This procedure has been used to microinject DNA fragments, arginase *(134,135)*, proteins, nucleic acids, ferritin, latex particles, bovine and human serum albumin and enzyme thymidine kinase *(131)* to various eukaryotic cells.

Advantages of this method include quantitative injection of materials into cells, simultaneous introduction of several materials into a large number of cells, minimal damage to cell, avoidance of degradation effects of lysosomal enzymes, and simplicity of technique. Disadvantages include a need for a larger size of fused cells, thus making them amenable to RES clearance, adverse effects of fusogens, unpredictable effects on cell resulting from co-introduction of various components. Hence, this method is limited to mainly cell biological applications rather than drug delivery *(132)*.

6. NOVEL APPROACHES

6.1. Erythrosomes

These are specially engineered vesicular systems that are chemically cross-linked to human erythrocytes support, upon which a lipid bilayer is coated. This process is achieved by modifying a reverse-phase evaporation technique. These vesicles have been proposed as useful encapsulation systems for macromolecular drugs *(136–138)*.

6.1.1. Nanoerythrosomes

These are prepared by extrusion of EGs to produce small vesicles with an average diameter of 100 nm. Daunorubicin was covalently conjugated to nanoerythrosomes using gluteraldehyde spacer. This complex was more active than free daunorubicin alone, both *in vitro* and *in vivo (139,140)*.

7. REFERENCES

1. **Telen, MJ.** The mature erythrocytes, in Winthrob's clinical hematology, (Lee, R., et al. eds.), 9th ed., Lea and Febiger, Philadelphia, 1993, pp. 101–133.
2. **Guyton, AC. and Hall, JE.** Red blood cells, anemia, and polycythemia, in textbook of medical physiology, 10th edition, W.B. Saunders, Philadelphia, 1996, pp. 425–433.
3. **Torotra, GJ. and Grabowski, SR.** The cardiovascular system: the blood, in principles of anatomy and physiology, 7th ed., Harper Collins College Publishers, New York, 1993, pp. 566–590.
4. **Lewis, DA. and Alpar, HO.** Therapeutic possibilities of drugs encapsulated in erythrocytes. *Int. J. Pharm.* 1984;22:137–146.
5. **Jain, S. and Jain, NK.** Engineered erythrocytes as a drug delivery system. *Ind. J. Pharm. Sci.* 1997;59:275–281.
6. **Vyas, SP. and Khar, RK.** Resealed erythrocytes in targeted and controlled drug delivery: novel carrier systems, CBS Publishers and Distributors, India, 2002, pp. 87–416.
7. **Jaitely, V., Kanaujia, P., Venkatesan, N., Jain, S., and Vyas, SP.** Resealed erythrocytes: drug carrier potentials and biomedical applications. *Ind. Drugs* 1996;33:589–594.
8. **Updike, SJ. and Wakamiya, RT.** Infusion of red blood cell-loaded asparaginase in monkey. *J. Lab. Clin. Med.* 1983;101:679–691.
9. **Alpar, HO. and Irwin, WJ.** Some unique applications of erythrocytes as carrier systems. *Adv. Biosci.* (series) 1987;67:1–9.
10. **Eichler, HC., Gasic, S., Daum, B., Bacher, S., and Steger, G.** In vitro drug release from human carrier erythrocytes. *Adv. Biosci.* (series) 1987;67:11–15.
11. **Summers, MP.** Recent advances in drug delivery. *Pharm. J.* 1983;230:643–645.
12. **Talwar, N. and Jain, NK.** Erythrocytes as carriers of primaquin preparation: characterization and evaluation. *J. Control. Release* 1992;20:133–142.
13. **Lewis, DA.** Red blood cells for drug delivery. *Pharm. J.* 1984;233:384–385.
14. **Alpar, HO. and Lewis, DA.** Therapeutic efficacy of asparaginase encapsulated in intact erythrocytes. *Biochem. Pharmacol.* 1985;34:257–261.
15. **Adriaenssens, K., Karcher, D., Lowenthal, A., and Terheggen, HG.** Use of enzyme-loaded erythrocytes in in vitro correction of arginase deficient erythrocytes in familiar hyperargininemia. *Clin. Chem.* 1976;22:323–326.
16. **Sprandel, U.** Towards cellular drug targeting and controlled release of drugs by magnetic fields. *Adv. Biosci.* (series) 1987;67:243–250.
17. **Eichler, HG., Gasic, S., Bauer, K., Korn, A., and Bacher, S.** In vivo clearance of antibody-sensitized human drug carrier erythrocytes. *Clin. Pharmacol. Ther.* 1986;40:300–303.
18. **Baker, R.** Entry of ferritin into human red cells during hypotonic hemolysis. *Nature* 1967;215:424–425.
19. **Ihler, GM. and Tsang, HCW.** Hypotonic hemolysis methods for entrapment of agents in resealed erythrocytes. *Methods Enzymol.* 1987;149:221–229.
20. **Vienken, J., Jeltsch, E., and Zimmermann, U.** Penetration and entrapment of large particles in erythrocytes by electrical breakdown techniques. *Cytobiologie* 1978;17:182–186.
21. **Jain, S., Jain, SK., and Dixit, VK.** Erythrocytes based delivery of isoniazid: preparation and *in vitro* characterization. *Ind. Drugs* 1995;32:471–476.
22. **Pitt, E., Lewis, DA., and Offord, R.** The use of corticosteroids encapsulated in erythrocytes in the treatment of adjuvant induced arthritis in the rat. *Biochem. Pharmacol.* 1983;132:3355–3358.
23. **Kinositav, K. and Tsong, TY.** Survival of sucrose-loaded erythrocytes in the circulation. *Nature* 1978;272:258–260.
24. **Zimmermann, U.** Cellular drug-carrier systems and their possible targeting in targeted drugs, (Goldberg, EP. ed.), John Wiley & Sons, New York, 1983, pp. 153–200.
25. **Schlegel, RA., McEvoy, L., Weiser, M., and Williamson, P.** Phospholipid organization as a determinant of red cell recognition by the reticuloendothelial system. *Adv. Biosci.* (series) 1987;67:173–181.
26. **Jenner, DJ., Lewis, DA., Pitt, E., and Offord, RA.** The effect of the intravenous administration of corticosteroids encapsulated in intact erythrocytes on adjuvant arthritis in the rat. *Br. J. Pharmacol.* 1981;73:212P–213P.

27. **Green, IR. and Widder, KJ.** Methods in enzymology, Academic Press, San Diego, 1987, 149 p.

28. **Gardos, G.** Akkumulation de kalium onen durch menschiche blutkorperchen. *Acta Physiol. Acad. Sci. Hung.* 1953;6:191–196.

29. **Iher, GM., Glew, RM., and Schnure, FW.** Enzyme loading of erythrocytes. *Proc. Natl. Acad. Sci. USA* 1973;70:2663–2666.

30. **Zimmermann, U.** Jahresbericht der kernforschungsanlage julich GmbH, Nuclear Research Center, Julich, 1973, pp. 55–58.

31. **Hamidi, M. and Tajerzadeh, H.** Carrier erythrocytes: an overview. *Drug Deliv.* 2003;10:9–20.

31a. **Magnani, M (ed.).** Erythrocyte engineering for drug delivery and targeting, Biotechnology intelligence unit 6, Plenum publishers, USA, 2003.

32. **Deloach, JR., Harris, RL., and Ihler, GM.** An erythrocyte encapsulator dialyzer used in preparing large quantities of erythrocyte ghosts and encapsulation of a pesticide in erythrocyte ghosts. *Anal. Biochem.* 102:220–227.

33. **Ihler, GM.** Erythrocyte carriers. *Pharmacol. Ther.* 1983;20:151–169.

34. **Magnani, M., Rossi, L., D'ascenzo, M., Panzani, I., Bigi, L., and Zanella, A.** Erythrocyte engineering for drug delivery and targeting. *Biotechnol. Appl. Biochem.* 1998;28:1–6.

35. **Pitt, E., Johnson, CM., Lewis, DA., Jenner, DA., and Offord, RE.** Encapsulation of drugs in intact erythrocytes: an intravenous delivery system. *Biochem. Pharmacol.* 1983;22:3359–3368.

36. **Deloach, JR. and Ihler, GM.** A dialysis procedure for loading of erythrocytes with enzymes and lipids. *Biochim. Biophys. Acta* 1977;496:136–145.

37. **Talwar, N. and Jain, NK.** Erythrocytes as carriers of metronidazole: in-vitro characterization. *Drug Dev. Ind. Pharm.* 1992;18:1799–1812.

38. **Updike, SJ., Wakarniya, RT., and Lightfoot, EN.** Asparaginase entrapped in red blood cells: action and survival. *Science* 1976;193:681–683.

39. **Bhaskaran, S. and Dhir, SS.** Resealed erythrocytes as carriers of salbutamol sulphate. *Ind. J. Pharm. Sci.* 1995;57:240–242.

40. **Rechsteiner, MC.** Uptake of protein by red cells. *Exp. Cell Res.* 1975;43:487–492.

40a. **Aquaro, S., Calio, R., Balzarini, J., Bellocchi, MC., Garaci, E., and Perno, CF.** Macrophages and HIV infection: therapeutical apporaches toword this reservior, *Antivir. Res.*, 2002;55:209–225.

41. **Field, WN., Gamble, MD., and Lewis, DA.** A comparison of treatment of thyroidectomized rats with free thyroxin and thyroxin encapsulated in erythrocytes. *Int. J. Pharm.* 1989;51:175–178.

42. **Tajerzadeh, H. and Hamidi, M.** Evaluation of the hypotonic preswelling method for encapsulation of enalaprilat in human intact erythrocytes. *Drug Dev. Ind. Pharm.* 2000;26:1247–1257.

43. **Bird, J., Best, R., and Lewis, DA.** The encapsulation of insulin in erythrocytes. *J. Pharm. Pharmacol.* 1983;35:246–247.

44. **Jain, S., Jain, SK., and Dixit, VK.** Magnetically guided rat erythrocytes bearing isoniazid: preparation, characterization and evaluation. *Drug Dev. Ind. Pharm.* 1997;23:999–1006.

45. **Klibansky, C. PhD.** thesis, Hebrew University, Jerusalem, Israel, 1959.

46. **Dale, GL., Villacorte, DG., and Beutler, E.** High yield entrapment of protein into erythrocytes. *Biochem. Med.* 1977;18:220–225.

47. **Benatti, U., Zocchl, E., Tonetti, M., Guida, L., and DeFlora, A.** Comparative tissue distribution and metabolism of free versus erythrocyte-encapsulated adriamycin in the mouse. *Adv. Biosci.* (series) 1987;67:129–136.

48. **Kravtozoff, R., Ropars, C., Laguerre, M., Muh, JP., and Chassaigne, M.** Erythrocytes as carriers for L-asparaginase: methodological and mouse in vivo studies. *J. Pharm. Pharmacol.* 1990;42:473–476.

49. **Jrade, M., Villereal, MC., Boynard, M., Dufaux, J., and Ropars, C.** Rheological approach to human red blood cell carriers desferrioxamine encapsulation. *Adv. Biosci.* (series) 1987;67:29–36.

50. **Berman, JD.** Antileishmanial activity of red cell encapsulated drugs. *Adv. Biosci.* (series) 1987;67:145–152.

51. **Deloach, JR., Andrews, K., Sheffield, CL., and Koths, K.** Subcutaneous administration of [35-S] r-IL-2 in mice carrier erythrocytes: alteration of IL-2 pharmacokinetics. *Adv. Biosci.* (series) 1987;67:183–190.

52. **Deloach, JR. and Doleskey, R.** Preparation and properties of microcytic carrier erythrocytes from sheep and goats. *Adv. Biosci.* (series) 1987;67:199–212.

53. **Zanella, A., Rossi, F., Sabionedda, L., et al.** Desferrioxamine loading of red cells for transfusion. *Adv. Biosci.* (series) 1987;67:17–27.

54. **Fiorelli, G., Fargion, S., Piperno, A., et al.** Transfusion of thalassemic patients with desferrioxamine loaded standard red blood cell units. *Adv. Biosci.* (series) 1987;67:47–54.

55. **Villareal, MC., et al.** Approach to optimization of inositol hexaphosphate entrapment into human red blood cells. *Adv. Biosci.* (series) 1987;67:55–62.

56. **Hurel, C., et al.** Optimization of desferrioxamine loading in red blood cells. *Adv. Biosci.* (series) 1987;67:37–46.

57. **Villareal, MC., Bailleul, C., Ropars, C., Nicolau, C., Casset, D., and Itti, R.** Modification of cardiac parameters in piglets after infusion of IHP-loaded red blood cells. *Adv. Biosci.* (series) 1987;67:81–88.

58. **Teisseire, B., Ropars, C., Villereal, MC., and Nicolau, C.** In vivo consequences of rightward shift of the hemoglobin dissociation curve. *Adv. Biosci.* (series) 1987;67:89–94.

59. **Jrade, M., Ropars, C.,VanVooren, C., and Chassaigne, M.** Technical aspects of human red blood cell carriers methodology. *Adv. Biosci.* (series) 1987;67:223–232.

60. **Garin, MI., Lopez, RM., Sanz, S., Pinilla, M., and Luque, J.** Erythrocytes as carriers for recombinant human erythropoietin. *Pharm. Res.* 1996;13:869–874.

60a. **Kinosita, K., Jr. and Tsong, TY.** Hemolysis of human erythrocytes by transient electric field. *Proc. Natl. Acad. Sci. USA* 1977a;74:1923–1941

61. **Davson, H. and Danielli, JF.** Dannen Conn, Hanfer Publishing Company, Germany, 1970, 80 p.

62. **Billah, MM., Finean, JB., Coleman, R., and Michell, RH.** Permeability characteristics of erythrocyte ghosts prepared under isoionic conditions by a glycol-induced osmotic lysis. *Biochim. Biophys. Acta* 1977;465(3):515–526.

63. **Bird, J., Best, R., and Lewis, DA.** The encapsulation of insulin in erythrocytes. *J. Pharm. Pharmacol.* 1983;35:246–247.

64. **Deuticke, B., Kim, M., and Zolinev, C.** The influence of amphotericin-B on the permeability of mammalian erythrocytes to nonelectrolytes, anions and cations. *Biochim. Biophys. Acta* 1973;318:345–359.

65. **Kitao, T., Hattori, K., and Takeshita, M.** Agglutination of leukemic cells and daunomycin entrapped erythrocytes with lectin *in vitro* and *in vivo*. *Experimentia* 1978;341:94–95.

66. **Lin, W., Mota de Freitas, D., Zhang, Q., and Olsen, KW.** Nuclear magnetic resonance and oxygen affinity study of cesium binding in human erythrocytes. *Arch. Biochem. Biophys.* 1999;369(1):78–88.

67. **Kinosita, K. and Tsong, TY.** Hemolysis of human erythrocytes by a transient electric field. *Proc. Natl. Acad. Sci. USA* 1977;74:1923–1927.

68. **Kinosita, K. and Tsong, TY.** Formation and resealing of pores of controlled sizes in human erythrocyte membrane. *Nature* 1977;268:438–441.

69. **Zimmermann, U., Pilwat, G., and Riemann, F.** Preparation of erythrocyte ghosts by dielectric breakdown of the cell membrane. *Biochim. Biophys. Acta* 1975;375(2):209–219.

70. **Tsong, TY. and Kinosita, K. Jr.** Use of voltage pulses for the pore opening and drug loading, and the subsequent resealing of red blood cells. *Bibl. Haematol.* 1985; 51:108–114.

71. **Ropars, C., Chassaigne, M., and Nicoulau, C.** Advances in the BioSciences, Pergamon Press, Oxford, 1987, 67 p.

72. **Zimmermann, U., Riemann, F., and Pilwat, G.** Enzyme loading of electrically homogenous human red blood cell ghosts prepared by dielectric breakdown. *Biochim. Biophys. Acta.* 1976;436:460–474.

73. **Mitchell, DH., James, GT., and Kruse, CA.** Bioactivity of electric field-pulsed human recombinant interleukin-2 and its encapsulation into erythrocyte carriers. *Biotechnol. Appl. Biochem.* 1990;12(3):264–275.

74. **Mouneimne, Y., Tosi, PF., Gazitt, Y., and Nicolau, C.** Electro-insertion of xeno-glycophorin into the red blood cell membrane. *Biochem. Biophys. Res. Commun.* 1989;159(1):34–40.

75. **Mangal, PC. and Kaur, A.** Electroporation of red blood cell membrane and its use as a drug carrier system. *Ind. J. Biochem. Biophys.* 1991;28(3):219–221.

76. **Schrier, SL., Bensch, KG., Johnson, M., and Junga, I.** Energized endocytosis in human erythrocyte ghosts. *J. Clin. Invest.* 1975;56(1):8–22.

76a. **Bassat, IB., Bensch, KG., and Schrier, SI.** Drug-induced erythrocyte membrane internalization. *J. Clin. Invest.* 1972;51(7):1833–1844.

77. **Schrier, SL.** Shape changes and deformability in human erythrocyte membranes. *J. Lab. Clin. Med.* 1987;110(6):791–797.

78. **DeLoach, JR.** Encapsulation of exogenous agents in erythrocytes and the circulating survival of carrier erythrocytes. *J. Appl. Biochem.* 1983;5(3):149–157.

79. **Li, LH., Hensen, ML., Zhao, YL., and Hui, SW.** Electrofusion between heterogeneous-sized mammalian cells in a pellet: potential applications in drug delivery and hybridoma formation. *Biophys. J.* 1996;71(1):479–486.

80. **Nicolau, C. and Gersonde, K.** Incorporation of inositol hexaphosphate lipid vesicles with erythrocytes. *Naturwissenschaften* 1979;66(11):563–566.

81. **Hamidi, M., Taherzadeh, H., Dehpour, AR., Rouini, MR., and Ejtemaee-Mehr, S.** In vitro characterization of human intact erythrocytes loaded by enalaprilat. *Drug Deliv.* 2001;8:231–237.

82. **Vyas, SP., Talwar, N., Karajgi, JS., and Jain, NK.** Erythrocyte based bioadhesive system for nasal delivery of propranolol. *J. Control. Release* 1993;23:231–237.

83. **Eichler, HG., Raffesberg, W., Gasic, S., Korn, A., and Bauer, K.** Release of vitamin B12 from carrier erythrocytes *in vitro*. *Res. Exp. Med.* 1985;185:341–344.

84. **Lewis, DA. and Desai, J.** The use of animal models in the encapsulation of drugs in erythrocytes. *Adv. Biosci.* (series) 1987;67:213–222.

85. **Deloach, JR.** Comparative encapsulation of cytosine arabinoside onophosphate in human and canine erythrocytes with in vitro drug efflux. *J. Appl. Biochem.* 1982; 4:533–541.

86. **Green, R., Lamon, J., and Curran, D.** Clinical trial of desferrioxamine entrapped in red cell ghosts. *Lancet* 1980;1:327–330.

87. **Harris, RC.** Enzyme replacement in red cells. *N. Eng. J. Med.* 1977;296:942–943.

88. **Beutler, E., Dale, GL., Guinto, DE., and Kuhl, W.** Enzyme replacement therapy in Gaucher's disease. Preliminary clinical trial of a new enzyme preparation. *Proc. Natl. Acad. Sci. USA* 1977;74:4620–4623.

89. **Kruse, CA., James, GT., Freehauf, CL., and Williams, CM.** Methotrexate loaded erythrocytes carriers: optimization their formation, their characterization, and their pharmacological efficiency in treating hepatoma 129 ascites tumors in mice. *Adv. Biosci.* (series) 1987;67:137–144.

90. **Deloach, JR. and Barton, C.** Circulating carrier erythrocytes: slow release vehicle for an antileukemic drug, cytosine arabinoside. *Am. J. Vet. Res.* 1982;43:2210–2212.

91. **Al-Achi, A. and Boroujerdi, M.** Pharmacokinetics and tissue uptake of doxorubicin associated with erythrocyte-membrane: erythrocyte ghosts versus erythrocyte-vesicles. *Drug Dev. Ind. Pharm.* 1990;16:2199–2219.

92. **Kitao, T., Hattori, K., and Takeshita, M.** Agglutination of leukemic cells and daunomycin entrapped erythrocytes with lectin in vitro and in vivo. *Experimentia* 1978;341:94–95.

93. **Hamidi, M., Tajerzadeh, H., Dehpour, AR., and Ejtemaee-Mehr, Sh.** ACE inhibition in rabbits upon administration of enalaprilat-loaded intact erythrocytes. *J. Pharm. Pharmacol.* 2001;53:1281–1289.

94. **McLaren, GD., Muir, WA., and Kellermeyer, RW.** Iron overload disorders. *Crit. Rev. Clin. Lab. Sci.* 1983;19:205–266.

95. **Alvarez, FJ., Jordan, JA., Calleja, P., et al.** Cross-linking treatment of loaded erythrocytes increases delivery of encapsulated substance to macrophages. *Biotechnol. Appl. Biochem.* 1998;27(pt 2):139–143.

95a. **Antonelli, A., Crinelli, R., Bianchi, M., et al.** Efficient inhibition of macrophage TNF-α production upon targeted delivery of K48R ubiquitin. *Br. J. Haematol.* 1999;104:475–481.

96. **Franco, L., Guida, L., Bruzzone, S., Zocchi, E., Usai, C., and De Flora, A.** The transmembrane glycoprotein CD38 is a catalytically active transporter responsible for generation and influx of the second messenger cyclic ADP-ribose across membranes. *FASEB J.* 1998;12(14):1507–1520.

97. **Alvarez-Guerra, M., Nazaret, C., and Garay, RP.** The erythrocyte Na^+, K^-, and Cl^- co-transporter and its circulating inhibitor in dahl salt-sensitive rats. *J. Hypertens.* 1998;10:1499–1504.

98. **Mishra, PR. and Jain, NK.** Surface modified methotrexate loaded erythrocytes for enhanced macrophage uptake. *J Drug Targeting* 2000;8(4):217–224.

99. **Deloach, J. and Ihler, G.** A dialysis procedure for loading erythrocytes with enzymes and lipids. *Biochim. Biophys. Acta* 1977;496(1):136–145.

100. **Zocchi, E., Tonetti, M., Polvani, C., Guida, L., Benatti, U., and De Flora, A.** *In-vivo* liver and lung targeting of adriamycin encapsulated in glutaraldehyde-treated murine erythrocytes. *Biotechnol. Appl. Biochem.* 1988;10:555–562.

101. **Gaudreault, RC., Bellemare, B., and Lacroix, J.** Erythrocyte membrane-bound daunorubicin as a delivery system in anticancer treatment. *Anticancer Res.* 1989;9(4):1201–1205.

102. **Tonetti, M., Astroff, B., Satterfield, W., De Flora, A., Benatti, U., and DeLoach, JR.** Construction and characterization of adriamycin- loaded canine red blood cells as a potential slow delivery system. *Biotechnol. Appl. Biochem.* 1990;12(6):621–629.

103. **DeLoach, JR., Wagner, GG., and Corrier, DE.** Pharmacokinetics of imidocarb dipropionate encapsulated in carrier erythrocytes and use of carrier cells for babesiosis chemotherapy. *J. Control. Release* 1989;9:243–248.

104. **Cannon, EP., Leung, P., Hawkins, A., Petrikovics, I., DeLoach, J., and Way, JL.** Antagonism of cyanide intoxication with murine carrier erythrocytes containing bovine rhodanese and sodium thiosulfate. *J. Toxicol. Environ. Health* 1994;41(3):267–274.

105. **Pei, L., Omburo, G., McGuinn, WD., et al.** Encapsulation of phosphotriesterase within murine erythrocytes. *Toxicol. Appl. Pharmacol.* 1994;124(2):296–301.

106. **Sprandel, U., Hubbard, AR., and Chalmers, RA.** In vivo life span of resealed rabbit erythrocyte 'Ghosts'. *Res. Exp. Med.* (Berl) 1980;177(1):13–17.

107. **Jain, SK. and Vyas, SP.** Magnetically responsive diclofenac sodium-loaded erythrocytes: preparation and in vitro characterization. *J. Microencapsul.* 1994;11(2):141–151.

108. **Flynn, G., McHale, L., and McHale, AP.** Methotrexate-loaded, photosensitized erythrocytes: a photo-activatable carrier/delivery system for use in cancer therapy. *Cancer Lett.* 1994;82(2):225–229.

109. **Chiarantini, L., Rossi, L., Fraternale, A., and Magnani, M.** Modulated red blood cell survival by membrane protein clustering. *Mol. Cell Biochem.* 1995;144(1):53–59.

110. **Price, RJ., Skyba, DM., Kaul, S., and Skalak, TC.** Delivery of colloidal particles and red blood cells to tissue through microvessel ruptures created by targeted micro-bubble destruction with ultrasound. *Circulation* 1998;98(13):1264–1267.

111. **Deloach, JR. and Droleskey, R.** Survival of murine carrier erythrocytes injected via peritoneum. *Comp. Biochem. Physiol.* 1986;83A:447–450.

112. **Kitao, T., Hattori, K., and Takeshita, M.** Agglutination of leukemic cells and daunomycin entrapped erythrocytes with lectin *in vitro* and *in vivo*. *Experimentia* 1978;341:94–95.

113. **Benatti, U., Zocchi, E., Tonetti, M., Guida, L., Polvani, C., and De Flora, A.** Enhanced antitumor activity of adriamycin by encapsulation in mouse erythrocytes targeted to liver and lungs. *Pharmacol. Res.* 1989;21(2):27–33.

114. **Magnani, M., Rossi, L., D'ascenzo, M., Panzani, I., Bigi, L., and Zanella, A.** Erythrocyte engineering for drug delivery and targeting. *Biotechnol. Appl. Biochem.* 1998;28:1–13.

115. **Fraternale, A., Rossi, L., and Magnani, M.** Encapsulation, metabolism, and release of 2-fluoro-Ara-AMP from human erythrocytes. *Biochim. Biophys. Acta* 1996;1291(2):149–154.

116. **Al-Achi, A. and Greenwood, R.** Human insulin binding to erythrocyte-membrane. *Drug Dev. Ind. Pharm.* 1993;19 (6):673–684.

116a. **Kogurea, K., Itoh, T., Okuda, O., Hayashi, K., and Ueno, M.** The delivery of protein into living cells by use of membrane fusible erythrocyte ghosts. *Int. J. Pharm.* 2000;210(1):117–120.

117. **Al-Achi, A. and Greenwood, R.** Erythrocytes as oral delivery systems for human insulin. *Drug Dev. Ind. Pharm.* 1998;24(1):67–72.

118. **Magnani, M., Laguerre, M., Rossi, L., et al.** Acetaldehyde dehydrogenase-loaded erythrocytes as bioreactors for removal of blood acetaldehyde, alcoholism. *Clin. Exp. Res.* 1989;13:849–859.

119. **Ihler, GW., et al.** Enzymatic degradation of uricase-loaded human erythrocytes. *J. Clin. Invest.* 1975;56:595–602.

120. **Tan, C.** L-asparaginase in leukemia. *Hosp. Pract.* 1972;7: 99–103.

121. **Ibels, LS. and Pollock, CA.** Lead intoxication. *Med. Toxicol.* 1986;1:387–410.

122. **Guyton, AC. and Hall, JE.** Transport of oxygen and carbon dioxide in the blood and body fluids. Textbook of medical physiology, W.B. Saunders, Philadelphia, 1996, pp. 513–523.

123. **Arnone, A. and Perutz, MF.** Structure of inositol hexaphosphate human deoxyhaemoglobin complex. *Nature* 1974;249:34–36.

124. **Teisseire, B., Ropars, C., Vallez, MO., Herigault, RA., and Nicolau, C.** Physiological effects of high-P50 erythrocyte transfusion on piglets. *J. Appl. Physiol.* 1985;58: 1810–1817.

125. **Baron, JF., Vicaut, E., Stucker, O., et al.** Isolated heart as a model to study the effects of the decrease in oxygen haemoglobin affinity. *Adv. Biosci.* (series) 1987;67:73–78.

126. **Woodson, R., Hoerl, C., and Borchardt, M.** P50 shifts and tissue oxygen pressure. *Adv. Biosci.* (series) 1987;67:79–80.

127. **Stucker, O., Vicaut, E., Villereal, MC., Ropars, C., Teisseire, BP., and Duvelleroy, MA.** Coronary response to large decreases of haemoglobin-O_2 affinity in isolated rat heart. *Am. J. Physiol.* 1985;249:H1224–H1227.

128. **Woodson, RD. and Auerbach, S.** Effect of increased oxygen affinity and anemia on cardiac output and its distribution. *J. Appl. Physiol.* 1982;53:1299–1306.

129. **Schlegel, RA. and Rechsteiner, MC.** Red cell-mediated microinjection of macromolecules into mammalian cells. *Methods Cell Biol.* 1978;20:341–354.

130. **Loyter, A., Zakai, N., and Kulka, RG.** Ultramicroinjection of macromolecules or small particles into animal cells. *J. Cell Biol.* 1975;66:292–305.

131. **Wille, W. and Willecke, K.** Retention of purified proteins in resealed human erythrocyte ghosts and transfer by fusion into cultured murine cells. *FEBS Lett.* 1976;65:59–62.

131a. **McClung, JK. and Kletzien, RF.** Analysis of BHK cell growth kinetics after microinjection of catalytic subunit of cyclic AMP-dependent protein kinase. *Mol. Cell Biol.* 1984;4(6):1079–1085.

132. **Furusawa, M., Nishimura. T., Yamaizumi, M., and Okada, Y.** Injection of foreign substances into single cells by cell fusion. *Nature* 1974;249:449–450.

133. **Schlegel, RA. and McEvoy, L.** Red cell-mediated microinjection. *Methods Enzymol.* (series) 1987;149:293–301.

134. **Kruse, CA., Spector, EB., Cederbaum, SD., Wisnieski, BJ., and Popjak, G.** Microinjection of arginase into enzyme-deficient cells with the isolated glycoprotein of sendai virus as fusogen. *Biochim. Biophys. Acta.* 1981;645:339–345.

135. **Kruse, A., James, GT., Cederbaum, SD., and Spector, EB.** Arginase-loaded erythrocyte carriers: their fusion to host cells with viral fusogenic proteins and subcellular localization of arginase. *Adv. Biosci.* (series) 1987;67:113–122.

136. **Cuppoletti, J., Mayhew, E., Zobel, CR., and Jung, CY.** Erythrosomes: large proteoliposomes derived from cross-linked human erythrocyte cytoskeletons and exogenous lipid. *Proc. Natl. Acad. Sci. USA* 1981;78(5):2786–2790.

137. **Jung, CY.** Methods in enzymology, Academic Press, New York, 1987, pp. 149–217.

138. **Vyas, SP. and Dixit, VK.** Pharmaceutical biotechnology 1, CBS Publishers and Distributors, New Delhi, 1999, 655 p.

139. **Moorjani, M., Lejeune, A., Gicquaud, C., Lacroix, J., Poyet, PC., and Gaudreault, R.** Nanoerythrosomes, a new derivative of erythrocyte ghost II: identification of the mechanism of action. *Anticancer Res.* 1996;16(5A): 2831–2836.

140. **Lejeune, A., Poyet, PC., Gaudreault, R., and Gicquaud, C.** Nanoerythrosomes, a new derivative of erythrocyte ghost: III. "Is phagocytosis involved in the mechanism of action?". *Anticancer Res.* 1997;17(5A):3599–3603.

9

Micellar Drug Delivery Systems

Dr. R.S.R. Murthy, M.PHARM, PhD

CONTENTS

1. INTRODUCTION

Drugs and other therapeutic compounds used in curing disorders are poorly soluble in aqueous media. Therefore, this makes the delivery of such compounds difficult and quite challenging. For success of therapy, delivery system has to be proven and acceptable. As more sophisticated synthetic compounds enter the field of therapy, delivery systems have to undergo changes and innovated to accommodate these. The development of effective delivery systems is crucial to the success of future drugs *(1)*. Micellar delivery systems can be exploited to deliver such complex and sophisticated molecules. Polymeric micelles formed in this method can also be used for solubilisation, stabilisation and delivery of challenging agents. It is also useful in encapsulation and delivery of hydrophobic drugs.

2. STRUCTURE OF MICELLE

Micelle is an aggregate of surfactant molecules dispersed in a liquid colloid. A typical micelle in aqueous solution forms an aggregate with the hydrophilic "head" regions in contact with surrounding solvent, sequestering hydrophobic tail regions in the micelle centre. Micelles are often globular and roughly spherical in shape (Fig.1), but ellipsoids, cylinders and bilayers are also possible. The shape and size of a micelle (Fig. 2) is a function of molecular geometry of its surfactant molecules and solution conditions such as surfactant concentration, temperature, pH and p*I*. Micelles can be spherical or non-spherical depending on hydrophilic segment of core block. If hydrophilic segment is longer than the core block, the shape of resulting micelles is spherical. Increasing the length of core segment beyond that of corona-forming chains gives the shape as non-spherical, rod like and lamellar *(2)*.

Individual surfactant molecules that are in colloid but are not part of a micelle are called "monomers". In water, the hydrophilic "heads" of surfactant molecules are always in contact with bulk solvent, regardless of whether the surfactants exist as monomers or as part of a micelle. However, the hydrophobic "tails" of surfactant molecules have less contact with water when they are part of a micelle. In a micelle, the hydrophobic tails of several surfactant molecules assemble into an oil-like core that has less contact with water. In contrast, surfactant monomers are surrounded by water molecules, which create a "cage" of molecules connected by hydrogen bonds. Micelles are formed when the concentration of surfactant is greater than critical micelle concentration (CMC), and the temperature of system is greater than critical micelle temperature, or

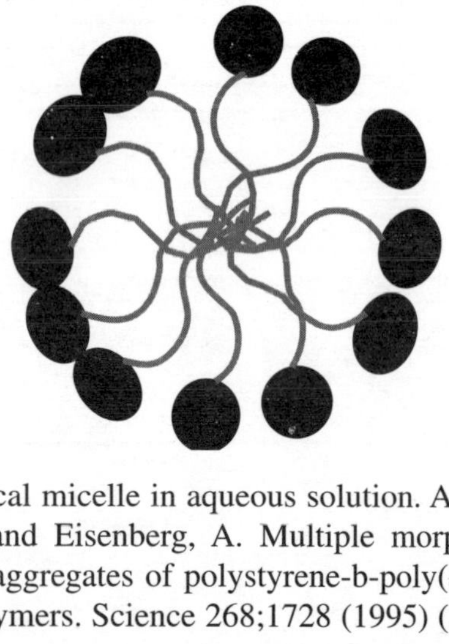

Fig. 1. Typical micelle in aqueous solution. Adapted from Zhang, L. and Eisenberg, A. Multiple morphologies of "crew-cut" aggregates of polystyrene-b-poly(acrylic acid) block copolymers. Science 268;1728 (1995) (2).

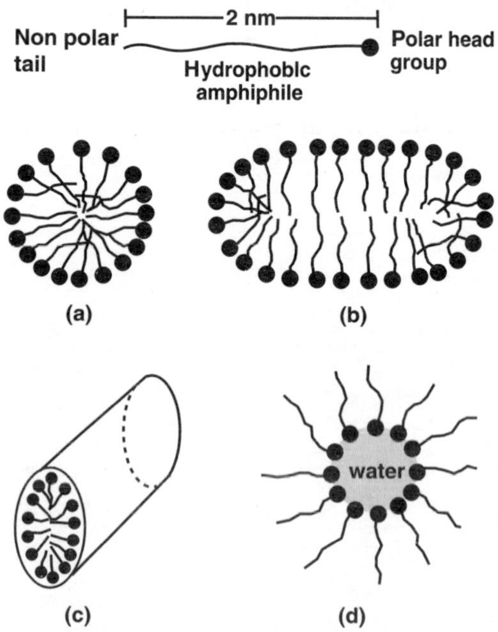

Fig. 2. Form of an amphiphile and several forms of micelle: **(a)** spherical, **(b)** disk, **(c)** rod, and **(d)** reversed. Adapted from Zhang, L. and Eisenberg, A. Multiple morphologies of "crew-cut" aggregates of polystyrene-b-poly(acrylic acid) block copolymers. Science 268;1728 (1995) (2).

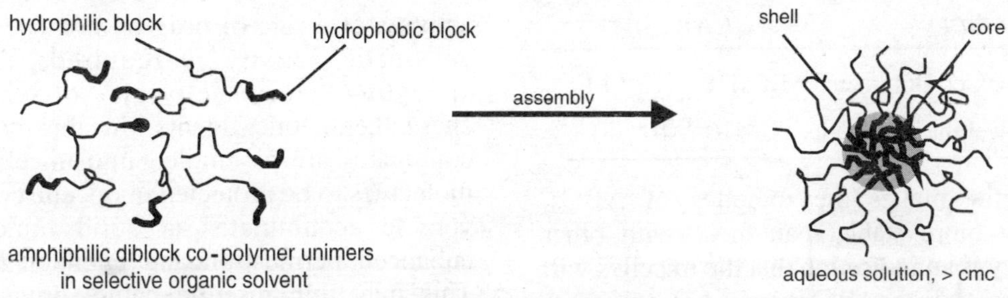

Fig. 3. Micellisation model for an amphiphilic AB—diblock co-polymer.

Krafft temperature. Thermodynamically, micelles can form spontaneously because of a balance between entropy and enthalpy. In water, the hydrophobic effect is driving force for micelle formation, despite the fact that assembling surfactant molecules together reduces their entropy. Broadly speaking, above CMC, the entropy required to assemble surfactant molecules is less than the entropy required for caging water molecules. Enthalpic considerations, such as electrostatic interactions that occur between charged (or ionic) surfactants are also important for micelle formation.

2.1. Reverse Micelle

In a non-polar solvent, exposure of hydrophilic head groups to surrounding bulk solvent is energetically unfavourable. In this case, the hydrophilic groups are sequestered in micelle core and hydrophobic groups remain solvent-exposed on the surface of micelle. These reverse micelles are extremely difficult to form from surfactants with charged head groups, because hydrophilic sequestration would create highly unfavourable electrostatic interactions.

2.2. Polymeric Micelle

Co-polymers with amphiphilic character, having a large solubility difference between hydrophilic and hydrophobic segments, are known to assemble in an aqueous milieu into polymeric micelles with a mesoscopic size range (upto 10 nm). These micelles have a fairly narrow size distribution and are characterised by their unique core-shell architecture (hence they are also called as "core-shell" nanoparticles), where hydrophobic segments are segregated from aqueous exterior to form an inner core surrounded by a hydrophilic segments. Compared with surfactant micelles, polymeric micelles are generally more stable, with a remarkably lowered CMC, and have a slower rate of dissociation, allowing retention of loaded drugs for a longer period of time and, eventually, achieving higher accumulation of a drug at target site. Furthermore, polymeric micelles have mesoscopic size range with a considerably narrow distribution.

Polymeric micelles can be formed by amphiphilic block co-polymers (ABCs). ABCs consist of at least two regions of distinct chemical nature that undergo phase separation as a result of chain association in solvents that selectively dissolve one of the blocks. This process results in formation of nanoscopic supra-molecular core/shell structures, i.e., polymeric micelles. One of the reasons for formation of ABCs into micelles is because of relative interactions between hydrophilic and hydrophobic blocks with one another and the surrounding medium. During micellisation process, the hydrophobic blocks associate to form the core region, whereas the hydrophilic segments position between core and external aqueous medium. Hence, the hydrophobic core is stabilised by hydrophilic shell, which serves as an interface between bulk aqueous phase and hydrophobic domain (Fig. 3). This unique architecture enables polymeric micelles to serve as nanoscopic depots or stabilisers for poorly water-soluble compounds. There has been great interest in use of polymeric micelles as drug carriers *(3–5)*.

Block co-polymer micelles are generally formed by self-assembly of either amphiphilic or oppositely charged co-polymers in aqueous medium. The hydrophilic and hydrophobic blocks form the corona and the core of micelles, respectively *(6)*. Polymeric micelles are formed in aqueous solutions by association of ABCs into nanoscopic core/shell structures at or above the CMC. Polymeric micelles are association colloids. ABCs and low molecular weight surfactants form micellar structures near or above CMC. The concentration of surfactant molecules added is crucial factor that determines the formation of micelles. At CMC, both the bulk and interface get saturated with monomers/unimers. Free energy changes at this phase and the change in standard free energy for micellisation process,

$$\Delta G^0_{\text{mic}} = RT \ln(\text{CMC})$$

where R is gas constant, T is temperature of system.

Class of surfactant	*CMC*
Amphiphilic block co-polymers (ABCs)	10^{-6}–10^{-7} M
Low molecular weight surfactants	10^{-3}–10^{-4} M

The above factor makes the micelles of ABCs, thermodynamically more stable than those with other surfactants. Stability is an indication that the micelles will not disassemble themselves. ABC micelles also possess kinetic stability leading to dissociation into monomers at slower process even under extreme dilutions *(7,8)*. This factor of kinetic stability during dilution gains a lot of importance while delivery of parenteral medications. For example, a less thermodynamically and kinetically stable carrier might release drug prematurely because of dissociation of micelle structure, whereas a more stable system might be preferred for long circulating, sustained-release delivery systems *(9)*.

ABCs have been used extensively in pharmaceutical applications ranging from sustained-release technologies to gene delivery. The utility of ABCs for delivery of therapeutic agents results from their unique chemical composition, which is characterised by a hydrophilic block that is chemically tethered to a hydrophobic block.

ABCs can be classified as per chemical nature of the core-forming hydrophobic blocks.

1. Poly(ethylene oxide)-block-poly(L-amino acid) (PEO-*b*-P[L-AA]).
2. Poly(ethylene oxide)-block-poly(ester).
3. Poly(ethylene oxide)-block-poly(propylene oxide)-block-poly(ethylene oxide), i.e., Pluronics.

2.3. Poly(Ethylene Oxide)-Block-Poly (L-Amino Acid)s

Polymeric micelles based on PEO-*b*-P(L-AA)s, are quite versatile because they may facilitate chemical modification to core-forming blocks and allow loading of therapeutic substances by both chemical and physical means. The hydrophobic portions of PEO-*b*-P(L-AA)s often contain functional groups that may be derivatised to enhance the properties of core-forming blocks with respect to drug delivery. Consequently, P(L-AA) block may offer possibility of post-polymerisation modification by chemical means *(10)*. Micelles based on poly(ethylene oxide)-block-poly(L-aspartate), PEO-*b*-P(L-Asp) have been used extensively for drug delivery. Because of carboxyl functionality imparted by P(L-Asp) block, PEO-*b*-P(LAsp) is useful for chemical conjugation of drugs *(11,12)*. Drug loaded in this manner, as polymer/drug conjugate, acts as a prodrug. For drug activity, cleavage of drug by non-specific hydrolysis or enzymatic activity is required. This approach is appealing for delivery of highly cytotoxic chemotherapeutic agents. In this case, polymer/drug conjugates are assembled into micelles, enabling drug molecules to be protected in micelle core until the carrier vehicle accumulates at solid tumour sites due to enhanced permeation and retention (EPR) effect *(11)*. This may minimise premature drug release and non-specific action towards healthy cells, yet still allow for drug release in tumour tissues. Utilising this approach with polymeric micelles may increase selectivity for tumour tissues via "passive" targeting.

Micelles based on PEO-*b*-P(L-Asp) have also been used for physical entrapment of drugs. The drug molecules show their pharmacological activity by getting partitioned out of the micellar structure.

For example: amphotericin B (AmB), a potent anti-fungal agent, as PEO-*b*-P(N-hexylstearate-L-aspartamide) micelles results in reduced hemolytic activity compared with free AmB *(13)*. Polymeric micelles based on PEO-*b*-poly(N-hexyl-L-aspartamide)-acyl esters solubilise AmB at high concentrations and result in sustained release of encapsulated drug *in vitro*.

Further, many drug molecules with poor water solubility, like indomethacin, doxorubicin, etc., also have been loaded onto micellar structures for their enhanced pharmacological activity. Reconstitutable solid polymeric micelle formulations also have been tried and tested for their efficacy. Micelles prepared from derivatives of PEO-*b*-PBLA have also shown promise as delivery vehicles. For example, PEG-*b*-P(C16-benzyl-L-aspartate) was prepared via an ester exchange reaction between PEO-*b*-PBLA and cetyl alcohol, and then used for incorporation of a water insoluble anti-cancer drug.

Uses:

1. To entrap water-insoluble drug molecules.
2. It is possible to customise the core-forming block of functional groups.
3. It is possible to prepare polyion complex (PIC) micelles. These can be used in anti-sense therapy or entrapment of enzymes.

These may be biodegradable and non-toxic. The poly(amide) backbone of poly(L-AA) may undergo hydrolysis and/or enzymatic degradation to yield biocompatible materials based on naturally occurring L-AA. Phase I clinical trials conducted in Japan suggest that doxorubicin (DOX) loaded into PEO-*b*-P(L-Asp) micelles containing a chemically conjugated DOX side chain is safe, with no overt signs of cardiotoxicity, liver toxicity or untoward infusion-related side effects.

2.4. Poly(Ethylene Oxide)-Block-Poly(Ester)

These type of core-forming blocks are less-suitable for chemical modification than other types. It is safe to be administered in human. ABCs containing poly(ester) core-forming blocks are often used for biomaterials and drug delivery applications. Aliphatic poly(ester) are susceptible to non-specific hydrolysis and, therefore, subject to degradation in aqueous media. For delivery purposes, some of the most commonly used poly(ester) includes poly(glycolic acid), poly(D-lactic acid), poly(D,L-lactic acid), co-polymers of lactide/glycolide and poly(e-caprolactone). The core-forming block of PEO-*b*-P(e-caprolactone), PEO-*b*-PCL, is semi-crystalline. It is possible to control the degree of crystallinity of PCL by altering the ratio of PEO to PCL.

Merits:

1. Biocompatible.
2. Biological activity is unaltered.
3. Sustained release of encapsulated materials is possible.
4. Micelles may act as long circulating drug carriers and allow for passive accumulation in tumour tissues via EPR effect.
5. Can be used to target tumour tissues.
6. Non-toxic *in vivo*.
7. Increases apparent solubility of poorly water-soluble drugs.
8. Can be used for site-specific delivery applications.
9. Glycoreceptors can be actively targeted.
10. Poly(ester) are often used in gel-forming systems.
11. It is used for delivery of therapeutic proteins.
12. It is used for delivery of small molecules.

2.5. Poly(Ethylene Oxide)-Block Poly(Propylene Oxide)-Block-Poly(Ethylene Oxide)

One more important class of ABCs used in drug delivery applications is Pluronics, also known as poloxamers. Pluronics are tri-block ABA-type co-polymers based on poly(ethylene oxide)-block-poly(propylene oxide)-block-poly(ethylene oxide), which are typically expressed as PEO*m*/2-*b*-PPO*n* *b*-PEO*m*/2, where *m* and *n* designate total average number of PEO and PPO repeat units, respectively. Pluronics are not cytotoxic at low concentrations. Pluronics are commercially available in different molecular weights and block ratios. The size of PPO block in structure show an impact on CMC and partitioning of hydrophobic molecules into Pluronic micelles making it easier to select the type for enhancing drug delivery properties. Pluronics inhibit efflux actions of P-glycoproteins (P-GP). The overexpression of P-GP in cancerous tissues is often linked to reduced accumulation of therapeutic agents at tumour sites *(14)*. P-GP-mediated multidrug resistance (MDR) is a mechanism through which tumours can become resistant to a variety of functionally and structurally diverse chemotherapies *(15)*. Pluronics have shown potential for suppression of MDR. Specifically, the effect of Pluronics on P-GP-mediated efflux is mediated primarily by unimers *(16)*. Pluronics micelles can be loaded with cytotoxic agents like MDR and non-MDR type of drugs. Therefore, the use of Pluronics can be a promising strategy for overcoming challenging drug delivery barriers like MDR and blood–brain barrier (BBB). Delivery of therapeutic agents to central nervous system by Pluronics can be made possible by inhibiting P-GP efflux transport system.

Example—delivery of digoxin and Pluronics P 85 together shows increase in delivery of digoxin across BBB *in vitro* by inhibiting P-GP-mediated drug transport and enhances delivery to brain. Pluronic P 85, both above and below CMC, has been used to increase transport of a number of therapeutic agents across a model BBB and Caco-2 cells.

The use of ultrasonic enhancement has been explored as a method for controlled, or targeted, delivery with Pluron micelles. This approach makes use of EPR effect to achieve selective accumulation at target, i.e., tumour site. Then, ultrasound is applied exclusively to tumour to yield localised drug delivery *(17)*. Marin *et al.* demonstrated that ultrasound enhances drug uptake *in vitro* by increasing both micelle uptake by HL-60 cells and the concentration of free drug in incubation medium *(18)* . This effect results in increased DOX uptake, even in MDR cells *(19)*. Like PEO-*b*-poly(ester) -*b*-PEO, Pluronics have been used in gelling systems. For instance, mixed Pluronic solutions containing F127 and F68 have been used for development of a thermosetting ophthalmic drug delivery device in order to increase ocular residence time *(20)*. Pluronics F127 and F68 have also shown promise for formulation of nystatin, a polyene macrolide antifungal agent *(21)*. Using Pluronics, it might be possible to attenuate the toxicity of nystatin via modulation of self-aggregation state of drug.

Uses of ABCs:

1. Used for delivery of therapeutic agents.
2. Can be used to form micelles.
3. Viable for solubilisation of hydrophobic compounds.
4. Drug can be incorporated by chemical, physical and/or electrostatic means.

5. Micelles formed by ABCs are stable on dilution and show prolonged circulation times.
6. They avoid RES uptake and increase blood residence time.
7. Drugs can be encapsulated into micelles by direct dissolution, dialysis, chemical complexation, oil-in-water (O/W) emulsion and various solvent removal procedures.
8. Loaded drugs are protected from physiological environment, which might prohibit non-specific and enzymatic hydrolysis, pH-dependent degradation, etc.
9. Drugs can be released in a controlled manner.
10. It has versatility to choose appropriate polymers and/or tailor ABCs to the task at hand, whether that is burst or sustained release, gene delivery, prolonged circulation, targeting, bioadhesion, etc.
11. ABCs can be used for targeting purposes.
12. ABCs can be used as a viable approach for stabilising substances during systemic circulation.

Block co-polymer micelles have capacity to increase the solubility of hydrophobic molecules stems from their unique structural composition, which is characterised by a hydrophobic core, sterically stabilised by a hydrophilic corona. The core serves as a reservoir in which drug molecules can be incorporated by means of chemical, physical or electrostatic interactions, depending on their physicochemical properties.

Another important property of block co-polymer micelles is its ability to target their payload to specific tissues through either passive or active means. These can be achieved by prolonging the residual time of micelles in systemic circulation. The size must also be sufficiently large to avoid renal excretion (>50 kDa), yet small enough (<200 nm) to bypass filtration by inter-endothelial cell slits in the spleen *(22)*. Micelles must be stable to fulfil these characteristics. To enhance the stability of micelles, the stability of carrier is very important. Genevie`ve Gaucher *et al.* have tried to enhance the effectivity of carriers used for micelles *(6)*.

Other method of classifying polymeric micelles or block co-polymer micelles is according to type of inter-molecular forces driving the segregation of core segment from the aqueous milieu. Among different methods of classification available, one method of classification generally adopted is as follows *(23,24)*:

1. Amphiphilic micelles (formed by hydrophobic interactions).
2. PIC micelles (PICM—from electrostatic interactions).
3. Micelles from metal complexation.

Most amphiphilic co-polymers employed for drug delivery purposes contain either a polyester or a poly(amino acid) derivative as hydrophobic segment.

1. Poly(lactic acid) (PLA).
2. Poly(q-caprolactone) (PCL).
3. Poly(glycolic acid).

All the above polyesters are biocompatible and biodegradable and structurally versatile, and are approved by Food and Drug Administration (FDA) for biomedical applications in human. Poly(aspartic acid) (PAsp), poly(glutamic acid) (PGlu), poly(L-lysine) (PLys) and poly(histidine) (PHis) are some of the poly (L-amino acid) (PAA) that can be used for drug delivery. The property of PAA segment is very important for polymers to self-assemble into amphiphilic micelles. They must either be electro-statically neutral or conjugated to hydrophobic moieties. The enzymatic degradability and degree of immunogenicity of PAA can be tailored by varying the chemical structure of PAA *(25)*. One more class of polymers, which can be employed to prepare amphiphilic micelles, is polyethers. Most of the polyethers of pharmaceutical interest belong to poloxamer family, i.e., co-polymers of (poly[ethylene glycol]-*b*-poly[propylene oxide]-*b*-poly[ethylene glycol]) (PEG-*b*-PPO-*b*-PEG) *(26)*. To better predict and control properties of a micellar system, it is crucial that the co-polymers utilised be well-defined. The nature of polymer to be synthesised will determine most appropriate polymerisation reaction to use (viz., anionic, ring-opening polymerisation [ROP] or radical polymerisation). The polymers can again be classified as diblock co-polymers and multiblock co-polymers (Fig. 4).

3. MICELLE PREPARATION

Preparation of micelles requires drug loading and the procedures of drug loading can be applied depending on physicochemical properties of block co-polymer *(27)*.

There are two classes of drug-loading procedures:

1. Direct dissolution—this involves dissolving block co-polymer along with the drug in an aqueous solvent. This procedure is mostly employed for

DIBLOCK CO-POLYMERS

1.

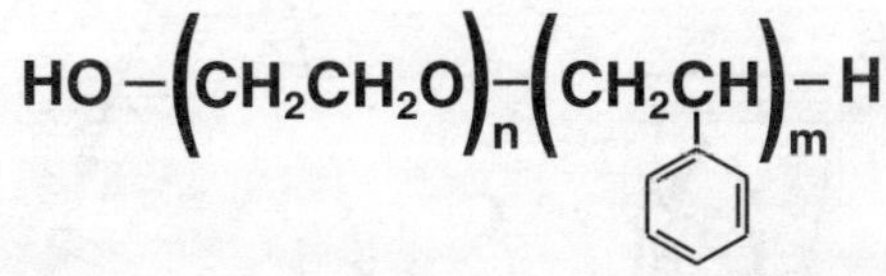

poly(ethylene oxide)-*b*-poly(styrene) block co-polymer

2.

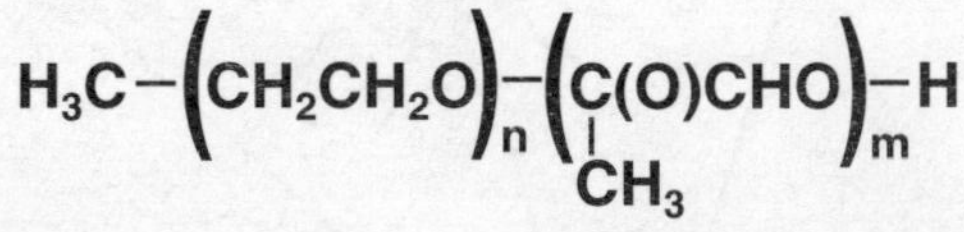

poly(ethylene oxide)-*b*-poly(D,L-lactide) block co-polymer

3.

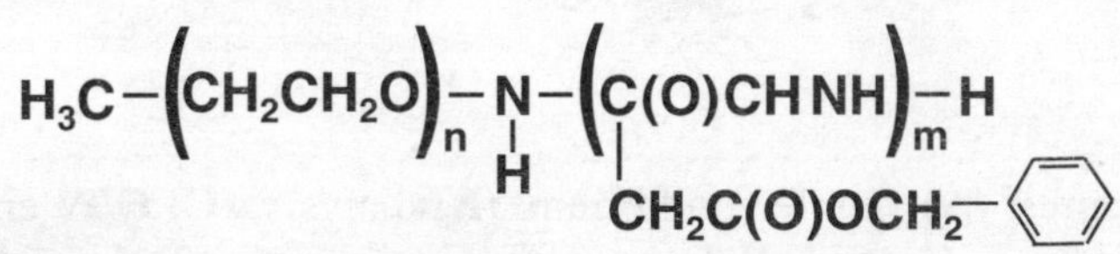

poly(ethylene oxide)-*b*-poly(β-benzyl L-aspartate) di-block co-polymer

TRI-BLOCK CO-POLYMERS

4.

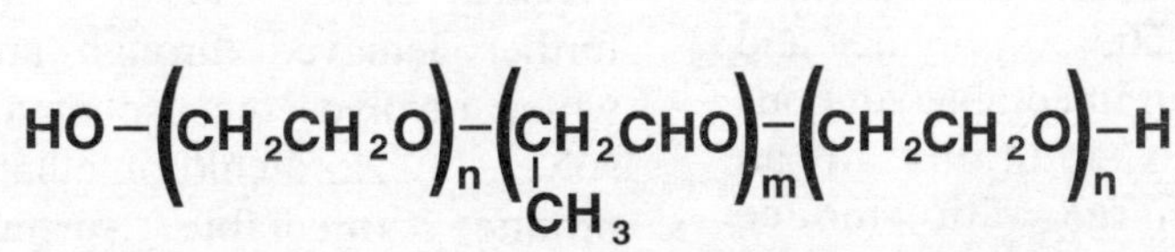

poly(ethylene oxide)-*b*-poly(propylene oxide)-*b*-poly(ethylene oxide) tri-block co-polymer

5.

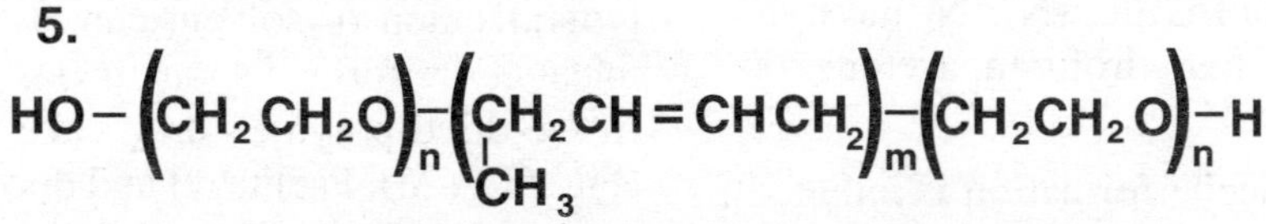

poly(ethylene oxide)-*b*-poly(isoprene)-*b*-poly(ethylene oxide) tri-block co-polymer

Fig. 4. Some examples of micelle-forming di- and tri-block co-polymers. (Reprinted from J. Control. Release, 73, Torchilin, VP., Structure and design of polymeric surfactant based drug delivery system, 137–172, 2001 with permission from Elsevier) *(69)*.

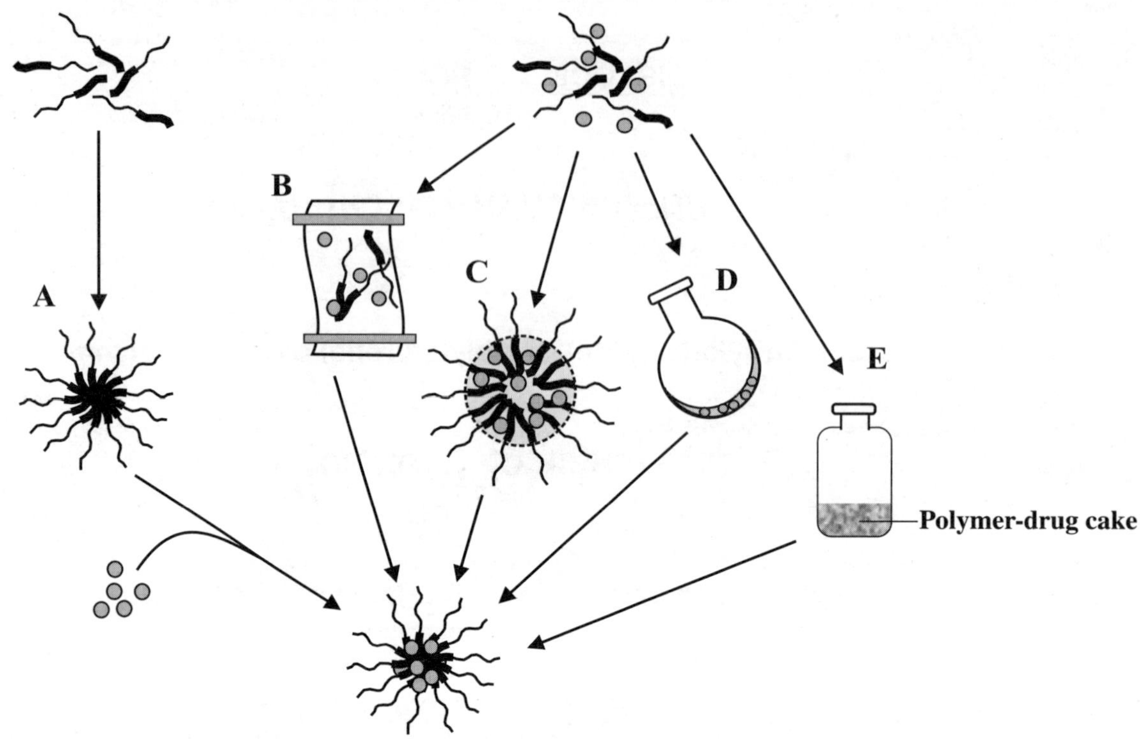

Fig. 5. Common drug-loading procedures: **(A)** simple equilibrium, **(B)** dialysis, **(C)** O/W emulsion, **(D)** solution casting, and **(E)** freeze-drying. (Reprinted From J. Control. Release, 109, Gaucher, G., Dufresne, MH., Sant, VP., Kang, N., Maysinger, D., and Leroux, JC. Block copolymer micelles: preparation, characterization and application in drug delivery, 169–188, 2005, with permission from Elsevier) *(6)*.

moderately hydrophobic co-polymers, such as poloxamers, and may require heating of aqueous solution to bring about micellisation via dehydration of core-forming segments. Direct dissolution method is also used to prepare PICM. The co-polymer and drug is dissolved separately in an injectable aqueous vehicle. Combination of two solutions in an appropriate drug–polymer charge ratio induce micelle formation.

2. This applies to amphiphilic co-polymers, which are not readily soluble in water. This is also for those types of substances for which an organic solvent common to both co-polymer and drug, is needed. For example, dimethylsulfoxide, N, N-imethyl-formamide, acetonitrile, tetrahydrofuran acetone or dimethylacetamide.

The mechanism by which micelle formation is induced depends on solvent-removal procedure. For water-miscible organic solvents, the co-polymer mixture can be dialysed against water, whereby slow removal of organic phase triggers micellisation. Alternatively, the solution-casting method entails evaporation of organic phase to yield a polymeric film where polymer–drug interactions are favoured. Re-hydration of film with a heated aqueous solvent produces drug-loaded micelles. Physical entrapment of a hydrophobic drug may be further achieved through an O/W emulsion process, which involves the use of a water-immiscible organic solvent (viz., dichloromethane and ethyl acetate). To produce injectable formulations, these require sterilisation and freeze-drying. This will ensure adequate shelf-life for the formulations. The figure-5 shows the different methods used for drug incorporation. One-step procedure based on dissolution of both polymer and drug in a water/tert-butanol mixture with subsequent lyophilisation of solvent can also be used. Drug-loaded micelles are formed spontaneously upon reconstitution of freeze-dried polymer–drug cake in an injectable vehicle (Fig. 5E) *(28)*. Paclitaxel and docetaxel, two hydrophobic anti-cancer agents were loaded by using this one-step method into a poly(N-vinyl-2-pyrrolidone and poly(D,L-lactide) (PVP-*b*-PDLLA) co-polymer, yielding stable spherical micelles with a monodisperse size distribution and a mean diameter of 30–60 nm *(6)*.

4. CHARACTERISATION OF MICELLAR SYSTEMS

1. Influence of solvent on dynamics of micellisation.
2. Solubilising capacity of solvent.
3. Mean micelle diameter and aggregation number after lyophilisation.
4. Process parameters and its effects on micellisation.
5. Nature and proportion of organic phase.
6. Affinity of organic phase for core-forming segment.
7. Method incorporated to prepare micelles.
8. Order of addition of liquid phases in preparation of micelles.

5. MICELLAR DRUG SOLUBILISATION

Polymeric micelles as solubilisers require selection of an appropriate hydrophobic core-forming polymer. Many important features, like stability, encapsulation efficiency and drug release kinetics, depend on interaction of drug and polymer. Surfactants and ABCs can greatly affect the aqueous solubility of compounds by providing a hydrophobic reservoir where they can partition. For example, doxorubicin depends on polymer–drug hydrophobic interactions, hydrogen-bonding interactions for encapsulation *(29)*. The loading efficiency of indomethacin changes, depending on hydrophobicity of various polylactones. The release profile of indomethacin from polymeric micelles also depends on same characteristic *(30)*. The nature of core-forming polyester influences the stability of paclitaxel-loaded polymeric micelles *(31)*.

6. MICELLE STABILITY

Micelles are prone to a lot of problems like dissociation and premature release of its payload into systemic circulation. Therefore, micelles must be physically stable and withstand these problems. Besides this, binding to proteins can disrupt micelle cohesion or trigger release of drug prematurely. This is because blood proteins tend to get adsorbed onto the surface of charged or hydrophobic foreign matter making faster clearance from blood stream. The impact of serum proteins on stability of micelles differs significantly according to nature and composition of block co-polymer *(32)*. Protein–drug interactions can lead to rapid dissociation of drug from its carrier. It can be seen that assessing the partitioning of drug between micellar system and aqueous medium containing protein may allow for a more accurate prediction of system's fate *in vivo*. The concentration of polymer is important for association into micelles and it is called as critical association concentration (CAC). The concentration of polymer depends on volume of distribution and rate of removal of vector from blood compartment. In comparison with low molecular weight surfactants, polymeric micelles exhibit significantly lower CAC values. This indicates greater thermodynamic stability. It is important to understand the dynamics of dissociation. This gives the understanding of stability and *in vivo* performance of polymeric micelles.

It is seen that the rate at which micelles tend to dissociate is related to composition, physical state and cohesion of micelle core. Micellar stability sometimes depends on the length of hydrophobic segment in amphiphilic co-polymer, with higher proportions of hydrophobic polymer conferring greater thermodynamic stability. It has been demonstrated by a steady-state pyrene fluorescence technique that increasing PDLLA proportion in PVP-*b*-PDLLA-*b*-PVP tri-block co-polymers from 27 to 55 mol% led to a decrease in CAC values from 19.9 to 5.1 mg/L *(33)*. At the same time, size exclusion chromatography has demonstrated that increase in the length of core-forming segment could reduce the leakage, while it increases resistance to dissociation *(34)*. Other studies have demonstrated that modification of properties of the core-forming blocks enhances hydrophobicity. For example, in the experiment conducted by Adams *et al.*, they developed PEG-*b*-poly(N-hexyl-L-aspartamide) co-polymers containing acyl side chains of varying lengths conjugated to aspartic acid core segments *(35)*. They found a good correlation between level of stearate substitution and stability of system.

The stability of micelles is also associated with physical state of polymer, which forms the core irrespective of whether it is amorphous or crystalline. Block co-polymer micelles comprised of a hydrophobic block with a glass transition temperature (T_g) exceeding 37°C possess frozen cores. This means molecular motions of chains in the core are constrained contributing to greater kinetic stability upon dilution *(27)*. In some cases, CAC was constant at a temperature range below T_g, it drastically increased at temperatures above Tg, suggesting enhanced core fluidity and a decrease in stability of micelles *(36)*. In some more studies, superior stability was reported from paclitaxel-loaded PEG-*b*-PDLLA vs PEG-*b*-P(DLLA-co-CL) micelles, resulting from reduced fluidity of PDLLA core (as determined by fluorescence intensity and anisotropy techniques) *(31)*. Stability of micelles depends on crystallinity. This can contribute greater drug retention properties by decreasing the rate of diffusion of drug from core. With a method reported by Slager *(37)*, the crystallinity and kinetic stability of block co-polymer micelles was increased. A time-dependent stability study by dynamic light scattering (DLS) revealed that these innovated micelles exhibited kinetic stability superior to that of their basic characteristic polymeric micelles. Slight improvement of stability of micellar system was observed with increase of PLA chains in co-polymer. Van der Waals interactions between PLA chains and stereo complexes enhanced the stability of micelles resulting in a more compact conformation and denser packing of polymer *(38)*.

The stability of micelles can be improved by cross-linking the shell or core of hydrophobic micelles. This shows decreased CAC or absence of CAC also *(49)*. The core of PEG-*b*-PCL micelles with paclitaxel was cross-linked by radical polymerisation of double bonds introduced into PCL blocks *(40)*. These cross-linked micelles showed significant increase in stability against dilution with aqueous solvents. This showed no collapse of micelles upon dilution. Another example can be given by trypsin-loaded PEG-*b*-P(Asp) PICM cross-linked with glutaraldehyde micelles prepared by Jaturanpinyo *et al. (41)*. These micelles showed very high stability against higher salt concentrations while preserving the activity of incorporated protein.

Strong cohesive forces between drug and polymer core segments can also confer the physical stability to system. Lee *et al.* demonstrated that PEG-*b*-PDLLA co-polymers with additional carboxylic acid groups could establish hydrogen bonds with incorporated drug papaverine *(42,43)*. These interactions resulted in a controlled release profile *in vitro* wherein the drug was released within 7 day against 10 h for micelles without COOH moieties.

A drug may otherwise be covalently conjugated to core-forming polymer through various linkers, which consist mainly of hydrolysable bonds (including esters *[12]*, amides *[44]*, carbamates *[45]* or pH-sensitive bonds such as h-thiopropionate *[46]*, hydrazones *[47]* and cis-acotinyl *[48]*). Li *et al.* found that higher the level of methotrexate ester conjugation, greater the micelle stability and slower the drug release from the carrier *(12)*.

The stability of PICM is also dictated by p*I*, or salt concentration, of aqueous solvent. The presence of salts in solution can shield electrostatic interactions between core-forming, oppositely charged polyions and trigger either micelle dissociation or structural changes. On the other hand, pH will have a bearing on the degree of ionisation of polyions and their mutual capacity to participate in coupling reactions. The composition of polyions influences the resistance of PICM to salt and pH variations. Among several polymers presenting pendant amino groups with different degrees of substitution, polycations with highest pK_a values formed the most stable PICM towards basification and an increase in p*I*. In this respect, PEG-*b*-P(AEMA), a co-polymer bearing primary amino groups, proved to be promising for the formulation of heparin *(49)*. In a parallel study, the susceptibility of PICM to dissociate in presence of salts was found to be inversely related to the length of core-forming polyions. PICM of PEG-*b*-poly(-nBA-co-MAA) and PLys of various chain lengths (viz., 1800, 8300 and 30,200) were prepared and submitted to escalating NaCl concentrations. Figure 6 illustrates how PICM of greater stability were formed when the length of polycation was increased. This phenomenon can be ascribed to co-operative electrostatic forces of greater magnitude for PICM of larger molecular weight.

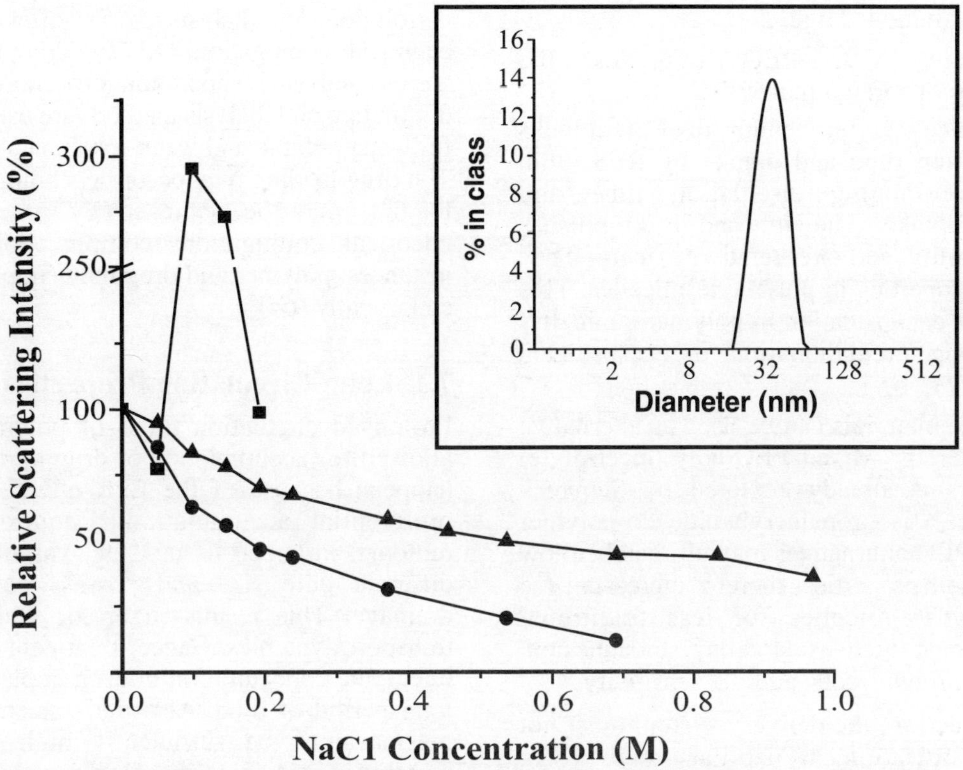

Fig. 6. Effect of pI on scattering intensity of stoichiometric PICM prepared from PEG45-*b*-P(nBA25-co-MAA26) and PLys 1880 (•), PLys 8300 (•) and PLys 30,200 (•). Scattering intensity is expressed relative to initial scattering count. The inset represents the size distribution of PEG45-*b*-P(nBA25-co-MAA26)/PLys 30,200 PICM at physiological p*I* (0.15 *M* NaCl). (Reprinted from J. Control. Release, 109, Gaucher, G., Dufresne, MH., Sant, VP., Kang, N., Maysinger, D., Leroux, JC. Block copolymer micelles: preparation characterization & application in drug delivery, 169–188, 2005, with permission from Elsevier) *(6)*.

7. STEALTH PROPERTIES OF POLYMERIC MICELLES

The presence of a non-ionic water-soluble shell as well as the scale (10–100 nm) of polymeric micelles are expected to restrict their uptake by mononuclear phagocyte system and allow for passive targeting of cancerous or inflammed tissues through EPR effect *(6)*. This is crucial for achieving prolonged residence time in blood compartment. RES uptake for polymeric micelles is a function of hydrophilicity and fulfilled by the hydrophilic shell as this is in direct contact with blood after parenteral administration. The hydrophilic block used for polymeric micelle drug delivery systems is poly(ethylene oxide)/poly(ethylene glycol). PEO is used for its low toxicity and can be used as a shell-forming material.

The other advantages of PEO can be listed as follows *(42)*:

1. Attachment of PEO chains to hydrophobic surfaces is particularly effective against protein adsorption.
2. It has minimal interfacial free energy with water.
3. It possesses high aqueous solubility.
4. It exhibits high mobility.

5. The exclusion volume is large.
6. The attachment with PEO improves the biocompatibility of foreign materials.

For polymeric micelles, the length of PEO blocks influences circulation time and uptake by RES, with longer chains prolonging circulation time and decreasing RES uptake. The attached PEO brushes impart steric stability and are relatively inert. They impart "stealth" properties to polymeric micelles. This makes it viable for encapsulation in polymeric micelles resulting in prolong circulation time of encapsulated medicinal agents *(11,50)*.

Other polymeric materials can be used as alternative shell-forming materials. Mixed PEO/poly (electrolyte) block co-polymers is already explored by Stepanek *(51)*. pH-sensitive N-isopropylacrylamide co-polymer can also be used. PEO alternatives may ultimately allow for tailoring of shell properties, thereby increasing the utility of polymeric micelles for less traditional delivery applications, such as targeting, bioadhesion, responsiveness to proteins/cells and pH sensitivity.

For prolonged action, the delivery system must not be removed by filtration in capillary beds *(52)*. Polymeric micelles are normally <100 nm in diameter. This makes them pass through microvasculature. Prolonged action requires the system to avoid renal excretion also. This helps in increased blood residence times of polymeric micelles. In most cases, the molecular weight of polymeric micelles is inrange of <106 g/mol *(37,38,53)*. Therefore, characteristically high molecular weight polymeric micelles should avoid renal clearance. Tumour vasculature is characterised by high permeability and decreased or defective lymphatic drainage *(54)*. It is possible for polymeric micelles to extravasate *in vivo* resulting in accumulation in pathological tissues that have poor lymphatic drainage *(54,55)*. The ability of macromolecules to accumulate somewhat selectively in tumour tissues has been termed EPR effect. The EPR effect has been exploited as a strategy for altering the biodistribution of encapsulated compounds by passively targeting polymeric micelles to solid tumours *(11)*. An additional advantage associated with small size of polymeric micelles is relative ease of sterilisation by filtration.

Several core-forming blocks have been studied for pharmaceutical applications. ABCs as discussed earlier can be divided into following three categories. The classification is based on chemical structure of core-forming block (Table 2). ABC micelle systems can further be subclassified depending on method of incorporating drugs. The methods generally used are direct dissolution *(56)*, dialysis *(57,58)*, oil/water emulsion *(59)*, chemical conjugation *(12,60)*, complexation *(61)* and various solvent evaporation procedures *(62,63)*. Direct dissolution and dialysis methods are used most commonly for water-soluble and water-insoluble ABCs, respectively. The drug loading may occur depending on method. Drug loading may be achieved by physical entrapment, chemical conjugation, complexation, etc. In some instances, polymer and drug may simply be administered congruently *(64)*.

7.1. Long Circulating Properties

Prolonged circulation times of polymeric micelles are allowed for accumulation of drug at required sites. This happens because of the EPR effect. This is called as preferential accumulation. Required sites may be tumours, inflamed tissues, etc. Vascular defects have a different pore size and possess defective lymphatic drainage. This results in erratic fluid and molecular transport dynamics. Cancer treatment by EPR-mediated effect, the concentration of drug in plasma must be for a long period of time. Also the concentration of drug in plasma must be sufficiently high *(65)*. The afore-mentioned principles are true theoretically but the fate of a dosage form *in vivo* is unpredictable and unknown. Same is the fact with drug-loaded polymeric micelles after administration. Studies reveal that when paclitaxel was formulated as micelles with PEG-*b*-PDLLA and delivered, the drug was released very fast from its carrier and the chains of PEG-*b*-PDLLA were found accumulated in kidney. They undergo extensive renal excretion *(31)*. If the carriers are intended for prolonged circulation, a lot of factors govern the result. Size distributions, steric hindrance, presence of a hydrophilic corona are the most important of several factors.

Considering PEG as an example, we can understand some facts required for prolonged circulation. PEG is most commonly used polymer for forming a shell. It is a synthetic polymer and approved by FDA for internal use. It is biocompatible and non-toxic in nature. PEG forms a dense brush of polymer chains stretching out from the core of micelle when mixed with water. PEG exhibits large exclusion volume, is highly water soluble and highly mobile *(9)*. These properties impart steric stability to micellar structure by minimising the interfacial free energy of micellar core and by impeding hydrophobic inter-micellar attractions *(66)*. 1_H-NMR analysis suggests that PEG chains anchored to a polyester core extend outwards into aqueous environment, displaying flexibility and mobility comparable with PEG molecules dissolved in water *(67)*. The hydrophilic corona is vital in preventing opsonin adsorption and subsequent clearance by mononuclear

Table 1. Block Co-Polymers Used for Drug and Gene Delivery

General class	*Incorporation mechanism*	*Core-forming block*	*Encapsulated compound*
Poly(L-amino acid)	Chemical conjugation	Poly(L-aspartate)	Doxorubicin
		Poly(2-hydroxyethyl-L-aspartamide)	Methotrexate
	Physical entrapment	Poly(β-benzyl-L-aspartate)	Indomethacin, KRN 5500, pyrene, Amphotericin B and doxorubicin
	Complexation	Poly(L-lysine)	Oligo-deoxy-nucleotide DNA
		Poly(L-aspartate)	Cisplatin and lysozyme
		Poly(L-lysine) succinate	Cisplatin
Polyester	Chemical conjugation	PLGA	Doxorubicin
	Physical entrapment	Poly(ε-caprolactone)	Indomethasone, FK506, dihydrotestosterone and nimodipine
		Poly(D-L-lactide)	Paclitaxel, doxorubicin
		PLGA	Doxorubicin
Pluronics	Physical entrapment	P 105	Ruboxyl, doxorubicin
		P 85	Doxorubicin, vinblastin, mitomycin-C, methotrexate, cisplatin, epirubicin, taxol, etoposide, valporoic acid and loperamide
		F 127, F 68	Nystatin
	Co-treatment	P 85	Digoxin, fluoroscein, rhodamine-123, taxol, doxorubicin, etoposide, valporoic acid and loperamide

phagocyte system in liver and spleen *(22)*. This is especially true for PICM, which might present cores with residual positive charges. Kursa *et al*. have shown that the neutral nature of PEG corona could effectively shield the cationic PEI and prevent non-specific interactions with negatively charged plasma proteins in biological environment, thereby ensuring prolonged circulation times *(68)*. Moreover, while PEG chains are usually between 1 and 15 kDa in length *(69)*, some data indicate that longer the chains and denser the hydrophilic brush, greater the resulting stealth effect and blood circulation times *(9)*. Peracchia *et al*. found that the conformation of PEG anchored to polymeric nanoparticles could influence protein adsorption and complement-mediated phagocytosis *(70)*. Indeed, PEG attached by both ends to nanoparticles formed a more compact conformational cloud which showed greater hindrance against blood protein adsorption. Lastly, the PEG chain end can be functionalised to tether ligands not only to actively target certain tissues in body but also to modify the properties of corona. Kataoka *et al*. prepared acetaldehyde-functionalised PEG-*b*-PDLLA micelles to which an anionic peptide ligand (tyrosyl-glutamic acid) was coupled to confer a negative surface charge for enhanced stealth properties *(71)*. Up to 25% of administered polymeric micelles were still circulating 24 h after intravenous injection, suggesting that elimination half-life of carrier resembled that of well established vectors such as PEGylated liposomes.

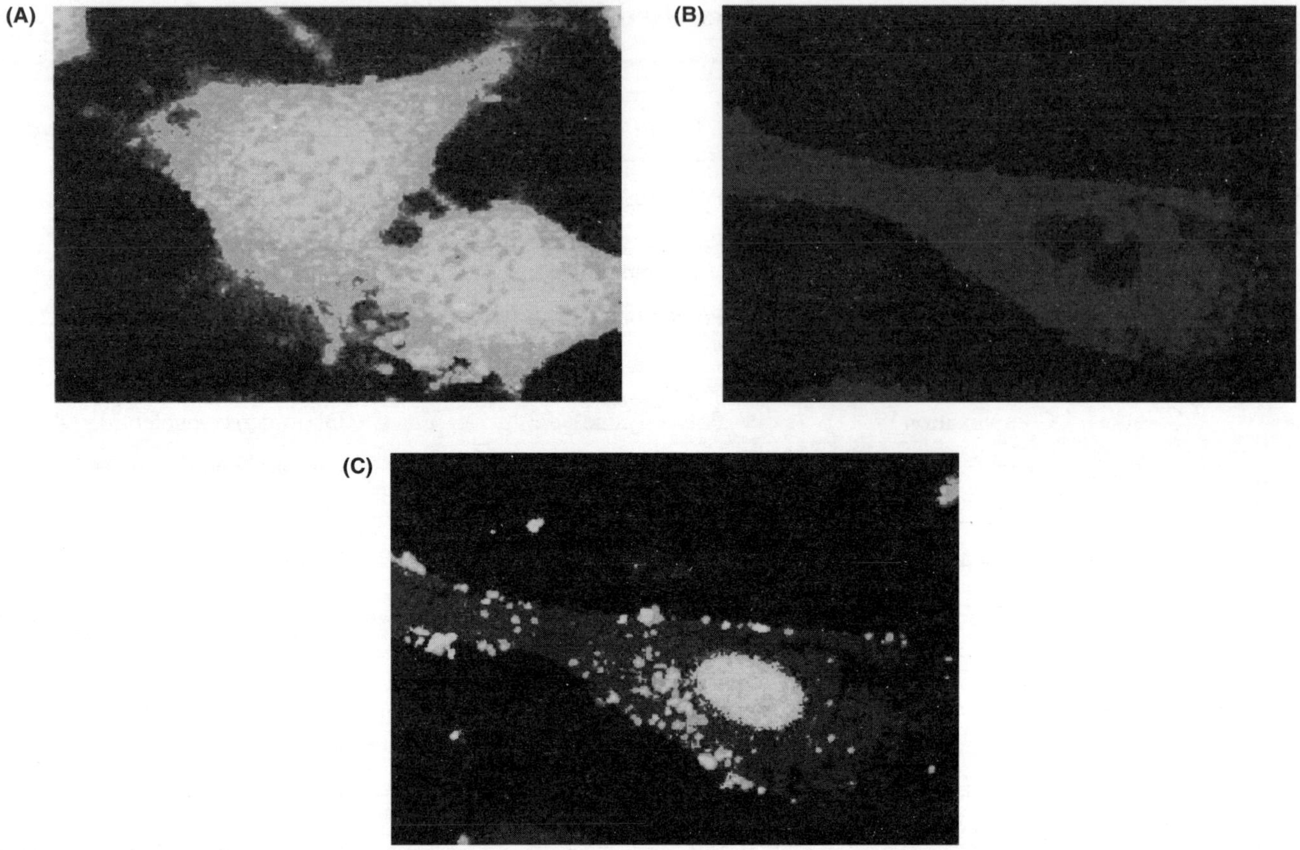

Fig. 7. CLSM of MCF-7 cells (human breast adenocarcinoma) showing **(A)** internalisation of free labelled drug, **(B)** lysosomes and **(C)** internalisation of labelled drug-loaded polymer micelles. Cells were analysed with confocal microscopy. Nuclei is stained blue, lysosomes with red and drug-loaded micelles localised in lysosomes in yellow (Reprinted from J. Control Release, 109, Gaucher, G., Dufresne, MH., Sant, VP., Kang, N., Maysinger, D., and Leroux, JC. Block copolymer micelles: preparation characterization and application in drug delivery, 169–188, 2005, with permission from Elsevier) *(6)*.

Studies have indicated that incorporation of a hydrophobic molecule into PEG-*b*-PCL polymeric micelles could significantly decrease its rate of cellular uptake. Labelling of block co-polymers with a fluorescent probe confirmed that nanocarriers were internalised as intact micelles, as opposed to free unimer chains *(72)*. Other analytical methods indicated that the micelles were predominantly localised in cytoplasm and distributed within several cytoplasmic organelles, but not in nucleus *(73)*. Block co-polymers gathered within sub-cellular compartments (lysosomes) but free drug gets diffused throughout the cytoplasm and nucleus (Fig. 7).

8. MICELLE IN SITE SPECIFIC DELIVERY

Targeting of micelles is very much an essential factor for maximum benefit of delivery system. Functionalisation of hydrophilic corona is the step that involves in modulating the biodistribution of polymeric micelles and to induce specific cellular uptake by receptor-mediated endocytosis. This is required for cellular specific targeting. Over-expression of specific protein receptors on surface of some tissues is a factor that has led to advancements of targeted drug delivery. Direct synthesis of hetero bifunctional block co-polymers or post-modification of a co-polymer with bifunctional spacer molecules tethers a ligand to outer shell of micelles *(74,75)*. Targeted micelles generally exhibit greater cellular uptake and improved *in vitro* efficacy than their unmodified counterparts. Table 3 highlight systems that demonstrate the potential of polymeric micelles for active targeting of drugs and other therapeutic compounds.

Table 2. Examples of Ligand Mediated Targeting *(6)*

Pilot molecules	*Polymers*	*Drug incorporated*	*References*
Glucose, galactose, lactose and mannose	PEG-*b*-PDLLA	N/A	*75–78*
Galactose	PEG-*b*-P(DMAEMA-co-VP	Plasmid DNA	*79*
Mannose	Poly(acrylic acid)-*b*-poly (methacrylate)	N/A	*80*
Lactose	PEG-*b*-PDLLA	N/A	*75,78*
Lactose	PEG-*b*-PDMAEMA	Plasmid DNA	*81*
Folate	PEG-*b*-PCL	Paclitaxel	*82*
Folate	PEG-*b*-PLGA, PEG-*b*-PLLA, PEG-*b*-PHis	Doxorubicin	*44,83*
Transferin	PEG-*b*-PEI	Plasmid DNA	*68*
		PT-Oligonucleotide	*84*
Epidermal growth factor	PEG-*b*-PEI	Plasmid DNA	*84*
HIV-1 Tat protein	Poly(acrylic acid)-*b*-poly (methacrylate)	N/A	*85*
Antigen-binding fragment of OV-TL16 antibody	PEG-*b*-PEI	Plasmid DNA	*86*

The approaches of targeting depend on various other factors as well. The micelles can be formulated as stimuli responsive polymeric micelles and these react depending on biological stimuli. The targeting rely on the fact that many pathological processes present either a slight increase in temperature or decrease in pH. For example—the pH of normal blood is 7.4 and pH of extracellular areas in tumourous tissues is around 6.8–7.0. The difference in pH is mainly due to higher rate of aerobic and anaerobic glycolysis compared with normal cells *(83)*. Cellular compartments, such as endosomes and lysosomes, exhibit even lower pH levels of about 5–6. Micelles designed to be pH sensitive undergo dissociation in response to decreased pH levels. This releases their payload (drug) as soon as they enter into cytoplasm or upon accumulation at tumour site. PEG-*b*-PDMAEMA-*b*-PDEAEMA tri-block co-polymers assemble into micelles in normal physiological pH. They also exhibit solubilisation of hydrophobic drug molecules. If the media is acidified, protonation of tertiary amine DEAEMA units occurs. This is followed by micellar dissociation and rapid release of drug at lower pH values. This was demonstrated *in vitro (87)*. The sensitivity of carrier to environmental differences depends on block co-polymer used to formulate the system. This can be tailored to the needs and pH values at which dissociation is needed or at the levels at which release of drug is intended. Polymeric micelles loaded with photosensitiser aluminium chloride phthalocyanine exhibited greater cytotoxicity against EMT-6 mouse mammary cells relative to control Cremophor EL formulation *(88)*. This enhanced activity was reduced in presence of chloroquine, a weak base impeding the acidification of endosomal/lysosomal compartments *(89)*, and was ascribed to the capacity of polymer to destabilise the endosomal membrane upon a pH-triggered conformational change *(56)*. Cross-linking of micelle core is a newly developed strategy aiming at augmenting the physical stability and circulation time of a drug delivery system. PICM may one day be applied to cytoplasmic delivery of genes and related compounds *(90)*. Intra-cellular drug delivery could be achieved through acid-sensitive linkers *(48,91)*. For example, Kataoka worked on developing environment-sensitive polymeric micelles based on PEG-*b*-PAsp-hydrazone-doxorubicin. *In vitro*, this system released drug at a pH-dependent rate, and optimal hydrazone cleaving pH was found corresponding to that of late endosomes and/or lysosomes (pH 5.0). Results from *in vivo* assays on mice bearing C26 tumours demonstrated enhanced therapeutic effect and reduced toxicity of micelle-incorporated drug *(92)*. Environment-responsive polymeric micelles can be a promising approach to oral delivery of hydrophobic drug molecules. The afore-mentioned strategy can be used to target drugs to basic environments in body following oral administration. It can also be used to increase the oral bioavailability of poorly water-soluble drugs *(93)*. The same can be used to release their cargo with response to exogenous stimuli as well. Ultrasounds have been successfully applied to trigger *in vitro* and *in vivo* release of drug from poloxamer micelles *(94–96)*. PNIPAM was incorporated in polymeric micelles to create thermo-responsive systems where the corona precipitated under local hyperthermia and initiated drug release. *In vitro* "on/off" control can be exercised over release of drug from co-polymer micelles via heating and cooling cycles *(97)*. The modification of composition of core-forming block can alter the thermo-sensitivity of micelles *(98)*.

9. CONCLUSION

These types of micellar delivery systems can be used in anticancer drug therapy. Polymeric micelles hold promise for the delivery of a large array of chemically diverse therapeutic compounds. Their utility in field of drug delivery is based on their characteristic self-assembly into core-shell nanostructures in aqueous milieu. In general, hydrophobic or electrostatic interactions are driving force behind the segregation of core from surrounding media. Apart from enhancing the water-solubility of many hydrophobic drugs, polymeric micelles can modify biodistribution of drugs through either passive or active targeting strategies. Designing vectors with sufficient physical stability to withstand dissociation upon dilution and ensure drug transport within the bloodstream to specific biological sites is of prime importance in achieving successful drug delivery. Issues of *in vivo* stability and drug retention, or lack thereof, have inevitably become focal points of research conducted on micellar systems.

REFERENCES

1. **Davis, SS. and Illum, L.** Drug delivery systems for challenging molecules. *Int. J. Pharm.* 1998;176:1–8.
2. **Zhang, L. and Eisenberg, A.** Multiple morphologies of "crew-cut" aggregates of polystyrene-b-poly(acrylic acid) block copolymers. *Science* 1995;268:1728–1731.
3. **Jones, M.C. and Leroux J.C.** Polymeric micelles: a new generation of colloidal drug carriers. *Eur. J. Pharm. Biopharm.* 1999;48:101–111.
4. **Rosler, A., Vandermeulen, GW., and Klok, H.A.** Advanced drug delivery devices via self-assembly of amphiphilic block copolymers. *Adv. Drug Deliv. Rev.* 2001;53:95–108.
5. **Kataoka, K., Kwon, G., Yokoyama, M., Okano, T., and Sakurai, Y.** Block copolymer micelles as vehicles for drug delivery. *J. Control. Release* 1992;24:119–132.
6. **Gaucher, G., Dufresne, MH., Sant, VP., Kang, N., Maysinger, D., and Leroux, JC.** Block copolymer micelles: preparation, characterization and application in drug delivery. *J. Control. Release* 2005;109:169–188.
7. **Yokoyama, M., Sugiyama, T., Okano, T., Sakurai, Y., Naito, M., and Kataoka, K.** Analysis of micelle formation of an adriamycin-conjugated poly(ethylene glycol)-poly(aspartic acid) block copolymer by gel permeation chromatography. *Pharm. Res.* 1993;10:895–899.
8. **Halperin, A. and Alexander, S.** Polymeric micelles: their relaxation kinetics. *Macromolecules* 1989;22:2403–2412.
9. **Adams, ML., Lavasanifar, A., and Kwon, GS.** Amphiphilic block copolymers for drug delivery. *J. Pharm. Sci.* 2003;92(7):1343–1355.
10. **Adams, ML. and Kwon, GS.** The effects of acyl chain length on the micelle properties of poly(ethylene oxide)-block-poly(N-hexyl-L-aspartamide)-acyl conjugates. *J. Biomater. Sci. Polym. Ed.* 2002;13:991–1006.
11. **Kwon, GS., Suwa, S., Yokoyama, M., Okano, T., Sakurai, Y., and Kataoka, K.** Enhanced tumor accumulation and prolonged circulation times of micelle-forming poly(ethylene oxide-aspartate) block copolymeradriamycin conjugates. *J. Control. Release* 1994;29:17–23.
12. **Li, Y. and Kwon, GS.** Methotrexate esters of poly (ethylene oxide)-block-poly(2-hydroxyethyl-Laspartamide). I. Effects of the level of methotrexate conjugation on the stability of micelles and on drug release. *Pharm. Res.* 2000;17:607–611.

13. **Lavasanifar, A., Samuel, J., and Kwon, GS.** Micelles self-assembled from poly(ethylene oxide)-blockpoly(N-hexyl stearate L-aspartamide) by a solvent evaporation method: effect on the solubilization and haemolytic activity of amphotericin B. *J. Control. Release* 2001;77:155–160.

14. **Venne, A., Li, S., Madeville, R., Kabanov, A., and Alakhov, V.** Hypersensitizing effect of Pluronic L61 on cytotoxic activity, transport, and subcellular distribution of doxorubicin in multiple drug-resistant cells. *Cancer Res.* 1996;56:3626–3629.

15. **Krishna, R. and Mayer LD.** Multidrug resistance (MDR) in cancer. Mechanisms, reversal using modulators of MDR and the role of MDR modulators in influencing the pharmacokinetics of anticancer drugs. Eur. *J. Pharm. Sci.* 2000;11:265–283.

16. **Batrakova, E., Lee, S., Li, S., Venne, A., Alakhov, V., and Kabanov, A.** Fundamental relationship between the composition of Pluronic block copolymers and their hypersensitization effect in MDR cancer cells. *Pharm. Res.* 1999;16:1373–1379.

17. **Rapaport, NY., Herron, JN., Pitt, WG., and Pitina, L.** Micellar delivery of doxorubicin and its paramagnetic analog, ruboxyl, to HL-60 cells: effect of micelle structure and ultrasound on the intracellular drug uptake. *J. Control. Release* 1999;58:153–162.

18. **Marin, A., Muniruzzaman, MD., and Rapoport, N.** Acoustic activation of drug delivery from polymeric micelles: effect of pulsed ultrasound. *J. Control. Release* 2001;71:239–249.

19. **Marin, A., Sun, H., Husseini, GA., Pitt, WG., Christensen, DA., and Rapoport, NY.** Drug delivery in Pluronic micelles: effect of high-frequency ultrasound on drug release from micelles and intracellular uptake. *J. Control. Release* 2002;84:39–47.

20. **Wei, G., Xu, H., Ding, PT., Li, SM., and Zheng, JM.** Thermosetting gels with modulated gelation temperature for ophthalmic use: the rheological and gamma scintigraphic studies. *J. Control. Release* 2002;83:65–74.

21. **Yu, B., Nichols, BC., Aramwit, P., and Kwon, G.** The effect of Pluronics1 F127 and F68 on the aggregation state and hemolytic activity of nystatin. *Biomaterials and Drug Delivery Toward New Millennium,* (Park, KD., Kwon, IC., Yuim N., Jeongm SY., and Park, K., eds.), Han Rim Won Publishing, Seoul, 2000, pp. 373–381.

22. **Kwon, GS.** Polymeric micelles for delivery of poorly watersoluble compounds. *Crit. Rev. Ther. Drug Carr. Syst.* 2003;20:357–403.

23. **Nishiyama, Y., Kato, Y., Sugiyama, Y., and Kataoka, K.** Cisplatin loaded polymer–metal complex micelle with time-modulated decaying property as a novel drug delivery system. *Pharm. Res.* 2001;18:1035–1041.

24. **Nishiyama, N., Okazaki, S., Cabral, H., Miyamoto, M., Kato, Y., Sugiyama, Y., Nishio, K., Matsumura Y., and Kataoka K.** Novel cisplatin-incorporated polymeric micelles can eradicate solid tumors in mice. *Cancer Res.* 2003;63:8977–8983.

25. **Lavasanifar, A., Samuel, J., and Kwon, GS.** Poly(ethylene oxide)- block-poly(l-amino acid) micelles for drug delivery. *Adv. Drug Deliv. Rev.* 2002;54:169–190.

26. **Kabanov, A., Batrakova, EV., and Alakhov, VY.** Pluronic block copolymers as novel polymer therapeutics for drug and gene delivery. *J. Control. Release* 2002;82:189–212.

27. **Allen, C., Maysinger, D., and Eisenberg, A.** Nano-engineering block copolymer aggregates for drug delivery. *Colloids Surf. B* 1999;163–227.

28. **Dufresne, MH., Fournier, E., Jones, M-C., Ranger, M., and Leroux, JC.** Block copolymer micelles—engineering versatile carriers for drugs and biomacromolecules, (Gurny, R., ed.), B.T. Gattefosse′, vol. 96, Gattefosse′, Saint-Priest, 2003, pp. 87–102.

29. **Shuai, X., Ai, H., Nasongkla, N., Kim, S., and Gao, J.** Micellar carriers based on block copolymers of poly(q-caprolactone) and poly(ethylene glycol) for doxorubicin delivery. *J. Control. Release* 2004;98:415–426.

30. **Lin, W.J., Juang, L.W., and Lin, C.C.** Stability and release performance of a series of pegylated copolymeric micelles. *Pharm. Res.* 2003;20:668–673.

31. **Burt, HM., Zhang, X., Toleikis, P., Embree, L., and Hunter, WL.** Development of copolymers of poly(d,l-lactide) and methoxypolyethylene glycol as micellar carriers of paclitaxel. *Colloids Surf. B* 1999;16:161–171.

32. **Liu, J., Zeng, F., and Allen, C.** Influence of serum protein on polycarbonate-based copolymer micelles as a delivery system for a hydrophobic anti-cancer agent. J. *Control. Release* 2005;103:481–497.

33. **Kang, N. and Leroux, J.C.** Triblock and star-block copolymer of N-(2-hydroxypropyl) methacrylamide or N-vinyl-2-pyrrolidone and d,l-lactide: synthesis and self-assembling properties in water. *Polymer* 2004;45:8967–8980.

34. **Jette, KK., Law, D., Schmitt, EA., and Kwon, GS.** Preparation and drug loading of poly(ethylene glycol)-block-poly(qcaprolactone) micelles through the evaporation of a cosolvent azeotrope. *Pharm. Res.* 2004;21:1184–1191.

35. **Adams, ML. and Kwon, GS.** Relative aggregation state and hemolytic activity of amphotericin B encapsulated by poly(ethylene oxide)-block-poly(N-hexyl-l-aspartamide)-acyl conjugate micelles: effects of acyl chain length. *J. Control. Release* 2003;87:23–32.

36. **Yamamoto, Y., Yasugi, K., Harada, A., Nagasaki, Y., and Kataoka, K.** Temperature-related change in the properties relevant to drug delivery of poly(ethylene glycol)-poly(d,l,lactide) block copolymer micelles in aqueous milieu. *J. Control. Release* 2002;82:359–371.

37. **Slager, J. and Domb, AJ.** Biopolymer stereocomplexes. *Adv. Drug Deliv.* Rev. 2003;55:549–583.

38. **Kang, N., Perron, ME., Prud'homme, RE., Zhang, Y., Gaucher, G., and Leroux, JC.** Stereocomplex block copolymer micelles: core-shell nanostructures with enhanced stability. *Nano. Lett.* 2005;5:315–319.

39. **Thurmond, KB., II, Huang, H., Clark, CG., Jr., Kowalewski, T., and Wooley, KL.** Shell cross-linked polymer micelles: stabilized assemblies with great versatility and potential. *Colloids Surf. B* 1999;16:45–54.

40. **Shuai, X., Merdan, T., Schaper, AK., Xi, F., and Kissel, T.** Corecross-linked polymeric micelles as paclitaxel carriers. *Bioconjug. Chem.* 2004;15:441–448.

41. **Jaturanpinyo, M., Harada, A., Yuan, X., and Kataoka, K.** Preparation of bionanoreactor based on core-shell structured polyion complex micelles entrapping trypsin in the core cross-linked with glutaraldehyde. *Bioconjug. Chem.* 2004;15:344–348.

42. **Lee, JH., Lee, HB., and Andrade, JD.** Blood compatibility of polyethylene oxide surfaces. *Prog. Polym. Sci.* 1995;20:1043–1079.

43. **Lee, J., Cho, EC., and Cho, K.** Incorporation and release behavior of hydrophobic drug in functionalized poly(d,l-lactide)-block-poly(ethylene oxide) micelles. *J. Control. Release* 2004;94:323–335.

44. **Yoo, HS. and Park, TG.** Folate receptor targeted biodegradable polymeric doxorubicin micelles. *J. Control. Release* 2004;96:273–283.

45. **Yoo, HS. and Park, TG.** Biodegradable polymeric micelles composed of doxorubicin conjugated PLGA-PEG block copolymer. *J. Control. Release* 2001;70:63–70.

46. **Oishi, M., Nagasaki, Y., Itaka, K., Nishiyama, N., and Kataoka, K.** Lactosylated poly(ethylene glycol)-siRNA conjugate through acid-labile h-thiopropionate linkage to construct pH-sensitive polyion complex micelles achieving enhanced gene silencing in hepatoma cells. *J. Am. Chem. Soc.* 2005;127:1624–1625.

47. **Hruby, M., Konak, C., and Ulbrich, K.** Polymeric micellar pH sensitive drug delivery system for doxorubicin. *J. Control. Release* 2005;103:137–148.

48. **Yoo, HS., Lee, EA., and Park, TG.** Doxorubicin-conjugated biodegradable polymeric micelles having acid-cleavable linkages. *J. Control. Release* 2002;82:17–27.

49. **Dufresne, MH. and Leroux, JC.** Study of the micellization behavior of different order amino block copolymers with heparin. *Pharm. Res.* 2004;21:160–169.

50. **Yokoyama, M., Okano, T., Sakurai, Y., Ekimoto, H., Skibazaki, C., and Kataoka, K.** Toxicity and antitumor activity against solid tumors of micelleforming polymeric anticancer drug and its extremely long circulation in blood. *Cancer. Res.* 1991;51:3229–3236.

51. **Stepanek, M., Podhajecka, K., Tesarova, E., and Prochazka, K.** Hybrid polymeric micelles with hydrophobic cores and mixed polyelectrolyte/nonelectrolyte shells in aqueous media. I. Preparation and basic characterization. *Langmuir* 2001;17:4240–4244.

52. **Moghimi, SM., Hunter, AC., and Murray, JC.** Longcirculating and target-specific nanoparticles: theory to practice. *Pharmacol. Rev.* 2001;53:283–318.

53. **Lavasanifar, A., Samuel, J., and Kwon, GS.** The effect of fatty acid substitution on the in vitro release of amphotericin B from micelles composed of poly(ethylene oxide)-block-poly(N-hexyl stearate- L-aspartamide). *J. Control. Release* 2002;79:165–172.

54. **Maeda, H., Wu, J., Sawa, T., Matsumara, Y., and Hori, K.** Tumor vascular permeability and the EPR effect in macromolecular therapeutics: A review. *J. Control. Release* 2000;65:271–284.

55. **Maeda, H., Sawa, T., and Konno, T.** Mechanism of tumor-targeted delivery of macromolecular drug, including the EPR effect in solid tumor and clinical overview off the prototype drug SMANCS. *J. Control. Release* 2001;74:47–61.

56. **Kwon, GS., Naito, M., Yokoyama, M., Okano, T., Sakurai, Y., and Kataoka, K.** Physical entrapment of adriamycin in AB block block copolymer micelles. *Pharm. Res.* 1995;12:192–195.

57. **Yokoyama, M., Fukushima, S., Uehara, R., Okamoto, K., Kataoka, K., Sakurai, Y., and Okano, T.** Characterization of physical entrapment and chemical conjugation of adriamycin in polymeric micelles and their design for in vivo delivery to a solid tumor. *J. Control. Release* 1998;50:79–92.

58. **Kwon, G., Naito, M., Yokoyama, M., Okano, T., Sakurai, Y., and Kataoka, K.,** Block copolymer micelles for drug delivery: loading and release of doxorubicin. *J. Control. Release* 1997;48:195–201.

59. **La, SB., Okano, T., and Kataoka, K.** Preparation and characterization of the micelle-forming polymeric drug indomethacin-incorporated poly(ethylene oxide)–poly (b-benzyl L-aspartate) block copolymer micelles. *Pharm. Sci.* 1996;85:85–90.

60. **Dorn, K., Hoerpel, G., and Ringsdorf, H.** Polymeric antitumor agents on a molecular and cellular level, (Gebelein, CG., Jr. and Carraher, CE., eds.), Bioactive Polymer Systems: An Overview, Plenum Press, New York, 1985, pp. 531–585.

61. **Harada, A. and Kataoka, K.** Formation of stable and mono diespersive polyion complex micelles in aqueous medium from poly(ethylene glycol)–poly(aspartic acid) block copolymer. *Pure Appl. Chem. A* 1997;34:2119–2133.

62. **Yokoyama, M., Satoh, A., Sakurai, Y., Okano, T., Matsumura, Y., Kakizoe, T., and Kataoka, K.** Incorporation of water-in-soluble anticancer drug into polymeric micelles and control of their particle size. *J. Control. Release* 1998;55:219–229.

63. **Pratten, MK., Lioyd, JB., Horpel, G., and Ringsdorf, H.** Micelle forming block copolymers: pinocytosis by macrophages and interaction with model membranes. *Macromol. Chem.* 1985;186:725–733.

64. **Batrakova, EV., Miller, DW., Li, S., Alakhov, VY., Kabanov, AV., and Elmquist, WF.** Pluronic P85 enhanced the delivery of digoxin to the brain: *in vitro* and *in vivo* studies. *J. Pharmacol. Exp. Ther.* 2001;296:551–557.

65. **Greish, K., Fang, J., Inutsuka, T., Nagamitsu, A., and Maeda, H.** Macromolecular therapeutics: advantages and prospects with special emphasis on solid tumour targeting. *Clin. Pharmacokinet.* 2003;42:1089–1105.

66. **Otsuka, H., Nagasaki, Y., and Kataoka, K.** PEGylated nanoparticles for biological and pharmaceutical applications. *Adv. Drug Deliv. Rev.* 2003;55:403–419.

67. **Hrkach, JS., Peracchia, MT., Domb, A., Lotan, N., and Langer, R.** Nanotechnology for biomaterials engineering: structural characterization of amphiphilic polymeric nanoparticles by 1H NMR spectroscopy. *Biomaterials* 1997;18:27–30.

68. **Kursa, M., Walker, GF., Roessler, V., et al.** Novel shielded transferrin–polyethylene glycol–polyethyleneimine/DNA complexes for systemic tumor-targeted gene transfer. *Bioconjug. Chem.* 2003;14:222–231.

69. **Torchilin, VP.** Structure and design of polymeric surfactantbased drug delivery systems. *J. Control. Release* 2001;73:137–172.

70. **Peracchia, MT., Vauthier, C., Passirani, C., Couvreur, P., and Labarre, D.** Complement consumption by poly(ethylene glycol) in different conformations chemically coupled to poly(isobutyl 2-cyanoacrylate) nanoparticles. *Life Sci.* 1997;61:749–761.

71. **Yamamoto, Y., Nagasaki, Y., Kato, Y., Sugiyama, Y., and Kataoka, K.** Long-circulating poly(ethylene glycol)–poly(d,l-lactide) block copolymer micelles with modulated surface charge. *J. Control. Release* 2001;77:27–38.

72. **Luo, L., Tam, J., Maysinger, D., and Eisenberg, A.** Cellular internalization of poly(ethylene oxide)-b-poly (q-caprolactone) diblock copolymer micelles. *Bioconjug. Chem.* 2002;13:1259–1265.

73. **Savic, R., Luo, L., Eisenberg, A., and Maysinger, D.** Micellar nanocontainers distribute to defined cytoplasmic organelles. *Science* 2003;300:615–618.

74. **Vinogradov, S., Batrakova, E., Li, S., and Kabanov, A.** Polyion complex micelles with protein-modified corona for receptormediated delivery of oligonucleotides into cells. *Bioconjug. Chem.* 1999;10:851–860.

75. **Jule, E., Nagasaki, Y., and Kataoka, K.** Surface plasmon resonance study on the interaction between lactose-installed poly(ethylene glycol)–poly(d,l-lactide) block copolymer micelles and lectins immobilized on a gold surface. *Langmuir* 2002;18:10,334–10,339.

76. **Yasugi, K., Nakamura, T., Nagasaki, Y., Kato, M., and Kataoka,** K. Sugar-installed polymer micelles: synthesis and micellization of poly(ethylene glycol)–poly(d,l-lactide) block copolymers having sugar groups at the PEG chain end. *Macromolecules* 1999;32:8024–8032.

77. **Nagasaki, Y., Yasugi, K., Yamamoto, Y., Harada, A., and Kataoka, K.** Sugar-installed block copolymer micelles: their preparation and specific interaction with lectin molecules. *Biomacromolecules* 2001;2:1067–1070.

78. **Jule, E., Nagasaki, Y., and Kataoka, K.** Lactose-installed poly(ethylene glycol)–poly(d,l-lactide) block copolymer micelles exhibit fast-rate binding and high affinity toward a protein bed simulating a cell surface. A surface plasmon resonance study. *Bioconjug. Chem.* 2003;14:177–186.

79. **Lim, DW., Yeom, YI., and Park, TG.** Poly(DMAEMA-NVP)-b-PEG-galactose as gene delivery vector for hepatocytes. *Bioconjug. Chem.* 2000;11:688–695.

80. **Joralemon, MJ., Murthy, KS., Remsen, EE., Becker, ML., and Wooley, KL.** Synthesis, characterization and bioavailability of mannosylated shell cross-linked nanoparticles. *Biomacromolecules* 2004;5:903–913.

81. **Wakebayashi, D., Nishiyama, N., Yamasaki, Y., et al.** Lactoseconjugated polyion complex micelles incorporating plasmid DNA as a targetable gene vector system: their preparation and gene transfecting efficiency against cultured HepG2 cells. *J. Control. Release* 2004;95:653–664.

82. **Park, EK., Lee, SB., and Lee, YM.** Preparation and characterization of methoxy poly(ethylene glycol)/poly (q-caprolactone) amphiphilic block copolymeric nanospheres for tumorspecific folate-mediated targeting of anticancer drugs. *Biomaterials* 2005;26:1053–1061.

83. **Lee, ES., Na, K., and Bae, YH.** Polymeric micelle for tumor pH and folate-mediated targeting. *J. Control. Release* 2003;91:103–113.

84. **Ogris, M., Walker, G., Blessing, T., Kircheis, R., Wolschek, M., and Wagner, E.** Tumor-targeted gene therapy: strategies for the preparation of ligand–polyethylene glycol–polyethylenimine/DNA complexes. *J. Control. Release* 2003;91:173–181.

85. **Becker, ML., Remsen, EE., Pan, D., and Wooley, KL.** Peptidederivatized shell-cross-linked nanoparticles: 1. Synthesis and characterization. *Bioconjug. Chem.* 2004;15:699–709.

86. **Merdan, T., Callahan, J., Petersen, H., et al.** Pegylated polyethylenimine-Fab' antibody fragment conjugates for targeted gene delivery to human ovarian carcinoma cells. *Bioconjug. Chem.* 2003;14:989–996.

87. **Tang, Y., Liu, SY., Armes, SP., and Billingham, NC.** Solubilization and controlled release of a hydrophobic drug using novel micelle-forming ABC triblock copolymers. *Biomacromolecules* 2003;4:1636–1645.

88. **Leroux, JC., Roux, E., Le Garrec, D., Hong, K., and Drummond, DC.** N-isopropyl acrylamide copolymers for the preparation of pH-sensitive liposomes and polymeric micelles. *J. Control. Release* 2001;72:71–84.

89. **Taillefer, J., Brasseur, N., van Lier, JE., Lenaerts, V., Le Garrec, D., and Leroux, JC.** In-vitro and in-vivo evaluation of pH-responsive polymeric micelles in a photodynamic cancer therapy model. *J. Pharm. Pharmacol.* 2001;53:155–166.

90. **Kakizawa, Y., Harada, A., and Kataoka, K.** Glutathione-sensitive stabilization of block copolymer micelles composed of antisense DNA and thiolated poly(ethylene glycol)-blockpoly(l-lysine): a potential carrier for systemic delivery of antisense DNA. *Biomacromolecules* 2001;2:491–497.

91. **Gillies, ER. and Fre_chet, JMJ. A** new approach towards acid sensitive copolymer micelles for drug delivery. *Chem. Commun.* 2003;1640–1641.

92. **Bae, Y., Nishiyama, N., Fukushima, S., Koyama, H., Yasuhiro, M., and Kataoka, K.** Preparation and biological characterization of polymeric micelle drug carriers with intracellular pH-triggered drug release property: tumor permeability, controlled subcellular drug distribution, and enhanced in vivo antitumor efficacy. *Bioconjug. Chem.* 2005;16:122–130.

93. **Sant, VP., Smith, D., and Leroux, JC.** Enhancement of oral bioavailability of poorly water-soluble drugs by poly(ethylene glycol)-block-poly(alkyl acrylate-co-methacrylic acid) self-assemblies. *J. Control. Release* 2005;104:289–300.

94. **Rapoport, NY., Christensen, DA., Fain, HD., Barrows, L., and Gao, Z.** Ultrasound-triggered drug targeting of tumors *in vitro* and *in vivo*. *Ultrasonics* 2004;42:943–950.

95. **Rapoport, N., Pitt, WG., Sun, H., and Nelson, JL.** Drug delivery in polymeric micelles: from *in vitro* to *in vivo*. *J. Control. Release* 2003;91:85–95.

96. **Rapoport, N.** Combined cancer therapy by micellarencapsulated drug and ultrasound. *Int. J. Pharm.* 2004;277:155–162.

97. **Chung, JE., Yokoyama, M., Aoyagi, T., Sakurai, Y., and Okano, T.** Thermo-responsive drug delivery from polymeric micelles constructed using block copolymers of poly(N-isopropyla-crylamide) and poly(butylmethacrylate). *J. Control. Release* 1999;62:115–127.

98. **Chung, JE., Yokoyama, M., and Okano, T.** Inner core segment design for drug delivery control of thermo-responsive polymeric micelles. *J. Control. Release* 2000;65:93–103.

10

Dendrimers

Dr. R.S.R. Murthy, M.PHARM, PhD
Mr. Prudhvi Rajn, M.PHARM

CONTENTS

1. INTRODUCTION

Dendrimers are a novel class of polymeric materials, which are highly branched, spherical, monodisperse macromolecules with a well-defined globular structure and high functionality. Dendrimer chemistry was first discovered in early 1978s by Fritz Vögtle and co-workers *(1)* and named as cascade molecules. In 1980 Donald Tomalia and co-workers synthesised first family of dendrimers *(2,3)*. The term "dendrimer" was originated from two words, the Greek word dendron, meaning tree and meros, meaning part. At the same time, Newkome's group reported synthesis of similar macromolecules *(4)*. They called them arborols from the Latin word "arbor" also meaning a tree, but "dendrimer" is the best established one.

2. STRUCTURE AND PROPERTIES

The three traditional macromolecular architectural classes (i.e., linear, cross-linked and branched) are widely recognised to generate rather polydisperse products of different molecular weights. In contrast, the synthesis of dendrimers offers the opportunity to generate monodisperse, structure-controlled macromolecular architectures similar to those observed in biological systems. Dendrimers are three-dimensional macromolecules with an initiator core, several branching units and multiple active terminal groups *(5,6)* (Fig. 1). Dendrimers are synthesised through a stepwise, repetitive reaction sequence from simple branched monomers. Each additional step of reaction leads to a higher generation dendrimer with double number of active sites (called end groups) and approximately double the molecular weight of previous generation. The uniqueness in dendrimer synthesis generates monodisperse symmetrical molecules with complete control on required composition and molecular weight. The diameter range is from about 1 to 13 nm, depending upon the number of generations in their synthesis.

The number of branch ends on a dendrimer increases exponentially as a function of generation, while the surface area of dendrimer increases with square of generation. Dendrimers of lower generations have highly asymmetric shape and possess more open structures as compared with higher generation dendrimers. As the chains growing from core molecule become longer and more branched (i.e., from fourth generation) dendrimers adopt a globular structure due to steric crowding of the branches at surface *(4,8)*. Dendrimers become densely packed as they extend out to periphery, which forms a closed membrane-like structure. When a critical branched state is reached, dendrimers cannot grow because of a lack of space. This is called the "starburst limit" *(8)*.

Dendrimers possess interior cavities surrounding the core, to which these dendrons are attached, represent well-defined nanoenvironments, which are protected from outside by the dendrimer surface (nanoscale containers) in case of higher generation

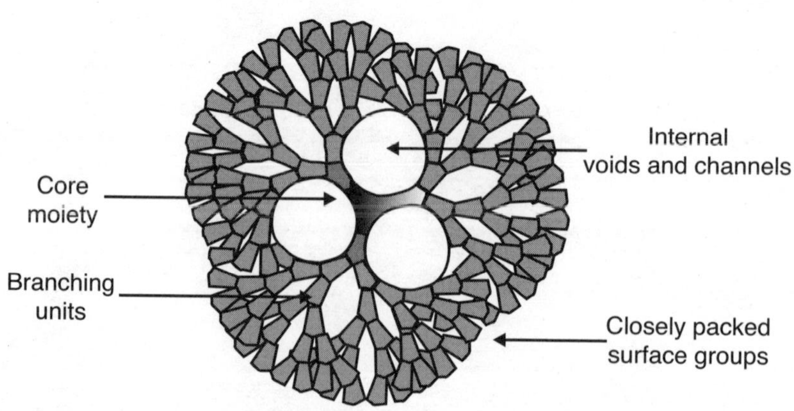

Fig. 1. A diagram of a dendrimer showing its unique structural characteristics (Reprinted from Prog. Polym. Sci., 23, Matthews. OA., Shipway, AN., and Stoddart, JF. Dendrimers—Branching out from curiosites into new technology, 1–56, 1998, with permission from Elsevier) *(6)*.

dendrimers. In periphery, dendrimer contains a homogenous, mathematically defined, surface functionality (nanoscaffold), which may be hydrophilic or hydrophobic depending on method of synthesis. These dendrimers with flexible surface groups can be tailored for specific applications. The dendrimer architecture, therefore, permits control over properties such as size, shape, density, polarity, reactivity and solubility *(5)*. Drug molecules can be loaded both in the interior of dendrimers as well as attached to surface groups.

3. GENERAL METHODS OF DENDRIMER SYNTHESIS

At present dendrimers are synthesised using several methods. These include divergent dendrimer growth, convergent dendrimer growth, growth using hypercores and branched monomers, double-exponential and mixed growth (Fig. 2) *(2–10)*.

3.1. Divergent Growth

In divergent method, the dendrimer grows outwards from a multi-functional core molecule *(2–4)*. The core is treated with an excess of first branched monomer reacting with all the core's reaction sites. This monomer with reactive groups further reacts with second monomer and gives rise to first generation. This process is repeated for several generations and a dendrimer is built as layer after layer. The divergent approach allows for attachment on the periphery of potentially functional molecules such as saccharides or peptides.

Advantages:
Large quantities of dendrimers can be produced because in each generation-adding step, the molar mass increases more than twice.

Disadvantages:
Divergent method requires excess monomer loading, particularly at higher generations. Incomplete growth steps and side reactions lead to isolation and characterisation of slightly imperfect samples.

Pure divergently grown dendrimers are virtually impossible to isolate from their side products and requires extremely efficient reactions in order to ensure low polydispersities.

Examples: polyamidoamine (PAMAM) dendrimer and polypropyleneimine dendrimers.

PAMAM dendrimers (Dendritech™, USA) were synthesised by Tomalia and were called as "Starburst™

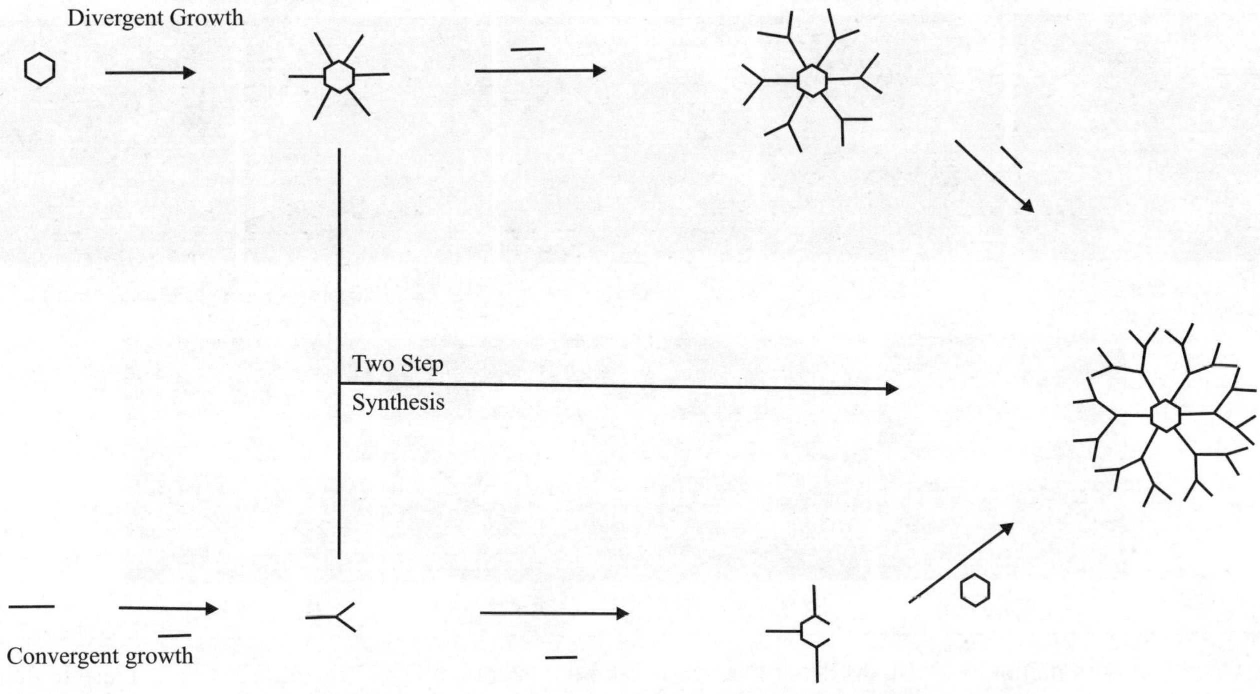

Fig. 2. Schematic representation of divergent and convergent growth.

dendrimers" (Fig. 3). The initiator core may be an ammonia or ethylenediamine (EDA) molecule (Fig. 4) in PAMAM dendrimers. The divergent synthesis of PAMAM dendrimers starts with an amine functional core unit that is reacted with methyl acrylate by Michael addition reaction *(2,4,11–13)*. This results in formation of two new branches per amine group with ester-terminated dendrimer, which is called "half-generation" dendrimer. Subsequent amidation of methyl ester with ethylene diamine gives a "full generation" amine-terminated dendrimer. Repetition of Michael addition and amidation steps gives the next higher "generation" dendrimer with increase in molecular weight, number of terminal functional groups and size (Fig. 5) *(14)*. The number of reactive surface sites is doubled with every generation and mass increases more than twice (Table 1) *(9)*. PAMAM dendrimers are biocompatable, non-immunogenic, water-soluble and possess terminal-modifiable amine functional groups for binding various targeting or guest molecules.

Polypropyleneimine dendrimers *(Astramo™) [Fig.6],* created by Meijer at DSM of the Netherlands) are synthesised by the divergent method starting from 1,4-diaminobutane *(15,16)*. They are grown by a reiterative sequence consisting of (1) a double Michael addition of acrylonitrile to primary amino groups followed by (2) hydrogenation under pressure in presence of Raney cobalt. Products are made up to generation 5.

3.2. Convergent Growth

In convergent approach, the dendrimer is constructed in reverse order, starting from the end groups and progressing inwards and finally attached to a multi-functional core molecule *(17)*. The convergent approach offers the opportunity to prepare "segregated" dendrimers and other interesting hybrid structures by employing the single reactive group at the focal point (or periphery).

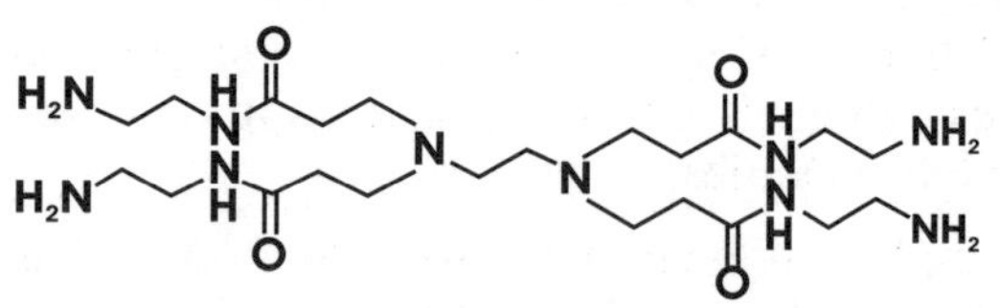

Fig. 3. Diagrammatic representation of PAMAM dendrimer.

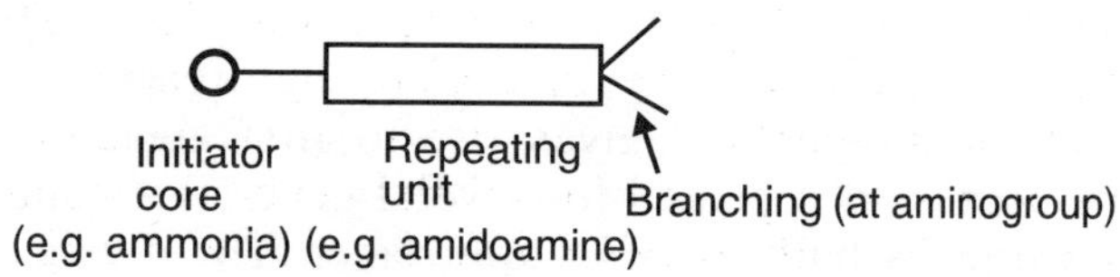

Fig. 4. PAMAM dendrimer with EDA core.

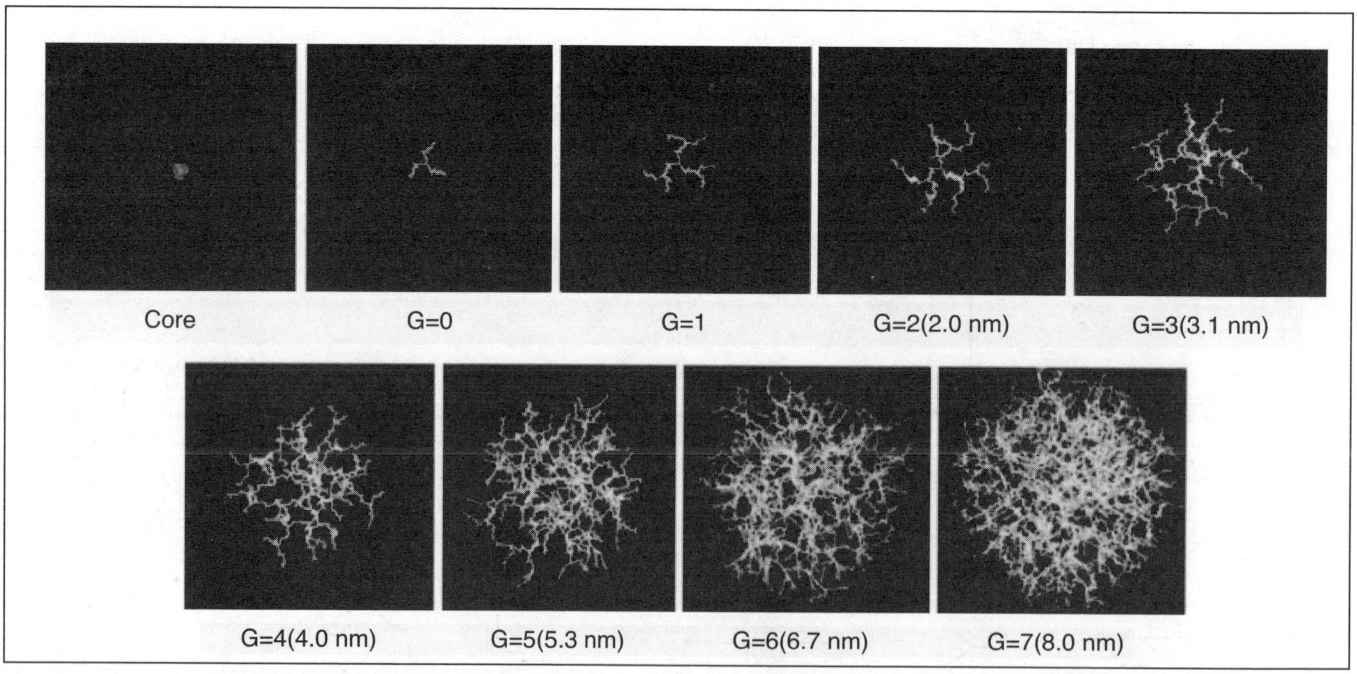

Fig. 5. Graphical presentation of PAMAM dendrimers from core to generation G = 7 showing linear increase in diameter and exponential growth of number of surface groups (Reprinted from Adv. Drug Deliv. Rev., 57, Svenson, S., Tomalia, DA, Dendrimers in biomedical applications-reflection on the field, 2106–2129, 2005, with permission from Elsevier) *(14)*.

Table 1. Theoretical Properties of PAMAM Dendrimers *(9)*

	Ammonia core		*EDA core*	
Generation	*Molecular mass*	*Number of terminal groups*	*Molecular mass*	*Number of terminal groups*
0	359	3	516	4
1	1043	6	1428	8
2	2411	12	3252	16
3	5147	24	6900	32
4	10619	48	14196	64
5	21563	96	28788	128
6	43451	192	57972	256
7	87227	384	116340	512
8	174779	678	233076	1024
9	349883	1536	466548	2048
10	700091	3072	933492	4096

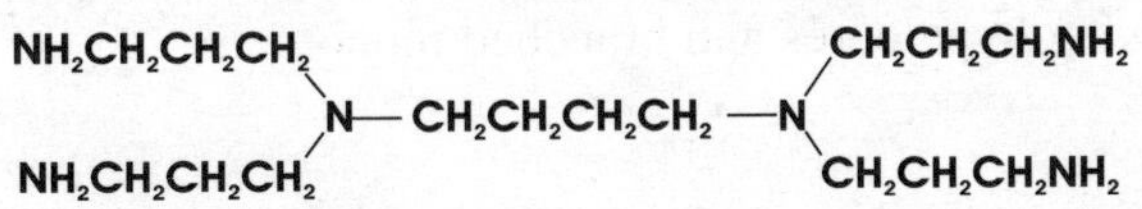

Fig. 6. Polypropyleneimine tetra-amine dendrimer.

Advantages of Convergent Method:
Using convergent synthesis, a nearly perfect dendrimer structure can be achieved, and drawbacks associated with divergent method likc structural defects due to side reactions, incomplete reactions, requirement of excess reagents to complete the reactions and difficulties in purification of final product can be overcome by convergent method. The growth reactions do not need to be as selective as in divergent synthesis and it is possible to selectively make changes to dendrimer as well.

Disadvantages of Convergent Method:
Low yields during synthesis of large structures and encounter of steric problems at their "focal points".

The number of steps required to build up a large structure is not reduced compared with divergent approach, yet a great deal of more starting material is required.

Examples: aromatic polyether dendrimers introduced by Frechet *(17)* and phenylacetylene dendrimers created by Jeffrey Moore *(18–22)*.

3.3. Growth Using Hypercores and Branched Monomers

Hypercores and branched monomers were developed by the Fréchet-group to reduce time required for dendrimer synthesis. These hypercore *(23)* and branched monomers *(24)* are pre-branched analogues of cores and monomers that are used in normal dendrimer synthesis. These pre-branched analogues are further linked together to get larger dendrimers in fewer steps, using advantages of both convergent and divergent methods. Frechet developed first-, second- and third generation hyper-cores for construction of polyether dendrimers. They synthesised fifth generation dendrimer (Fig. 7) by reaction of first generation hypercore and fourth generation wedge.

Advantages:
Facilitates synthesis of large dendrimers with relatively few steps.

Faster synthesis compared with conventional methods.

Disadvantages:
Hypercore synthesis may not be suitable for divergent synthesis.

3.4. Double-Exponential and Mixed Growth

Double-exponential growth is latest breakthrough in dendrimer synthesis. The method is based on an AB2 monomer with protecting units at functional groups

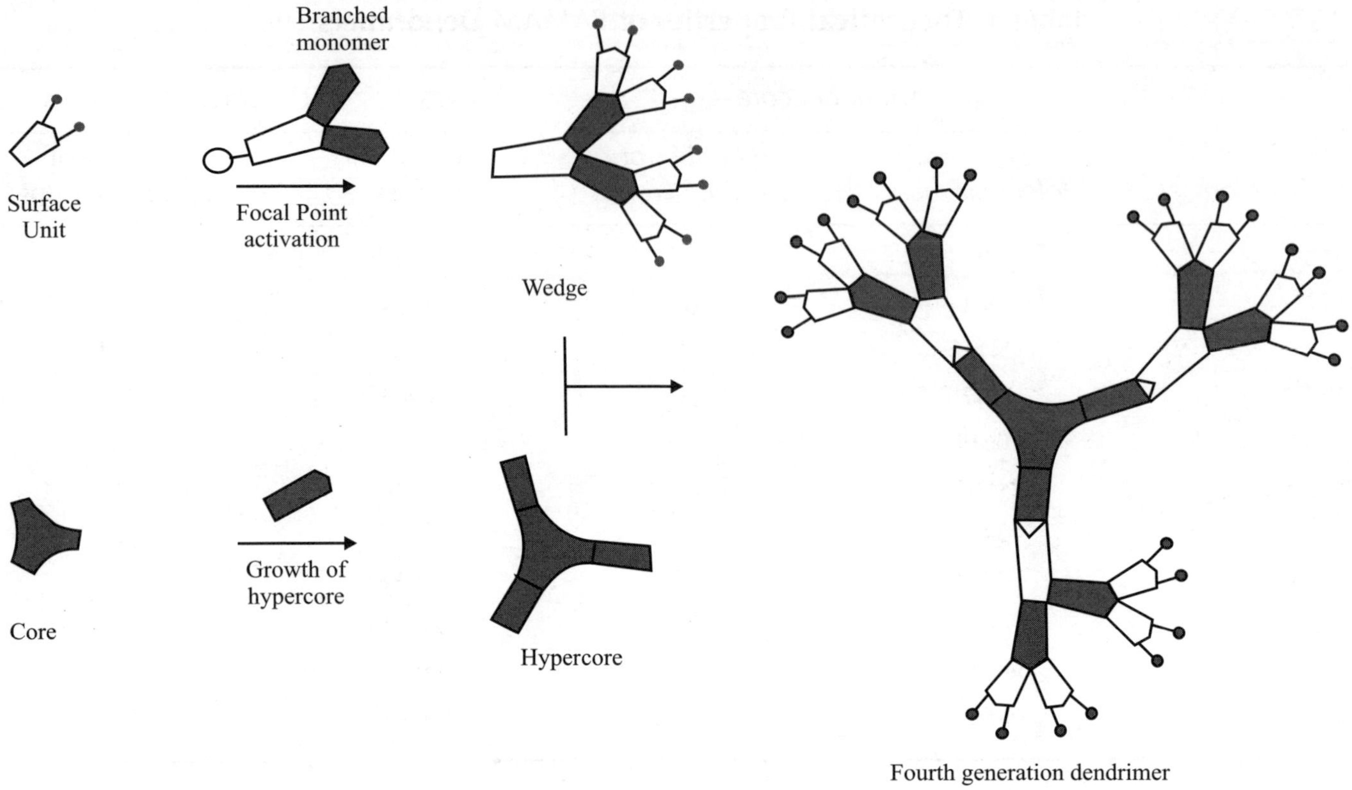

Fig. 7. Schematic representation of dendrimer growth using hypercores and branched monomers.

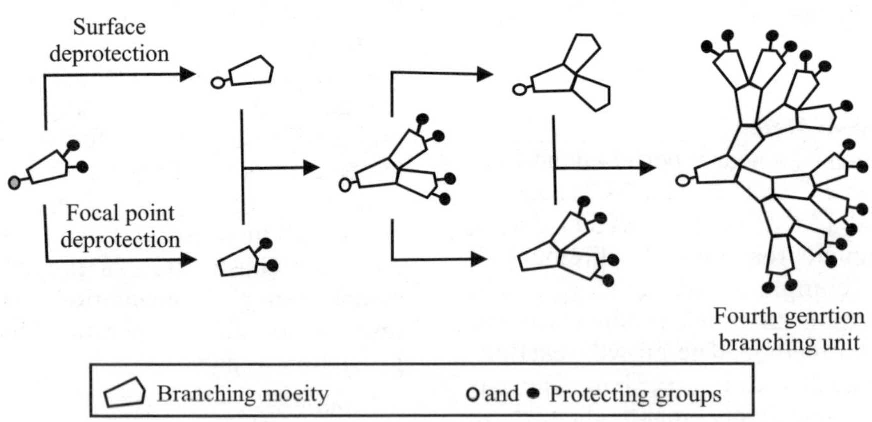

Fig. 8. Schematic representation of double exponential and mixed growth.

named A and B. This allows preparation of monomers for convergent as well as divergent growth from one single raw material. A and B are then reacted to result in an orthogonally protected trimer, which in turn can be used to repeat the growth process (Fig. 8). Shankai and co-workers were the first researchers, who described this type of synthesis. The term "double exponential" was given by Moore *et al. (25–28).*

Advantages:

More refined than traditional methods.

Facilitates synthesis of large dendrimers with relatively few steps.

Disadvantages:

Growth is so fast that it can be repeated only two or perhaps three times before further growth becomes impossible.

4. CHARACTERISATION OF DENDRIMERS

The following is tabulated data of different parameters of dendrimers and their characterisation using suitable analytical techniques (Table 2).

Table 2. Characterisation of Dendrimers Using Suitable Analytical Techniques

S. no.	*Characterisation*	*Technique*
1	Chemical and structural analysis like purity, imperfections, impurities, average molecular weight, polydispersity and surface functionality	Ultraviolet-visible spectroscopy ^{1}H and ^{13}C nuclear magnetic resonance *(29,30)* Size-exclusion chromatography—multi-angle laser light scattering *(30)* Capillary electrophoresis Polyacrylamide gel electrophoresis *(30–34)* Matrix-assisted laser desorption ionisation-time-of-flight mass spectrometry *(35–39)* Small angle X-ray and neutron scattering *(40–46)* Fourier transform (FT)-Raman spectroscopy *(47)* High-performance liquid chromatography (HPLC) *(48–50)* Electron paramagnetic resonance *(51)* Electron spin resonance *(52)* spectroscopy
2	Separation of different generations of dendrimers, quantitative estimation of the amount of "structural errors" in first generations and analysis of generational homogeneity of dendrimers	Capillary zone electrophoresis *(53)* Dynamic coating capillary electrophoresis *(54)*
3	Surface morphology and imaging	Transmission electron microscopy—for larger generations *(3,11,55,56)*. Atomic force microscopy *(31,57)*
4	Calculation of radii of gyration, hydrodynamic radii and polydispersities	Gel permeation chromatography *(58)*
5	Characterisation of three-dimensional structures	Molecular dynamic simulations
6	Structural changes in drug–dendrimer complex	X-ray diffraction and FT-infrared spectroscopy *(59)*

5. APPLICATIONS OF DENDRIMERS

Many potential applications of dendrimers are based on their unparalleled molecular uniformity, multi-functional surface and presence of internal cavities. These specific properties make dendrimers suitable for a variety of high technology uses including biomedical and industrial applications.

5.1. Biomedical Applications

Particulate carriers with well-defined sizes and shapes are of well-known interest in certain medical applications such as drug delivery, gene transfection and imaging. The superior control over architectural design of dendrimers, their size, shape, branching length/density and their multi-functionality, clearly makes them as ideal carriers for afore-mentioned applications (Fig. 9).

5.1.1 Delivery of Encapsulated Drugs

The interior cavities surrounding the core and core to which the dendrons are attached (nanoscale containers) are well suited for host–guest interaction and encapsulation of guest molecules. The utility of internal

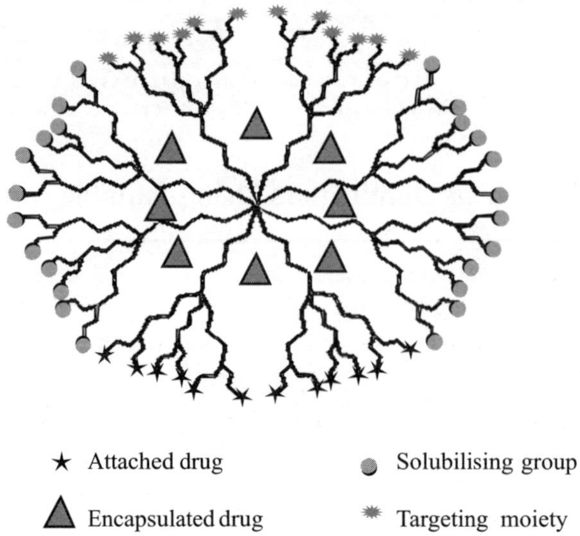

Fig. 9. Schematic drawing of an ideal dendrimer-based multi-functionalised drug delivery system *(60)*.

Table 3. Drugs Encapsulated in Dendrimers

Drug/agent encapsulated	*Application*	*References*
Anthracene	Solubility enhancement	*70*
Benzoic acid	Solubility enhancement	*65*
5-Flurouracil	Controlled release	*71*
Ibuprofen	Solubility enhancement and controlled release	*68,72*
Flurbiprofen	Solubility enhancement and controlled release	*73*
Ketoprofen	Solubility enhancement and controlled release	*74*
Nicotinic acid	Solubility enhancement and controlled release	*74*
Indomethacin	Solubility enhancement and controlled release	*63,75,76*
Methotrexate	Solubility enhancement and controlled release	*77,78*
Rhodamine B	Fluorescence and radio labelling	*79*
Rose Bengal	Encapsulation and controlled release	*66*

void volume of dendrimers to encapsulate hydrophobic guest molecules and drugs has been demonstrated by several research groups *(8,56,61–67)*. Some of the reported drugs encapsulated in dendrimers are shown in the Table 3. Meijer and co-workers were the first to entrap guest molecules (Rose Bengal dye *[66]*) in a dendritic molecule by using tert-butyloxycarbonyl groups to produce bulky, sterically crowded amino acid derivatives on surface of poly(propyleneimine) dendrimers. The Rose Bengal molecules can be liberated by acid hydrolysing outer shell to yield original flexible dendrimer. The number of guests that can be entrapped in dendritic box depends on shape of guest and the architecture of box and its cavities. A dendritic box may be suitable for drug delivery if the rigid shell can be selectively removed under physiological conditions. PEGylated dendrimers with their amphiphilic characteristics can hold hydrophobic guest molecules in dendrimer core and enhances water solubility of hydrophobic drugs *(68)*. Polyethylene glycol's (PEG) arm length and arm number at the surface impact the

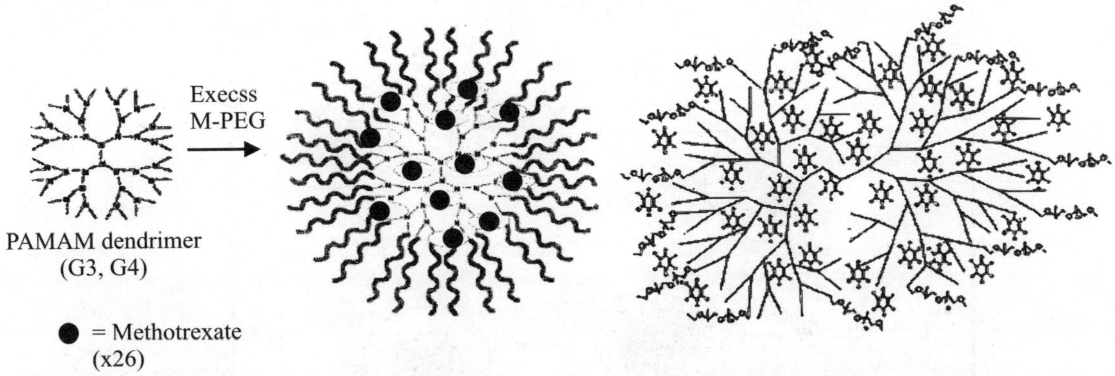

Fig. 10. Schematic representation of methotrexate encapsulated PEG–PAMAM dendrimer *(13)*.

Table 4. Drugs Covalently Attached to Dendrimers

Drug/agent covalently attached	*Application*	*References*
Antibodies	Radio labelling	*90*
5-Flurouracil	Controlled release	*71*
5-Aminosalicylic acid	Colon-specific delivery	*91*
Methotrexate	Enhancement of solubility and in controlled release	*77*
Platinate/*cis*-platin	Targeted delivery for treatment of cancer	*92*
Polyoxyethylene glycol	Targeted delivery for treatment of cancer	*93*

encapsulation of drugs as well as dendrimer generation. Kojima and his colleagues investigated the encapsulation of anti-cancer drugs within PEGylated PAMAM dendrimers *(69)* (Fig. 10).

5.1.2. Delivery of Covalently Linked Drugs

The surface of dendrimers provides an excellent platform for attachment of cell-specific ligands, solubility modifiers and stealth molecules reducing the interaction with macromolecules from body defense system and imaging tags. The ability to attach any or all of these molecules in a well-defined and controllable manner onto a robust dendritic surface clearly differentiates dendrimers from other carriers such as micelles, liposomes, emulsion droplets and engineered particles (Table 4). Modified dendrimers can be used to carry drug molecules to a specific location and release them in a controlled way *(80,81)*. Attachment of PEG to dendrimer surface can provide one additional ending group for coupling reaction. These additional end groups can be utilised for liganding of drugs. Yang and Lopina have developed synthetic approaches to synthesise penicillin-conjugated PEG–PAMAM star polymers. Dendrimers modified with folic acid (Fig. 11) and carbohydrates as cell-specific carriers are well-suited for targeted, cancer-specific drug delivery of cytotoxic substances (Fig. 12) *(82–89)*.

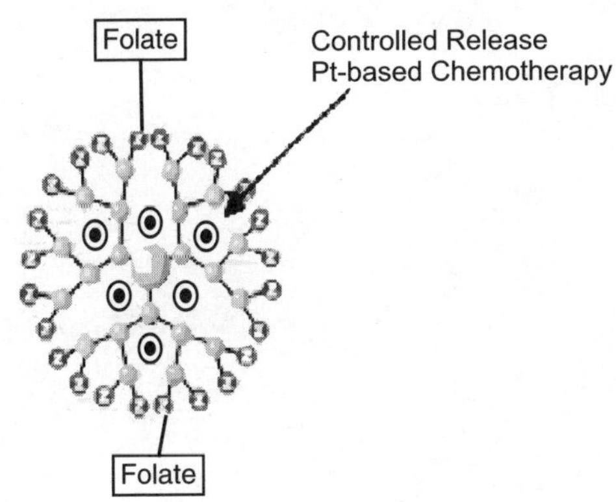

Fig. 11. Platinum encapsulated—folate PAMAM dendrimer—as a controlled release Pt based chemotherapy (94).

5.1.3. In Gene Delivery

Dendrimers have been studied as effective agents for delivery of genetic materials in gene transfection

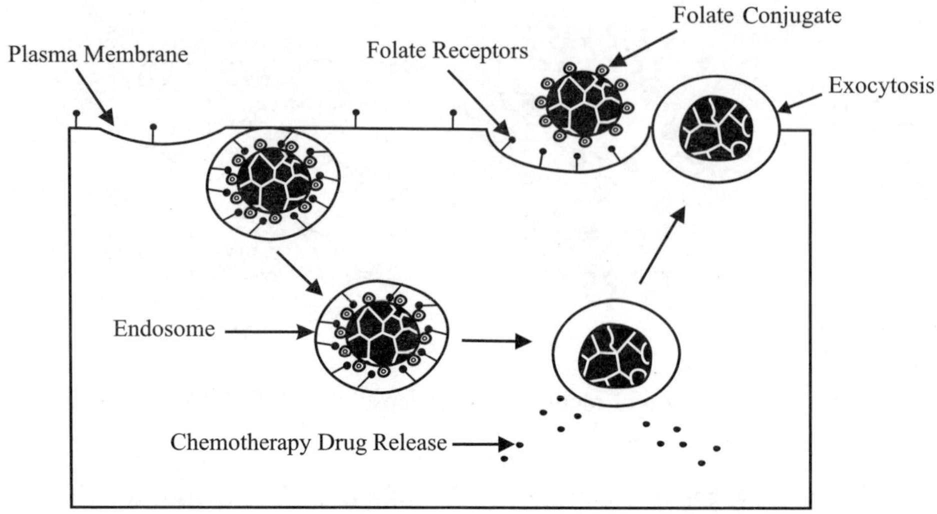

Fig. 12. Dendrimer-based receptor-mediated endocytosis hypothesis for Pt chemotherapy.

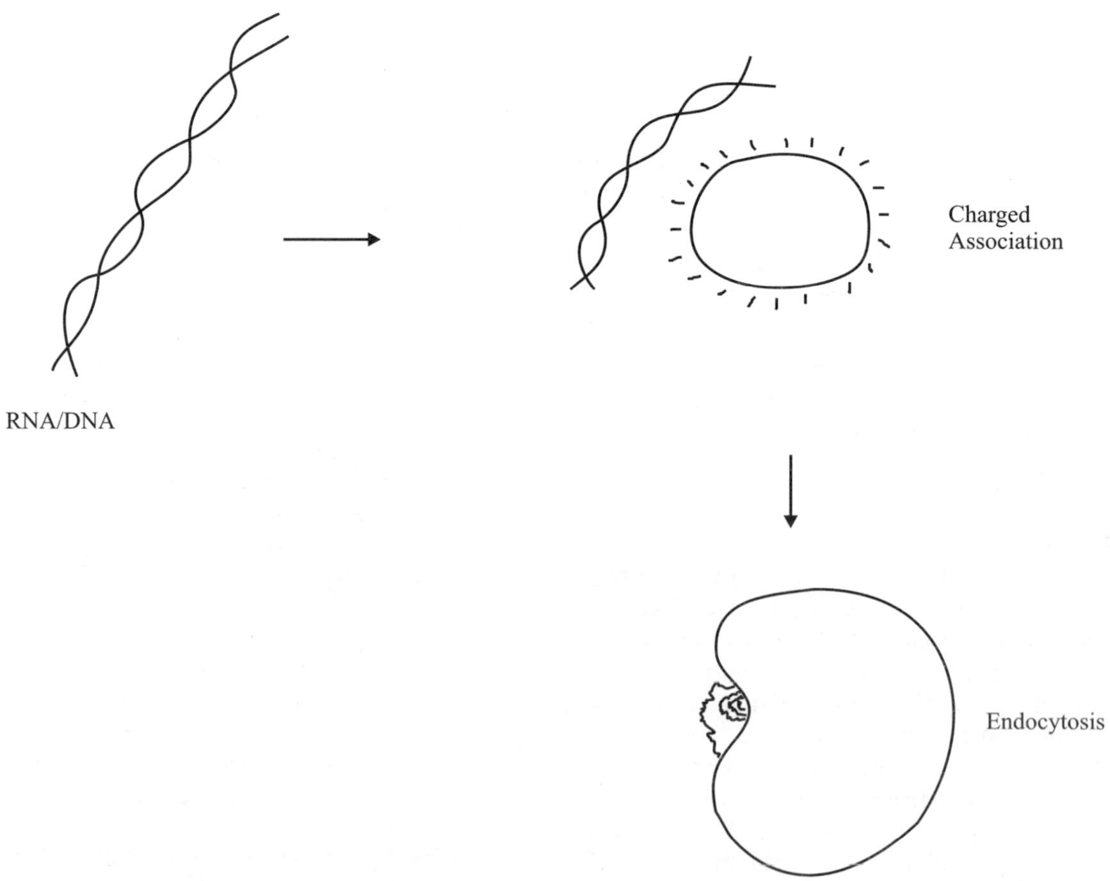

Fig. 13. Dendrimers as DNA transfection agents and their cellular uptake.

and targeting efficacy *in vitro.* Cationic dendrimers can form complexes with negatively charged DNA and once a polycation–DNA complex is formed, the overall positive charge of complex allows interaction with negatively charged cell surface groups. This interaction may result in adsorptive endocytosis (Fig. 13 and 14) and membrane destabilisation resulting in effective internalisation of DNA *(95).* However, the

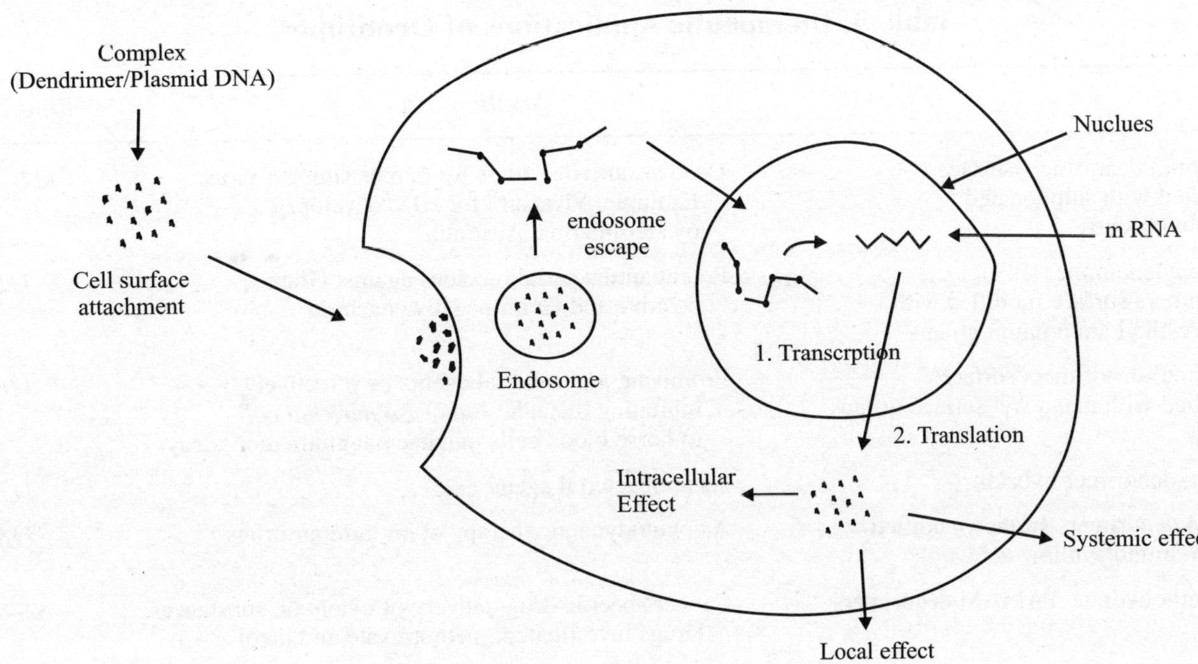

Fig. 14. Dendrimer-based receptor-mediated endocytosis hypothesis in gene transfection.

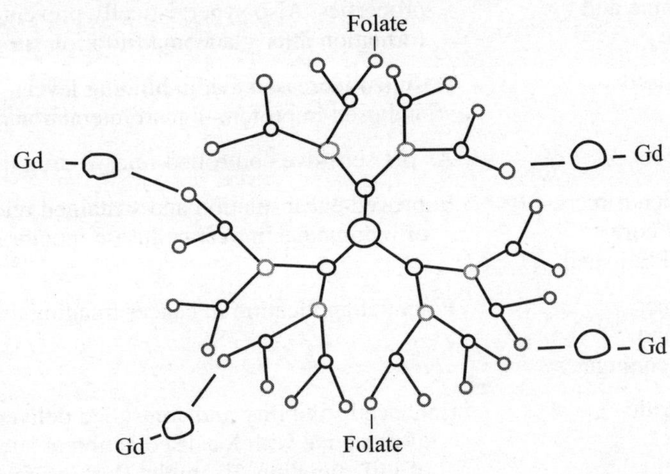

Fig. 15. Gadolinium–folate conjugated PAMAM dendrimers complex—as target-specific MRI contrast agents.

transfection efficiency depends on size and amount of dendrimer in DNA–dendrimer complex.

PAMAM dendrimers are highly effective and most investigated for gene delivery *(96–99)*. PAMAM dendrimers give no indication of inducing an immune response, show low *in vitro* cytotoxicity and stabilise polynucleic acids against nucleases.

5.1.4. Dendrimer Complex's as Diagnostic Reagents

Dendrimer–antibody conjugates are used in an immunoassay for rapid and sensitive detection of markers indicative of heart attacks.

In biosensor systems (systems containing reactive molecules and dyes).

In magnetic resonance imaging by conjugating with paramagnetic ions as contrast agents. Example: gadolinium–folate conjugated PAMAM dendrimers complex *(101,102)*.

5.1.5. Dendrimers as Biomimetic Artificial Proteins

Based on their dimensional length scaling, narrow size distribution and other biomimetic properties, dendrimers are often referred to as artificial proteins. Within PAMAM family, they closely match the

Table 5. Therapeutic Applications of Dendrimers

Dendrimer	*Application*	*References*
Poly(lysine) dendrimers surface modified with sulphonated naphthyl groups	Used as antiviral drugs for herpes simplex virus. Example: VivaGel® for HIV, developed by star pharma, Australia	*111–114*
Poly(propyleneimine) (PPI) dendrimers surface modified with tertiary alkyl ammonium groups	Potent antibacterial biocides against Gram-positive and Gram-negative bacteria	*115*
Poly(lysine) dendrimers surface modified with mannosyl surface groups	Promising antibacterial agents by effectively inhibiting the adhesion of *Escherichia coli* to horse blood cells in a haemagglutination assay	*116*
Chitosan–dendrimer hybrids	As antibacterial agent	*117*
PAMAM dendrimers surface modified with 5-aminolevulinic acid	As photodynamic therapy of antitumour drugs	*118*
Folate/carbohydrate–PAMAM dendrimers	Cancer-specific drug delivery of cytotoxic substances. Drugs investigated: methotrexate and taxol	*82–89*
PEG–PAMAM dendrimers	To improve solubility and biocompatibility. Drugs investigated: adriamycin and methotrexate	*69,82*
Anionic PAMAM dendrimers (G = 3.5) conjugated to D (+)-glucosamine and D (+)-glucosamine-6-sulphate	Revealed immunomodulatory and antiangiogenic properties. Also synergistically prevented scar tissue formation after glaucoma filtration surgery	*119*
PAMAM dendrimers functionalised with biotin.	Resulted increased avidin binding levels, and used in protein–ligand interactions	*120*
Quarternised PPI dendrimers	As pH-sensitive controlled-release drug delivery materials	–
Dual functional polyaryl ether dendrimers with a hydrophobic polyether core surrounded by a hydrophilic PEG shell	Improved encapsulation and sustained release of indomethacin over cellulose membranes	–
Radiolabelled antibody–dendrimer conjugates like ^{125}I-labelled and boronated MoAb–dendrimer conjugates	Potential application in cancer imaging and therapy	*121,122*
PAMAM–drug complexes dendritic nanostructures	Enhanced solubility and controlled delivery of bioactive with localised action at site of inflammation. Example: flurbiprofen (FB). Enhanced solubility, Permeability to A549 lung epithelial cells and controlled release. Example: ibuprofen	*72–123*

sizes and contours of many important proteins and bioassemblies *(103–107)*. Example: ammonia-core PAMAM dendrimers *(108–110)*.

Third, fourth and fifth generations have same size as insulin (3 nm), cytochrome C (4 nm) and haemoglobin (5.5 nm).

Fifth and sixth generations have diameters approximately equivalent to thickness of lipid bilayer membranes (~5.5 nm) of biological cells.

And second generation dendrimer have same width (2.4 nm) of DNA duplexes.

(Table 5) is tabulated data for different types of dendrimers investigated and their applications.

5.2. Industrial Applications

5.2.1. Size Standards

The exceptionally uniform molecular size of various generations of PAMAM dendrimers makes them excellent size standards for calibration of analytical instruments *(124)*.

5.2.2. Nanocomposites

Recent studies showed that PAMAM dendrimers form stable interior molecular nanocomposites with metal cations, zero-valent metals, other electrophilic ligands and semi-conductor particles. These materials are actively being investigated in electronics, opto-electronics and catalysis.

5.2.3. Organosilane Coatings

PAMAM dendrimers are the basis of poly(amidoamine)-organosilane (PAMAMOS) coating technology. PAMAMOS coatings are tough, transparent, flexible coatings, which have many of the same attributes of PAMAM dendrimers in coating form. They are being investigated for applications in micro-electronics.

5.2.4. Inkjet Inks and Toners

PAMAM dendrimers, at low additive levels, improve water resistance and adhesion of inks to a variety of porous or non-porous substrates such as paper, glass, plastic or metal. Their water and alcohol solubility permit formulation of low volatile organic compound inks. These polymers exhibit Newtonian flow behaviour for shear stability in these formulations. In toners, they impart good admix and flow characteristics, stable properties and high image quality.

6. COMMERCIAL PRODUCTS

Dendrimer-based products (and those in pipeline) include, for example, the world's first drug based on dendrimers, developed by Australian-based Starpharma, a topical vaginal microbicide called VivaGel®, prevents infection by HIV and other sexually transmitted diseases during intercourse. The microbicide is first and currently the only dendrimer-based pharmaceutical to be allowed to proceed into clinical trials by Food and Drug Administration. VivaGel® completed a Phase I human clinical trial in 2006, and Starpharma expects to bring VivaGel® to market by 2008.

Principle of VivaGel®:
"VivaGel®" microbicide gel is based on antiviral properties of SPL7013, a lysine-based dendrimer with naphthalene disulphonic acid surface groups. The dendrimers (ball-and-stick structures) in VivaGel® prevent HIV infection by binding to receptors on virus surface *(114)*. This interaction keeps HIV from infecting T cells.

Superfect® transfection reagent from Qiagen: The proven activated dendrimer for transfection of a broad range of cell lines *(125)*.

Superfect reagent consists of activated-dendrimer molecules with a defined spherical architecture. Branches radiate from a central core and terminate at charged amino groups, which can then interact with negatively charged phosphate groups of nucleic acids. Superfect reagent assembles DNA into compact structures (Fig. 16) ("Superfect–cDNA interaction" *[124]*) that bind to cell surface and are taken into cell by non-specific endocytosis. The reagent buffers the pH of endosome, leading to pH inhibition of endosomal nucleases, which ensures stability of Superfect–cDNA complexes. Due to highly controlled chemical synthesis, the activated-dendrimer molecules in Superfect reagent have a precise size and a defined shape. This ensures consistent transfection complex formation and reproducible transfection results.

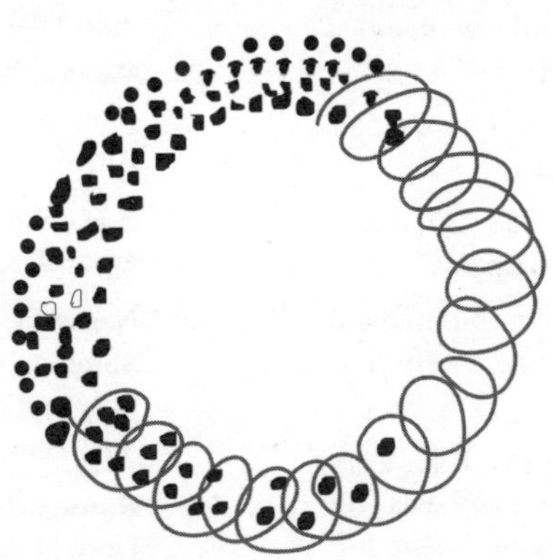

Fig. 16. Model of Superfect-cDNA complex *(124)*.

Stratus CS® (Dade Behring, Illinois): instrument for cardiac analysis, diagnoses a heart attack in 15 min by detecting certain protein biomarkers that are released in blood stream as a result of heart muscle damage. Developed by Dade Behring, one of the world's largest medical diagnostic firms.

The US Army Research Laboratory is developing a dendrimer-based anthrax detection agent, dubbed "Alert Ticket".

ExxonMobil owns patent 5,906,970 on a "flow improver" based on dendrimer technology—an additive that will increase the flow of oil in cold temperatures.

REFERENCES

1. **Buhleier, E., Winfried, W., and Vögtle, F.** "Cascade" and "Nonskid-Chain-like" syntheses of molecular cavity topologies. *Synthesis* 1978;1978:155–158.
2. **Tomalia, DA., Baker, H., Dewald, JR., et al.** A new class of polymers: starburst-dendritic macromolecules. *Polym. J.* 1985;17:117–132.
3. **Tomalia, DA., Naylor, AM., and Goddard III, WA.** Starburst dendrimers: molecular-level control of size, shape, surface chemistry, topology and flexibility from atoms to macroscopic matter. *Angew. Chem. Int. Ed. Engl.* 1990;29:138–175.
4. **Newkome, GR., Yao, ZQ., Baker, GR., and Gupta, VK.** Cascade molecules: a new approach to micelles, A [27]-arborol. *J. Org. Chem.* 1985;50:2003–2006.
5. **Cagin, T., Wang, G., Martin, R., and Goddard, WA.** Molecular modeling of dendrimers for nanoscale applications. *Nanotechnology* 2000;11(2):77–84.
6. **Matthews, OA. and Shipway, AN.** Dendrimers—branching out from curiosities into new technologies. *Prog. Polym. Sci.* 1998;23:1–56.
7. **Shipway, AN.** URL: http://www.ninger.com/dendrimer/, 1997.
8. **Naylor, AM., Goddard, WA., Kiefer, GE., and Tomalia, DA.** Starburst dendrimers: 5. Molecular shape control. *J. Am. Chem. Soc.* 1989;111:2339–2341.
9. **Klajnert, B. and Bryszewska, M.** Review: dendrimers: properties and applications. *Acta Biochimica. Polonica.* 2001;48(1):199–208.
10. **Hodge, P.** Polymer science branches out. *Nature* 1993; 362:18–19.
11. **Tomalia, DA., Baker, H., Dewald, J., et al.** Dendritic molecules: synthesis of starbrust dendrimers. *Macromolecules* 1986;19:2466–2468.
12. **Tomalia, DA. and Dewald, JR.** US Patent No. 4 507 466, 4 587 329, 1985, assigned to Dow Chemical Company.
13. **Tomalia, DA. and Dewald, JR.** US Patent No. 4 568 737, 4 587 329, 4 599 400, 4 631 337., Dow Chemical Company.
14. **Svenson, S. and Tomalia, DA.** Dendrimers in biomedical applications-reflections on the field. *Adv. Drug Deliv. Rev.* 2005;57:2106–2129.
15. **de Brabander-van den Berg, EMM. and Meijer, EW.** Poly (propylene imine) dendrimers: large scale synthesis by heterogeneously catalyzed hydrogenations. *Angew. Chem. Int. Ed. Engl.* 1993;32:1308–1311.
16. **Kabanov, VA., Sergeyev, VG., Pyshkina, OA., et al.** Interpolyelectrolyte complexes formed by DNA and astramol poly(propylene imine) dendrimers. *Macromolecules* 2000;33:9587–9593.
17. **Hawker, CJ. and Frechet, JMJ.** Preparation of polymers with controlled molecular architecture. A new convergent approach to dendritic macromolecules. *J. Am. Chem. Soc.* 1990;112: 7638–7647.
18. **Zhang, J., Moore, JS., Xu, Z., and Aguirre, RA.** Nanoarchitectures. 1. Controlled-synthesis of phenylacetylene sequences. *J. Am. Chem. Soc.* 1992;114:2273–2274.
19. **Zhang, J. and Moore, JS.** Nanoarchitectures. 3. Aggregation of hexa (phenyl-acetylene) macrocycles in solution: a model system for studying interactions. *J. Am. Chem. Soc.* 1992; 114:9701–9702.
20. **Xu, Z. and Moore, JS.** Rapid construction of large-size phenylacetylene dendrimers up to 12.5 nanometers in molecular diameter. *Angew. Chem.* 1992;105:1394; *Angew. Chem. Int. Ed. Engl.* 1992;32:1354–1357.
21. **Xu, Z., Kyan, B., and Moore, JS.** Stiff dendritic macromolecules based on phenylacetylenes. *Adv. Dendritic Macromolecules*, (Newkome, GR., ed.), vol. 1, JAI Press, Greenwich CT, pp. 69–104.
22. **Xu, Z., Kahr, M., Walker, KL., Wilkins, CL., and Moore, JS.** Phenylacetylene dendrimers by the divergent, convergent and double-stage convergent methods. *J. Am. Chem. Soc.* 1994;116:4537–4550.
23. **Wooley, KL., Hawker, CJ., and Frechet, JMJ.** Hyperbranched macromolecules via a novel double-stage convergent growth approach. *J. Am. Chem. Soc.* 1991;113:4252–4261.
24. **Wooley, KL., Hawker, CJ., and Frechet, JMJ.** A branched-monomer approach for the rapid synthesis of dendimers. *Angew. Chemie-Int. Ed. Engl.* 1994;33:82–85.
25. **Nagasaki, T., Ukon, M., Arimori, S., and Shinkai, S.** "Crowned" arborols. *J. Chem. Soc. Chem. Commun.* 1992;608–610.
26. **Nagasaki, T., Kimura, O., Ukon, M., Arimori, S., Hamachi, I., and Shinkai, S.** Synthesis, metal-binding properties and polypeptide solubilization of "crowned" arborols. *J. Chem. Soc. Perkin. Trans.* 1994;1:75–81.
27. **Kawaguchi, T., Walker, KL., Wilkins, CL., and Moore, JS.** Double exponential dendrimer growth. *J. Am. Chem. Soc.* 1995;117:2159–2165.

28. **Frechet, JMJ., Gitsov, I., Grubbs, RB., et al.** Proceedings of the american chemical society division of polymeric materials: science and engineering. 1995;73:271–272.

29. **Majoros, IJ., Keszler, B., Woehler, S., Bull, T., and Baker, Jr. JR.** Acetylation of poly (amidoamine) dendrimers. *Macromolecules* 2003;36:5526–5529.

30. **Shi, X, Banyai, I., Islama, MT., Lesniaka, W., Davisa, DZ., Baker, JR., Jr., and Balogha, LP.** Generational, skeletal and substitutional diversities in generation one poly(amidoamine) dendrimers. *Polymer* 2005;46(9):3022–3034.

31. **Shi, X., Patri, A., Lesniak, W., et al.** Analysis of poly (amidoamine)–succinamic acid dendrimers by slab–gel electrophoresis and capillary zone electrophoresis. *Electrophoresis* 2005;26:2960–2967.

32. **Shi, X., Patri, A., Lesniak, W., et al.** Electrophoretic mobility and molecular distribution studies of poly (amidoamine) dendrimers of defined charges. *Electrophoresis* 2006;27:1758–1767.

33. **Sharma, A., Mohanty, DK., Desai, A., and Ali, R.** A simple polyacrylamide gel electrophoresis procedure for the separation of polyamidoamine dendrimers. *Electrophoresis* 2003;24:2733–2739.

34. **Sharma, A., Desai, A., Ali, R., and Tomalia, D.** Polyacrylamide gel electrophoresis separation and detection of polyamidoamine dendrimers possessing various cores and terminal groups. *J. Chromatogr. A* 2005;1081:238–244.

35. **Leon, JW. and Fréchet, JMJ.** Analysis of aromatic polyether dendrimers and dendrimer-linear block copolymers by matrix-assisted laser desorption ionization mass spectrometry. *Polym. Bull.* 1995;35:449–455.

36. **Walker, KL., Kahr, MS., Wilkins, CL., Xu, Z., and Moore, JS.** Analysis of hydrocarbon dendrimers by laser desorption time of flight and fourier transform mass spectrometry. *J. Am. Soc. Mass Spectrom.* 1994;5:731–739.

37. **Schwartz, BL., Rockwood, AL., Smith, RD., Tomalia, DA., and Spindler, R.** Detection of high molecular weight starburst dendrimers by electrospray ionization mass spectrometry. *Rapid Commun. Mass Spectrom.* 1995;9:1552–1555.

38. **Kallos, GJ., Lewis, S., Zhou, J., Hedstrand, DM., and Tomalia, DA.** Molecular weight determination of a polyamidoamine starburst polymer by electrospray ionization mass spectrometry. *Rapid Commun. Mass Spectrom.* 1991;5:383.

39. **Woller, EK., Cloninger, MJ., and Mannose.** Functionalization of a sixth generation dendrimer. *Biomacromolecules* 2001; 2:1052–1054.

40. **Silke, R., Tadeusz, P., and Volker, U.** Structure of star-burst dendrimers: a comparison between small angle X-ray scattering and computer simulation results. *J. Chem. Phy.* 2004;121(8):3840–3853.

41. **Huang, QR., Dubin, PL., Lal, J., Moorefield, CN., and Newkome, GR.** Small-angle neutron scattering studies of charged carboxyl-terminated dendrimers in solutions. *Langmuir* 2005;21(7):2737–2742.

42. **Ramzi, A., Scherrenberg, R., Brackman, J., Joosten, J., and Mortensen, K.** Intermolecular interactions between poly (propylene-imine) dendrimers: small-angle neutron scattering. *Am. Phys. Soc. Annu. March Meet.* 1998;16–20.

43. **Kuklin, AI., Ozerin, AN., Islamov, AKh., et al.** Complementarity of small-angle neutron and X-ray scattering methods for the quantitative structural and dynamical specification of dendritic macromolecules. *J. Appl. Crystallogr.* 2003;36(3–1):679.

44. **Ozerin, AN., Svergun, DI., Volkov, VV., et al.** The spatial structure of dendritic macromolecules. *J. Appl. Crystallogr.* 2005;38(6):996.

45. **Bauer, BJ., Hammouda, B., Barnes, JD., Briber, RM., and Tomalia, DA.** Abstracts of papers of the american chemical society. 1994;208:383-PMSE.

46. **Bauer, BJ., Briber, RM., Hammouda, B., and Tomalia, DA.** Abstracts of papers of the american chemical society. 1992;204:225-PMSE.

47. **Furer, VL., Majoral, JP., Caminade, AM., and Kovalenko, VI.** Elementoorganic dendrimes characterization by Raman spectroscopy. *Polymer* 2004;45:5889–5895.

48. **Islam, MT., Majoraos, IJ., and Baker, JR., Jr.** HPLC analysis of PAMAM dendrimer based multifunctional devices. *J. Chromatogr. B Anal. Technol. Biomed. Life Sci.* 2005;822:21–26.

49. **Islam, MT., Shi, X., Balogh, L., and Baker, JR., Jr.** HPLC separation of different generations of poly (amidoamine) dendrimers modified with various terminal groups. *Anal. Chem.* 2005;77(7):2063–2070.

50. **Shi, X., Bi, X., Ganser, TR., et al.** HPLC analysis of functionalized poly (amidoamine) dendrimers and the interaction between a folate–dendrimer conjugate and folate binding protein. *Analyst* 2006;131:842–848.

51. **Ottaviani, MF., Bossmann, S., Turro, NJ., and Tomalia, DA.** Characterization of starburst dendrimers by the EPR technique. 1. Copper complexes in water solution. *J. Am. Chem. Soc.* 1994;116:661–671.

52. **Ottaviani, MF. and Turro, NJ.** Characterization of dendrimer structures by ESR techniques, advanced ESR methods in polymer research, (Schlick, S. ed.), John Wiley & Sons, Inc., 2006, pp. 279–306.

53. **Ebber, A., Vaher, M., Peterson, J., and Lopp, M.** Application of capillary zone electrophoresis to the separation and characterization of poly(amidoamine) dendrimers with an ethylenediamine core. *J. Chromatogr. A* 2002;949(1 and 2): 351–358.

54. **Sedlakova, P., Svobodova, J., Miksik, I., and Tomas, H.** Separation of poly(amidoamine) (PAMAM) dendrimer generations by dynamic coating capillary electrophoresis. *J. Chromatogr. B Anal. Technol. Biomed. Life Sci.* 2006;841 (1 and 2):135–139.

55. **Jackson, CL., Chanzy, HD., Booy, FP., et al.** Visualization of dendrimer molecules by transmission electron microscopy (TEM): staining methods and cryo-TEM of vitrified solutions. *Macromolecules* 1998;31:6259–6265.

56. **Newkome, GR., Moorefield, CN., Baker, GR., Saunders, MJ., and Grossman, SH.** Unimolecular micelles. *Angew. Chemie-Int. Ed. Engl.* 1991;30:1178–1180.

57. **Li, J., Piehler, LT., Qin, D., Baker, JR., Jr., Tomalia, DA., and Meier, DJ.** Visualization and characterization of poly (amidoamine) dendrimers by atomic force microscopy. *Langmuir* 2000;16:5613–5616.
58. **Hester, RD. and Mitchell, PH.** A new universal GPC calibration method. *J. Polym. Sci. Chem. Ed.* 1980;18:1727–1738.
59. **Popescu, MC., Filip, D., Vasile, C., et al.** Characterization by fourier transform infrared spectroscopy (FT-IR) and 2D IR correlation spectroscopy of PAMAM dendrimer. *J. Phy. Chem. B.* 2006;110(29):14,198–14,211.
60. **Sakthivel, T. and Florence, AT.** Dendrimers and dendrons: facets of pharmaceutical nanotechnology. *Drug Deliv. Technol.* 2003;3:73–78.
61. **Patri, AK., Majoros, I., and Baker, JRJ.** Dendritic polymer macromolecular carriers for drug delivery. *Curr. Opin. Chem. Biol.* 2002;6:466–471.
62. **Esfand, R. and Tomalia, DA.** Poly (amidoamine) (PAMAM) dendrimers: from biomimicry to drug delivery and biomedical applications. *Drug Discov. Today* 2001;6:427–436.
63. **Liu, M. and Frechet, JM.** Designing dendrimers for drug delivery. *Pharm. Sci. Technol. Today* 1999;2:393–401.
64. **Beezer, AE., King, ASH., Martin, IK., Mitchel, JC., Twyman, LJ., and Wain, CF.** Dendrimers as potential drug carriers; encapsulation of acidic hydrophobes within water soluble PAMAM derivatives. *Tetrahedron* 2003;59:3873–3880.
65. **Twyman, LJ., Beezer, AE., Esfand, R., Hardy, MJ., and Mitchell, JC.** The synthesis of water soluble dendrimers, and their application as possible drug delivery systems. *Tetrahedron Lett.* 1999;40:1743–1746.
66. **Jansen, JFGA., deBrabander-van den Berg, EMM., and Meijer, EW.** Encapsulation of guest molecules into a dendritic box. *Science* 1994;266:1226–1229.
67. **Jansen, JFGA., Meijer, EW., and deBrabander-van den Berg, EMM.** The dendritic box: shape-selective liberation of encapsulated guests. *J. Am. Chem. Soc.* 1995;117: 4417–4418.
68. **Milhem, OM., Myles, C., McKeown, NB., Attwood, D., and D' Emanuele, A.** Polyamidoamine starburst dendrimers as solubility enhancers. *Int. J. Pharm.* 2000;197(1 and 2): 239–241.
69. **Kojima, C., Kono, K., Maryama, K., and Takagishi, T.** Synthesis of polyamidoamine dendrimers having poly(ethylene) glycol grafts and their ability to encapsulate anticancer drugs. *Bioconjug. Chem.* 2000;11:910–917.
70. **Hawker, CJ., Wooley, KL., and Fréchet, JMJ.** Unimolecular micelles and globular amphiphiles: dendritic macromolecules as novel recyclable solubilization agents. *J. Chem. Soc. Perkin. 1* 1993;1287–1297.
71. **Zhuo, RX., Du, B., and Lu, ZR.** In vitro release of 5-fluorouracil with cyclic core dendritic polymer. *J. Control. Release* 1999;57(3):249–257.
72. **Kolhe, P., Misra, E., Kannan, RM., Kannan, S., and Lieh-Lai, M.** Drug complexation, in vitro release and cellular entry of dendrimers and hyperbranched polymers *Int. J. Pharm.* 2003;259(1 and 2):143–160.
73. **Asthana, A., Chauhan, AS., Diwan, PV., and Jain, NK.** Poly(amidoamine) (PAMAM) dendritic nanostructures for controlled site-specific delivery of acidic anti-inflammatory active ingredient. *AAPS Pharm. Sci. Tech.* 2005;6(3): E536–E542.
74. **Yiyun, C., Tongwen, X., and Rongqiang, F.** Polyamidoamine dendrimers used as solubility enhancers of ketoprofen. *Eur. J. Med. Chem.* 2005;40(12):1390–1393.
75. **Chauhan, AS., Jain, NK., Diwan, PV., and Khopade, AJ.** Solubility enhancement of indomethacin with poly(amidoamine) dendrimers and targeting to inflammatory regions of arthritic rats. *J. Drug Target* 2004;12(9 and 10):575–583.
76. **Chauhan, AS., Sridevi, S., Chalasani, KB., et al.** Dendrimer-mediated transdermal delivery: enhanced bioavailability of indomethacin. *J. Control. Release* 2003;90(3):335–343.
77. **Patri, AK., Kukowska-Latallo, JF., and Baker, JR.** Targeted drug delivery with dendrimers: comparison of the release kinetics of covalently conjugated drug and non-covalent drug inclusion complex. *Adv. Drug Deliv. Rev.* 2005;57(15): 2203–2214.
78. **Gurdag, S., Khandare, J., Stapels, S., Matherly, LH., and Kannan, RM.** Activity of dendrimer-methotrexate conjugates on methotrexate-sensitive and resistant cell lines. *Bioconjug. Chem.* 2006;17(2):275–283.
79. **Khopade, AJ., Caruso, F., Tripathi, P., Nagaich, S., and Jain, NK.** Effect of dendrimer on entrapment and release of bioactive from liposomes. *Int. J. Pharm.* 2002;232(1 and 2):157–162.
80. **Neerman, MF., Chen, HT., Parrish, AR., and Simanek, EE.** Reduction of drug toxicity using dendrimers based on melamine. *Mol. Pharm.* 2004;1(5):390–393.
81. **Shiyoshi, Y., Tatsuo, N., Akira, O., et al.** Superfluorescence action from rhodamine-cored dendrimer. *Colloids Surf.* 2002;198:433–438.
82. **Kono, K., Liu, M., and Frechet, JMJ.** Design of dendritic macromolecules containing folate or methotrexate residues. *Bioconjug. Chem.* 1999;10:1115–1121.
83. **Quintana, A., Raczka, E., Piehler, L., et al.** Design and function of a dendrimer-based therapeutic nanodevice targeted to tumour cells through the folate receptor. *Pharm. Res.* 2002;19:1310–1316.
84. **Shukla, S., Wu, G., Chatterjee, M., et al.** Synthesis and biological evaluation of folate receptor targeted boronated PAMAM dendrimers as potential agents for neutron capture therapy. *Bioconjug. Chem.* 2003;14:158–167.
85. **Bezouska, K., Pospisil, MF., Vannucci, LF., et al.** Design, functional evaluation and biomedical applications of carbohydrate dendrimers (glycodendrimers). *Rev. Mol. Biotechnol.* 2002;90:269–290.
86. **Roy, R.** Syntheses and some applications of chemically defined multivalent glycoconjugates. *Curr. Opin. Struc. Biol.* 1996;6:692–702.
87. **Rockendorf, N. and Lindhorst, TK.** Glycodendrimers. *Top. Curr. Chem. Dendrimers IV* 2001;217:201–238.
88. **Veprek, P. and Jezek, J.** Peptide and glycopeptide dendrimers: part II. *J. Pept. Sci.* 1999;5:203–220.

89. **Andre, S., Pieters, RJ., Vrasidas, I., et al.** Wedgelike glycodendrimers as inhibitors of binding of mammalian galectins to glycoproteins, lactose maxiclusters, and cell surface glycoconjugates. *Chem. Bio. Chem.* 2001;2:822–830.

90. **Roberts, JC., Adams, YE., Tomalia, DA., Mercer-Smith, JA., and Lavallee, DK.** Using starburst dendrimers as linker molecules to radiolabel antibodies. *Bioconjug. Chem.* 1990;1(5):305–308.

91. **Wiwattanapatapee, R., Lomlim, L., and Saramunee, K.** Dendrimers conjugates for colonic delivery of 5-aminosalicylic acid. *J. Control. Release* 2003;88(1):1–9.

92. **Malik, N., Evagorou, EG., and Duncan, R.** Dendrimer-platinate: a novel approach to cancer chemotherapy. *Anticancer Drugs* 1999;10:767–776.

93. **Bhadra, D., Bhadra, S., Jain, S., and Jain, NK.** A PEGylated dendritic nanoparticulate carrier of fluorouracil. *Int. J. Pharm.* 2003;257:111–124.

94. **Berry, R.** CEO, Dendrimer technology: a nanoscale delivery platform for the identification and treatment of cancer. *Dendritic Nanotechnologies* 2005; www.foresight.org/-conference2005/presentations/berry.pdf.

95. **Haensler, J. and Szoka, FC.** Polyamidoamine cascade polymers mediate efficient transfection of cells in culture. *Bioconjug. Chem.* 1993;4:372–379.

96. **Braun, CS., Vetro, JA., Tomalia, DA., Koe, GS., Koe JG., and Middaugh, CR.** Structure/function relationships of polyamidoamine/DNA dendrimers as gene delivery vehicles. *J. Pharm. Sci.* 2005;94:423–436.

97. **Luo, D., Haverstick, K., Belcheva, N., Han, E., and Saltzman, WM.** Poly (ethylene glycol)-conjugated dendrimer for biocompatible and high efficient DNA delivery. *Macromolecules* 2002;35:3456–3462.

98. **Kim, TI., Seo, HJ., Choi, JS., et al.** PAMAM–PEG–PAMAM: novel triblock copolymer as a biocompatible and efficient gene delivery carrier. *Biomacromolecules* 2004;5:2487–2492.

99. **Schatzlein, AG., Zinselmeyer, BH., Elouzi, A., et al.** Preferential liver gene expression with polypropylenimine dendrimers. *J. Control. Release* 2005;101:247–258.

100. **Fornari, M.** Dendrimers–modeling of multibranched structures. Presentation at "Materials Design Using Simulation Symposium, International Materials Research Conference"–Cancun, August 2003, www.phy.cmich.edu/-people/fornari/web/cancun03.pdf.

101. **Wiener, EC., Auteri, FP., Chen, JW., et al.** Molecular dynamics of ion-chelate complexes attached to dendrimers. *J. Am. Chem. Soc.* 1996;118:7774–7782.

102. **Bryant, LH., Brechbiel, MW., Wu, C., Bulte, JWM., Herynek, V., and Frank, JA.** Synthesis and relaxometry of high-generation (G=5, 7, 9, and 10) PAMAM dendrimer-DOTA-gadolinium chelates. *J. Magn. Reson. Imaging* 1999;9:348–352.

103. **Hecht, S. and Frechet, JMJ.** Dendritic encapsulation of function: applying nature's site isolation principle from biomimetics to materials science. *Angew. Chem. Int. Ed. Engl.* 2001;40:74–91.

104. **Jiang, DL. and Aida, T.** A dendritic iron porphyrin as a novel haemoproteinmimic: effects of the dendrimer cage on dioxygenbinding activity. *Chem. Commun.* 1996;1523–1524.

105. **Dandliker, PJ., Diederich, F., Zingg, A., et al.** Dendrimers with porphyrin cores: synthetic models for globular heme proteins. *Helv. Chim. Acta* 1997;80:1773–1801.

106. **Weyermann, P., Gisselbrecht, JP., Boudon, C., Diederich, F., and Gross, M.** Dendritic iron porphyrins with tethered axial ligands: new model compounds for cytochromes. *Angew. Chem. Int. Ed. Engl.* 1999;38:3214–3219.

107. **Arima, H., Kihara, F., Hirayama, F., and Uekama, K.** Enhancement of gene expression by polyamidoamine dendrimer conjugates with α-, β-, and γ-cyclodextrins. *Bioconjug. Chem.* 2001;12:476–484.

108. **Hudde, T., Rayner, SA., Comer, RM., et al.** Activated polyamidoamine dendrimers, a non-viral vector for genetransfer genetransfer to the cornial endothelium. *Gene Ther.* 1999;6:939–943.

109. **Eichman, JD., Bielinska, AU., Kukowska-Latallo, JF., and Baker, JR, Jr.** The use of PAMAM dendrimers in the efficient transfer of genetic material into cells. *Pharm. Sci. Technol. Today* 2000;3:232–245.

110. **Singh, P.** Terminal groups in starburst dendrimers: activation and reactions with proteins. *Bioconjug. Chem.* 1998;9:54–63.

111. **Bourne, N., Stanberry, LR., Kern, ER., Holan, G., Matthews, B., and Bernstein, DI.** Dendrimers, a new class of candidate topical microbicides with activity against herpes simplex virus infection. *Antimicrob. Agents Chemother.* 2000;44:2471–2474.

112. **Gong, Y., Matthews, B., Cheung, D., et al.** Evidence of dual sites of action of dendrimers: SPL-2999 inhibits both virus entry and late stages of herpes simplex virus replication. *Antivir. Res.* 2002;55:319–329.

113. **Witvrouw, M., Fikkert, V., Pluymers, W., et al.** Polyanionic (i.e., polysulfonate) dendrimers can inhibit the replication of human immunodeficiency virus by interfering with both virus adsorption and later steps (reverse transcriptase/integrase) in the virus replicative cycle. *Mol. Pharmacol.* 2000;58: 1100–1108.

114. **Halford, B.** Dendrimers branch out. *Chem. Eng. News* 2005;83(24):30–36.

115. **Chen, CZ., Beck-Tan, NC., Dhurjati, P., Van Dyk, TK., LaRossa, RA., and Cooper, SL.** Quaternary ammonium functionalized poly (propylene imine) dendrimers as effective antimicrobials: structure–activity studies. *Biomacromolecules* 2000;1:473–480.

116. **Nagahori, N., Lee, RT., Nishimura, S., Page, D., Roy, R., and Lee, YC.** Inhibition of adhesion of type 1 fimbriated *Escherichia coli* to highly mannosylated ligands. *Chem. Bio. Chem.* 2002;3:836–844.

117. **Sashiwa, H. and Aiba, SI.** Chemically modified chitin and chitosan as biomaterials. *Prog. Polym. Sci.* 2004;29: 887–908.

118. **Battah, SH., Chee, CE., Nakanishi, H., Gerscher, S., MacRobert, AJ., and Edwards, C.** Synthesis and biological studies of 5-aminolevulinic acid-containing dendrimers for photodynamic therapy. *Bioconjug. Chem.* 2001;12:980–988.

119. **Shaunak, S., Thomas, S., Gianasi, E., et al.** Polyvalent dendrimer glucosamine conjugates prevent scar tissue formation. *Nature. Biotechnol.* 2004;22:977–984.

120. **Hong, MY., Yoon, HC., and Kim, HS.** Protein–ligand interactions at poly (amidoamine) dendrimer monolayers on gold. *Langmuir* 2003;19:416–421.

121. **Barth, RF., Adams, DM., Soloway, AH., Alam, F., and Darby, MV.** Boronated Starburst® dendrimer-monoclonal antibody immunoconjugates: evaluation as a potential delivery system for neutron capture therapy. *Bioconjug. Chem.* 1994; 5:58–66.

122. **Wu, G., Barth, RF., Yang, W., et al.** Site-specific conjugation of boron-containing dendrimers to anti-EGF receptor monoclonal antibody cetuximab (IMC-C225) and its evaluation as a potential delivery agent for neutron capture therapy. *Bioconjug. Chem.* 2004;15:185–194.

123. **Kannan, S., Kolhe, P., Raykova, V., et al.** Effect of dendrimer end functionality on the cytotoxicity and the cellular drug delivery in lung epithelial cells. *J. Biomater. Sci. Polym. Ed.* 2004;15(3):311–330.

124. http://www.dendritech.com/applications.html., accessed on 24th July, 2007.

125. http://www1.qiagen.com/literature/brochures/tfbr/1020182_BRO_TF_0302WW.pdfhttp://www.ebiotrade.com/buyf/productsf/qiagen/301305.htm., accessed on 24th July, 2007.

11

Particulate Drug Delivery-Summary, Conclusions and Future Perspectives

An increasing number of newly developed drugs are poorly soluble; in many cases drugs are poorly soluble in both aqueous and organic media excluding the traditional approaches of overcoming such solubility factors and resulting in bioavailability problems. An alternative and promising approach is production of drug particles to overcome these problems. The major advantages of this technology are its general applicability to most drugs and its simplicity.

Micro- and nanoparticles are solid colloidal suspensions in which mean particle size is >1 or <1 μm, respectively. Under morphological point of view, two different types of particles can be distinguished: capsules and spheres. Sphere systems are usually characterizsed by a porous matrix in which drugs are contained, while capsule systems are formed by a core containing drugs surrounded by a shell. Polymeric particles are prepared from natural or synthetic polymers and, depending on preparation method and polymer used, micro- or nanocapsules and micro-or nanospheres can be distinguished. Polymeric particles have become very important because of their ability to deliver a variety of drugs to different areas of body for sustained periods of time. Off late, great interests are focused on much smaller carriers (e.g., nanoparticle) that are able to ensure fine drug delivery opportunities both in terms of efficacy and selectivity.

Concerning the materials used for preparation of these colloidal carriers, natural polymers (i.e., proteins, polysaccharides, and waxes) are not widely used because they present a huge variability in their purity and defined physicochemical properties. Furthermore, they often require a cross-linking procedure that may cause an alteration of encapsulated drug. For these reason, mainly synthetic polymers have received attention and have been largely investigated for potential use in drug delivery devices. The use of a large series of polymers is restricted and limited by their bioacceptability, which is also influenced by colloidal particle mean size. In fact, the diameter of smallest blood capillary is approximately 4 μm, thus nanoparticles should have a smaller diameter than this to traverse all capillaries. As a general consideration, choice of macromolecular polymer to be used as a nanoparticle matrix, should be based on biocompatibility, physicochemical properties of drug, as well as on the therapeutic goal to be reached. In this colloidal carrier, drugs can be adsorbed, attached, dissolved, entrapped, and/or encapsulated. Micro- and nanoparticles can be used to deliver both hydrophobic and hydrophilic molecules, proteins, vaccines, biological macromolecules. They can also be formulated for targeted delivery to all organs or made for long-term systemic circulation.

Other class of particulate system,—the dendrimers, are a novel class of polymeric materials, which are highly branched, spherical, monodisperse macromolecules with a well-defined globular structure and high functionality. They possess interior cavities surrounding core and core to which these dendrons are attached represent well-defined nanoenvironments, which are protected from outside by dendrimer surface (nanoscale containers) in case of higher generation dendrimers. In the periphery, dendrimer contains a homogenous, mathematically defined, surface functionality (nano-scaffold), which may be hydrophilic or hydrophobic depending on method of synthesis. The dendrimer architecture therefore not only permits control over properties such as size, shape, density, polarity, reactivity and solubility but also allow loading of drug molecules both in interior of dendrimers as well as attached to surface groups.

Erythrocytes are potential biocompatible vectors for different bioactive substances, including drugs. These can be used successfully as biological carriers of drugs, enzymes and peptides. Erythrocytes loaded with drugs and other substances allow for different release rates to be obtained. Encapsulation in erythrocytes significantly changes the pharmacokinetic properties of drugs in both animals and humans, enhancing liver and spleen uptake and targeting reticuloendothelial system.

Particulate drug delivery technology has made considerable advances, bringing even few clinical products to market. However, major needs for drug delivery devices are still unmet and drugs used to treat some very important classes of diseases have yet to benefit from these technological successes. The central focus of any novel delivery devices including particulate system is "control of drug release". This can be achieved if: (1) the size of device can be modulated as accurately as possible; (2) the device can be produced with certain reproducibility; (3) the device is stable enough for administration purpose; (4) the device is biocompatible; (5) the rate of drug delivery should be independent of surrounding environment. Till date, it is possible to adopt a lot of innovative approaches to modulate physicochemical properties of delivered drug, the administration route, and therapeutic aims. Many aspects of these drug delivery devices require an improvement to be applied to clinical use, but considering *in vitro* and *in vivo* results, they seem to be very much promising. From the appearance of first drug delivery device till date, a constant improvement has been made, i.e, from microtechnology we have passed to nanotechnology, and from an non specific drug delivery, we have passed to a selective drug delivery. New challenges for future are feasibility of scaling-up processes to bring to market quickly, innovative therapeutic entities and the possibility of obtaining multifunctional devices that will be able to fulfill different biological and therapeutic requirements.

Index*

D

E

F

G

H

I

K

L

M

N

O

P

Q

R

T

U

V

W

Z